# EXPLICATIVE CASES OF CONTROVERSIAL ISSUES IN NEUROSURGERY

Edited by **Francesco Signorelli**

**Explicative Cases of Controversial Issues in Neurosurgery**
Edited by Francesco Signorelli

**Published by InTech**

Janeza Trdine 9, 51000 Rijeka, Croatia



**Publishing Process Manager** Bojan Rafaj

**Technical Editor** Teodora Smiljanic

**Cover Designe**r InTech Design Team

Additional hard copies can be obtained from orders@intechopen.com

Explicative Cases of Controversial Issues in Neurosurgery, Edited by Francesco Signorelli
p. cm.
ISBN 978-953-51-0623-4

For EU product safety concerns:
IN TECH d.o.o., Prolaz Marije Krucifikse Kozulić 3, 51000 Rijeka, Croatia,
info@intechopen.com or visit our website at intechopen.com.

# Meet the editor

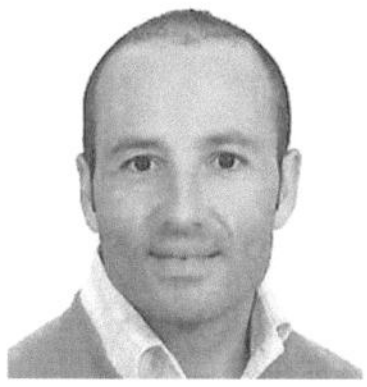

Professor Francesco Signorelli is an Italian board certified neurosurgeon. He was trained in neurosurgery at the University Hospital of Naples, Italy. He was fellow in neurosurgery in London and Southampton, UK, and fellow in vascular neurosurgery and skull base neurosurgery at the Notre Dame Hospital of the University of Montreal, Canada. In 2007 he was appointed associate professor of neurosurgery at the University Hospital of Catanzaro, Italy. He has recently rejoined the staff of the neurosurgical and neurovascular department at the "P. Wertheimer" Hospital for Neurology and Neurosurgery in Lyon, France, where he is also involved in teaching medical students and trainees in neurosurgery and neuroradiology. His surgical practice has canvassed the spectrum of neurosurgery, together with his scientific activity, with over 50 articles in peer-reviewed journals, and several book chapters and review articles. He is member of national and international neurosurgical associations and of the "Association pour le Développement Médical au Vietnam", a French humanitarian association. His current major interests are vascular neurosurgery and brain tumors in eloquent areas. Surgical and endovascular treatment of brain vascular malformations is a significant portion of his practice.

# Contents

# Preface

Neurosurgery is a rapidly developing field of medicine. Therefore, staying keeping track of the advancements in the field is paramount for trainees as well as fully trained neurosurgeons. This book, fully available online, is a part of our effort of improving availability of medical information for anyone who needs to keep up-to-date.

Medical information need to be free and we strongly support this objective. Nevertheless, the biggest risk open access is inaccuracy for lack of control so in order to overcome this, each chapter of the book has been carefully reviewed to provide the reader with the complete, accurate and reliable information.

We wish to offer our appreciation to our colleagues who consistently contributed to the genesis of this book and shared their expertize with the readers.

We welcome any suggestion and feedback the reader will give us through the web site of the publisher.

Finally, I wish to thank Vanessa, my wife, and Alice, my daughter: your support always goes beyond my expectations.

**Francesco Signorelli,**
Lyon,
France

# Section 1

## Anaesthesia and Neurocritical Care

# Trigeminocardiac Reflex in Neurosurgery – Current Knowledge and Prospects

Amr Abdulazim[1], Martin N. Stienen[1], Pooyan Sadr-Eshkevari[2], Nora Prochnow[1], Nora Sandu[4], Benham Bohluli[3] and Bernhard Schaller[4]
[1]*Department of Neuroanatomy and Molecular Brain Research, Ruhr-University Bochum, Bochum,*
[2]*Farzan Clinical Research Institute,Teheran,*
[3]*Department of Oral and Maxillofacial Surgery, Tehran Azad School of Dental Medicine, Tehran,*
[4]*Department of Neurosurgery, University of Paris, Paris,*
[1]*Germany*
[2,3]*Iran*
[4]*France*

## 1. Introduction

Sudden development of cardiac arrhythmia as far as cardiac arrest, arterial hypotension, apnea and gastric hypermobility as manifestations of the trigeminocardiac reflex (TCR) were initially described in 1870 by Kratschmer *et al.* (Kratschmer, 1870) after nasal mucosa manipulation in cats and rabbits. In 1908, Aschner and Dagnini presented the oculocardiac reflex (OCR) - nowadays considered as initial description of a peripheral subtype of TCR - which gained broad attention by ophthalmologist (Blanc, et al., 1983). In 1977 Kumada *et al.* (Kumada, et al., 1977) described similar autonomic "trigeminal depressor" responses after low frequency electrical stimulation within portions of the trigeminal complex in anaesthetized or decerebrated rabbits, indicating that not only peripheral but also central stimulation of parts of the trigeminal pathway results in autonomic reflex responses. In 1988 the term "trigeminocardiac reflex" was introduced by the anaesthetists Shelly and Church (Shelly and Church, 1988). In 1999, Schaller *et al.* (Schaller, et al., 1999) initially described the occurrence of central TCR in human after stimulation of central parts of the trigeminal nerve during cerebellopontine angle and brain stem surgery. It was then Schaller who merged the two entities of peripheral and central TCR to a common concept, which is now generally accepted.

This chapter introduces the TCR, which has gained broad attention in the field of neurosurgery. In the past years, TCR has been reported to occur during several other neurosurgical procedures such as transsphenoidal surgery (Schaller, 2005a), Jannetta microvascular decompression (Schaller, 2005b), percutaneous radiofrequency thermocoagulation and percutaneous microcompression of the trigeminal ganglion (Meng, et al., 2008), neuroendovascular approaches in neurosurgery (Amiridze, et al., 2009, Lv, et al.,

2010, Lv, et al., 2007, Ong, et al., 2010), and during aneurysm clipping (Spiriev, et al., 2011a). As the TCR may have decisive impact on the surgical course as well as the postoperative functional outcome of neurosurgical patients with skull-base pathologies, the awareness of the TCR is essential for everyone involved in the treatment of those patients. Therefore, in the following chapter we provide the current knowledge on TCR with respect to its risk and predisposing factors, its clinical implementation in neurosurgery, preventive and therapeutical means and its influence on functional outcome. Above that, we delineate the role of the TCR as an oxygen-conserving reflex and present future aspects on TCR research.

## 2. Definition

The trigeminocardiac reflex is considered to be a brainstem reflex, and has currently been defined as a decrease in heart rate (HR) and mean arterial blood pressure (MABP) of more than 20% as compared with baseline values before application of the stimulus and coinciding with the surgical manipulation at or around any branches of the trigeminal nerve (Schaller, 2005a, Schaller, et al., 2007). However, this definition seems to be problematic as the 20% benchmark is somewhat arbitrary and implies that alterations of less than this value are not defined as TCR, which blurs the true incidence and leads to an underestimation of TCR in daily operative clinical practice. Anyway, from a statistical point of view, such a definition makes sense and therefore should be used for large series having in mind that the incidence might be underestimated by this definition. Thus, it seems more reasonable to define the TCR as any cardiac reflex triggered upon stimulation of the trigeminal nerve anywhere throughout its course. Clinically, however, TCR might be best described as sudden onset of relative bradycardia upon the stimulation of the trigeminal nerve, anywhere throughout its course. This seems to be a rather inclusive and simplified definition for TCR. Any abrupt autonomic reflex response, additional to or without a cardiac response, upon stimulation of the trigeminal nerve anywhere throughout its course may be subsumed as trigeminovagal reflex (TVR). As for the further classification, subtypes of TCR may be defined based on triggerpoints at the proximity of the central nervous system or at peripheral nerve branches. Central (proximal) TCR is triggered upon stimulation of the intracranial course of the trigeminal nerve, namely from the Gasserian ganglion to the brainstem. Peripheral (distal) TCR is elicited upon stimulation of the trigeminal nerve anywhere throughout its course outside the cranium to the Gasserian ganglion. Peripheral TCR is further subdivided based on the branch of the affected trigeminal nerve distinguishing ophthalmocardiac reflex (OCR) and maxillomandibulocardiac reflex (MCR).

## 3. Etiology and pathophysiology

Stimulation of any of the trigeminal branches or nerve endings is suggested to send the afferent signal via the Gasserian ganglion to the sensory nucleus of the trigeminal nerve within the vicinity of the floor of the fourth ventricle. Small internuncial nerve fibers of the reticular formation connect the afferent to the efferent pathway, originating from the motor nucleus of the vagal nerve. The efferent pathway sends depressor fibers to the myocardium, thus complementing the reflex arc (Figure 1) (Lang, et al., 1991, Schaller, 2004). As cardiac responses to TCR are still maintained in decerebrated animals, its circuitry is considered to be located in the brainstem (Elsner and Gooden, 1983, Schaller, 2004). Experimental results

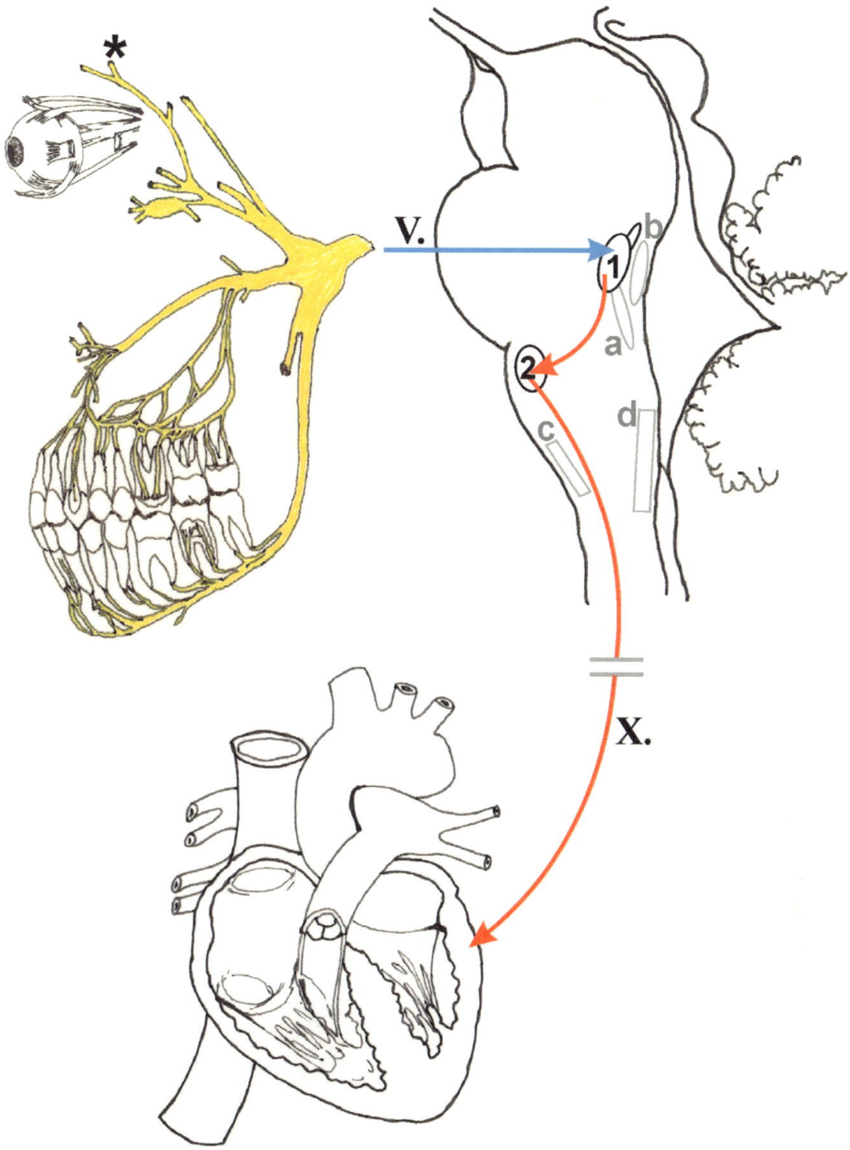


Fig. 1. The anatomy of trigeminocardiac reflex arc representing the three branches of the trigeminal nerve namely ophthalmic nerve (CN V1) responsible for OCR mediation, maxillary (CN V2) and mandibular (CN V3) nerves responsible for what the authors of the present review intend to call maxillomandibulocardiac reflex (MCR). The asterisk shows the origin of anterior ethmoidal nerve, a branch of the ophthalmic nerve, which descends into and innervates the nasal mucosa and is suggested to be responsible for the diving reflex (DR). The Gasserian ganglion, CN V root (blue arrow), the main sensory nucleus of CN V (1), internuncial fibers (upper red arrow), motor nucleus of CN X (2), and vagal myocardial depressor fibers (lower red arrow) complement the reflex arc. Further, the parabrachial nucleus (a), trigeminal nucleus caudalis (b), dorsal medullary reticular field (c), and rostral ventrolateral medulla (d) are shown for they are putatively involved in the reflex circuitry.

suggest that the TCR response is initially mediated from the trigeminal nucleus caudalis, with subsequent inclusion of the parabrachial nucleus, the rostral ventrolateral medulla oblongata, the dorsal medullary reticular field, and the paratrigeminal nucleus (Ohshita, et al., 2004, Schaller, B., et al., 2009a, Schaller and Buchfelder, 2006). However, regarding the afferent pathway, there are marked differences between subtypes of TCR, which also lead to different reflex arcs. Whereas the peripherally stimulated *TCR* is relayed via the spinal nucleus of the trigeminal nerve to the Kölliker-Fuse nucleus, the centrally stimulated *TCR* is conveyed via the nucleus of the solitary tract to the lateral parabrachial nucleus (Schaller, B., et al., 2009a). Previous studies have revealed that peripheral stimulation (anterior ethmoidal nerve in the nasal mucosa) co-actives vagal and sympathetic nerves, resulting in both sympathetically mediated peripheral vasoconstriction (hypertension) and parasympathetically mediated bradycardia (Dutschmann and Herbert, 1996, McCulloch, et al., 1999). This is in contrast to central stimulation of TCR where profound activation of the cardiac vagal branch and distinct inhibition of the inferior cardiac sympathetic nerve is observed (Nalivaiko, et al., 2003, Schaller, B., et al., 2009a).

### 3.1 Subtypes of TCR

Based on the common definition of the TCR, Schaller has included different peripherally and centrally stimulated subtypes into the TCR concept (**Table 1**) (Cornelius, et al., 2010).

#### 3.1.1 Oculocardiac Reflex (OCR)

OCR has frequently been the substrate of case series reporting severe bradycardia or asystole caused by ocular surgery (Blanc, et al., 1983). Most commonly OCR occurs in strabismus surgery, resulting from traction on the extraocular muscles. However, it can also be observed during other operations and manipulations of ocular and periocular structures innervated by the ophthalmic division of the trigeminal nerve (Anderson, 1978, Blanc, et al., 1983, Chesley and Shapiro, 1989, Kerr and Vance, 1983, Robideaux, 1978, Schaller, 2004, Stott, 1989).

#### 3.1.2 Maxillomandibulocardiac Reflex (MCR)

As thoroughly reviewed by Lang *et al.* (Lang, et al., 1991) and Bohluli *et al.* (Bohluli, et al., 2009), bradycardic reflex responses have also been observed and described for the maxillary and mandibulary divisions of the trigeminal nerve during maxillofacial surgery.

#### 3.1.3 Diving Reflex (DR)

DR constitutes an intrinsic brain stem reflex that is characterized by breath-holding, slowing of the HR, reduction of limb blood flow and gradually rises of the MABP. It is elicited by the combination of water touching the face and the either voluntary or involuntary (reflex) arrest of breathing (Gooden, 1994). Functionally, the DR has been demonstrated to be a mechanism for conserving oxygen (Gooden, 1993, 1994).

#### 3.1.4 Central vs. peripheral

Both OCR and MCR are considered to represent peripheral physiological subtypes of TCR. The literature supports the hypothesis of differentially induced peripheral and central TCR (Schaller, 2004, 2005a, Schaller, B., et al., 2009a, Schaller, et al., 1999, Schaller, et al., 2007).

OCR for example is well associated with bradycardia but, in contrast to central TCR, not with hypotension (Blanc, et al., 1983, Schaller, et al., 1999). Likewise, MCR has mainly been observed without accompanying hypotension, even though this understanding has been challenged by a recent study indicating decent decrease of MABP in MCR (Bohluli, et al., 2009, Bohluli, et al., 2010). From a physiologic point of view, TCR and DR seem to be closely linked, for they both underlie similar brainstem reflex arcs. The bradycardic efferent responses of both reflexes are attributed to centers located in the medulla oblongata and are mediated by parasympathetic pathways. Equally, peripheral vasoconstriction is conducted via efferent sympathetic pathways (Cornelius, et al., 2010, Khurana, et al., 1980, Schaller, B., et al., 2009a, Schaller, et al., 1999). However, in TCR the MABP decreases, whereas it gradually increases in DR as similarly observed for peripheral TCR (Schaller, B., et al., 2009a, Schaller, et al., 2008a). These findings suggest that DR might constitute a further peripheral subform of TCR and is a phylogenetic old reflex that is only present in aberrant form in adults (Cornelius, et al., 2010, Schaller, B., et al., 2009a, Schaller, et al., 2008a).

| | Peripheral TCR | | | Central TCR |
|---|---|---|---|---|
| | Ophthalmocardiac Reflex | Maxillomandibulo-cardiac Reflex | Diving Reflex | |
| Triggered by | pressure on ocular bulb, traction on extrinsic muscles of the eye, intraorbital injections or haematomas, acute glaucoma, stretching of the eyelid's muscles | maxillary and mandibulary branches and innervated tissues | stimulation of anterior ethmoidal nerve in the nasal mucosa | stimulation of central divisions of the trigeminal nerve including Gasserian ganglion |
| Afferent path | LCN/SCN -> CG -> O -> GG -> MSN $V^{th}$ -> SIF | VII/VIII -> GG -> MSN $V^{th}$ -> SIF | AEN -> GG -> Sp5C -> KF -> SIF | TN -> GG -> NTS -> LPBN -> SIF |
| Efferent path | MN $X^{th}$ -> CDN | MN $X^{th}$ -> CDN | MN $X^{th}$ -> CDN | MN $X^{th}$ -> CDN |
| Heart Rate | Bradycardia | Bradycardia | Bradycardia | Bradycardia |
| Respiration | Apnea | Apnea | Apnea (Gooden, 1993, 1994) | Apnea |
| Mean arterial blood pressure | Normotension | Normotension/ Hypotension | Hypertension | Hypotension |

*LCN* long ciliary nerves; *SCN* short ciliary nerves; *CG* ciliary ganglion; *O* ophthalmic branch of the $V^{th}$ cranial nerve; *GG* Gasserian ganglion; *MSN $V^{th}$* main sensory nucleus of the $V^{th}$ nerve; *SIF* short internuncial fibres; *MN $X^{th}$* motor nucleus of the $X^{th}$ nerve; *CDN* cardiac depressor nerve; *AEN* anterior ethmoidal nerve; *Sp5C* spinal trigeminal nucleus, pars caudalis; *KF* Kölliker-Fuse nucleus; *TN* trigeminal nerve; *NTS* nucleus tractus solitarii; *LPBN* lateral parabrachial nucleus

Table 1. Summary of the trigeminocardiac reflex subtypes according to points of elicitation, afferent and efferent paths, heart rate, respiratory alterations, and mean arterial blood pressure changes.

### 3.2 TCR as an oxygen-conserving reflex

Beside the clinical implementation, the TCR must be seen as a physiological and phylogenetically-inherited oxygen conserving reflex as it induces an increased cerebral blood flow (CBF) without changing cerebral metabolic rates of oxygen and glucose (Sandu, et al., 2010, Schaller, B.J., et al., 2009). An increase in CBF without change of cerebral metabolic rates provides the brain with oxygen rapidly and efficiently. Cerebrovascular vasodilatation may therefore possibly be a secondary response to amend hypoxia and trigeminovagally induced hypotension. Carbon dioxide ($CO_2$) which is increased in hypno/apneic states might be a main contributor in inducing the TCR and the subsequent protective cerebral vasodilatation, as described for oxygen conserving reflexes (Wolf, 1966). Previous studies in the anatomical circuitry of the TCR and oxygen conserving reflexes revealed the activation of brainstem areas which overlap with those described for hypoxic vasodilatation (Schaller, 2004). The latter was initially supposed to be elicited by direct effect of hypoxia on blood vessels and stimulation of arterial chemoreceptors (Schaller, 2004). TCR therefore needs to be reconsidered in terms of brain hypoxia prevention. That would, theoretically, open the door for TCR as a treatment option - for example in inducing tolerance for hypoxemia during stroke and similar ischemic conditions.

## 4. Epidemiology

As the TCR has been demonstrated to be triggered at any point throughout the course of the trigeminal nerve it can be observed during several different surgical approaches in the fields of craniofacial- and neurological surgery which involve manipulation of structures innervated by the trigeminal nerve or the trigeminal nerve itself.

### 4.1 Risk factors and predisposition

Generally accepted predisposing factors for the occurrence of intraoperative TCR constitute hypercapnia, hypoxemia, light general anaesthesia, young age (higher resting vagal tone in children), as well as strong and/or long-lasting provoking stimulus. Interestingly, bilateral stimulation of trigeminally innervated structures or of trigeminal nerve fibers results in a more profound reflex than observed in unilateral stimulation (Bauer, et al., 2005). Even though the previously mentioned risk factors are based on research done nearly 30 years ago, they could again be identified in our recent publications on this topic. In addition, Spiriev *et al.* (Spiriev, et al., 2010, Spiriev, et al., 2011b) observed perioperative TCR on the basis of a subdural empyema or exposure to $H_20_2$, indicating that chemical or inflammatory stimuli may constitute predisposing factors. Even antecedent transient ischemic attacks less than six weeks before an operation represent a significant risk factor for subsequent intraoperative occurrence of the TCR (Nothen, et al., 2010). Furthermore drugs, including potent narcotic agents like sufentanil and alfentanil, beta-blockers and calcium channel blockers, have been reported to predispose for TCR as they inhibit the sympathetic nervous system (potent narcotics), decrease the sympathetic response of the heart (beta-blockers) and cause peripheral arterial vasodilatation resulting in reduced HR and MABP (Arasho, et al., 2009, Blanc, et al., 1983, Bohluli, et al., 2009, Campbell, et al., 1994, Lang, et al., 1991, Lubbers, et al., 2010, Schaller, et al., 1999). However, evidence for impact of those drugs is low, as effects could not be confirmed in newer literature.

Based on these findings, we have developed the concept that most risk factors lead to a sensitization of the trigeminal nerve and make it more prone to trigger TCR during intraoperative stimulation (Schaller, B., et al., 2009a, Spiriev, et al., 2011b). However, as predisposing drugs actively influence the balance of the autonomic outflow, we believe, that their effect is rather exerted via modulation of the efferent reflex pathway than in the reduction of the reception threshold of the afferent pathway.

## 5. Clinical presentation

Clinically, TCR has gained enormous attention and importance due to its potentially life-threatening complication which may include sudden onset of bradycardia culminating in asystole, asystole without preceding bradycardia or apnea (Campbell, et al., 1994, Schaller, 2004). During several different surgical procedures, including ocular- and orbital cavity surgery, maxillofacial surgery and various neurosurgical procedures, TCR has been observed subsequently to manipulation of either peripheral or central parts of the trigeminal nerve, thus affecting the ongoing operation and requiring immediate and appropriate intervention to serve the patient from devastating cardiovascular deterioration. In the following section the neurosurgical procedures in which TCR has been described and thus in which TCR needs to be attended are introduced.

### 5.1 Cerebellopontine angle surgery

In 1999, Schaller *et al.* (Schaller, et al., 1999) for the first time reported TCR after stimulation of central parts of the trigeminal nerve during surgery in the cerebellopontine angle, and thus introduced TCR to the neurosurgical community. A total of 125 patients who underwent surgery in the cerebellopontine angle due to neoplasms were monitored with respect to the occurrence of autonomic cardiovascular responses consistent with TCR. Indeed, 11% of the patients showed responses most likely attributable to TCR. While dissecting the tumor near the trigeminal nerve at the brainstem, the patient's HR and MABP decreased significantly. The mean HR fell 38% from a mean of 76 beats/minute before manipulation to a mean of 47 beats/minute during the procedure, and returned to a mean of 77 beats/minute after manipulation. The MABP fell 48% from a mean of 84 mmHg before manipulation to 44 mmHg during the procedure, and returned to 82 mmHg after manipulation. Both HR and MABP returned to normal (pre-manipulative) values after the dissection. In three cases, there was an asystole, with duration of 30 to 70 seconds and a return to a normal cardiac rhythm within 90 to 180 seconds after termination of the surgical manipulation (Schaller, et al., 1999). In each of the 14 cases, the surgical manipulation of the trigeminal nerve near the brainstem elicited a specific and unequivocal effect (sudden bradycardia and arterial hypotension). Elimination of the inducing stimulus, such as manipulations near or at the trigeminal nerve, resolved the effect and repetition of the stimulus lead to the same effect each time (Schaller, et al., 1999).

### 5.2 Transsphenoidal surgery

To determine the nature and the extent of TCR during transsphenoidal surgery, Schaller *et al.* (Schaller, 2005a) reviewed a consecutive series of 117 patients with immunohistochemically and/or electronmicroscopically diagnosed and transsphenoidally operated pituitary adenomas with special emphasize on incidence and risk factors of TCR.

The incidence for TCR in this series was 10% with lacking statistical difference between TCR- and non-TCR subgroups for the parameters age, gender, tumor histology, or the duration and distribution of preoperative symptoms. During the preparation of the nasal septum none of the patients revealed TCR. However, a significant decrease in HR and MABP was observed during lateral tumor resection near the cavernous sinus. The mean HR decrease was 43% from a mean of 78 ± 13 beats/minute before manipulation to a mean of 45 ± 13 beats/minute. The mean MABP decrease was 54% from a mean of 86 ± 8 mmHg before to 40 ± 13 mmHg during the manipulation. Within ten minutes after cessation of the stimulus and without administration of anticholinergics HR and MABP values returned to 77 ± 9 beats/minute and 82 ± 8 mmHg. The post-procedural values were not significantly different from preoperative baseline values. Two patients revealed asystole lasting 25-63 sec and a sinus rhythm resumed within 75-135 sec after the end of the surgical manipulation. The follow-up of these two patients was uneventful. Interestingly, TCR occurred significantly more often in patients with invasive adenomas grade III/IV, according to Hardy's classification as modified by Wilson (83% versus 22%; $p < 0.001$) (Hardy, 1969, Wilson, 1983). On the basis that TCR occurred during preparation near the cavernous sinus and was associated with more invasive adenomas, which potentially invade or compress the cavernous sinus, Schaller *et al.* (Schaller, 2005a) concluded that TCR has to be elicited by structures passing the cavernous sinus. In the absence of parasympathetic fibers and with the first and second branch of the trigeminal nerve running through the cavernous sinus (branches of the trigeminal nerve innervate the cavernous sinus wall), it seems most likely that the observed autonomic response was due to TCR. This has been underlined by Abou-Zeid *et al.* (Abou-Zeid, et al., 2009), who reported the case of a patient who needed to be reoperated due to a residual pituitary adenoma adjacent to the left cavernous sinus wall. During the dissection of a small amount of tumor that was noted to be extending through the left cavernous sinus wall the patient became profoundly bradycardic and developed a 30 sec period of asystole, which rapidly reversed on the application of atropine. The bradycardia and the transient asystole also in this patient are most likely related to manifestation of TCR.

### 5.3 Microvascular trigeminal decompression (Jannetta procedure)

After TCR had been demonstrated to occur during surgery in the cerebellopontine angle and in the pituitary region, the question about the relevancy of TCR in other neurosurgical approaches necessitating preparation and manipulation of and around the trigeminal nerve remained. Thus, Schaller (Schaller, 2005b) reviewed the consecutive case histories of 28 patients who received microvascular trigeminal decompression for trigeminal neuralgia. 18% of the patients in this study displayed TCR during the course of surgery. In the time of preparation around the trigeminal nerve, the patient's HR and MABP decreased significantly. The mean HR fell 46% from a mean of 72 beats/minute before manipulation to a mean of 39 beats/minute during the procedure, returning to a mean of 75 beats/minute after manipulation. The MABP fell 57% from a mean of 81 mmHg before manipulation to 35 mmHg during the procedure, returning to 84 mmHg after manipulation. One patient developed a 33 sec lasting asystole which returned to normal cardiac rhythm within 83 sec after completion of surgical manipulation. All cases of TCR occurred while separating microvascular structures from the sensoria radix of the trigeminal nerve (Schaller, 2005b). This emphasizes that the trigeminal nerve route forms the afferent pathway of the observed autonomic responses in this study.

### 5.4 Aneurysmal clipping

Most recently, Spiriev *et al.* (Spiriev, et al., 2011a) have reported a patient who presented with subarachnoid hemorrhage (SAH) (Hunt and Hess 2, Fischer III) following the rupture of an aneurysm of the posterior communicating artery-internal carotid artery junction (PcomA-ICA). After the sylvian fissure had been opened, the carotid and optic cisterns were approached and a careful dissection around the supraclinoid portion of the ICA with target to ambient cistern was performed. During the latter maneuver the aneurysm ruptured demanding temporary clipping of the parent vessel. After placing clips on the ICA, the patient experienced a 30 sec lasting sudden heart arrest (Spiriev, et al., 2011a). Taking into consideration that trigeminal terminals are found on all vessels of the circle of Willis and their distal branches throughout the adventitia and that the cell bodies of the supratentorial meningeal and cortical vessels lie within the ophthalmic division of the trigeminal ganglion it is possible that the observed response on the manipulation represents TCR (Simons and Ruskell, 1988). Spiriev *et al.* (Spiriev, et al., 2011a) reviewed the literature with reference to the occurrence of underlying TCR in aneurysm clipping procedures and found three further cases where cardiovascular responses are also most likely on the basis of TCR (Ganjoo, et al., 2010, Murakawa, et al., 2002, Takenaka, et al., 2006). Still, it has to be emphasized, that cardiac dysfunction including myocardial infarction is observed in up to 30% of SAH patients and has been discussed to result from excessive activity of the autonomous nervous system of unknown origin (Seule, et al., 2010). Since onset of the asystole was clearly associated with clip placement and not with the rebleeding in this patient however, the case presented by Spiriev *et al.* rather presents TCR than cardiac dysfunction associated with SAH.

## 6. Diagnosis

Generally, there may be several different reasons for miscellaneous intraoperative cardiovascular alterations. As for declaring the occurrence of TCR one have to consider its current definition which presumes an abrupt drop of HR and MABP of more than 20% compared to baseline values and coinciding with manipulation at or around the trigeminal nerve itself or structures innervated by it. Additionally, cessation of traction needs to result in a spontaneous increase of HR and MABP values and the phenomenon has to recur when traction is repeated. Another means to prove TCR and to exclude other causes of cardiovascular alterations is blocking the nerves that conduct the afferent path of the reflex, which needs to result in alleviation of the reflex response.

## 7. Prevention and treatment options

The risk of TCR always needs to be considered if an intervention in the territory of the trigeminal nerve is performed. The surgeon should notify the anaesthesiologist if he directly approaches the nerve or any of its branches. Direct trauma to nervous tissue should be reduced to a minimum as smooth and gentle manipulations are less likely to evoke TCR. Intraoperative factors such as light anaesthesia, hypercapnia, hypoxia and acidosis should be corrected before the beginning of the surgical manipulation as they potentiate TCR (Schaller, B., et al., 2009a). A thorough and constant monitoring of the HR and MABP during the surgical procedure allows the surgeon to immediately interrupt his surgical maneuvers once hemodynamic deteriorations from TCR occur. This has mostly been shown to be sufficient in causing a cessation of the reflex and in restoring normal HR and blood pressure levels, without the need to administer anticholinergics (Arasho, et al., 2009, Bohluli, et al., 2009, Schaller, B., et al., 2009a). However, if bradycardia and hypotension appear to be refractory to immediate pause of the manipulation, intravenous administration of anticholinergics (atropine and/or glycopyrrolate) should be initiated (Bohluli, et al., 2009, Matturri, et al., 2005, Prabhakar, et al., 2006, Schaller, B., et al., 2009a, Schaller, B., et al., 2009b). Notably, bradycardia and hypotension in TCR may not only result from excessive vagal stimulation but also from reduction of the sympathetic tone. In these cases, the patient will not respond to vagolytics and application of epinephrine has been shown to be efficacious, also stressing that the TCR contains a sympathetically mediated component (Arasho, et al., 2009, Prabhakar, et al., 2008). Refractory TCR requiring immediate cardiac life support have been reported previously but seem to be rare (Campbell, et al., 1994, Prabhakar, et al., 2008). Recent studies have shown that local anaesthetic infiltration or block of the nerve(s) which constitute the afferent path, may accomplish a prophylaxis of the peripheral TCR (Gupta, et al., 2007, Misurya, et al., 1990, Shende, et al., 2000). Peribulbar block using bupivacaine in patients operated for retinal detachment significantly reduced the incidence and attenuated the severity of the reflex (Shende, et al., 2000). In comparison to topical local anaesthetic application in children undergoing strabismus surgery, peribulbar block was efficacious in reflex prophylaxis (Gupta, et al., 2007). Misurya *et al.* studied the effectiveness of peripheral cardiac muscarinic receptor blockade using intravenous atropine sulphate and the conduction of the afferent limb at the ciliary ganglion with retrobulbar xylocaine hydrochloride. They found, that each method was capable of reducing the rate of the OCR to 10%-20% and that the reflex was completely suppressed when both methods were combined (Misurya, et al., 1990). Still, what seems to be feasible and effective for peripheral TCR is not applicable to central TCR. This might be attributable to the fact that central TCR is elicited by central divisions near the brainstem and that, unlike peripheral TCR, its reflex circuitry is located nearly completely intrinsic to the latter (Schaller, B., et al., 2009a, Schaller, et al., 1999). From a mechanistic perspective, central manipulation of the trigeminal nerve may cause a radiated traction of the brainstem itself or of the nerve's outlet resulting in the activation of the intrinsic central reflex arc. Thus, a peripheral block of the trigeminal nerve or any of its branches would be obsolete and inefficacious in preventing the central TCR.

## 8. Outcome and prognosis

The occurrence of the TCR during a surgical procedure may significantly influence the course of the operation and threaten the patient. But despite its abrupt onset and drastic deteriorations of HR and MABP, intraoperative TCR can sufficiently be kept under control when considered adequately and managed appropriately. However, TCR does not only have significant impact on the intraoperative course but it has moreover been shown to influence the postoperative functional outcome. For example, occurence of intraoperative TCR is correlated with postoperative ipsilateral tinnitus and decline of auditory function (Gharabaghi, et al., 2006, Schaller, et al., 2008b). Gharabaghi *et al.* (Gharabaghi, et al., 2006) have prospectively studied 100 patients scheduled for vestibular schwannoma surgery for their postoperative auditory function in correlation to the occurrence of TCR. TCR occurred in 11% of the patients and hearing function could be preserved in 47% of all patients. However, only 11.1% of the patients in the TCR group *vs.* 51.4% in the non-TCR group experienced a preserved auditory function postoperatively (Gharabaghi, et al., 2006). On the basis of these results, Acioly *et al.* (Acioly, et al., 2010) studied if intraoperatively monitored deteriorations of the brain auditory evoked potentials (BAEP) during surgery of the cerebellopontine angle were directly connected to the occurrence of TCR. The authors were able to identify distinct BAEP alterations as predictive parameters for the risk of postoperative hearing impairment. While a definite causality of BAEP deteriorations to TCR could not be substantiated by this study, they were at least likely to result from TCR as BAEP changes in this study were not associated with previously described eliciting factors (Acioly, et al., 2010). Likewise, Schaller *et al.* (Schaller, et al., 2008b) reported the impact of TCR on postoperative ipsilateral tinnitus in patients undergoing vestibular schwannoma surgery. This retrospective study included 36 patients, with TCR occurring in a total of 17% of the patients. Overall, 22% of the investigated patients experienced postoperative ipsilateral tinnitus, whereas its incidence was up to 60% among the TCR group and just 17% among the non-TCR group (Schaller, et al., 2008b). These studies outline the putative role of TCR in affecting postoperative functional outcome, while the question regarding the pathophysiological mechanism remains unanswered. Possible explanations include changes in the vascular supply of the auditory apparatus. It is hypothesized, that in schwannoma patients an already impaired vascular supply of the medullo-pontine brainstem region due to tumor compression may be critically exaggerated by the sudden TCR-induced hypotension (Gharabaghi, et al., 2006). Substantiation for this hypothesis derives from the observation of BAEP deteriorations after TCR that are thought to be of vascular origin as they occur minutes after the eliciting reflex (Acioly, et al., 2010). Therefore, postoperative consequences are currently believed to derive from deterioration of the vascular supply.

## 9. Expert suggestions

Recently, TCR has been appreciated in the field of clinical neuroscience as its appearance may fundamentally affect patient's surgical and clinical courses. As a consequence, there are many reports and studies on TCR dealing with its clinical implementation and influence on functional outcome. These reports emphasize that knowledge on TCR, its clinical and surgical consideration and recognition, and its appropriate management is essential for neurosurgical patient care. Furthermore, the role of TCR as physiological reflex besides its detrimental role in skull base surgery has largely remained unappreciated. It seemingly plays an important yet not fully understood physiological role with respect to saving the brain from ischemic states and providing oxygen. Besides, TCR has found to be a putatively oxygen-conserving, neuroprotective reflex and is considered to be a valuable tool in prevention of brain hypoxia, for example in inducing intraischemic tolerance for hypoxemia during stroke. This very aspect underlines the great importance of the TCR for practice in clinical neurology and cardiovascular therapy as it might open the door for putative future treatment options.

## 10. References

Abou-Zeid, A.H., Davis, J.R., Kearney, T. & Gnanalingham, K.K. (2009). Transient asystole during endoscopic transsphenoidal surgery for acromegaly: an example of trigeminocardiac reflex. *Pituitary*, 12, 4, 373-4, 1573-7403 (Electronic) 1386-341X (Linking)

Acioly, M.A., Carvalho, C.H., Koerbel, A., Lowenheim, H., Tatagiba, M. & Gharabaghi, A. (2010). Intraoperative brainstem auditory evoked potential observations after trigeminocardiac reflex during cerebellopontine angle surgery. *J Neurosurg Anesthesiol*, 22, 4, (Oct), 347-53, 1537-1921 (Electronic) 0898-4921 (Linking)

Amiridze, N., Zoarski, G., Darwish, R., Obuchowski, A. & Solovevchic, N. (2009). Embolization of a Cavernous Sinus Dural Arteriovenous Fistula with Onyx via Direct Puncture of the Cavernous Sinus through the Superior Orbital Fissure: Asystole Resulting from the Trigeminocardiac Reflex. A Case Report. *Interv Neuroradiol*, 15, 2, (Jul 29), 179-84, 1591-0199 (Print) 1591-0199 (Linking)

Anderson, R.L. (1978). The blepharocardiac reflex. *Arch Ophthalmol*, 96, 8, (Aug), 1418-20, 0003-9950 (Print) 0003-9950 (Linking)

Arasho, B., Sandu, N., Spiriev, T., Prabhakar, H. & Schaller, B. (2009). Management of the trigeminocardiac reflex: facts and own experience. *Neurol India*, 57, 4, (Jul-Aug), 375-80, 0028-3886 (Print) 0028-3886 (Linking)

Bauer, D.F., Youkilis, A., Schenck, C., Turner, C.R. & Thompson, B.G. (2005). The falcine trigeminocardiac reflex: case report and review of the literature. *Surg Neurol*, 63, 2, (Feb), 143-8, 0090-3019 (Print) 0090-3019 (Linking)

Blanc, V.F., Hardy, J.F., Milot, J. & Jacob, J.L. (1983). The oculocardiac reflex: a graphic and statistical analysis in infants and children. *Can Anaesth Soc J*, 30, 4, (Jul), 360-9, 0008-2856 (Print) 0008-2856 (Linking)

Bohluli, B., Ashtiani, A.K., Khayampoor, A. & Sadr-Eshkevari, P. (2009). Trigeminocardiac reflex: a MaxFax literature review. *Oral Surg Oral Med Oral Pathol Oral Radiol Endod*, 108, 2, (Aug), 184-8, 1528-395X (Electronic) 1079-2104 (Linking)

Bohluli, B., Bayat, M., Sarkarat, F., Moradi, B., Tabrizi, M.H. & Sadr-Eshkevari, P. (2010). Trigeminocardiac reflex during Le Fort I osteotomy: a case-crossover study. *Oral Surg Oral Med Oral Pathol Oral Radiol Endod*, 110, 2, (Aug), 178-81, 1528-395X (Electronic) 1079-2104 (Linking)

Campbell, R., Rodrigo, D. & Cheung, L. (1994). Asystole and bradycardia during maxillofacial surgery. *Anesth Prog*, 41, 1, 13-6, 0003-3006 (Print) 0003-3006 (Linking)

Chesley, L.D. & Shapiro, R.D. (1989). Oculocardiac reflex during treatment of an orbital blowout fracture. *J Oral Maxillofac Surg*, 47, 5, (May), 522-3, 0278-2391 (Print) 0278-2391 (Linking)

Cornelius, J.F., Sadr-Eshkevari, P., Arasho, B.D., Sandu, N., Spiriev, T., Lemaitre, F. & Schaller, B. (2010). The trigemino-cardiac reflex in adults: own experience. *Expert Rev Cardiovasc Ther*, 8, 7, (Jul), 895-8, 1744-8344 (Electronic) 1477-9072 (Linking)

Dutschmann, M. & Herbert, H. (1996). The Kolliker-Fuse nucleus mediates the trigeminally induced apnoea in the rat. *Neuroreport*, 7, 8, (May 31), 1432-6, 0959-4965 (Print) 0959-4965 (Linking)

Elsner, R. & Gooden, B. (1983). Diving and asphyxia. A comparative study of animals and man. *Monogr Physiol Soc*, 40, 1-168, 0079-2020 (Print) 0079-2020 (Linking)

Ganjoo, P., Navkar, D.V. & Tandon, M.S. (2010). Complete heart block complicating intracranial aneurysm surgery in a pregnant patient. *Neurol India*, 58, 1, (Jan-Feb), 146, 0028-3886 (Print) 0028-3886 (Linking)

Gharabaghi, A., Koerbel, A., Samii, A., Kaminsky, J., von Goesseln, H., Tatagiba, M. & Samii, M. (2006). The impact of hypotension due to the trigeminocardiac reflex on auditory function in vestibular schwannoma surgery. *J Neurosurg*, 104, 3, (Mar), 369-75, 0022-3085 (Print) 0022-3085 (Linking)

Gooden, B.A. (1993). The evolution of asphyxial defense. *Integr Physiol Behav Sci*, 28, 4, (Oct-Dec), 317-30, 1053-881X (Print) 1053-881X (Linking)

Gooden, B.A. (1994). Mechanism of the human diving response. *Integr Physiol Behav Sci*, 29, 1, (Jan-Mar), 6-16, 1053-881X (Print) 1053-881X (Linking)

Gupta, N., Kumar, R., Kumar, S., Sehgal, R. & Sharma, K.R. (2007). A prospective randomised double blind study to evaluate the effect of peribulbar block or topical application of local anaesthesia combined with general anaesthesia on intra-operative and postoperative complications during paediatric strabismus surgery. *Anaesthesia*, 62, 11, (Nov), 1110-3, 0003-2409 (Print) 0003-2409 (Linking)

Hardy, J. (1969). Transsphenoidal microsurgery of the normal and pathological pituitary. *Clin Neurosurg*, 16, 185-217,

Kerr, W.J. & Vance, J.P. (1983). Oculocardiac reflex from the empty orbit. *Anaesthesia*, 38, 9, (Sep), 883-5, 0003-2409 (Print) 0003-2409 (Linking)

Khurana, R.K., Watabiki, S., Hebel, J.R., Toro, R. & Nelson, E. (1980). Cold face test in the assessment of trigeminal-brainstem-vagal function in humans. *Ann Neurol*, 7, 2, (Feb), 144-9, 0364-5134 (Print) 0364-5134 (Linking)

Kratschmer, F. (1870). Influence of reflexes of the nasal mucosa on breathing and circulatory. *Sber Akad Wis Wien*, 62, 147 - 170,

Kumada, M., Dampney, R.A. & Reis, D.J. (1977). The trigeminal depressor response: a novel vasodepressor response originating from the trigeminal system. *Brain Res*, 119, 2, (Jan 7), 305-26, 0006-8993 (Print) 0006-8993 (Linking)

Lang, S., Lanigan, D.T. & van der Wal, M. (1991). Trigeminocardiac reflexes: maxillary and mandibular variants of the oculocardiac reflex. *Can J Anaesth*, 38, 6, (Sep), 757-60, 0832-610X (Print) 0832-610X (Linking)

Lubbers, H.T., Zweifel, D., Gratz, K.W. & Kruse, A. (2010). Classification of potential risk factors for trigeminocardiac reflex in craniomaxillofacial surgery. *J Oral Maxillofac Surg*, 68, 6, (Jun), 1317-21, 1531-5053 (Electronic) 0278-2391 (Linking)

Lv, X., Li, Y., Jiang, C. & Wu, Z. (2010). The incidence of trigeminocardiac reflex in endovascular treatment of dural arteriovenous fistula with onyx. *Interv Neuroradiol*, 16, 1, (Mar), 59-63, 1591-0199 (Print) 1591-0199 (Linking)

Lv, X., Li, Y., Lv, M., Liu, A., Zhang, J. & Wu, Z. (2007). Trigeminocardiac reflex in embolization of intracranial dural arteriovenous fistula. *AJNR Am J Neuroradiol*, 28, 9, (Oct), 1769-70, 0195-6108 (Print) 0195-6108 (Linking)

Matturri, L., Ottaviani, G. & Lavezzi, A.M. (2005). Sudden infant death triggered by dive reflex. *J Clin Pathol*, 58, 1, (Jan), 77-80, 0021-9746 (Print) 0021-9746 (Linking)

McCulloch, P.F., Faber, K.M. & Panneton, W.M. (1999). Electrical stimulation of the anterior ethmoidal nerve produces the diving response. *Brain Res*, 830, 1, (May 29), 24-31, 0006-8993 (Print) 0006-8993 (Linking)

Meng, Q., Zhang, W., Yang, Y., Zhou, M. & Li, X. (2008). Cardiovascular responses during percutaneous radiofrequency thermocoagulation therapy in primary trigeminal neuralgia. *J Neurosurg Anesthesiol*, 20, 2, (Apr), 131-5, 1537-1921 (Electronic) 0898-4921 (Linking)

Misurya, V.K., Singh, S.P. & Kulshrestha, V.K. (1990). Prevention of oculocardiac reflex (O.C.R) during extraocular muscle surgery. *Indian J Ophthalmol*, 38, 2, (Apr-Jun), 85-7, 0301-4738 (Print) 0301-4738 (Linking)

Murakawa, T., Jin, T. & Matsuki, A. (2002). [A case of ventricular fibrillation during emergency clipping operation for cerebral aneurysm]. *Masui*, 51, 2, (Feb), 203-5, 0021-4892 (Print) 0021-4892 (Linking)

Nalivaiko, E., De Pasquale, C.G. & Blessing, W.W. (2003). Electrocardiographic changes associated with the nasopharyngeal reflex in conscious rabbits: vago-sympathetic co-activation. *Auton Neurosci*, 105, 2, (May 30), 101-4, 1566-0702 (Print) 1566-0702 (Linking)

Nothen, C., Sandu, N., Prabhakar, H., Filis, A., Arasho, B.D., Buchfelder, M. & Schaller, B.J. (2010). Trigemino-cardiac reflex and antecedent transient ischemic attacks. *Expert Rev Cardiovasc Ther*, 8, 4, (Apr), 509-12, 1744-8344 (Electronic) 1477-9072 (Linking)

Ohshita, N., Nakajo, N. & Takemura, M. (2004). Characteristics of the trigeminal depressor response in cats. *J Neurosci Res*, 76, 6, (Jun 15), 891-901, 0360-4012 (Print) 0360-4012 (Linking)

Ong, C.K., Ong, M.T., Le, K., Power, M.A., Wang, L.L., Lam, D.V., Parkinson, R.J. & Wenderoth, J.D. (2010). The trigeminocardiac reflex in Onyx embolisation of intracranial dural arteriovenous fistula. *J Clin Neurosci*, 17, 10, (Oct), 1267-70, 1532-2653 (Electronic) 0967-5868 (Linking)

Prabhakar, H., Ali, Z. & Rath, G.P. (2008). Trigemino-cardiac reflex may be refractory to conventional management in adults. *Acta Neurochir (Wien)*, 150, 5, (May), 509-10, 0942-0940 (Electronic) 0001-6268 (Linking)

Prabhakar, H., Anand, N., Chouhan, R.S. & Bithal, P.K. (2006). Sudden asystole during surgery in the cerebellopontine angle. *Acta Neurochir (Wien)*, 148, 6, (Jun), 699-700; discussion 700, 0001-6268 (Print) 0001-6268 (Linking)

Robideaux, V. (1978). Oculocardiac reflex caused by midface disimpaction. *Anesthesiology*, 49, 6, (Dec), 433, 0003-3022 (Print) 0003-3022 (Linking)

Sandu, N., Spiriev, T., Lemaitre, F., Filis, A. & Schaller, B. (2010). New molecular knowledge towards the trigemino-cardiac reflex as a cerebral oxygen-conserving reflex. *ScientificWorldJournal*, 10, 811-7, 1537-744X (Electronic) 1537-744X (Linking)

Schaller, B. (2004). Trigeminocardiac reflex. A clinical phenomenon or a new physiological entity? *J Neurol*, 251, 6, (Jun), 658-65, 0340-5354 (Print) 0340-5354 (Linking)

Schaller, B. (2005a). Trigemino-cardiac reflex during transsphenoidal surgery for pituitary adenomas. *Clin Neurol Neurosurg*, 107, 6, (Oct), 468-74, 0303-8467 (Print) 0303-8467 (Linking)

Schaller, B. (2005b). Trigemino-cardiac reflex during microvascular trigeminal decompression in cases of trigeminal neuralgia. *J Neurosurg Anesthesiol*, 17, 1, (Jan), 45-8, 0898-4921 (Print) 0898-4921 (Linking)

Schaller, B., Cornelius, J.F., Prabhakar, H., Koerbel, A., Gnanalingham, K., Sandu, N., Ottaviani, G., Filis, A. & Buchfelder, M. (2009a). The trigemino-cardiac reflex: an update of the current knowledge. *J Neurosurg Anesthesiol*, 21, 3, (Jul), 187-95, 1537-1921 (Electronic) 0898-4921 (Linking)

Schaller, B., Probst, R., Strebel, S. & Gratzl, O. (1999). Trigeminocardiac reflex during surgery in the cerebellopontine angle. *J Neurosurg*, 90, 2, (Feb), 215-20, 0022-3085 (Print) 0022-3085 (Linking)

Schaller, B., Sandu, N., Filis, A., Ottaviani, G., Rasper, J., Noethen, C. & Buchfelder, M. (2009b). Trigemino-cardiac reflex: the trigeminal depressor responses during skull base surgery. *Clin Neurol Neurosurg*, 111, 2, (Feb), 220, 1872-6968 (Electronic) 0303-8467 (Linking)

Schaller, B.J. & Buchfelder, M. (2006). Trigemino-cardiac reflex in skull base surgery: from a better understanding to a better outcome? *Acta Neurochir (Wien)*, 148, 10, (Oct), 1029-31; discussion 1031, 0001-6268 (Print) 0001-6268 (Linking)

Schaller, B.J., Filis, A. & Buchfelder, M. (2008a). Trigemino-cardiac reflex in humans initiated by peripheral stimulation during neurosurgical skull-base operations. Its first description. *Acta Neurochir (Wien)*, 150, 7, (Jul), 715-7; discussion 717-8, 0942-0940 (Electronic) 0001-6268 (Linking)

Schaller, B.J., Rasper, J., Filis, A. & Buchfelder, M. (2008b). Difference in functional outcome of ipsilateral tinnitus after intraoperative occurrence of the trigemino-cardiac reflex in surgery for vestibular schwannomas. *Acta Neurochir (Wien)*, 150, 2, (Feb), 157-60, 0942-0940 (Electronic) 0001-6268 (Linking)

Schaller, B.J., Sandu, N., Cornelius, J.F., Filis, A. & Perez-Pinzon, M.A. (2009). Oxygen-conserving implications of the trigemino-cardiac reflex in the brain: the molecular basis of neuroprotection? *Mol Med*, 15, 5-6, (May-Jun), 125-6, 1528-3658 (Electronic) 1076-1551 (Linking)

Schaller, B.J., Weigel, D., Filis, A. & Buchfelder, M. (2007). Trigemino-cardiac reflex during transsphenoidal surgery for pituitary adenomas: methodological description of a prospective skull base study protocol. *Brain Res*, 1149, (May 29), 69-75, 0006-8993 (Print) 0006-8993 (Linking)

Seule, M.A., Stienen, M.N., Cadosch, D., Fournier, J.Y., Lussmann, R., Hildebrandt, G. & Gautschi, O.P. (2010). [Aneurysmal subarachnoid hemorrhage - therapy and complications]. *Anasthesiol Intensivmed Notfallmed Schmerzther*, 45, 1, (Jan), 8-17, 1439-1074 (Electronic) 0939-2661 (Linking)

Shelly, M.P. & Church, J.J. (1988). Bradycardia and facial surgery. *Anaesthesia*, 43, 422,

Shende, D., Sadhasivam, S. & Madan, R. (2000). Effects of peribulbar bupivacaine as an adjunct to general anaesthesia on peri-operative outcome following retinal detachment surgery. *Anaesthesia*, 55, 10, (Oct), 970-5, 0003-2409 (Print) 0003-2409 (Linking)

Simons, T. & Ruskell, G.L. (1988). Distribution and termination of trigeminal nerves to the cerebral arteries in monkeys. *J Anat*, 159, (Aug), 57-71, 0021-8782 (Print) 0021-8782 (Linking)

Spiriev, T., Kondoff, S. & Schaller, B. (2011a). Trigeminocardiac reflex during temporary clipping in aneurismal surgery: first description. *J Neurosurg Anesthesiol*, 23, 3, (Jul), 271-2, 1537-1921 (Electronic) 0898-4921 (Linking)

Spiriev, T., Sandu, N., Arasho, B., Kondoff, S., Tzekov, C. & Schaller, B. (2010). A new predisposing factor for trigemino-cardiac reflex during subdural empyema drainage: a case report. *J Med Case Reports*, 4, 391, 1752-1947 (Electronic) 1752-1947 (Linking)

Spiriev, T., Tzekov, C., Kondoff, S., Laleva, L., Sandu, N., Arasho, B. & Schaller, B. (2011b). Trigemino-cardiac reflex during chronic subdural haematoma removal: report of chemical initiation of dural sensitization. *JRSM Short Rep*, 2, 4, 27, 2042-5333 (Electronic)

Stott, D.G. (1989). Reflex bradycardia in facial surgery. *Br J Plast Surg*, 42, 5, (Sep), 595-7, 0007-1226 (Print) 0007-1226 (Linking)

Takenaka, I., Aoyama, K., Iwagaki, T., Ishimura, H. & Kadoya, T. (2006). Development of torsade de pointes caused by exacerbation of QT prolongation during clipping of cerebral artery aneurysm in a patient with subarachnoid haemorrhage. *Br J Anaesth*, 97, 4, (Oct), 533-5, 0007-0912 (Print) 0007-0912 (Linking)

Wilson, C. (1983). Surgical management of endocrine-active pituitary adenomas, *Oncology of the nervous system*, M. Walker, 117-150 Martinus Nijhoff, Boston

Wolf, S. (1966). Sudden death and the oxygen-conserving reflex. *Am Heart J*, 71, 6, (Jun), 840-1, 0002-8703 (Print) 0002-8703 (Linking)

2

# Anesthesiologic Management for Awake Craniotomy

Roberto Zoppellari, Enrico Ferri and Manuela Pellegrini
*Departement of Anesthesia and Intensive Care,*
*S. Anna University Hospital, Ferrara*
*Italy*

## 1. Introduction

The term "awake craniotomy" comprises the entire spectrum of surgical-anesthesiological techniques developed to allow intra-operative brain mapping during surgery in or near eloquent brain areas , in order to minimize the risk of postoperative functional sequelae.

Indeed, when dealing with brain lesions located in functional areas, such as sensorimotor, language or vision, neurosurgeons aim at removing the maximum amount of lesion minimizing the risk of producing neurological deficits so as to avoid impairing patient's quality of life. As a matter of fact, in the span of a few millimetres around the margin of the resection, as well as within the lesion to be removed, one can find eloquent sites whose function is better explored on an awake individual. In fact the collaboration of an awake patient is crucial to guide the surgeon in sparing the function while being as most radical as possible in removing the tumour.

No consensus exists about the optimal anesthetic regimen to follow, among the many proposed that allow intra-operative brain mapping. They range from local anesthesia to conscious sedation or general anesthesia with an "awake" intraoperative phase. The choice is based on the institution past experience and on different surgical needs and is generally tailored on patients characteristics and procedure durations [7, 39].

Independently of the technique chosen, the anaesthesiologist should be able to provide adequate analgesia and comfort during each surgical step and should prevent nausea, vomiting and seizures, while maintaining respiratory, haemodynamic and neurologic homeostasis [6]. Obviously, preoperative evaluation and patients selection are crucial for the success of this type of surgery [37].

The aim of this chapter is to evaluate the application of different anesthesiological regimens and related intraoperative complications in awake craniotomy for resection of lesions located in eloquent brain areas.

## 2. Indications and contraindications of specific anesthesiological techniques

Traditionally, awake craniotomy can be performed with 3 different anesthesiological techniques [39]. The "Asleep-Awake-Asleep" (AAA) technique [21] consists of 3 phases: at first general anesthesia is induced and the patient is intubated or ventilated through a laryngeal mask (LMA) and kept asleep until the brain is exposed; then anesthesia is discontinued and the tracheal tube or LMA removed and the patient is allowed to fully awake for brain mapping and monitoring of neurological functions to be spared. When brain mapping needs to be alternated with lesion removal, e.g. when subcortical pathways are in or near the lesion, patients are kept awake also during surgical resection; then anesthesia is induced again, the patient re-intubated or the LMA reinserted and surgery is completed. In the so called "Asleep-Awake" (AA) technique [24], after completion of the tumour resection the patient is let awake or just lightly sedated until the end of surgery. The third technique, called "Monitored Anesthesia Care" (MAC) consists of sedation and analgesia, titrated to the different surgical phases, and requires the anaesthesiologist to accurately choose from an armamentarium of different drugs and to combine them and their dosages in order to achieve the desired level of sedation [3, 13, 27]. This technique does not require the use of tracheal tube or LMA and is centred on the association between a good loco-regional anesthesia of the scalp and the use of short acting, easy titratable anaesthetics [26].

Hans considers three main reasons for performing awake craniotomy. First, no real benefit is expected from general anesthesia. The second reason is to avoid any interference between anesthetics and the electrical activity of the brain. The last and most important reason is the opportunity to take advantage of the awake state of the patient and of his capacity to co-operate during selected neurosurgical procedures (removal of lesions involving Broca's and Wernicke's speech areas or vascular lesions in or near other eloquent areas) [17].

Each anesthetic technique requires, beyond respiratory and hemodynamic control, adequate anesthesia/sedation, analgesia, and should not interfere with electrophysiologic mapping and measurements, or cognitive testing.

### 2.1 The Asleep-Awake-Asleep technique (AAA)

The asleep-awake-asleep technique (AAA), described above, has the advantages of a good airway control, implemented through tracheal intubation or LMA, and a deep sedation that leads the patient to feel less psychological stress and discomfort and not to feel pain. However, the AAA finds its main limitations in the fact that patients have to endure more physical stress associated with intubation, mechanical ventilation and longer hospital stays [35].

During the awake period all airway devices have to be removed to enable verbal communication and patient collaboration. This manoeuvre may induce airway irritation and coughing, leading to patient movement and intracranial pressure increase with brain bulging. Reinsertion of the airway devices at the end of surgery may be cumbersome, especially for the rigid head pin-fixation [7]. Another major drawback is the residual effect of the anesthetic used in the asleep phase on the cortical functions that are being evaluated during the awake period. Short-acting, easily titratable anesthetics should be used for this purpose [13].

### 2.2 The Asleep-Awake (AA) technique

An evolution of the technique described above, AA consists of avoiding to induce anesthesia again at the end of the procedure, thus bypassing the problems related to reinsertion of the ventilation device [7]. Of course this entails providing sedation and analgesia for closure, thus it sums the particularities of both AAA and monitored anaesthesia care, described below.

### 2.3 Monitored anesthesia care

Monitored anesthesia care includes sedation with short-acting anesthetics titrated during the different phases of surgical procedure and local anesthetic infiltration of the scalp.The anesthesiologist thus provides adequate analgesia and full cooperation of the patient, addresses clinical problems and provides psychological support to patients [36].

This method requires proper planning and the ability to convert the planned analgesia and sedation into general anesthesia, if necessary. Maintaining the optimal sedation level and adequate intra-operative management of the airways are the main skills required by this technique. The former is crucial, since over-sedation results in an uncooperative patient and respiratory depression, whereas under-sedation makes the patient extremely uncomfortable, anxious and restless [13]. Fundamental is the performance of a scalp block to reduce the need for opioids and thus the risks of respiratory depression [9, 10].

The combination of remifentanil and propofol has been successfully used in spontaneously breathing patients undergoing awake craniotomy [17, 23]. Remifentanil has a very short context-sensitive half life and allows rapid control of the depth of anaesthesia and great haemodynamic stability [39] while propofol is associated with a decreased incidence of convulsions [19], although both drugs tend to produce respiratory depression with subsequent hypercarbia and hypoxia [7, 19, 39].

Airway instrumentation may be deemed necessary by respiratory depression, uncontrollable seizures or sudden neurological deterioration. This risk is obviously increased by patient's co-morbidities, such as morbid obesity and/or obstructive sleep apnoea syndrome (OSAS) [17]. The latter condition is often associated to cardiovascular disorders, such as arterial hypertension, ischemic heart disease, atrial fibrillation and stroke [33], and is considered an absolute exclusion criteria by some authors [37]. Recently, some experiences have been reported on the use of continuous positive airway pressure in patients with OSAS undergoing awake craniotomy [15, 22].

Obesity, as well as obstructive lung disease, is not an absolute contraindication [37], but a balance between the possible benefits and risks has to be done in each case [3]. In a retrospective chart review of 332 propofol-based awake craniotomies for epilepsy surgery using the AAA technique, Skucas found BMI higher than 30 to be a consistent risk factor for haemoglobin desaturation, requiring a secured airway [42].

Therefore, predictors of difficult airway management must be thoroughly searched for and anticipated, and are to be taken into serious account when selecting the anesthesiological management.

## 3. Preoperative planning

A specific and focused clinical assessment is extremely important and must consider the following aspects [6, 36]. Preoperative airway evaluation is essential given the difficulty of managing airway complications and the possibility of obstruction during the surgical procedure. Ease of mask airway, Mallampati score, and other predictors of difficulty with laryngoscopy, intubation and any history of past anesthesia must be extensively reviewed. The anesthesiologist must be prepared to emergent laryngoscopy, perhaps in a difficult position because of surgical drapes or pinions, and ensure all necessary equipment is immediately at hand. As discussed above, the opinion of the authors is that OSAS is to be considered as an absolute exclusion criterion [37]. Patients with epilepsy should be carefully evaluated for both type and frequency of seizures, verifying the regimen and serum levels of preoperative therapy. A patient may receive an oral loading dose of phenytoin or other antiepileptic drugs, depending on the frequency of seizures.

Peripheral access sites and the need for an arterial line and urinary catheter placement should be assessed during the preoperative examination.

Obesity, gastroesophageal reflux, dysphagia and chronic cough or wheezing may be relative contraindications depending on severity [36].

Evaluation of brain swelling is also important, because intracranial pressure control during spontaneous breathing is much harder compared to the mechanical ventilation setting.

Steroids, for example dexamethasone, must be considered in these cases, also to prevent nausea and vomiting, in combination with specific anti-emetic drugs, such as metoclopramide or ondansetron [17].

Other factors including tumour size, haemorrhagic risk and hemodynamic stability are considered in agreement with the surgeon.

A key role in preoperative evaluation is assessment of psychological state of patient and of his level of anxiety. Perks et al found that anxiety was common in neurosurgical patients, the incidence ranging between 60% and 92%, it was higher for female patients and regarded mostly surgical procedure and postoperative neurological deficits [34].

Berkenstadt in his review describes the administration of clonidine at a dose of 2-3 mcg $kg^{-1}$ orally one hour before entering operating room to induce mild sedation, haemodynamic stability, as well as analgesic and anti-emetic effects with a lower incidence of cognitive deficits[3].

An adequate preoperative and explanatory conversation turns out to be essential to gain patients' confidence. Patient must be informed about potential risks, safety measures, stages of procedure, and all that will occur in operating room. In a study on patient perceptions of awake brain tumour surgery, Whittle found that the procedure was well tolerated if fully explained preoperatively [45]. In this study about 20% of patients did not recall being awake although they were cooperative, 20% had more than minor discomfort, about 30% were anxious, and 15% experienced fear.

The anesthesiologist must not conceal sounds (monitor alarms, cranial drilling, elektroknife, ultrasonic surgical aspirator) or discomforts (unchangeable position, aphasia during cortical mapping) from the patient, who must understand that these discomforts are necessary to the procedure. The anesthesiologist must work in team with the neurosurgeon and speech therapist and motivate the patient, this being one major factor determining how successful the surgical procedure will be.

Selecting a patient who is able to cooperate in an unfamiliar and stressful environment for an extended period of time is crucial. As a matter of fact, it has been claimed that the only absolute contraindication to the awake technique is an uncooperative patient [39].

## 4. Key steps of the procedure

Every patient scheduled for awake craniotomy has to be referred to the anaesthesiologist some days before surgery, to be evaluated, informed and reassured about the procedure.

Preoperative evaluation concerns mainly the possibility of maintaining airway patency during sedation for the craniotomy. In particular, the risk of obstructive sleep apnoea and criteria for difficult intubation or ventilation are considered respectively absolute and relative exclusion criteria.

On the day of surgery, in the operating room, a peripheral venous line is inserted while ECG, SpO2 and non invasive blood pressure monitoring is set up. Supplemental oxygen is delivered through nasal prong with end tidal carbon dioxide and respiratory rate monitoring.

### 4.1 Monitored Anesthesia Care (MAC)

Usually, if pre-anesthesia has not been administered on the ward, midazolam 20 mcg $kg^{-1}$ and clonidine 1 mcg $kg^{-1}$ are administered intravenously. Emergency intubation equipment has to be readily available. Under light sedation an arterial line is generally set up in the radial artery, and a Foley urinary catheter may be inserted. Some key points have to be respected for the success of the technique.

1. The patients' position on the surgical table must be adjusted to be comfortable for several hours.
2. It is important to assure a good analgesia and sedation during the positioning of the Mayfield headrest and the craniotomy. Paramount is the combination of an extensive local anesthesia and intravenous sedative and analgesics, to reduce the need for opioids administration, thus minimizing the risk of oversedation. For this purpose the performance of a good scalp block (supraorbital, zygomatic-temporal, auricolotemporal, lesser and greater occipital nerves, see table 1) with ropivacaine or levo-bupivacaine is fundamental. The block must be reinforced with local anesthetic infiltration of the headpin sites and of the surgical incision line. For analgesia and sedation the anesthesiologist will chose short acting drugs, which guarantee proper titration and the rapid shift through the various phases of the procedure and above all the lack of interference with the electro-cortical stimulation and cognitive tests. Sedation depth and analgesia must be systematically assessed using a sedation score and the Visual Analogue Scale or a numeric rating scale respectively. During the head fixation and the craniotomy, sedation is titrated to obtain a Ramsay score between 3 and 4.
3. After the dura opening, sedation has to be terminated at least 15 minutes prior to intraoperative monitoring and patients maintained fully awake and cooperative until the end of brain mapping or tumour removal, depending on the type and purpose of surgery. In case of pain arising during this phase, paracetamol 1g and eventually remifentanil 0.025-0.05 mcg $kg^{-1}$ $min^{-1}$ can be administered.
4. In the end patients are sedated again to obtain a Ramsay score between 2 and 4, as in the first part of the procedure. Sedation is withdrawn after removing the Mayfield headrest.

5. Postoperative analgesia can be achieved with a combination of intravenous analgesics and the repetition of the scalp block using a long lasting local anesthetic. Prevention of nausea and vomiting is another key factor in order to accomplish the patients' comfort and satisfaction.

### 4.2 Asleep-Awake-Asleep (AAA) and Asleep-Awake (AA)

In the case of AAA or AA techniques, the first part of the intervention is performed under general anesthesia. This guarantees immobility and maximum patient comfort, while assuring adequate oxygenation and ventilation. Airway control is nowadays generally achieved by LMA [8, 14, 39].

The key-points in these techniques are emergence from anesthesia and re-introduction of the ventilation device (AAA only). Emergence must be smooth, considering that the patient has to maintain rigid head fixation. For the same reason the AAA technique is made difficult by reinsertion of LMA. A recent report addresses the advantages of using the LMA-Supreme [31].

As discussed below, both techniques may take advantage from the use of short-acting anesthetics, whose fast offset allows rapid neurologic evaluation and reliable brain mapping [8,24,39]. This is exceedingly true for the AA technique in which drugs titration is crucial to afford the last part of surgery under sedation without airway control.

### 4.3 Drugs

Tumour resection, unlike epilepsy surgery, does not require routine intraoperative electro-corticography. This increases the choice of anaesthetic agents use. Anyway, the target controlled infusion (TCI) of propofol, associated to remifentanil-based analgesia, accurately titrated on the surgical stimula, are a reasonable choice and proved to be feasible and safe. TCI infusion allows brain mapping to be performed earlier after the suspension of sedation [3, 17, 23, 24, 26, 39]. Non pharmacologic measures such as frequent reassurance and holding the patient's hand cannot be overemphasised.

Dexmedetomidine is a selective alpha-2 adrenoreceptor agonist that has been shown to provide sedation and analgesia without significant respiratory depression. It also has a sparing effect on analgesia requirement. Dexmedetomidine has been used successfully in this setting, although some concerns of impaired neurocognitive testing after stopping infusion have been cast. Hypotension and bradycardia are common side effects of the drug [41].

| | |
|---|---|
| supraorbital | lesser occipital nerve |
| zygomatic-temporal | greater occipital nerve |
| auricolotemporal | |

Table 1. Nerves blocked when performing the scalp block

## 5. Postoperative care

The occurrence, level and duration of acute post operative pain in neurosurgical patients is not precisely known, because of a lack of clinical studies. A lot of analgesics could be used for post-craniotomy pain control, although no one is free from disadvantages. The opiates can cause nausea, vomit and respiratory depression with consequent cerebral blood flow and intracranial pressure increase. Non-steroidal anti-inflammatory drugs are not commonly used as they are associated to an increased intracranial risk of haemorrhage [16].

Scalp infiltration seems to be an effective procedure in the reduction of postoperative pain, caused mainly by the surgical wound [5]. Grossman et al [16] evaluated the efficacy of infiltrating the wound with lidocaine and bupivacaine associated to a single intravenous dose of metamizole for the control of postoperative pain in patients undergoing awake craniotomy. The majority of patients did not ask for extra analgesia during the first 12 postoperative hours, which are reported to be the most painful after craniotomy [16].

Scalp infiltration or surgical wound infiltration with local anesthetics have been successfully associated also with paracetamol for postoperative analgesia [20, 25, 45].

When not associated to regional anesthesia, paracetamol alone does not appear sufficient for postoperative analgesia. In this case the addition of tramadol or nalbuphine to paracetamol seems to be necessary, with the drawback of a greater incidence of nausea and vomiting [44].

Postoperative nausea and vomiting (PONV), in patients submitted to craniotomy, represent indeed another frequent post-operative complication that asks for an indispensable treatment. Manninen indicates a comprehensive incidence of 38% with a predominance in younger compared to adult patients [28]. The frequency of PONV seems to be lower in patients submitted to awake craniotomy compared to those submitted to craniotomy under general anaesthesia. This fact is likely due to the greater use of opioids, particularly morphine, either pre or post-operatively [29]. The most used antiemetic is ondansetron 4-8 mg, but metoclopramide (10 mg), droperidol (0.625 mg) or dexamethasone (4-16 mg) have all been used [18, 29, 39, 45].

## 6. Complications and their treatment

Anesthesia for awake craniotomy is challenging. The risk of complications either anesthesia-related or caused by surgical stimulation has been clearly outlined by many authors [7, 10, 24, 27, 38, 39, 42]. Seizures are reported to be a common intraoperative complication during awake craniotomy for tumour resection [7, 27] and can be seen both in awake and in asleep patients. As reported by Conte et al, intraoperative seizures' incidence can be as high as 30% in an asleep-awake technique, but those requiring medical intervention are 6-7% [8]. Other authors report an overall incidence of intraoperative seizures lower than 8% in tumour awake surgery [10, 39] but all patients in these series received prophylactic anticonvulsants. This high variability might also be explained by differences in seizures definition, by different level of intraoperative electrophysiological monitoring, current intensity and stimulator used, by different anesthesia or underlying patients pathology (tumour vs. intractable epilepsy or both), and seizure control [8, 24]. Usually, seizures occur during mapping or tumour resection and are of short duration and self-limiting [27]. It can be the case of focal seizures, whose therapy mainly consists of the irrigation of the surgical field with ice cold Ringer's lactate solution [40]. Generalized seizures not responding to ice cold irrigation can require the administration of benzodiazepines or propofol, which is much safer in an intubated and mechanically ventilated patient [7]. Although its pro- and anti-convulsant properties are still under debate, propofol sedation during epilepsy surgery is popular and does not appear to interfere with electrocorticography, provided it is suspended at least 15 minutes before recording [19]. Preoperative prophylaxis with phenytoin or other antiepilectic drugs is advocated by some authors [8].

Monitored anesthesia care is an approach that does not include airway control, thus it is vulnerable to ventilation impairment, ranging from respiratory depression to airway obstruction. Their common endpoint are hypoxia and hypercarbia, leading to brain swelling. Hypoxia and hypoventilation are commonly related to over-sedation [13]. Nonetheless, Skucas and Artru , analyzing intraoperative complications in 322 patients undergoing awake craniotomy for epilepsy surgery, indicate that only 5 patients (1.5%) showed an oxygen saturation below 90% [42].

The immediate management of airway obstruction includes decreasing sedation level, jaw thrust or instrumentation of the airways. Emergency airway devices should be immediately available throughout the procedure. Intubation under direct vision, blind nasal intubation, fiberoptic-assisted intubation and different kinds of LMA are among the possible options that have to be planned before the surgical procedure [41].

Hypertension is reported with varying incidence by different authors, although by some of them invasive blood pressure monitoring was used inconsistently [42] or even never used [10, 39]. It occurs mainly as a consequence of painful stimula, such as application of the Mayfield headrest [3, 42], generally without negative sequelae to the patients. Therefore, it seems reasonable to seek for a better anticipation of these stimuli with proper analgesia supplements. Remifentanil appears the drug of choice for its favourable kinetic profile and it demonstrated to provide good haemodynamic control during particularly noxious portions of craniotomy procedures [3, 11, 12, 23]. Reluctance to provide sufficient anesthesia that might cause apnoea has been addressed [24] and occasionally intravenous antihypertensive agents may be needed [41]. Beta-blockers such as labetalol and esmolol are the most commonly used drugs for arterial pressure increase [36]. Urapidil has also been used successfully for treating hypertension during awake craniotomy [38].

Nausea and vomiting are annoying for the patient and can make him/her agitated and uncooperative. Many studies on awake craniotomy with different techniques report an incidence varying from 0 to 9% [4, 10, 24, 27, 39, 42]. The use of propofol associated to low dose of opioids has been advocated as the cause of a minor incidence of nausea/vomiting with awake craniotomy compared to general anesthesia [29]. The use of antiemetics can minimize its incidence, but it is not always successful because this complication is often directly related to surgical manipulation (e.g. during dural opening, mesial temporal and basal frontal lobes or amygdala manipulation, major intracranial vessels handling) or to inadequate analgesia and hypovolemia [18, 46].

Other anesthesia-related complications are shivering, pain and poor cooperation. Shivering must be prevented by warming the patient. Clonidine, dexmedetomidine, meperidine, tramadol, nefopam, and ondansetron can be used for shivering prevention or treatment [1]. Since this type of procedure is very long, forced posture may create pain. The administration of analgesics such as paracetamol, or the titration of the ongoing analgesia and the possibility of small movements are all useful for intra-operative management. Poor cooperation and agitation may occur at any step of the procedure. They can be related to anxiety, pain, over sedation, seizures, and inadequate intra-operative psychological support [36].

Venous air embolism is a rare but possible adverse event in awake craniotomy [2, 43]. Its occurrence must be kept in mind any time there is a pressure gradient between the surgical site and the right atrium. It is a typical complication of neurosurgical cases performed in the sitting position, with a highly variable incidence (10-80%) [32]. During awake craniotomy, spontaneous breathing raises even more the pressure gradient between surgical site and right atrium, therefore favouring air suction [36]. However, awake craniotomy is typically performed in the lateral or supine positions, and its incidence in this setting has been reported as low as 0.64%[2]. Diagnosis can be made with precordial Doppler [2, 30]. Complications can be prevented by reducing the gradient between surgical field and heart and by elevating venous pressure raising the legs above the heart level and hydrating the patient [30]. Patients with patent foramen ovale should be carefully evaluated for the risk of paradoxical cerebral air embolism [30].

## 7. Outcome and prognosis

In a prospective observational study Klimek assumed that awake craniotomy (AC) and craniotomy performed under general anesthesia (GAC) may be associated with different levels of stress and consequently different inflammatory responses and release of plasma interleukins [25]. The authors have considered two groups of 20 patients each, undergoing respectively AC and GAC. The results obtained from pre-intra-and post operative determinations of circulating levels of IL-6, IL-8 and IL-10 suggested that awake function-controlled craniotomy does not cause a significantly different inflammatory response than craniotomy performed under general anesthesia. Postoperative pain was significantly lower in the AC group compared to the GAC group at 12 hours [25]. Hol et al prospectively evaluated two groups of patients undergoing awake craniotomy with a propofol-remifentanil based sedation or craniotomy under general anesthesia, to compare the plasma amino acid profiles in the two groups as an index of physical and emotional stress and pain [20]. They found a significantly higher phenylalanine/tyrosine ratio, suggesting a grater oxidative stress, in the general anesthesia group, which had also a longer hospitalization and experienced greater pain [20].

Monitored anesthesia care, performed combining regional scalp anesthesia with a propofol-remifentanil sedation regimen, accomplishes the noteworthy result of obtaining an optimal sedation level throughout the entire surgical procedure, using minimal doses of opioids and propofol. We prospectively studied 70 patients undergoing awake surgery for lesions located near eloquent brain areas. As shown in the picture below, remifentanil infusion rate, propofol concentration at the effect site and Ramsay sedation score showed a related trend throughout the procedure (fig. 1) when using our technique, pointed out in the paragraph "Expert Suggestions". At the time of the scalp block the mean Ramsay score was 2.4 ± 0.46, remifentanil infusion rate was 0.045 ± 0.03 mcg $kg^{-1}$ $min^{-1}$ and the mean propofol concentration at the effect site was 0.14 ± 0.12 mcg $ml^{-1}$. At the time of the bone flap removal the mean infusion rate of remifentanil was 0.07 ± 0.03 mcg $kg^{-1}$ $min^{-1}$ and the mean propofol concentration at the effect site was 0.5 ± 0.28 mcg $ml^{-1}$ with a mean Ramsay score of 3.5 ± 0.6. At the starting of intra-operative monitoring (IOM) remifentanil and propofol had been stopped 10 minutes before: propofol concentration at the effect site was 0.11 ± 0.06 mcg $ml^{-1}$ and Ramsay score was 2.1 ± 0.24.

All patients completed successfully the intervention under monitored anaesthesia care. No patient required admission to our ICU. Complications were transient and easily controlled. Hypertension was the most common intraoperative adverse event, occurring in 40% of patients, and it was treated by intravenous labetalol or urapidil boluses. The other three most common intraoperative complications were nausea (18.6%), oxygen desaturation lasting > 30 seconds (15.7%) and short duration seizures (14.3%). All complications were easily handled: nausea was treated with ondansetron 4 mg intravenously, seizures with cold irrigation of the cortex, and oxygen desaturation, being almost constantly the consequence of oversedation, was treated by lowering propofol or remifentanil infusion. None of these events did affect the course of surgery. Postoperative pain, assessed at 2-6-12-24 hours postoperatively, was <= 3 on a Numeric Rating Scale.

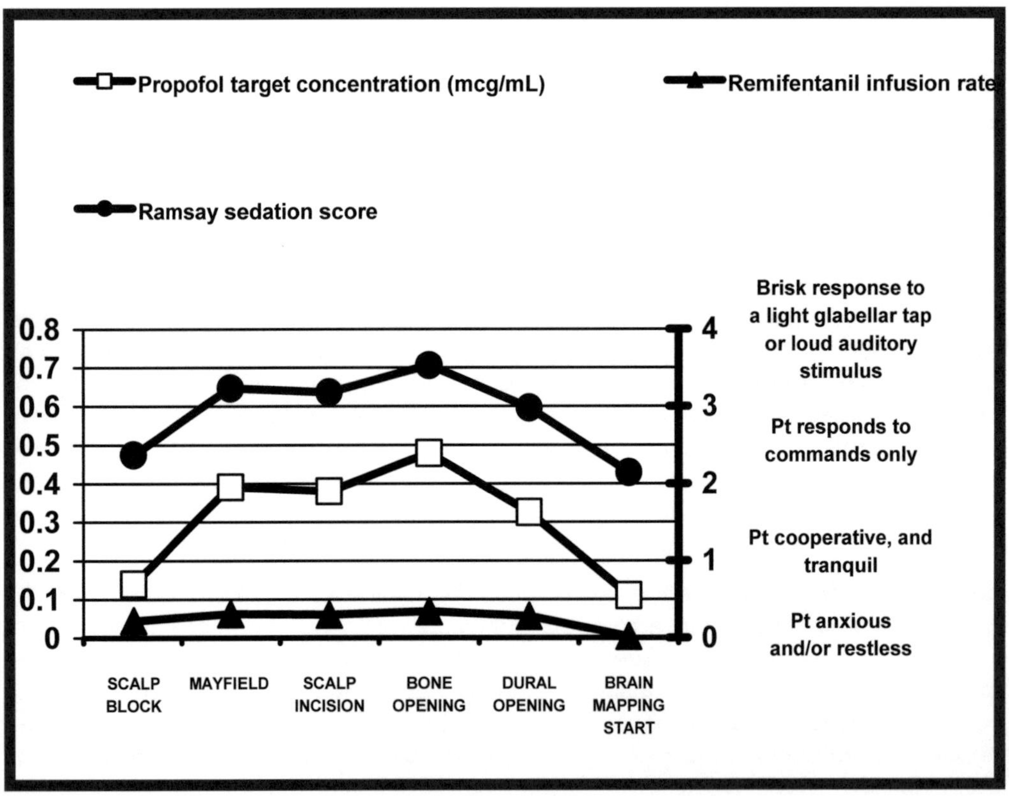


Fig. 1. Remifentanil infusion rate, propofol concentration at the effect site and Ramsay sedation score on 70 consecutive patients undergoing awake surgery for lesions located near eloquent brain areas.

## 8. Expert suggestions

Preoperative assessment is the step in which the relationship between patient and anesthesiologist has to be set. Having the same doctor evaluating the patient preoperatively and performing anesthesia the day of surgery contributes to create this relationship, that is crucial for the outcome. Clear explanations, reassurance and constant feedback are the mainstay of psychological assistance that these patients deserve before and during surgery.

Airway is the main concern on the debate on the choice of anesthesia regimen, among monitored anesthesia care and asleep-awake-asleep or asleep-awake. To date, no study definitely demonstrates that one technique is superior to the others. Each institution has to develop its own protocol, as a function of past experience and results. A good rule is that the anesthesiologist should have the skills to shift from a technique to the other in any case that require general anesthesia to be instituted.

Our technique entails intravenous midazolam 20 mcg $kg^{-1}$ and clonidine 1 mcg $kg^{-1}$ at the arrival in the operating room, then sedation with propofol TCI and analgesia with remifentanil starts, while the anesthesiologist blocks the nerves of the scalp with ropivacaine 1 %. The Mayfield headrest is positioned by preventively anaesthetizing the headpin sites with lidocaine and the surgical incision line is infiltrated with mepivacaine 1% with 1:200,000 epinephrine.

Propofol TCI is then set to reach an effect site concentration around 0.5 mcg $ml^{-1}$ (range 0.2 to 1.5) and remifentanil between 0.075 and 0.1 mcg $Kg^{-1}$ $min^{-1}$. This should provide an adequate sedation without respiratory depression during bone and dura mater opening. This phase is very challenging for the anesthesiologist because haemodynamic and respiratory derangements are very likely to occur during the deepening of sedation. A Ramsay sedation score of 3 to 4 is the goal and accurate titration of propofol and remifentanil is the key rule to accomplish it.

At the end of dura mater opening, brain mapping starts and no interference by sedation is allowed in order to test patients' neurologic function. Ten minutes in our experience are enough to allow for propofol washout since infusion is stopped. Remifentanil low context-sensitive half-time (CSHT), independent of infusion time, provides complete washout in about three minutes.

Should patients require supplemental analgesia or light sedation to tolerate the fixed position on the operating table during brain mapping, remifentanil up to 0.05 mcg $Kg^{-1}$ $min^{-1}$ can be administrated without impairing intraoperative neurophysiologic monitoring.

Patients are maintained fully awake and cooperative until the end of tumour removal, especially if it needs to be alternated to brain mapping, and then sedated again with propofol TCI and remifentanil to obtain a Ramsay score between 2 and 4, as in the first part of the procedure.

## 9. Explicative cases

### Case 1

A 52-year-old man, American Society of Anaesthesiology (ASA) physical status 2, underwent awake craniotomy under monitored anaesthesia care for a left temporoparietooccipital grade III anaplastic olygodendroglioma placed in the rolandic area. He was on phenytoin for a former epileptic episode. He had no other relevant data on his medical history. Weight was 75 kg and Body Mass Index (BMI) was 25. The day of surgery he was prepared as described above. The procedure went on uneventfully until sedation was resumed for closure. At this time propofol effect-site concentration was 0.6 mcg $ml^{-1}$ and remifentanil dosage was 0.15 mcg $Kg^{-1}$ $min^{-1}$ and $SpO_2$ decreased below 90% for a time frame > 30 seconds. Patient's Ramsay score was 4, he was stimulated intensely and allowed to breath deeply pure oxygen through a facial mask for some minutes, regaining rapidly $SpO_2$ > 95%. This event induced to lower remifentanil infusion rate to 0.1 mcg $Kg^{-1}$ $min^{-1}$, after which no respiratory complications were seen until the end of surgery. Total operating room time was 475 minutes; propofol effect site concentration and remifentanil infusion rate reached 0.8 mcg $ml^{-1}$ and 0.2 mcg $Kg^{-1}$ $min^{-1}$ respectively during skin incision and bone opening, two among the most painful phases of craniotomy. At that point $PaCO_2$ was 43.2 mmHg.

Comment: Oversedation occurred because painful stimulation was expected to occur and analgesia and sedation were probably resumed too promptly compared to the onset of surgical stimulation. In fact an even higher dosage of the same drugs did not produce the same effect during the opening phase, when it was adequate to pain. Lowering remifentanil infusion rate and breathing pure oxygen through a facial mask for a few minutes are simple maneuvers that immediately resolved the complication. Excellent view and access to patient face is crucial to prevent more serious events.

**Case 2**

A 58-year-old man, ASA physical status 2, weight 70 kg (BMI 23.7) was scheduled to undergo awake craniotomy for a recidivating left frontotemporal astrocytoma. His past medical history revealed gastritis and craniotomy for the same tumour one year before. Surgery was foreseen to last 10 hours, and the patient, although willing to collaborate, was deemed not able to cope with such a long procedure due to anxiety. Therefore he was candidate for the asleep-awake technique. Anesthesia was induced with propofol 100 mg and remifentanil 0.1 mcg $Kg^{-1}$ $min^{-1}$ in neutral supine position, an i-gel® supraglottic airway device # 3 was inserted and lungs were mechanically ventilated to maintain a $PaCO_2$ around 35 mmHg (Vt 700 ml; RR 13 breaths per min). Mayfield headrest was positioned after performing the scalp block, then he was flipped to right lateral position, and the opening phase took place. Anesthesia was maintained with propofol 2.5-3 mcg $ml^{-1}$ at the effect site and remifentanil 0.15-0.2 mcg $Kg^{-1}$ $min^{-1}$. Three hours later, upon completion of dura opening, anesthesia was discontinued, the patient was awakened and the LMA removed. Fifteen minutes later brain mapping started. Intraoperative monitoring was carried out without complications for the following 2 hours, then the patient became very anxious and restless, and he claimed to be very tired and not to be able to complete the last part of the procedure in the awake state. A shift to "asleep-awake-asleep" was decided and anaesthesia was induced again. Reinsertion of i-gel® airway device was smooth despite the lateral position. I-gel® was chosen because insertion and tight adherence to the laryngeal framework in a non-supine patient could have been cumbersome using a standard LMA. Four hours later, surgery ended and the patient was successfully awakened.

Comment. This case is described to show how one should be able to modify his standard technique to adapt it to different settings. Airway management is one of the major drawbacks of AAA, and the anesthesiologist should be familiar with a large spectrum of devices to choose from in each particular case.

## 10. Acknowledgement

We would like to thank Dr. Anna Matina for her precious help.

## 11. References

[1] Alfonsi P. Postanesthetic shivering. Epidemiology, pathophysiology and approaches to prevention and management. Drugs 2001; 61: 2193-205.

[2] Balki M, Manninen PH, McGuire GP, El-Beheiry H, Bernstein M. Venous air embolism during awake craniotomy in a supine patient. Can J Anesth 2003; 50 (8): 835-8.

[3] Berkenstadt H, Perel A, Hadani M, Unofrievich I, Ram Z. Monitored anesthesia care using remifentanil and propofol for awake craniotomy. J Neurosurg Anesthesiol 2001; 13 (3): 246-9.

[4] Blanshard HJ, Chung F, Manninen PH, Taylor MD, Bernstein M. Awake craniotomy for removal of intracranial tumor: considerations for early discharge. Anesth Analg 2001; 92: 89-94.

[5] Bloomfield E.L, Schubert A, Secic M , Barnett G, Shutway F, Ebrahim Z.Y. The Influence of scalp infiltration with bupivacaine on hemodynamics and postoperative pain in adult patients undergoing craniotomy. Anesth Analg 1998; 87: 579-82.

[6] Bonhomme V, Born JD, Hans P. Anaesthetic management of awake craniotomy. Ann Fr Anesth Reanim 2004; 23: 389-94.

[7] Conte V, Baratta P, Tomaselli P, Songa V, Magni L, Stocchetti N. Awake neurosurgery: an update. Minerva Anestesiol 2008; 74: 289-92.

[8] Conte V, Magni L, Songa V, Tomaselli P, Ghisoni L, Magnoni S, Bello L, Stocchetti N. Analysis of propofol/remifentanil infusion protocol for tumour surgery with intraoperative brain mapping. J Neurosurg Anesthesiol 2010; 22:119–127.

[9] Costello TG, Cormack JR. Anaesthesia for awake craniotomy: a modern approach. J Clin Neurosci. 2004; 11: 16–9.

[10] Danks RA, Aglio LS, Gugino LD, Black PM. Craniotomy under local anesthesia and monitored conscious sedation for the resection of tumours involving eloquent cortex. J Neurooncol 2000; 49 (2):131-9.

[11] Egan T, Lemmens HJM, Fiset P, Hermann DJ. Pharm D, Muir K.T, Stanski D.R, Shafer S.L. The pharmacokinetics of the new short-acting opioid remifentanil (GI87084B) in healthy adult male volunteers. Anesthesiology: 1993; 79 (5): 881-92.

[12] Egan, Talmage D. Pharmacokinetics and pharmacodynamics of remifentanil: an update in the year 2000. Curr Opin Anaesthesiol 2000; 13 (4): 449-55.

[13] Frost E, Booij L. Anesthesia in the patient for awake craniotomy. Curr Opin Anaesthesiol 2007; 20 (4): 331-5.

[14] Gadhinglajkar S, Sreedhar R, Abraham M. Anesthesia management of awake craniotomy performed under asleep–awake–asleep technique using laryngeal mask airway: report of two cases. Neurol India 2008; 56: 65–7.

[15] Gonzales J, Lombard FW, Borel CO. Pressure support mode improves ventilation in «asleep-awake-asleep» craniotomy. J Neurosurg Anesthesiol 2006; 18 (1): 88.

[16] Grossman R, Ram Z, Perel A, Yusim Y, Zaslansky R, Berkenstadt H. Control of postoperative pain after awake craniotomy with local intradermal analgesia and metamizol. Isr Med Assoc J 2007; 9 (5): 380–2.

[17] Hans P, Bonhomme V. Anesthetic management for neurosurgery in awake patients. Minerva Anestesiol 2007; 73 (10): 507-12.

[18] Herrick IA, Craen RA, Gelb AW, Miller LA, Kubu CS, Girvin JP, Parrent AG, Eliasziw M, Kirkby J. Propofol sedation during awake craniotomy for seizures: patient-controlled administration versus neurolept analgesia. Anesth Analg 1997; 84 (6): 1285-91.

[19] Herrick IA, Craen RA, Gelb AW, McLachlan RS, Girvin JP, Parrent AG, Eliasziw M, Kirkby J. Propofol sedation during awake craniotomy for seizures: electrocorticographic and epileptogenic effects. Anesth Analg1997; 84 (6): 1280-4.

[20] Hol JW, Klimek M, van der Heide-Mulder M, Stronks D, Vincent AJ, Klein J, Zijlstra FJ, Fekkes D. Awake craniotomy induces fewer changes in the plasma amino acid profile than craniotomy under general anesthesia. J Neurosurg Anesthesiol 2009; 21: 98–107.

[21] Huncke K, Van de Wiele B, Fried I, Rubinstein E. The Asleep-Awake-Asleep anesthetic technique for intraoperative language mapping. Neurosurgery 1998; 42 (6): 1312-6.

[22] Huncke T, Chan J, Doyle W, Kim J, Bekker A. The use of continuous positive airway pressure during an awake craniotomy in a patient with obstructive sleep apnea. J Clin Anesth 2008; 20 (4): 297-9.

[23] Johnson KB, Egan TD. Remifentanil and propofol combination for awake craniotomy: case report with pharmacokinetic simulations. J Neurosurg Anesthesiol 1998; 10 (1): 25-9.

[24] Keifer JC, Dentchev D, Little K, Warner DS, Friedman AH, Borel CO. A retrospective analysis of a remifentanil/propofol general anesthetic for craniotomy before awake functional brain mapping. Anesth Analg. 2005; 101 (2): 502-8.

[25] Klimek M, Hol JW, Wens S, Heijmans-Antonissen C, Niehoff S, Vincent AJ, Klein J, Zijlstra FJ. Inflammatory profile of awake function-controlled craniotomy and craniotomy under general anesthesia. 2009; 2009: 670480.

[26] Lobo, Francisco MD; Beiras, Aldara MD. Propofol and remifentanil effect-site concentrations estimated by pharmacokinetic simulation and bispectral index monitoring during craniotomy with intraoperative awakening for brain tumour resection. J Neurosurg Anesthesiol 2007, 19 (3): 183-9.

[27] Manninen PH, Balki M, Lukitto K. Bernstein M. Patient satisfaction with awake craniotomy for tumour surgery: a comparison of remifentanil and fentanyl in conjunction with propofol. Anesth Analg 2006; 102: 237-42.

[28] Manninen PH, Raman SK, Boyle K , EI-Beheiry H. Reports of Investigation. Early postoperative complications following neurosurgical procedures. Can J Anesth 1999; 46 (1): 7-14.
[29] Manninen PH, Tan TK. Postoperative nausea and vomiting after craniotomy for tumour surgery: a comparison between awake craniotomy and general anesthesia. J Clin Anesth 2002; 14 (4): 279-83.
[30] Mirski MA, Lele AV, Fitzsimmons L, Toung T. Diagnosis and treatment of vasculair air embolism. Anesthesiology 2007; 106 (1) : 164-77.
[31] Murata H, Nagaishi C, Tsuda A, Sumikawa K. Laryngeal mask airway Supreme for asleep-awake-asleep craniotomy. Br. J. Anesth. 2010; 104 (3): 389-90.
[32] Palmon SC, Moore LE, Lundberg J, Toung T. Venous Air Embolism: A Review. J Clin Anesth 1997; 9 (3): 251-7.Parati G, Lombardi C, Narkiewicz K. Sleep apnea: epidemiology, pathophysiology and relation to cardiovascular risk. Am J Physiol Regul Integr Comp Physiol 2007; 293 (4): R1671-83.
[34] Perks A, Chakravarti S, Manninen P. Preoperative Anxiety in Neurosurgical Patients. J Neurosurg Anesthesiol 2009; 21 (2): 127-30.
[35] Peruzzi P, Bergese SD, Viloria A, Puente EG, Abdel-Rasoul M, Chiocca EA. A retrospective cohort-matched comparison of conscious sedation versus general anesthesia for supratentorial glioma resection. J Neurosurg 2011; 114 (3): 633-9.
[36] Piccioni F, Fanzio M. Management of anesthesia in awake craniotomy. Minerva Anestesiol 2008; 74 (7-8): 393-408.
[37] Picht T, Kombos, HJ, Brock M, Suess O. Multimodal protocol for awake craniotomy in language cortex tumour surgery. Acta Neurochir 2006; 148: 127-38.
[38] Saltarini M, Zorzi F. Awake craniotomy. Minerva Anestesiol 2005; 71 (suppl 1, n 10): 183-5.
[39] Sarang A, Dinsmore J. Anaesthesia for awake craniotomy-evolution of a technique that facilitates awake neurological testing. Br J Anaesth 2003; 90 (2): 161-5.
[40] Sartorius CJ, Berger MS. Rapid termination of intraoperative stimulation-evoked seizures with application of cold Ringer's lactate to the cortex. Technical note. J. Neurosurg 1998; 88: 349-51.
[41] See JJ, Lew TW, Kwek TK, Chin KJ, Wong MF, Liew QY, Lim SH, Ho HS, Chan Y,Loke GP, Yeo VS. Anaesthetic management of awake craniotomy for tumour resection. Ann Acad Med Singapore 2007; 36 (5): 319-25.
[42] Skucas AP, Artru AA. Anesthetic complications of awake craniotomies for epilepsy surgery. Anesth Analg 2006; 102: 882-7.
[43] Suarez S, Ornaque I, Fábregas N, Valero R, Carrero E. Venous Air Embolism During Parkinson Surgery in Patients with Spontaneous Ventilation. Anesth Analg 2010; 110: 1138-45.
[44] Verchére E, Grenier B, Abdelghani M, Siao D, Mussa S, Maurette P. Postoperative Pain Management After Supratentorial Craniotomy. J Neurosurg Anesthesiol 2002; 14 (2): 96-101.
[45] Whittle IR, Midgley S, Georges H, et al. Patient perceptions of "awake" brain tumour surgery. Acta Neurochir 2005; 147: 275-7.

[46] Zorzi F, Saltarini M, Bonassin P, Vecil M, De Angelis P, De Monte A. Anesthetic management in awake craniotomy. Signa Vitae 2008; 3 (1) S: 28 – 32.

3

# Anaesthetic Management of Patients Undergoing Intraventricular Neuro-Endoscopic Procedures

A.F. Kalmar[1] and F. Dewaele[2]
*[1]University Medical Centre Groningen*
*[2]Ghent University Hospital*
*[1]The Netherlands*
*[2]Belgium*

## 1. Introduction

Endoscopic neurosurgery has a long history of solid progression of over a century (Enchev et al., 2008). In this period, several neuroendoscopic procedures were described, but although steady technical improvements increased the endoscopic functionality and indications, poor magnification and illumination kept neuroendoscopy difficult and unreliable, keeping it out of routine practice until the end of the 1980's. Only after the invention of new lenses, electronics and fiberoptics allowed for the manufacturing of a new generation of endoscopes granting brighter illumination and improved resolution, neuroendoscopy came forward as routine treatment in neurosurgery (Li et al., 2005). Initially, neuroendoscopy was almost exclusively performed for endoscopic third ventriculostomy (ETV) for the treatment of obstructive hydrocephalus, and still the majority of neuroendoscopies is performed for ETV. Recently however, it is increasingly used for the management of all types of neurosurgically treatable disorders (Enchev & Oi, 2008), either as a primary surgical approach or as an adjunct, such that endoscopic procedures are common in most neurosurgical departments. A continued evolution of technological advances, introduction of robotic technology, steerable endoscopes and novel neurosurgical techniques are expected to increase its applications even further. These newly implemented surgical practices offer improved treatment options, commonly referred to as 'minimally invasive' in many clinical conditions. Since endoscopic techniques allow for intracranial interventions with minimal damage to healthy brain tissue, these advances are obviously a major benefit. Additionally, some interventions have a better outcome when performed endoscopically. However, in several of these interventions, direct surgical manipulation of cerebral structures and particularities of the endoscopic techniques are a constant hazard since they can severely disturb intracranial pressure, cerebral perfusion and oxygenation. This perturbation of cerebral homeostasis may imply important risks for irreversible brain damage, and severe haemodynamical effects which, if not taken proper care of, make these surgical improvements much less minimal invasive than previously supposed. A proper understanding of the physiological changes induced by and during these procedures is essential for optimal patient care. Neuroendoscopy has been successfully used for third ventriculostomy, tumor biopsy or resection, cyst fenestration or removal, evacuation of intraventricular haemorrhage and plexus coagulation. The technique has had its greatest application in the treatment of noncommunicating hydrocephalus by third ventriculostomy (Shubert et al., 2006). The surgeon establishes a connection between the third ventricle and the prepontine subarachnoid space by endoscopically fenestrating the floor of the third ventricle to allow the cerebrospinal fluid to flow directly from the third ventricle to the basal subarachnoid spaces, thus bypassing the aqueduct and the CSF pathways of the posterior fossa.

## 2. Key steps of the procedure

In most cases patients are positioned in the supine or semisitting position with the head flexed, so that the burr hole is located at the apex. This helps to minimize loss of CSF and air entrapment into the ventricles or the subdural space (Amini & Schmidt, 2005). During neuroendoscopy, the endoscope is operated carefully in order to minimize brain tissue damage and to allow precise manipulation of the working instruments. The presence of the shaft through the brain tissue mandates absolute immobility of the patient during the procedure. To ensure this precondition, the patient's head is fixated with neurological head pins in most cases. After infiltration with a local anaesthetic, a burr hole is made at an appropriate location for access to the intended trajectory. For endoscopic third ventriculostomy, this is mostly a right precoronal burr hole, 2-3 cm lateral to the midline. In most cases, this will provide a direct trajectory from the entry site through the foramen of Monro into the third ventricle. Then preferably a rigid endoscope is introduced through the frontal cortex into the lateral ventricle (Caemaert et al., 1992), the mandrins of the irrigation channel(s) and of the working channel are retracted. Then the endoscope is advanced into the lateral ventricle and through the foramen of Monro into the third ventricle. A connection between the third ventricle and the subarachnoid space is established by endoscopically fenestrating the floor of the third ventricle. The floor of the third ventricle is perforated bluntly, often using the tip of a Fogarty balloon catheter or coagulation probe. The initial fenestration is then enlarged to approximately a 4-mm opening by inflating the Fogarty catheter. After fenestration, the cerebrospinal fluid can drain into the basal cistern, bypassing the aqueductal stenosis. If an imperforate membrane of Liliequist is present beneath the floor of the third ventricle, which would obstruct CSF outflow, it can be opened under direct vision with a glass fiber or balloon catheter (Amini & Schmidt, 2005). During fenestration of the ventricle, there is a risk of injury to the basilar artery, which can result in fatal haemorrhage or brainstem infarction. Adequate visualization often requires continuous irrigation of the ventricles with warmed normal saline or preferably lactated ringers accompanied by drainage of cerebrospinal fluid and irrigating fluid through the scope or the burr hole. Therefore, the inlet irrigation tubes are connected to the rinsing fluid bags, either with or without pressurising equipment for active rinsing. If any significant haemorrhage occurs in the ventricle as a result of the procedure, copious irrigation must be possible until the haemorrhage is cleared. The unrestrained efflux of rinsing fluid needs to be assured in order to prevent uncontrolled intracranial hypertension during heavy rinsing. In order to prevent increased hydrostatic pressure caused by the shaft of the endoscope, an outflow tube is often connected to the outlet of the endoscope and its distal end is fixed at the same level as the burr hole, so that there is no siphoning effect or raised ICP.

## 3. State of the art anaesthesia

The anaesthetic goals should center on intraoperative immobilization, cardiovascular stability, and rapid emergence for early neurologic examination. Sharp increases in intracranial pressure must be detected and treated immediately. In this view, adequate monitoring and good communication with the neurosurgeons is essential.

### 3.1 Preoperative planning

Patients presenting for ventriculostomy may have prior shunt placements with existing shunt tubing routed from the cranium to peritoneal, pleural (rarely), or central vascular locations. Patients may present with symptoms of elevated intracranial pressure (ICP) such as vomiting, headache, confusion or obtundation. Prolonged nausea and vomiting may have caused dehydration or electrolyte abnormalities requiring correction prior to surgery. The patient's neurologic status and examination should be documented prior to induction (Shubert et al., 2006). Hydrocephalus is often part of multisystem congenital syndromes, with associated risks such as higher risk for urinary tract infections or impaired renal function. Premedication with anxiolytics or narcotics should be titrated very carefully, since the procedures are usually very short and fast postoperative neurologic assessment is desirable. Therefore, benzodiazepines or other agents that may contribute to prolonged postoperative sedation are preferably avoided (Fàbregas & Craen, 2010).

### 3.2 Anaesthetic technique

Intravenous and volatile hypnotics are both routinely used for neurosurgery. However, in published studies inhalation anaesthesia was the predominant technique of choice. Nitrous oxide should not be used in order to avoid elevations in ICP (Derbent et al., 2006), because of the additional risk with venous air embolism (Ganjoo et al., 2010) and the risk of diffusion into and expansion of ventricular air bubbles (Shubert et al., 2006). Mild hyperventilation can be performed in order to decrease intracranial brain volume. Because rapid emergence is of prime concern, we would recommend the use of remifentanil during the procedure, combined with either intravenous or volatile hypnotics. Adequate care for thermoregulation must be taken since patients - especially small children - are at risk for hypothermia during neuroendoscopy, mainly because of large exchanges of irrigating fluid and ventricular CSF and by the wetting of drapes (Ambesh & Kumar, 2000). Prophylaxis against postoperative nausea and vomiting is advisable because the elevated ICP is often associated with increased gastric acid secretion, and may additionally increase the risk of vomiting. Prophylactic analgesics should be given before emergence of narcosis. A combination of a low dose of opiates (such as morphine 0.03mg/kg) and paracetamol in most cases provides adequate analgesic effect without compromising neurologic evaluation. Non-steroidal anti-inflammatory drugs are generally discouraged because of haemostatic concerns.

### 3.3 Intraoperative monitoring

Most authors recommend invasive blood pressure monitoring by an indwelling arterial catheter in all patients, including children. We would also strongly suggest continuous measurement of the ICP and CPP. Active rinsing of the ventricles can unexpectedly increase the ICP very severely. The principal reasons for induced intracranial hypertension are high flow rinsing (used to improve visibility during bleeding or to maintain access in collapsing ventricles ) and obstruction of the outflow channel by tissue debris , blood clots or kinking of outflow tubes. These increases in ICP must be detected as soon as possible to prevent severe complications such as cardiovascular instability (Fabregas et al., 2002, Handler et al., 1994) , herniation syndromes, retinal bleeding (Boogaarts et al., 2008 ; Hoving et al., 2009) and excessive fluid resorption (Kalmar et al., 2009). Aside from these unambiguous complications animal research showed that awakening without apparent neurological deficit does not preclude histological damage (Kalmar et al. 2009). It is possible that the same could apply for humans. Beat-to-beat monitoring of the arterial blood pressure offers the most reliable warning sign for a developing Cushing reflex, which is a sign of decreased CPP (Kalmar et al., 2005a). This CPP should at all time be maintained above 40mmHg. Transcranial doppler is the fastest and most reliable method to show abrupt decreases in cerebral blood flow due to increased ICP (Kalmar et al., 2005b). Because of its high sensitivity to impaired cerebral blood flow, it may be considered as basic monitoring, although practical objections limit its routine use during neuroendoscopy.

### 3.4 Active rinsing and Intracranial hypertension

Two strategies to ensure sufficient efflux of rinsing fluid are commonly used. The first option is to use a peel-away sheath with a diameter just slightly larger than the endoscope to provide a working porthole into the anatomy. Aside from allowing easy insertion and reduced tissue damage during endoscope manipulation, it allows for egress of irrigation fluid (Amini & Schmidt, 2005). Most surgeons however do not use an extra sheath. Effusion capacity of the rinsing fluid is consequently largely restricted to the outflow channel of the endoscope, in which case substantial intracranial pressure can emerge, mandating adequate ICP monitoring (Fàbregas et al., 2001; Kalmar et al, 2005a). The manipulation of intraventricular fluid volume and pressure by controlling the rinsing inflow and outflow is sometimes advocated as a particular advantage. A surgical skill consists of deliberately increasing the intracranial pressure as a surgical intervention to expand collapsed ventricles. It is also proposed as an instrument to control haemorrhage. In the latter case, controlled increase of the intracranial pressure at least above the venous pressure, and even higher are advocated as a tool to tamponade venous or maybe even arteriolar bleeding. This allows for more delicate procedures to be performed endoscopically. Especially during complex operations, such as tumour resections characterized by frequent bleedings with each „bite" during the piece-by-piece removal, it allows to quickly regain visibility. An increase in ICP can be tolerated up to a certain level, and it is often inevitable while providing adequate rinsing to improve visibility. However, the rinsing activity and ICP increases have to be performed in a controlled manner. Particularly in these situations, meticulous ICP monitoring, monitoring of the haemodynamical status and optimal communication between the anaesthetist and neurosurgeon are critical (Kalmar et al., 2005a). Although the technique of "pressure feeding" the rinsing fluid (i.e. using pressurised rinsing fluid) is preferred by many surgeons to provide sufficient rinsing capacity, others prefer to perform the endoscopic procedure with a steady state inflow pressure using "gravity feed" (i.e. only using gravity as a driving pressure of the rinsing fluid) to avoid barotrauma to the brain ventricles. However, even in case of "gravity feed", a rinsing fluid bag at a level of 100 cm above the head still could cause an ICP of ~76mmHg in case of completely obstructed outflow. In case of a sudden severe increase of intracranial pressure, the surgeon should immediately stop the rinsing and remove any instrument out of the working channel. This mostly wide channel is an additional way out for the accumulated rinsing fluid.

### 3.5 Intracranial pressure and the Cushing reflex

Endoscopic third ventriculostomy is associated with a wide range of haemodynamic effects caused by direct stimulation of brain structures, and by changes in intracranial pressure. Several mechanisms have been postulated to elucidate the neurological origin of these changes, but no indiscriminate anatomical source of the reflexes has yet been determined (Fàbregas et al., 2010). The manifestation of haemodynamical reflexes during endoscopic neurosurgery described in literature differs between authors. Historically, the "Cushing reflex" was first described by Harvey Cushing in 1901 as a simultaneous occurrence of hypertension, bradycardia and apnoea following intracranial hypertension (Cushing 1901). This observation however, was based on his experiences as a neurosurgeon, where he treated patients that were referred some time after an intracranial bleeding or with longer lasting intracranial hypertension (hydrocephalus, tumors). Although Heymans showed in 1928 in animal research that there is an initial short-lasting tachycardia before the onset of bradycardia (Heymans 1928), it is only since the introduction of neuro-endoscopy, this has become of clinical relevance. Relying on the experience in relatively slow-evolving processes like a chronic subdural hematoma, hydrocephalus or cerebral tumors, many clinicians still consider bradycardia and hypertension as the first hemodynamic sign of hyperacute intracranial hypertension. In the literature describing the "Cushing reflex" during neuro-endoscopy, the observation of hypertension is ubiquitous. However, several groups observed mostly hypertension and bradycardia as a predominant sign (El-Dawlatly 2008 , Fàbregas 2001), while others (Van Aken 2003, Kalmar 2005a) systematically observed hypertension combined with an initial tachycardia, which only occasionally evolves into bradycardia. It is very conceivable that the differences in these observations are a result of variations in surgical practice. Additionally, direct pressure on certain anatomical regions seems mainly to provoke bradycardia (Baykan et al., 2005), while isolated intracranial hypertension seems rather to induce tachycardia (Kalmar et al., 2009). Al-Dawlatly suggests that the possible absence of tachycardia found in many studies may be due to the protocol that allows the irrigation fluid to vent out during the procedure without noticeable accumulation in the third ventricle. (Al-Dawlatly et al., 2008). In our experience, we frequently observe bradycardia at the moment of balloon inflation close to the brainstem. In order to prevent this, we retract the balloon somewhat into the third ventricle during dilatation of the bottom of the third ventricle. In an analysis focusing on the incidence of bradycardia, Al-Dawlatly postulated that bradycardia recorded in a small series was due to direct stimulation of the floor of the third ventricle (Al-Dawlatly et al., 1999). The most notable difference in surgical method is that for instance in the department of Van Aken & Kalmar, high-pressure rinsing is preferred as a surgical technique for rinsing, bleeding control and ventricular dilatation. Therefore, more swift and higher increases in intracranial pressure may occur which may explain the differences in clinical observations. In several neurosurgical centers however, gravitational flow, without the use of pressure bags, is preferred as a method to prevent very high ICP values. In our personal experience however, while endoscopic third ventriculostomy procedures can in most cases be performed with free flow gravitational rinsing, since bleeding is unusual and rather limited, procedures like tumor resection or biopsies are much more at risk for severe bleeding and therefore mandate higher rinsing flows requiring high-pressure rinsing. During such events, it is useful for the surgeon to be attentive to the beeps of the anaesthesia monitor. Changes in heart rate during neuroendoscopy are very informative for acknowledgement of the consequences of increased ICP or direct stimulation of brain structures, in which case immediate action can prevent serious complications. Typical hemodynamic reflexes such as bradycardia, tachycardia or hypertension associated with ETV are transient and will respond to simple surgical manoeuvres such as reducing or stopping the inflow and retraction of the working instrument to allow egress of irrigant fluids through the working channel (Fàbregas et al., 2010). Since extensive manipulation of cerebral structures during difficult surgical procedures often coincides with higher rinsing flows, it is impossible to clearly differentiate the cause of these haemodynamic changes between direct stimulation of the brainstem and a genuine Cushing reflex. In an animal model of sudden increases in ICP devoid of any direct stimulation of brain structures severe bradycardia was never observed in the initial hypertensive phase. The haemodynamic reflex induced by isolated intracranial hypertension always consisted of hypertension, and the absence of bradycardia did not even exclude a CPP of zero. In many cases, a severe tachycardia is the only and very distinct constituent of the induced Cushing reflex (Kalmar 2009). Moreover, in this animal model, significant rinsing fluid resorption was observed at high rinsing pressures, resulting in considerable decrease in hematocrit. Many of the animals succumbed from pulmonary edema. However, these observations of exceptional fluid resorption or pulmonary complications were never reported in human cases. Interestingly, although cerebral ischaemia was present for several minutes, many of the animals recovered without any apparent clinical signs of cerebral insult while histological analysis showed signs of ischaemic injury with an increased number of pinocytic neurons in the hippocampus. This indicates that a normal awakening of the patient after an apparently uneventful narcosis may not exclude important CPP suppression and even ischaemic injury.

### 3.6 ICP monitoring

Several strategies to measure ICP are recommended in the literature. ICP measurements with an ICP tip sensor through the working channel have been used, but this may interfere with the surgical procedure (Vassilyadi & Ventureyra, 2002). An intraparenchymal ICP tip sensor will provide reliable measurements, but it is invasive and therefore less acceptable as a routine practice (Prabhakar et al., 2007). An epidurally placed ICP tip sensor is a less invasive, but a less reliable method. Although considered the gold standard, pressure measurement via a separately inserted ventricular catheter is generally unfeasible and difficult to justify. Alternatively, an ICP Tipsensor can be advanced with the endoscope into the ventricles. This provides reliable ICP-readings but bears an additional risk of tissue damage and is quite expensive. Fàbregas proposed measuring the ICP by means of a fluid-filled catheter connected to a stopcock connected to the irrigation lumen of the neuroendoscope (inflow channel) and attached to a pressure transducer zeroed at the skull base (Fàbregas et al, 2000). This "Pressure Inside the Neuroendoscope" correlates with the epidural pressure (Salvador et al., 2010) and with manifestations of the Cushing reflex (Fàbregas et al., 2010 ; Kalmar et al.,2005a). Alternatively, the outlet of the endoscope-flushing system can be connected by a long pressure tube to a pressure transducer for continuous monitoring of the ICP (Kalmar et al., 2005a). The level of foramen of Monro was used as the zero reference point. A major pitfall in using the outflow channel to measure the ICP, is that blockage in the outflow lumen results in a severe underestimation of the true intracranial pressure. Measuring the ICP via the rinsing channels of the endoscope is preferred in literature, although it is not convincingly determined whether the inflow or outflow point is the most appropriate location. ICP monitoring is thus important, but the optimal location of monitoring is controversial. Since fluids flow down pressure gradients, and flowing fluids generate dynamic resistances, measurement at the rinsing inlet and outlet may at higher rinsing speeds correlate poorly with ventricular measurements. An In-vitro study comparing "ventricular" pressure with pressure at the rinsing inlet and outlet shows very significant respective over- and underestimations of the true "intracranial pressure" of up to 50mmHg at high rinsing flows (Dewaele et al., 2011). Measurement via a capillary tube or electronic tip sensor advanced through the rinsing inlet channel of the endoscope provides reliable ICP measurements and may - based on these in vitro observations - be proposed as best practice. Still, in order to minimally hinder rinsing capacity, only very thin catheters can be advanced through the rinsing channel. However convincing, no human studies have presently been published to confirm these in-vitro findings in clinical practice.

### 3.7 Irrigation fluid

Lactated Ringer solution at body temperature is the most frequently used irrigation fluid(Fábregas & Craen; 2010). A few studies suggest a significant disturbance of the CSF composition when using saline as rinsing fluid, especially after long procedures. To avoid intraoperative and postoperative complications arising from the use of irrigating fluids, some surgeons take care to limit the loss of CSF and to use irrigation only when necessary (Cinalli et al., 2006).

## 4. Complications

The incidence of complications can vary widely depending on the procedure. For endoscopic third ventriculostomy, an incidence of 0 to 31.2% is reported with a mortality rate of 1%. The most frequent intraoperative complications are haemostatic problems and infection. However, injury of the basilar artery complex is the most feared intraoperative complication and can cause massive intraventricular and subarchnoid hemorrhage, hemiparesis and midbrain damage (Jones & Kwok, 1994). Meningeal irritation, headache and high fever from an inflammatory response to irrigating fluid can occur (Oka et al., 1996). Uncontrolled intracranial pressure can cause retinal bleeding, resulting in Terson syndrome (Boogaarts et al., 2008; Hoving et al., 2009). Neurological morbidity can be very diverse, and can often be explained by the approach and technique, although a specific incident that is responsible for the postoperative defect is mostly unappreciated. For example, although gaze palsy is reported as a complication in 0.60% of patients, in no case was injury of the oculomotor nerve described as an intraoperative incident (boeras & Sgouros, 2011). Many studies report transient neurological dysfunctions, which can be explained by the mechanics of the operation, such as short memory disturbances caused by irritation of the fornix by scratching of the endoscope to the wall of the lateral ventricle at the level of the foramen of Monro.

## 5. Postoperative care and longterm outcome

Transient neurologic deficits such as delayed emergence, confusion, memory loss, transient papillary dysfunction or transient hemiplegia - are the most common postoperative complication occurring in 8–38% of patients (Fàbregas et al., 2000). In an extensive meta-analysis of 2985 cases of ETV, Bouras & Sqouros described that in the immediate postoperative period after ETV, CNS infections (meningitis, ventriculitis) are recorded in 1.81% of the patients. In 2 cases, a CSF infection is reported to have evolved to sepsis. Cerebrospinal fluid leaks are recorded in 1.61% of cases. Postoperative hemorrhagic complications are reported in 0.81% of the patients. These consist of subdural hematoma, intraventricular hemorrhage, intracerebral hematoma and epidural hematoma. Subdural hygromas were recorded in 0.27% of the patients. The rate of systemic complications was 2.34%. Among them, hyponatremia, systemic infections, and deep vein thrombosis were the most frequent (Bouras & Sqouros, 2011). Particularly, hypothalamic or pituitary stalk injury can occur, resulting in diabetes insipidus or the syndrome of inappropriate secretion of antidiuretic hormone (SIADH) (Grant & Mclone, 1997). These cases are often not permanent, but in case of doubt, plasma and urine electrolytes should be observed. In case of diabetes insipidus, desmopressin 1-4µg IV (adult dose) can be administered. In case of postoperative polyuria, appropriate diagnostic measures must be performed accordingly. Patients can develop transient fever due to aseptic irritation of the ependyma or to manipulation of the hypothalamus. Convulsions have been reported by several authors, with one case resulting from pneumoencephalus. Persisting high ICP can occur postoperatively, requiring additional diagnostic measures. Respiratory arrest has been reported in infants during the first hours after neuroendoscopy, necessitating the use of apnea monitors (Shubert et al., 2006). Preferably, patients are kept in the neurosurgical care unit overnight for close surveillance of vital signs, level of consciousness, change of papillary size, polyuria or other complications.

In a review of Bouras & Sqouros, overall permanent morbidity of ETV was calculated to be 2.38%. Neurological morbidity (1.44%) includes gaze palsy (0.60%), decreased consciousness (0.34%), hemiparesis (0.34%), and memory disorders (0.17%). Hormonal morbidity (0.94%) comprised diabetes insipidus (0.64%), weight gain (0.27%), and precocious puberty (0.04%).

The overall mortality rate was 0.28%, all of them in the postoperative period because of sepsis or hermorrhagic incidents. Global good long-term outcome after ETV is between 70-80% in most series (Gangemi et al., 2007)

## 6. Explicative cases

In 2003, a 56 year old woman presenting with a subependymal tumour in the right lateral ventricle, was being operated on for an endoscopical biopsy and resection. Haemodynamic monitoring consisted of invasive arterial blood pressure (IABP), NIBP, ECG, pulse oximetry, and ICP-monitoring at the outflow-channel of the endoscope. After an uneventful induction and maintenance of narcosis with propofol, remifentanil and cisatracurium, classical patient positioning and introduction of the endoscope, the surgical procedure for tumour removal was performed.

Because of minor bleeding from the tumour surface, rinsing was performed more elaborately than usual. The heart rate and IABP revealed stable haemodynamics but without any other warning signs, an isolated increase in blood pressure of 30 mmHg was observed within less than ten seconds, followed by the onset of distinct tachycardia from 65 up to 105 bpm and a further increase of the systolic blood pressure to 180mmHg within a few seconds. Although monitoring showed a low ICP-level, the surgeon was informed of a high probability of severe intracranial hypertension, who instantly removed an instrument from the working channel in order to provide an additional outflow channel. Immediately, a flood of rinsing fluid gushed out of the working channel of the endoscope. Within fifteen seconds, the heart rate and IABP were stabilizing and after two minutes they had returned to normal levels. The procedure was resumed and completed without further events and the patient recovered without complications.

Interestingly, the collected rinsing fluid showed a lot of tumour debris floating, which probably had obstructed the outflow channel of the endoscope. This explains the inaccurately low ICP-level on the monitor.

This case shows the importance of adequate haemodynamic monitoring and comprehension of the Cushing reflex during neuroendoscopy. If in such a case the haemodynamic changes are perceived as a sign of arousal, pain or idiopathic hypertension, the patient would be treated incorrectly, while the intracranial pressure would covertly increase to deleterious levels. On the other hand, swift adequate action may have prevented severe complications. Both for the anaesthetist and the neurosurgeon, it is important to be constantly aware of sudden changes in heart rate and blood pressure. Therefore, the sound level of the monitor should be adequately high. During active rinsing, especially with presence of tissue debris in the rinsing fluid, the surgeon should be particularly attentive to such changes and act accordingly.

## 7. Expert suggestion

For stable anaesthesia and fast recovery in optimal conditions, we rely on balanced total intravenous anaesthesia with propofol TCI 2-5 µg/ml and remifentanil TCI 2-6 ng/ml. As a rinsing fluid, Ringer's lactate solution at body temperature is favourable in order to maximally preserve electrolyte homeostasis. Monitoring of the intracranial pressure is currently performed at either the inflow or outflow channel of the endoscope with both having their drawbacks. Optimal pressure monitoring will likely progress towards noninvasive transendoscopic ICP measurement but this remains to be investigated more thoroughly. We expect most accurate ICP measurement via a capillary through the rinsing inlet channel. Studies on this topic are being performed currently. As emphasized many times, it is imperative to have beat-to-beat information on changes in blood-pressure and heart rate whenever sudden increases in ICP are possible. Since even gravitational rinsing with the rinsing fluid positioned at only 1 meter above the patient can cause an ICP of 76mmHg, every endoscopy holds such a risk. Therefore we always use invasive blood pressure monitoring, but advanced noninvasive alternatives for beat-to-beat haemodynamic monitoring may become a fine alternative.

In the postoperative period, short term memory can be disturbed due to tissue damage and irritation of the fornix at the level of the foramen of Monro, caused by friction of the endoscopic shaft. In order to limit this complication, we favour using an endoscope with a diameter of 6mm.

## 8. References

Ambesh SP, Kumar R. Neuroendoscopic procedures: anesthetic considerations for a growing trend: a review. J Neurosurg Anesthesiol 2000; 12:262–270.

Amini A, Schmidt RH. Endoscopic third ventriculostomy in a series of 36 adult patients. Neurosurg Focus. 2005;19:E9.

Baykan N, Isbir O, Gerçek A, Dagçnar A, Ozek MM.Ten years of experience with pediatric neuroendoscopic third ventriculostomy. J Neurosurg Anesthesiol. 2005;17:33-7.

Boogaarts H, Grotenhuis A. Terson's syndrome after endoscopic colloid cyst removal. Minim Invasive Neurosurg 2008; 51: 303–5

Bouras T, Sgouros S. Complications of endoscopic third ventriculostomy. J Neurosurg Pediatr. 2011;7:643-9.

Caemaert J, Abdullah J, Calliauw L, Carton D, Dhooge C, van Coster R. Endoscopic treatment of suprasellar arachnoid cysts. Acta Neurochir. 1992;119:68-73.

Cinalli G, Spennato P, Ruggiero C, Aliberti F, Zerah M, Trischitta V, Cianciulli E, Maggi G. Intracranial pressure monitoring and lumbar puncture after endoscopic third ventriculostomy in children. Neurosurgery 2006; 58:126–136.

Cushing, H. Concerning a definite regulatory mechanism of the vasomotor centre which controls blood pressure during cerebral compression. Bull Johns Hopkins Hosp. 1901; 126: 289–292.

Derbent A, Ersahin Y, Yurtseven T, Turhan T. Hemodynamic and electrolyte changes in patients undergoing neuroend procedures. Childs Nerv Syst 2006; 22: 253–257.

Dewaele F, Kalmar AF, Van Canneyt K, Vereecke H, Absalom A, Caemaert J, Struys MM, Van Roost D. Pressure monitoring during neuroendoscopy: new insights. Br J Anaesth. 2011; 107: 218-24.

El-Dawlatly AA, Murshid W, El-Khwsky F. Endoscopic third ventriculostomy: a study of intracranial pressure vs. haemodynamic changes. Minim Invasive Neurosurg. 1999; 42: 198-200.

El-Dawlatly A, Elgamal E, Murshid W, Alwatidy S, Jamjoom Z, Alshaer A. Anesthesia for third ventriculostomy. A report of 128 cases. Middle East J Anesthesiol. 2008 Feb;19(4):847-57.

Enchev Y, Oi S. Historical trends of neuroendoscopic surgical techniques in the treatment of hydrocephalus. Neurosurg Rev. 2008; 31: 249-62.

Handler MH, Abbott R, Lee M. A near-fatal complication of endoscopic third ventriculostomy: case report. Neurosurgery 1994; 35: 525–7

Heymans C. The control of heart rate consequent to changes in the cephalic blood pressure and in the intracranial pressure. Am J Physiol 1928; 85: 498–505

Hoving EW, Rahmani M, Los LI, Renardel de Lavalette VW. Bilateral retinal hemorrhage after endoscopic third ventriculostomy: iatrogenic Terson syndrome. J Neurosurg 2009; 110: 858–60

Fàbregas N, López A, Valero R, Carrero E, Caral L, Ferrer E.. Anesthetic management of surgical neuroendoscopies: usefulness of monitoring the pressure inside the neuroendoscope. J Neurosurg Anesthesiol. 2000; 12: 21–28

Fàbregas N, Valero R, Carrero E, Tercero J, Caral L, Zavala E, Ferrer E.Episodic high irrigation pressure during surgical neuroendoscopy may cause intermittent intracranial circulatory insufficiency. J Neurosurg Anesthesiol. 2001; 13: 152-7.

Fabregas N, Craen RA. Anaesthesia for minimally invasive neurosurgery. Best Pract Res Clin Anaesthesiol 2002; 16:81–93

Fàbregas N, Craen RA. Anaesthesia for endoscopic neurosurgical procedures. Curr Opin Anaesthesiol. 2010; 23: 568-75.

Gangemi M, Mascari C, Maiuri F, Godano U, Donati P, Longatti PL. Long-term outcome of endoscopic third ventriculostomy in obstructive hydrocephalus. Minim Invasive Neurosurg. 2007 Oct;50(5):265-9.

Ganjoo P, Sethi S, Tandon MS, et al. Perioperative complications of intraventricular neuroendoscopy: a 7-year experience. Turk Neurosurg 2010; 20: 33–38.

Jones RF, Kwok BC, Stening WA, Vonau M. Neuroendoscopic third ventriculostomy. A practical alternative to extracranial shunts in non-communicating hydrocephalus. Acta Neurochir Suppl. 1994; 61: 79-83.

Kalmar AF, Van Aken J, Caemaert J, Mortier EP, Struys MM. (2005a). Value of Cushing reflex as warning sign for brain ischaemia during neuroendoscopy. Br J Anaesth. 2005; 94: 791-9.

Kalmar AF, Van Aken J, Struys MM. (2005b). Exceptional clinical observation: total brain ischemia during normal intracranial pressure readings caused by obstruction of the outflow of a neuroendoscope.J Neurosurg Anesthesiol 2005; 17: 175–6

Kalmar AF, De Ley G, Van Den Broecke C, Van Aken J, Struys MM, Praet MM, Mortier EP. Influence of an increased intracranial pressure on cerebral and systemic haemodynamics during endoscopic neurosurgery: an animal model.. Br J Anaesth 2009; 102: 361–8

Li KW, Nelson C, Suk I, Jallo GI. Neuroendoscopy: past, present, and future. Neurosurg Focus. 2005; 19: E1.

Oka K, Yamamoto M, Nonaka T, Tomonaga M. The significance of artificial cerebrospinal fluid as perfusate and endoneurosurgery. Neurosurgery 1996; 38: 733–736.

Prabhakar H, Rath GP, Bithal PK, Suri A, Dash H. Variations in cerebral haemodynamics during irrigation phase in neuroendoscopic procedures. Anaesth Intensive Care. 2007; 35: 209-12.

Salvador L, Valero R, Carazo J, Caral L, Rios J, Carrero E, Tercero J, de Riva N, Hurtado P, Ferrer E, Fábregas N. Pressure inside the neuroendoscope: correlation with epidural intracranial pressure during neuroendoscopic procedures.J Neurosurg Anesthesiol. 2010; 22: 240-6.

Schubert A, Deogaonkar A, Lotto M, Niezgoda J, Luciano M. Anesthesia for minimally invasive cranial and spinal surgery. J Neurosurg Anesthesiol. 2006; 18: 47-56.

van Aken J, Struys M, Verplancke T, de Baerdemaeker L, Caemaert J, Mortier E. Cardiovascular changes during endoscopic third ventriculostomy. Minim Invasive Neurosurg. 2003; 46: 198-201.

Vassilyadi M, Ventureyra EC. Neuroendoscopic intracranial pressure monitoring. Childs Nerv Syst 2002; 18: 147–148.

# 4

# Neurocritical Care

Mainak Majumdar
*Critical Care Physician, Peninsula Health, Victoria*
*Australia*

## 1. Introduction

Neurocritical care is at the forefront of bringing effective new therapies to patients with life threatening neurological diseases. Neurocritical care units have evolved from neurosurgical units focused primarily on postoperative monitoring to units that provide comprehensive medical and specialized neurological support for patients with life-threatening neurological diseases. In addition to standard interventions, areas of expertise unique to neurocritical care include management of intracranial pressure, hemodynamic augmentation to improve cerebral blood flow, therapeutic hypothermia, and advanced neuromonitoring. Neurointensivists defragment care by focusing on the interplay between the brain and other systems, and by integrating all aspects of neurological and medical management into a single care plan. Outcomes research has established that victims of traumatic brain injury and hemorrhagic stroke experience reduced mortality, better functional outcomes, and reduced length of stay when cared for by neurointensivists in a dedicated neurointensive care unit (Rincon & Mayer 2007). This chapter aims to provide an overview of global organ support of the critically ill neurosurgical patient.

## 2. Critical care for neurosurgical patients

The neurocritical care unit provides a venue where advanced monitoring enables optimisation of oxygen and metabolite delivery to the neurons by aggressive, often invasive interventions within a controlled environment.

### 2.1 Brain monitoring

The word "monitor" originates from the Latin *monere* (to warn). Monitoring merely provides warning of pathology and may track its progression long before it becomes clinically obvious thus allowing earlier aggressive management of underlying disease and assessment of response to therapy. The superiority of any one mode of monitoring over another has never been proven.

Available forms of brain monitoring include

Measurement of intra cranial pressure (ICP): ICP has traditionally been measured by a ventricular drain connected by a fluid coupled system to an external strain gauge.

Currently, available options include systems with micro strain gauges or fibreoptics built into the tip. Catheters may be placed in the parenchyma, subarachnoid, epidural or subdural spaces in addition to the ventricles. Generally, parenchymal catheters with micro strain gauges in the tip have good correlation with ventricular drain pressures. Subarachnoid, subdural and epidural catheters are thought to be less accurate.

Micro strain gauge and fibreoptic catheters need to be calibrated prior to insertion and cannot be recalibrated in situ. Theoretical concerns have been raised about measurement drift and resulting inaccuracy of measurement. There is little by way of published literature and the actual device selection is guided by institutional preference.

Measurement of cerebral blood flow: Transcranial Doppler monitoring is an easily available, reproducible, non invasive and inexpensive means of measuring cerebral blood flow by measuring flow velocity in the middle cerebral artery (MCA). It has been used to assess for cerebral vasospasm, to assess cerebral autoregulation (Reinhard et al, 2010) and diagnose traumatic dissection of the internal carotid artery (Bouzat et al, 2010).

Measurement of brain oxygenation: Jugular venous oxymetry (SjO2) has been used to assess oxygen delivery to the brain. Both low (<55%) and high (>75%) SjO2 have been associated with poor outcomes. The arterio jugular difference in oxygen content has been measured to assess cerebral oxygen extraction.

Brain tissue oxygenation (PBrO2) can be directly measured by placing catheters into affected areas of the brain to detect focal ischaemia. PBrO2<15 mmH is associated with poor neurologic outcome.

Near infra red spectroscopy (NIRS) has been mooted as a non invasive measure of regional transcranial oxygen saturation (rSO2). Though promising, its routine use in neurocritical care is potentially impeded by the presence of scalp wounds, hematoma and intracranial catheters.

Assessment of metabolic state: Cerebral microdialysis catheters placed directly into brain tissue have been used to measure levels of brain metabolites. The commonly measured ones are glucose, lactate, glutamate, pyruvate and lactate/pyruvate ratio. The use of these devices is uncommon outside of larger academic centres. Given the paucity of correlation with outcomes data, their routine use cannot currently be recommended.

Assessment of electrical activity: This has traditionally been done using electroencephalography (EEG). Its widespread use in critical care has been impeded by difficulties in the interpretation of EEGs by non neurologists.

Bispectral index (BIS) is a processed EEG monitoring tool that evaluates brain electrical activity for zero (flat line EEG) to 100 (awake patient). It is not in routine use currently in critical care environments.

Somatosensory evoked potentials (SEP) have been validated for prognostication after hypoxic brain injury. Delayed N20 bilaterally has been shown to correlate with poor neurologic outcome.

### 2.2 Management of ICP

ICP in normal subjects is usually less than 10 mmHg. It is generally accepted that active treatment for elevated ICP should be initiated for sustained rises in ICP to greater than 20 mmHg. The definitive treatment of elevated ICP remains, of course, management of the underlying pathology.

The following sequence of events is a suggested escalating way of medically managing elevated ICP to return it to <20mmHg. It is useful to simultaneously maintain a cerebral perfusion pressure (CPP) >60 mmHg, where CPP is the difference between mean arterial pressure (MAP) and ICP

- If the patient is not already intubated, consideration should be given to intubating and mechanically ventilating the patient to facilitate deep sedation
- The patient should be nursed 30-45° head up, if possible with head in neutral position and ties around the neck (eg. endotracheal tube tapes, cervical collars) loosened or repositioned if possible
- Ventilation titrated to normoxia ($SaO2>90$ mmHg, $PaO2>70$ mmHg) and normocapnia (PCO2 35-45 mmHg)
- Liberal opiate analgesia
- Liberal sedation targeting Richmond Agitation and Sedation Scale (RASS) -4 or lower.
- Neuromuscular blockade if frequent shivering or coughing
- Prompt treatment of any seizure activity
- Addition of phenobarbitone
- Hyperosmolar therapy (either 0.5-1 gm/kg of mannitol or 3% NaCl to target serum sodium ~150)
- Hyperventilation to PCO2<25 mmHg
- At this stage, consideration should be given to immediate evacuation of any mass lesions. Consideration should also be given to placing a ventricular catheter to drain CSF.
- Induction of hypothermia
- Consideration should be given at this stage to extreme measures like decompressive craniotomy or thiopentone infusion

### 2.3 Sedation, analgesia and neuromuscular blockade

A variety of drugs are commonly used to sedate and treat pain in critically ill ventilated patients.

It is inhumane to deny analgesia to a patient for fear of clouding neurologic signs. Adequate analgesia minimises noxious stimuli which may contribute to elevated ICP, ventilator dyssynchrony and reactive hypertension. In addition, opiates have sedative properties and can be used alone for sedation or in combination with other sedative agents. Morphine is traditionally the drug of choice. The author's practice is to be liberal with opiates and wherever possible, to use patient controlled analgesia. Fentanyl and sufentanyl have been associated with small but definite rises in ICP. To minimise this, they may be administered slowly intravenously. Regular administration of paracetamol may reduce opiate requirements. In a peri operative setting, non steroidal anti inflammatories may be used with caution, allowing for the impact on kidneys, gastrointestinal tract and platelet function.

Sedation allows tube tolerance in most intubated critical care patients. In a neurosurgical setting, sedation is neuroprotective and reduces cerebral oxygen demand and cerebral metabolism. The commonly available agents available for sedation are benzodiazepines and propofol. Given the association between benzodiazepines and increased delirium, the author's preferred first line agent is propofol, where haemodynamics permit. Caution needs to be exercised where more than 5 mg/kg/hour is being infused for more than 24 hours. Midazolam infusion is a reasonable alternative and, where clinically indicated, the two may be combined. The author's practice is to give daily sedation breaks as soon as clinically feasible. Alpha blockers like clonidine or dexmedetomidine should be considered for emergence delirium and as adjuncts to analgesia. Barbiturates are not routinely used for sedation in an ICU setting.

Neuro muscular blockade may be necessary for ongoing shivering, coughing or movement causing significant rise in ICP. It may also be needed to facilitate procedures and intra and/or inter hospital transport. This needs to be balanced against the association between neuromuscular blockade and the development of critical illness polymyoneuropathy which, in turn, can worsen outcomes prolong time on ventilator, ICU stay and hospital stay. The author's practice is to use small doses of non depolarising agents (vecuronium or atracurium) when clinically indicated.

### 2.4 Seizure management and prophylaxis

Craniotomies, especially supratentorial ones, are associated with a high incidence of post operative seizures. Depending on the reason for surgery, up to 50% patients have at least one seizure treated postoperatively (Shaw & Foy, 1991). There are no formal guidelines for routine seizure prophylaxis after neurosurgery in general.

Prophylactic anticonvulsants should not be used routinely in patients with newly diagnosed brain tumours. Anti convulsants should be tapered and discontinued after the first postoperative week in patients who have not had seizures (Glantz et al, 2000).

In traumatic brain injury, anticonvulsants are indicated to decrease the incidence of early post traumatic seizures (within 7 days of trauma). Early post traumatic seizures are not associated with worse outcomes. Phenytoin has been shown to reduce the incidence of early post traumatic seizures. Valproate has an effect comparable to phenytoin in reducing early post tramatic seizures but may be associated with higher mortality (Brain Trauma Foundation Guidelines, 3rd ed). Routine use of anticonvulsants is not recommended later than 1 week following head injury to prevent late post traumatic seizures and does not reduce their incidence.

### 2.5 Hyperosmolar therapy

Hyperosmolar therapy is often used to treat elevated ICP. It may buy time to do diagnostic (eg. imaging) or therapeutic (eg. evacuation of mass lesion) interventions. In the absence of ICP monitoring, its use should be restricted to patients with signs of transtentorial herniation or deteriorating neurologic state not attributable to extra cranial causes.

The two agents in common use are mannitol and hypertonic saline.

Mannitol in the dose range of 0.25-1 gm/kg as a bolus is effective in reducing ICP. While it has been used as prolonged therapy for raised ICP, there is lack of evidence to recommend repeated regular administration of mannitol over several days. Serum osmolarity should be monitored when mannitol is being administered, especially if repeated doses are being considered. While mannitol acts by increasing serum osmolarity, there is significant risk of acute kidney injury at high serum osmolarities. While there is no absolute threshold for a particular patient, osmolarities of more than 320 mOsm/L are likely to be hazardous. In the neurosurgical patient with a compromised blood brain barrier, theoretical concerns have also been raised regarding mannitol causing osmotic oedema in the injured areas of the brain, further compromising perfusion to these areas.

Hypertonic saline acts by osmotic mobilisation of water and reduction of total cerebral water content. It is usually well tolerated, cheap and easy to titrate off serum sodium levels, which are routinely measured in most intensive care units. Caution must be exercised in its liberal use in patients with chronic hyponatremia due to the risk of inducing central pontine myelinolysis. There is not enough strong evidence at present to make recommendations regarding the concentration or method of administration of hypertonic saline for treatment of raised ICP. As unmeasured hyperosmolar particles (such as mannitol) are not introduced to the serum, adequate osmolar monitoring is readily available from the serum sodium level. The author's practice is to use 20 ml aliquots of 3% NaCl aiming for a serum sodium level ~150 mmol/L.

There is a paucity of data on the safety and efficacy of combined hyperosmolar therapy with mannitol and hypertonic saline.

### 2.6 Induced hypothermia

Mild induced hypothermia (core temperature 32-34°C) has been thought to offer neuroprotection by reducing cerebral oxygen demand, altering the inflammatory cascade and reducing ICP.

There is no clear evidence that induced hypothermia reduces mortality in a neurosurgical population. In patients undergoing temporary clipping for aneurysm surgery, hypothermia was not associated with improved neurologic outcomes (Hindman et al 2010). A multi centre trial is currently under way to assess 6 month functional outcome after induction of hypothermia in patients with brain trauma (North American Brain Injury Study: Hypothermia IIR, Clifton et al, 2009).

## 3. Extracranial organ support in the neurocritical care unit

Critically unwell neurosurgical patients also need ongoing management of other organ systems and management of other non brain pathologies. Critical care interventions on extra cranial organs have implications for cerebral circulation and metabolism. Appropriate care also minimises secondary injury to the brain after primary insults like trauma.

### 3.1 Respiratory support

Mechanical ventilation has rapidly evolved in recent years, guided primarily by improved understanding of pathophysiology. Neurosurgical patients heavily rely on ventilation for support, and less commonly, for therapy. Meeting ventilation needs of these patients while minimising ventilator induced lung injury can be challenging (Johnson et al, 2007).

The purpose of ventilator support may loosely be divided into those of optimising systemic arterial oxygenation ($PaO_2$) and oxygen saturation ($SaO_2$) and regulating partial pressure of carbon dioxide in arterial blood ($PaCO_2$).

Hypoxia ($PaO_2$<60 and/ or $SaO_2$<90) is associated with poor neurologic outcomes in patients with acute brain injuries (Young et al 2010). The duration of hypoxia itself is an independent predictor of mortality (Jones et al 1994). The physiologic response to cerebral hypoxia is increased cerebral blood flow. In the context of elevated intracranial pressure, the resultant increase in intracranial blood volume is likely to exacerbate intracranial hypertension. This can be rapidly corrected by ventilating to normoxia (SaO2>90, PaO2>70) and often requires intubation and mechanical ventilation.

While primary insults like trauma cause areas of focal hypoperfusion of the brain, there is no conclusive evidence supporting attempts to achieve supra normal $PaO_2$ to improve local oxygen delivery. Extreme hyperoxemia may be detrimental in patients with severe traumatic brain injury (Davis et al 2009). Certainly, among patients admitted to intensive care after resuscitation from cardiac arrest, hyperoxia ($PaO_2$>300) is associated with increased risk of in hospital mortality (Kilgannon et al, 2010).

Historically, aggressive hyperventilation to induce hypocapnia ($PaCO_2$<25) has been advocated to reduce intracranial pressures (ICP). While hyperventilation certainly reduces ICP, the mechanism by which this occurs is cerebral vasoconstriction, reducing cerebral blood flow and ultimately, compromising blood flow to brain tissue. Prophylactic hyperventilation is no longer recommended and this intervention should be limited to being a temporising measure in the management of intractably elevated ICP. Its benefits may be outweighed by risks in the first 24 hours after acute brain insult when perfusion to the brain is poor and, where available, should be used in conjunction with monitoring of cerebral perfusion like jugular venous saturation ($JvSO_2$). (Brain trauma foundation guidelines edition 3). Hypercapnia (PCO2>50) causes cerebral vasodilation, increasing cerebral blood volume and thereby ICP. The optimal strategy would be to aim for normocapnia ($PaCO_2$ 35-45).

Positive end expiratory pressure (PEEP) improves oxygenation and forms part of routine lung protective ventilation strategies. Traditionally, concerns have been raised regarding the use of PEEP in ventilating neurosurgical patient as it may increase ICP and, by extension, reduce cerebral perfusion pressure (CPP). Low levels of PEEP to improve alveolar recruitment have been shown to not change ICP (Mascia et al 2005). Increasing PEEP to as high as 15 cmH2O to improve oxygenation was paradoxically associated with decreases in ICP and improved CPP (Huynh et al 2002).

Reasonable goals of ventilation would be to achieve SaO2>90, PaO2>70, PCO2 35-45. Lung protective ventilator strategies (low tidal volumes 6-8 ml/kg, judicious use of PEEP) would meet the ventilatory requirements of the majority of neurosurgical patients. Additional measures such as loosening tapes securing endotracheal tubes and optimum head positioning and head elevation to prevent jugular outflow obstruction would be of benefit to maintaining adequate CPP.

### 3.2 Cardiovascular support

The goal of all resuscitation is the delivery of oxygen and metabolites to end organs. Hypotension, defined as a systolic blood pressure less than 90 mmHg, has been shown to worsen outcomes from acute brain injury. Even isolated episodes of in hospital hypotension have been associated with increased mortality and morbidity (Jones et al, 1994). Due to ethical considerations, there is no Class I evidence on the effect of haemodynamic resuscitation on outcomes. However, raising the blood pressure improves outcome in proportion to the efficacy of the resuscitation (Vassar et al 1993).

The ideal fluid for volume resuscitation remains controversial. 0.9% NaCl remains the most commonly used fluid for this purpose, probably for reasons of familiarity, cost and ease of use. There is little conclusive evidence to support colloid over crystalloid therapy. The SAFE study suggested similar outcomes from fluid resuscitation with saline or 4% albumin. A post hoc analysis of the SAFE study data suggested higher mortality rates associated with fluid resuscitation with albumin compared to saline in patients with traumatic brain injury (SAFE study investigators, 2007). A multi centre randomised trial is currently under way comparing outcomes of resuscitation with saline and starch.

It is reasonable to use vasopressors and inotropes as needed to defend MAP and, by extension, CPP. There is no conclusive evidence to prove the superiority of any vasoactive agent over another. The use of these drugs is often determined by local critical care practice. The author's vasopressor of choice is noradrenaline.

The systolic blood pressure of 90 mmHg itself is a statistical rather than a physiological threshold. It makes more sense to try and approximate the patient's baseline blood pressure with hemodynamic therapies than chase an artificial statistical target. The author's practice is to stay within 20% of the patient's baseline blood pressure, where known.

Cerebral perfusion is reliant more on the systemic mean arterial pressure (MAP) and ICP. The MAP may be a more meaningful end point of resuscitation to aim for. Autoregulation of blood flow breaks down in most vascular beds below ~60 mmHg. Thus, assuming a "normal" ICP of 10 $cmH_20$ and intact cerebral vasculature, a MAP of 70 mmHg would be a reasonable initial target. Clearly, the above caveats are not necessarily true for many neurosurgical patients and, in the presence of ICP monitoring, the MAP can be titrated to maintain a CPP>60 mmHg. Alternately, in the presence of cerebral oxygenation monitoring (eg. JvSO2), the MAP can be titrated to adequate cerebral oxygenation.

There is no conclusive evidence for elevating MAP to supra normal targets. This may well be hazardous in the context of trauma or recent surgery, with concomitant disruption of the blood brain barrier and cannot be recommended in routine neuro critical care practice.

### 3.3 Nutrition

There is no disease process that benefits from lack of nutritional support. Critically unwell patients are hypercatabolic and at risk of losing significant lean body mass in the absence of nutritional support. Current practice would be to attempt to initiate nutrition early (within 72 hours) aiming to establish full calorific replacement within 7 days. Clearly this would be modified for patients presenting with evidence of poor nutritional state at baseline. Enteral nutrition, by gastric or jejunal routes, is the preferred route. In the event of inability to access the gut or failure to establish enteral nutrition within a reasonable time frame, parenteral nutrition should be considered.

Patients with traumatic brain injuries often have gastroparesis. Many drugs routinely administered in a critical care setting further alter gut motility. This is particularly true of opiates. Prokinetics (eg metoclopramide 10-20 mg 6 hourly) should be considered early in the establishment of enteral nutrition.

Reasonable goals of nutrition support should aim for 25-30 kcal/kg/day, of which 0.5-2 gm/kg/day should be protein content and 30-40% non protein content should be lipids. It is important to also supplement fat and water soluble vitamins and trace elements.

### 3.4 Glycemic control

Hyperglycemia is common in critically ill patients and is associated with morbidity and mortality in varying groups of patients.

In 2001, the Leuven Intensive Insulin Therapy Trial was published (van den Berghe et al, 2001), suggesting dramatic reductions in mortality in critically ill surgical patients with tight glycaemic control (target blood sugar 4.4-6.1 mmol/L). Subsequent studies failed to replicate these findings. Concerns were also raised regarding the risks of hypoglycaemia, increased resource use and the difficulty of achieving tight normoglycemia in critically ill patients.

The NICE-SUGAR study (Finfer et al, 2009) suggested blood glucose levels less than 10 mmol/L resulted in lower mortality than a target of 4.5-6 mmol/L. The author's current practice is to aim for a blood sugar level of 5-10 mmol/L.

### 3.5 Stress ulcer prophylaxis

Stress ulcers are a known complication of a variety of critical illnesses. They occur as a consequence of hypoperfusion of the mucosa of the upper gastro intestinal tract. It is common practice to provide prophylaxis to decrease the incidence of clinically significant bleeding.

The most commonly used classes of drugs used for this purpose are H2 antagonists, proton pump inhibitors and sucralfate. To a large extent, the agent used is dictated by local critical care practice.

H2 antagonists have been shown to be more effective than sucralfate, antacids and placebo in preventing stress ulcers (Stollman & Metz, 2005). However, concerns have been raised regarding the association between acid suppressive treatment and ventilator associated pneumonia (Cook et al, 1998). Ranitidine has been associated more strongly with nosocomial pneumonia than sucralfate (Messori et al, 2000). Further concerns have been raised regarding encephalopathy and cytochrome P450 induction by H2 antagonists. Omeprazole was shown to reduce clinically significant gastrointestinal bleeding compared to ranitidine (Levy et al, 1997). A recent single centre study found a higher association of nosocomial pneumonia with pantoprazole compared to ranitidine in cardiac surgical patients (Miano et al, 2009). Both H2 antagonists and proton pump inhibitors have been associated with increased risk of developing community and hospital acquired Clostridium difficile associated disease (CDC, 2005).

In keeping with the above, a recent systematic review was unable to find the most appropriate form of prophylaxis for neurocritical care patients (Schirmer et al, 2011). The most sensible approach appears to be aggressive haemodynamic resuscitation to improve mucosal perfusion in the upper gastrointestinal tract and the establishment of early enteral nutrition, where possible. It is standard Australian practice to prescribe stress ulcer chemoprophylaxis and both H2 antagonists and proton pump inhibitors are commonly used.

### 3.6 Thromboprophylaxis

Critically ill neurosurgical patients are at high risk of developing venous thromboembolism. The incidence of deep vein thrombosis (DVT) in patients with traumatic brain injury is estimated to be as high as 20% (Brain Trauma Foundation Guidelines, 3rd ed.). Pulmonary emboli (PE) are associated with high rates of mortality and morbidity in hospitalised patients. Treatment of PE in neurosurgical patients is often complicated by uncertainty regarding the safety of anticoagulation soon after craniotomy or intracranial haemorrhage. It makes sense to try and prevent DVT than have to treat the PE.

Options for DVT prophylaxis are mechanical (graduated compression stockings and sequential calf or foot compression devices) or chemical (low dose heparin or low dose low molecular weight heparin). Recent studies have failed to prove the superiority of low molecular weight heparins over low dose unfractionated heparin (Cook et al 2011, Goldhaber et al 2002)

Mechanical interventions have low risk of complications and should be offered to all patients. Caution needs to be exercised in patients with severe peripheral vascular disease and limb trauma may preclude their use in some cases.

Both low molecular weight heparin and unfractionated heparin have been shown to be effective for prophylaxis of venous thromboembolism in elective neurosurgery (Ioro & Agnelli, 2000). In traumatic brain injury, the risk versus benefit analysis must be made on a case by case basis. There appears to be little difference in the incidence of DVT or PE in patients receiving chemical prophylaxis after 72 hours of admission compared to those receiving prophylaxis earlier than 72 hours (Kim et al, 2002). In the event that chemical prophylaxis cannot be initiated within 72 hours of admission, consideration should be given to a vena caval filter.

## 4. Prognostication in neurocritical care

The outcome of critically ill neurosurgical patients after significant brain insult remains uncertain. Patients may survive to a cognitively impaired dependent state or worse, in a minimally conscious or persistently vegetative state with resultant implications for resource use.

Prediction of outcome involves making probability statements that depend on a logical relationship between outcome and features encapsulated in antecedent data. It still remains impossible to predict with certainty the outcomes of an individual patient.

In a neurocritical care population, the groups most widely studied in this context are those with traumatic brain injury and hypoxic brain injury.

### 4.1 Traumatic brain injury

The brain trauma foundation has published prognostic parameters for traumatic brain injury. The following factors have been considered

- Glasgow Coma Scale (GCS) score: If the initial GCS is reliably obtained and not tainted by pre hospital medications or intubation, there is increasing probability of poor outcome with a low GCS in a continuous stepwise manner. Approximately 20% patients with initial GCS 3 will survive and 8-10% will have a functional survival.
- Age: There is increasing probability of poor neurologic outcome with age, with a significant rise in poor outcomes in age>60 years.
- Bilaterally absent pupillary light reflex is a predictor of poor neurologic outcome
- Hypotension (systolic BP<90 mmHg) alone has a positive predictive value (PPV) of 67% for poor neurologic outcome. In conjunction with hypoxia (SaO2<90%), the PPV for hypotension rises to 79%
- Presence of abnormalities on initial CT study: Compressed or absent basal cisterns, traumatic subarachnoid haemorrhage and midline shift at the level of the foramen of Monro are predictive of poor neurological outcomes.
- The Marshall score (Marshall et al, 1991) was developed from the Trauma Coma Data Bank (TCDB) for estimating the severity of diffuse axonal injuries seen on CT (Table 1). Marshall scores of 3 or higher are associated with dramatically higher incidence of mortality.

| Grade | Definition |
|---|---|
| I | No visible intracranial pathology seen on CT scan |
| II | Cisterns present; midline shift 0–5 mm and/or lesion densities present; no high or mixed density lesion >25 cc |
| III | Cisterns compressed or absent with midline shift 0–5 mm; no high or mixed density lesion >25 mm |
| IV | Midline shift >5 mm; no high or mixed density lesion >25 cc |

Table 1.

### 4.2 Hypoxic brain injury

Attempts have been made to identify prognostic factors for poor outcomes in patients with hypoxic brain injuries at up to 3 days after admission (Levy et al, 1985 and Zandbergen et al, 2006). The American Academy of Neurology has published guidelines for prediction of outcomes in comatose survivors of cardiopulmonary resuscitation (Wijdicks et al 2006).

Development of myoclonus status epilepticus within the 1$^{st}$ day, bilaterally absent cortical response on somatosensory evoked potentials (delayed N20) at day 1-3, serum neuron specific enolase (NSE) >33micrograms/L at day 1-3, absent pupillary or corneal reflexes on day 3 or extensor or absent motor response to stimulus on day 3 are predictive of poor neurologic outcomes.

Burst suppression or generalised epileptiform activity on EEG was predictive of poor outcome but with insufficient prognostic accuracy. Imaging (CT, MRI, PET) and duration of CPR were not reliable predictors of poor outcome.

## 5. Determination of brain death

Death has always had immense cultural and religious significance for human societies across the world. Until the Renaissance, there was no biological understanding of death. William Harvey's seminal paper "On the Motion of the Heart and Blood in Animals" in the 17th century laid the foundation to the understanding of death as irreversible cessation of cardiovascular function. In 1959, Wertheimer et al first described "death of the central nervous system" as a syndrome of coma, areflexia and apnoea. Later that year, Mollaret and Goulon coined the term "coma depasse" to describe this syndrome.

Brain death is defined as irreversible cessation of brain function. Prior to the diagnosis of brain death being made, the following preconditions must be met

- Definite clinical and/ or neuro imaging evidence of acute brain pathology consistent with irreversible loss of neurologic function (eg. traumatic brain injury, intracranial haemorrhage, hypoxic ischaemic encephalopathy)
- Normothermic (temperature >35°C), normotensive (systolic BP>90 mmHg, MAP>60 mHg) patient
- Severe electrolyte (specifically sodium, magnesium, calcium, phosphate), metabolic (blood sugar, renal and hepatic functions) and endocrine disturbances ruled out
- Effect of sedative drugs ruled out
- Intact neuromuscular function

For further clinical testing, the following are also essential

- Ability to adequately examine brainstem reflexes including at least one ear and one eye
- Ability to safely perform apnoea testing, which may be precluded by severe hypoxia or high cervical spine injury

If the preconditions are met, brain death may be diagnosed by

- Clinical examination OR
- Demonstration of absence of intra cranial blood flow

Clinical examination consists of

- Absence of responsiveness for a period of observation AND
- Absence of brainstem reflexes to clinical examination AND
- Apnoea despite arterial pH<7.3, $PaCO_2$>60 mmHg

The American Academy of Neurology (AAN) guidelines (Wijdicks et al, 2010) comment that there is lack of evidence for a minimally acceptable observation period. The Australasian guidelines currently recommend a minimum 4 hour period of observation for unresponsiveness (The ANZICS Statement on Death and Organ donation).

It is common practice in Australasia for clinical testing to be carried out independently by 2 senior clinicians to confirm the diagnosis of brain death. This has been challenged in recent times and, under the current AAN guidelines, confirmatory clinical testing by an independent clinician is no longer required.

If clinical testing is inconclusive or cannot be carried out, Australasian practice would be to demonstrate absence of intra cranial blood flow by

- 4 vessel (both carotid arteries, both vertebral arteries) intra arterial angiography with digital subtraction to demonstrate lack of blood flow above the level of the carotid siphon (anterior circulation) and the foramen magnum (posterior circulation)
- Technetium 99m labelled hexamethyl propylene amine oxime (Tc-99m HMPAO) radionuclide scan demonstrating absence of intra cranial perfusion
- Single photon emission computerised tomography (SPECT)
- CT angiography 60 seconds after contrast bolus at the level of Circle of Willis demonstrating contrast enhancement of the external carotid but not of middle cerebral artery cortical branches, P2 segment of posterior cerebral arteries, pericallosal arteries and internal cerebral veins

There is no documented case of a person who fulfils the preconditions and criteria for brain death ever subsequently developing any return of brain function.

## 6. Illustrative cases

### 6.1 Traumatic brain injury

A 32 year old man was brought in by ambulance to the Emergency Department after being assaulted in a pub.

At scene, he was noted to eye open to voice, localise to noxious stimuli and had incoherent speech. His heart rate was 98 and regular and his systolic blood pressure was 110 mmHg. The paramedics at the scene had basic life support skills only. Two large bore intravenous cannulae were inserted, fluid resuscitation with 0.9% NaCl commenced and the patient transferred with spinal precautions to the nearest trauma centre, about 5 minutes away.

On arrival to hospital, he was moaning and unresponsive to pain. His haemodynamic status remained unchanged.

In the trauma room, he was intubated with in line manual stabilisation, a cervical collar was applied and the head supported with sandbags and tape. He was ventilated with 100% oxygen to a $PCO_2$ of 35-40 and sedated with morphine and midazolam. Primary and secondary surveys revealed no major limb, thorax, abdominal, pelvic or spinal trauma. There was no clinical evidence of base of skull fracture and his pupils were equal and reactive. He was taken for a non contrast CT of his head and neck. His cervical spine was intact and he was diagnosed as having an acute subdural haemorrhage about 15 mm in thickness over the left temporoparietal hemisphere with 5 mm midline shift. Subarachnoid blood was also noted.

In the operating room, the subdural haemorrhage was evacuated with a craniotomy and an external ventricular drain (EVD) inserted. The patient was transferred to the intensive care unit intubated and ventilated.

Over the next 24 hours, he remained deeply sedated with a combination of benzodiazepines, propofol and opiates and needed intermittent neuromuscular blockade with vecuronium. He required repeated drainage of CSF through his EVD and several administrations of 3% NaCl to keep his ICP <20 mmHg. His MAP was manipulated with noradrenaline to maintain a CPP >60 mmHg. His pupils remained equal and reactive and normothermia and euglycemia maintained. In terms of extracranial organ support, he was ventilated to normocapnoea and $SaO_2$ were maintained >92% at all times, with PEEP of 5 $cmH_2O$. Apart from manipulation of MAP to maintain CPP >60mmHg, he remained cardiovascularly stable and his ECG remained unchanged from normal sinus rhythm. Enteral nutrition was commenced through an orogastric tube. Ranitidine was given intravenously for gut protection. Only mechanical thromboprophylaxis with sequential calf compressors was provided.

Over the subsequent 72 hours, the ICP remained stable at less than 20 mmHg and sedation was lightened. Pupils remained equal and no seizure activity was noted. The CT showed no further progression of brain pathology and some resolution of cerebral oedema. There were no other extracranial organ support issues. On day 5, the EVD was removed. On day 7, on sedation break, the patient was noted to eye open to voice, appropriately follow simple commands and cough to endotracheal suction. The patient was extubated and discharged to the neurosurgical ward for ongoing management.

### 6.2 Posterior fossa bleed

A 54 year old man with a background history of treated hypertension and a known posterior fossa arterio venous malformation presented to the Emergency Department with a decreased level of consciousness after complaining of a headache, slurred speech and unsteady gait. A CT scan revealed a large posterior fossa bleed from the AV malformation.

The haematoma was emergently evacuated, the posterior fossa was decompressed and an external ventricular drain inserted. The patient was transferred to the intensive care unit.

He was sedated with propofol and morphine, ICP maintained at <20 mmHg and the MAP was manipulated with noradrenaline to sustain a CPP >60 mmHg. Normocapnoea, normothermia, normoxia, normotension and euglycemia were maintained and routine postoperative cares were provided. His care was complicated by a rebleed in the posterior fossa on day 3 needing further decompression and ongoing sedation and CSF drainage. The ICP finally stabilized on day 6, a subsequent CT was satisfactory, the EVD was removed and on day 8, on sedation break, the patient was noted to be eye opening to voice and following simple commands. He was extubated the next day but needed to be re intubated soon after for inability to clear secretions.

His stay was further complicated by a nosocomial pneumonia and a tracheostomy was performed to facilitate liberation from the ventilator over several days. There was reasonable recovery of motor and intellectual function, however, he failed attempts at decannulation due to inability to cough and clear secretions adequately. Interestingly, he was also noted to have central alveolar hypoventilation needing ventilator support during sleep (Ondine's curse). A tracheostomy was left in situ and the patient transferred to a chronic ventilation service under the care of the respiratory medicine team.

## 7. Conclusion

Neurocritical care is a relatively new sub speciality of medicine. Critical care physicians in these units defragment the care of critically ill neurosurgical patients, often with other organ pathologies, by

- optimising treatment of the underlying brain pathology
- preventing of secondary injury to neurons
- providing global extracranial organ support

The critical care unit itself provides a venue for advanced monitoring allowing

- continuous monitoring of respiratory and haemodynamic function
- continuous monitoring of ICP, allowing ongoing defence of CPP
- monitoring of cerebral perfusion and cerebral tissue oxygenation

This enables targeted aggressive invasive organ support to prevent or minimise secondary neuronal injury. Reasonable goals of resuscitation include

- CPP>60 mmHg
- PBrO2>15 mmHg
- SjO2 55-75%
- MAP>70 mmHg, ideally titrated to CPP if ICP measurement in situ or within 20% of patient's baseline MAP, if known
- $SaO_2$>90%
- $PO_2$>70 mmHg
- $PCO_2$ 35-45 mmHg
- Temperature 36-37°C
- Blood sugar 5-10 mmol/L
- Urine output> 30 ml/hour (or at least 0.5 ml/kg/hour)

Early aggressive management and prevention of secondary tissue injury in close coordination with neurosurgical teams is thought to improve neurologic outcomes for critically ill neurosurgical patients.

There is now accumulating evidence of outcomes after critical illness. In neurosurgical populations, significant advances have been made in identifying indicators of poor outcome. A thorough understanding of these factors and their significance arms the bedside clinician in prognosticating for individual patients in their care.

It is now about half a century since brain death as a phenomenon has been recognised. It is interesting that the diagnostic criteria and clinical examination to determine brain death have remained largely unchanged for over 30 years. Accumulating experience with various modalities of neuroimaging allow newer, more elegant ways of demonstrating absence of cerebral perfusion and are increasingly being used to diagnose brain death.

## 8. Acknowledgment

I would like to acknowledge the input and encouragement of my critical care, neurosurgical and neurology colleagues. I thank my family for their patience and forbearance during the writing of this chapter.

There are no conflicts of interest to declare in the writing of this chapter.

## 9. References

Brain Trauma Foundation Guidelines 3rd edition, available from http://tbiguidelines.org

Bouzat P.; Francony G.; Brun J.; Lavagne P.; Picard J.; Broux C.; Declety P.; Jacquot C.; Albaladejo P.; Payen J.F. (2010) *Detecting traumatic internal carotid artery dissection using transcranial doppler in head injured patients* Intensive Care Med 36 :1514-1520

Centers for Disease Control and Prevention (CDC) (2005) *Severe clostridium difficile associated disease in populations previously at low risk- four states* MMWR Morb Mortal Weekly Rep 54(47) :1201-05

Clifton G.L.; Drever P.; Valadka A.; Zygun D.; Okonkwo D. (2009) *Multicentre trial of early hypothermia in severe brain injury* J Neurotrauma 26(3) :393-397

Cook D.; Meade M.; Guyatt G; Walter S.; PROTECT investigators (2011) *Dalteparin versus unfractionated heparin in critically ill patients* N Engl J Med 364(14) :1305-14

Cook D.; Guyatt J.; Marshall J.; Leasa D.; Fuller H.; Hall R. (1998) *A comparison of sucralfate and ranitidine for the prevention of upper gastrointestinal bleeding in patients requiring mechanical ventilation* N Engl J Med 338 :791-7

Davis D.P.; Meade W.; Sise M.J.; Kennedy F.; Simon F.; Tominaga G.; Steele J.; Coimbra R. (2009). *Both hypoxemia and extreme hyperoxemia may be detrimental in patients with severe traumatic brain injury* J Neurotrauma 26(12) :2217-23

Finfer S.; Bellomo R.; Boyce N.; French J.; Myburgh J.; Norton R. (2004) *A comparison of albumin and saline for fluid resuscitation in the intensive care unit* N Engl J Med 350(22) :2247-56

Glantz M.J.; Cole B.F.; Forsyth P.A.; Recht L.D.; Wen P.Y.; Chamberlain M.C.; Grossman S.A.; Cairncross J.G. (2000) *Practice parameter : anticonvulsant prophylaxis in patients with newly diagnosed brain tumours : report of the quality standards subcommittee of the American Academy of Neurology* Neurology 54 :1886-93

Goldhaber S.Z.; Dunn K.; Gerhard- Herman M.; Park J.K.; Black P.M. (2002) *Low rate of venous thromboembolism after craniotomy for brain tumor using multimodality prophylaxis* Chest 122(6) :1933-37

Hindman B.J.; Bayman E.O.; Pfisterer W.K.; Torner J.C.; Todd M.M.; the IHAST investigators (2010) *No association between intraoperative hypothermia or supplemental protective drug and neurologic outcomes in patients undergoing temporary clipping during cerebral aneurysm surgery Anesthesiology* 112 :86-101

Huynh T.; Messer M.; Sing R.F.; Miles W.; Jacobs D.G.; Thomason M.H. (2002) *Positive end-expiratory pressure alters intracranial and cerebral perfusion pressure in severe traumatic brain injury* J Trauma 53(3) : 488-92

Ioro A.; Agnelli G. (2000) *Low molecular weight heparin and unfractionated heparin for prevention of venous thromboembolism in neurisurgery : a meta analysis* Arch Intern Med 160(15) :2327-32

Johnson, V.E.; Huang J.H & Pilcher W.H. (2007). *Special cases : mechanical ventilation of neurosurgical patients* Crit Care Clin 23(2) :275-90,x

Jones P.A.; Andrews P.J.; Midgley S.; Anderson S.I.; Piper I.R.; Tocher J.L. et al (1994). *Measuring the burden of secondary insults in head- injured patients during intensive care* J Neurosurg Anesthesiol 6(1) :4-14

Kilgannon J.H.; Jones A.E.; Shapiro N.I.; Angelos M.G.; Milcarek B.; Hunter K.; Parillo J.E.; Trzeciak S. (2010) Association between arterial hyperoxia following resuscitation from cardiac arrest and in- hospital mortality JAMA 303(21) :2165-71

Kim J.; Gearhart M.M.; Zurick A.; Zuccarello M.; James L.; Luchette F.A. (2002) *Preliminary report on the safety of heparin for deep vein thrombosis prophylaxis after head injury* J Trauma 53(1) :38-42

Levy D.E.; Caronna J.J.; Singer B.H.; Lapinski R.H.; Frydman H.; Plum F. (1985) *Predicting outcome from hypoxic ischaemic coma* JAMA 253 :1420-26

Levy M.J.; Seelig C.B.; Robinson N.J.; Ranney J.E. (1997) *Comparison of omeprazole and ranitidine for stress ulcer prophylaxis* Dig Dis Sci 42(6) :1255-59

Marshall L.F.; Gantille T.; Klauber M.R. (1991) *The outcome of severe closed head injury* J Neurosurg (Suppl) 75 :28-36

Mascia L.; Grasso S.; Fiore T.; Bruno F.; Bernardino M.; Ducati A. (2005) *Cerebro- pulmonary interactions during the application of low levels of positive end- expiratory pressure* Intensive Care Med 31(3) :373-9

Messori A.; Trippoli S.; Valani M.; Gorini M.; Corrado A. (2000) *Bleeding and pneumonia in intensive care patients given ranitidine and sucralfate for prevention of stress ulcer : meta-analysis of randomised controlled trials* BMJ 321 : 1103-06

Miano T.A.; Reichert M.G.; Houle T.T.; MacGregor D.A.; Kincaid E.H.; Bowton D.L. (2009) *Nosocomial pneumonia risk and stress ulcer prophylaxis : A comparison of pantoprazole versus ranitidine in cardiothoracic surgery patients* Chest 136(2) :440-47

Mollaret P. & Goulon L. (1959) *Le coma depasse (memoire preliminaire)* Rev Neurol (Paris) 101 :3-15

Myburgh J.; Cooper D.J.; Finfer S.; Bellomo R.; Norton R.; Bishop N.; Kai Lo S.; Vallance S. (2007) *Saline or albumin fluid resuscitation in patients with traumatic brain injury* N Engl J Med 357(9) :874-84

Reinhard M.; Neunhoffer G.; Gerds T.A.; Niesen W.G.; Buttler K.J.; Timmer J.; Schmidt B.; Czosnyka M.; Weiller C.; Hetzel A. (2010) *Secondary decline of cerebral autoregulation is assosciated with worse outcome after intra cerebral haemorrhage* Intensive Care Med 36 :264-271

Rincon, F. & Mayer S.A. (2007). *Neurocritical care : a distinct discipline?* Curr Opin Crit Care 13(2) : 115-21

Schirmer C.M.; Kornbluth J.; Hellman C.B.; Bhardwaj A. (2011) *Gastrointestinal prophylaxis in neurocritical care* Neurocrit Care Jul 12 [Epub ahead of print]

Shaw M.D.M.; Foy P.M. (1991) *Epilepsy after craniotomy and the place of prophylactic anticonvulsant drugs : discussion paper* J R Soc Med 84(4) :221-23

Stollman N.; Metz D.C. (2005) *Pathophysiology and prophylaxis of stress ulcer in intensive care unit patients* J Crit Care 20(1) :35-45

The Australian and New Zealand Intensive Care Society (ANZICS) Statement on Death and Organ Donation, Edition 3.1 (2010), available from http://www.anzics.com.au/death-and-organ-donation

Vassar M.J; Perry C.A.; Holcroft J.W. (1993) *Prehospital resuscitation of hypotensive trauma patients with 7.5% NaCl versus 7.5% NaCl with added dextran : a controlled trial* J Trauma 34(5) :622-32

Wijdicks E.F.M.; Hijdra A.; Young G.B.; Bassetti C.L.; Wiebe S. (2006) *Practice parameter : Prediction of outcome in comatose survivors after cardiopulmonary resuscitation (an evidence based review)* Neurology 67(2) :203-10

Wijdicks E.F.M.; Varelas P.N.; Gronseth G.S.; Greer D.M. (2010) *Evidence based guideline update : Determining brain death in adults* Neurology 74 :1911-18

Young N.; Rhodes J.K.; Mascia L.; Andrews P.J. (2010). *Ventilatory strategies for patients with acute brain injury* Curr Opin Crit Care 16(1) :45-52

Zandbergen E.G.J; Hijdra A.; Koehlman J.H.T.M.; Hart A.A.M.; Vos P.E.; Verbeek M.M.; de Haan R.J. (2006) *Prediction of poor outcomes within the first 3 days of postanoxic coma* Neurology 66(1) :62-68

# Section 2

## General Topics

# 5

# Decompressive Craniectomy for Refractory Intracranial Hypertension

Michal Bar[1], Stefan Reguli[2] and Radim Lipina[2]
[1]*Department of Neurology, Faculty Hospital and Faculty of Medicine University of Ostrava*
[2]*Department of Neurosurgery , Faculty Hospital, Ostrava, Czech Republic*

## 1. Introduction

Clinical and experimental data from the past two decades show that Decompressive Craniectomy (DC) is an effective treatment which reduces mortality within patients with refractory intracranial hypertension. Massive cerebral ischemic infarction and traumatic brain injury are the most frequent indication of DC. Since the conservative medical treatment of intracranial hypertension is ineffective in many patients, the idea of decompressive surgery of temporary release of swollen brain outside the cranium has been developed at the beginning of the last century. The first decompressive hemicraniectomy for traumatic brain injury was done in 1901 by Kocher. (Merenda & DeGeorgia, 2010) Harvey Cushing started using DC for the treatment in the cases on inoperable brain tumors and later also in the cases of traumatic diffuse brain edema and vascular malformations. (Kahar et al,2009) Decompressive surgery was first reported as a potential treatment for large hemispheric infarction in case reports as early as 1956. (Scarcella, 1956)

The results of experimental studies using rat models and prospective studies with acute stroke patients have provided further support for decompressive surgery strategy in patients with intracranial refractory hypertension. On the basis of these facts three randomized prospective studies with patients with malignant supratentorial infarction were started in the first decade of 21st century. The pooled analysis of these studies proved reduction of mortality without an increasing number of disabled people. Based on the pooled analysis of DECIMAL, HAMLET and DESTINY, the European Stroke Association (ESO) issued some new guidelines for malignant supratentorial brain ischemia treatment. (European Stroke Organization guidelines, 2008) The recommendations for the decompressive surgery for traumatic brain injury are not so unambiguous. (Servadei, 2011) DC is recommended in children patients in some specific situations and nowadays it is not recommended in adults routinely. Also in some other cases which lead to intracranial hypertension development, DC is performed only on the basis of the individual approach of the doctor to the patient, often after consulting the family. Generally, we can say that DC remains the only one option of intracranial hypertension (ICH) of various etiology treatment when the conservative treatment fails.

## 2. Patophysiology of intracranial hypertension

The syndrome of intracranial hypertension appears when the intracranial pressure (ICP) arises up to more than 20-25mmHg. Sustained ICP values of greater than 40-45 mm Hg indicate severe life-threatening state .The possible causes of increased ICP are shown in table No1. The high ICP reduces the cerebral blood perfusion and space occupying lesion causes mass effect which then leads to brain tissue displacements and herniation. There are four most common types of herniations; the subfalcial, temporal lobe tentorial (uncal herniation) , cerebellar - foramen magnum and cerebellar -tentorial herniation . (fig 1) Temporal uncal herniation and both types of cerebellar herniations can lead to compression of brainstem and a rapid alteration of consciousness , anisocoria , decerebrate posturing and alteration of breathing (atactic or cluster type of breathing) followed by apnoe and cardiac arrest in the end.

| |
|---|
| mass effect such as malignant ischemic stroke with edema, contusions, subdural or epidural hematoma, brain tumor etc. |
| generalized brain swelling without mass effect can occur in ischemic-anoxia states, traumatic brain edema ,acute liver or renal failure, hypertensive encephalopathy, status epilepticus etc. |
| increasing venous pressure can be due to venous sinus thrombosis or heart failure. |
| obstruction of cerebrospinal fluid flow or malfunction of its absorption can occur in hydrocephalus or in meningeal disease (e.g., infecious, carcinomatous or subarachnoidal hemorrhage). |
| idiopathic or unknown cause (idiopathic intracranial hypertension , pseudotumor cerebri) |

Table 1. The causes of increased intracranial pressure (ICP)

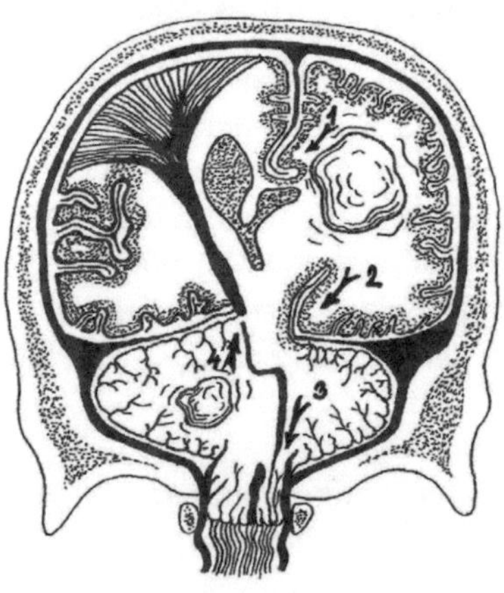


Legend: 1.subfalcinal herniation 2. temporal lobe tentorial (uncal) herniation 3. cerebellar – foramen magnum herniation 4. cerebellar –tentorial herniation

Fig. 1. The types of cerebral herniation, mass shifts associated with a parietal lobe and cerebellar tumor (Adams & Victor, 1997)

## 3. Conservative treatment of intracranial hypertension

Several types of the conservative treatment for reducing intracranial hypertension of various causes to prevent midline shift or herniation have been proposed in the past decades such as management of the airway, breathing and circulation (ABCs), osmotherapy, sedation, steroids, hyperventilation , and induced therapeutic hypothermia . (Sankhyan, 2010; Jüttler et al 2007) Osmotherapy (glycerol and mannitol) has been tested in several randomized and nonrandomized clinical trials of acute stroke, but none of these proved its effect on the clinical outcome. A systematic Cochrane review of these trials in acute stroke suggests a favourable effect of glycerol treatment on short-term survival, but no long-term efficacy. (Hofmeijer et al, 2003) The lack of proven benefit on long-term survival does not support the routine use of glycerol and mannitol in patients with acute ischemic stroke. None of the randomized trials in patients with ischemic stroke which would prove efficacy on their favourable outcome has been carried out. So far none of these terapeutic conservative strategies are recommended on level A or B for the treatment of ICH in space occupying ischemic stroke.

In traumatic brain injury (TBI) the recommendations are summarized in the Brain Trauma Foundation Guidelines. (Bullock et al, 2006) Hyperosmolar agents currently in clinical use for TBI are mannitol and hypertonic saline. Mannitol is widely used and its use is advocated in two circumstances. First, a single administration can have short term beneficial effects, during which further diagnostic procedures (e.g., CT scan) and interventions (e.g., evacuation of intracranial mass lesions) can be accomplished. Second, mannitol has been used as a prolonged therapy for raised ICP. (Bullock et al , 2006). There is a level II evidence that mannitol is effective for control of raised intracranial pressure (ICP) at doses of 0.25 gm/kg to 1 g/kg body weight. Arterial hypotension (systolic blood pressure < 90 mm Hg) should be avoided. (Bullock et al, 2006)

Current evidence is not strong enough to make recommendations on the use, concentration and method of administration of hypertonic saline for the treatment of traumatic intracranial hypertension.

## 4. Indications

The most common diagnosis, where DC is performed, are ischemic stroke and traumatic brain injury. Less frequently DC has been successfully reported in relation with the treatment of refractory intracranial hypertension in other diagnosis such as intracranial venous thrombosis, subarachnoidal hemorrhage , spontaneus intracerebral hemorhage , encephalitis , tumours and in encephalopathy related to Reye´s syndrom. (Schimer et al, 2008) Generally there are no fixed threshold value for surgery such as intracranial pressure value, midline shift size, expansion volume size, perfusion pressure etc. The indication for surgery is in most cases based on the individual approach of the clinician towards the patient.

### 4.1 Decompressive cranietomy for acute stroke

#### 4.1.1 Malignant supratentorial ischemic infarction

4.1.1.1 Rationale and randomized trials

The incidence of ischemic stroke in various European countries is between 183-349 /100 000 and e.g. in the Czech Republic it is 219/100 000. (Bamford et al 1990, Bar et al, 2010)

Generally, the massive hemispheric infarctions constitute approximately 5-10 % of all types of ischemic strokes and have a mortality rate of 50% to 80%. The prevalence of malignant supratentorial infarction with space-occupying edema is 1-10% of patients with territory of Middle Cerebral Artery (MCA) infarction. (Hacke et al, 1996) There is no clear evidence which patients with MCA ischemic stroke develop malignant infarction. Oppenhiem et al demonstrated that the infarction volume 145 cm3 and more on diffusion weighed images on magnetic resonance (DWI MRI) and the clinical status of more than 20 points in the National Institute of Health Stroke Scale (NIHSS) are strong predictors of malignant supratentorial infraction development. (Oppenhiem et al 2000)

The clinical picture of cerebral infarction in the territory of the middle cerebral artery is preliminary shown by a severe neurological deficit (severe hemiparesis or hemiplegia, gaze palsy, aphasia and or dysarthria). In the period of the next 2 to maximum of 5 days from the stoke onset, approximately 10% of patients develop brain edema. Mass effect subsequently leads to transtentorial uncal herniation and coning. In the clinical picture there occurs consciousness deterioration in the first place which is not typical for uncomplicated brain ischemia of MCA. In the another progression of the uncal herniation there develops unilateral (ipsilateral) hemiparesis (in the clinical picture there already dominates quadriparesis) with the ipsilateral and later also bilateral mydriasis. Another intracranial pressure increase leads to apnoe and cardiac arrest. Despite the best medical treatments such as hyperventilation, osmotherapy, barbiturate coma, and induced hypothermia, mortality is estimated to be between 50% and 78%. (Gupta et al, 2004)

There have been many studies published up until the year 2004 giving evidence of the benefit of decompressive hemicraniectomy in the reduction in mortality. Gupta et al analysed 15 studies with the total number of 129 patients who fulfilled the criteria for entering the analysis. In his analysis he proved the reduction in mortality of 25-30% in operated patients (Table 2). (Gupta et al, 2004)

Craniectomy reduced mortality in patients with malignant MCA stroke, but it was not still clear which patients may avoid severe disability after the procedure. These studies were not randomized and with retrospective design in most of them and therefore Cochrane´s review from 2002 concluded there was no evidence to recommend DC to treat intracranial hypertension following ischemic stroke. (Morley NC, 2002). Many other studies doubted the effect of decompression mainly in patients at their old age and with their left hemisphere affected. The predictors of the favourable outcome were not set and therefore it was not clear which patients should be candidates for decompressive surgery. These controversies and never ending discussion among stroke experts led to the start of three randomized studies in the end.

The clinical effect of decompressive surgery on functional outcome has been studied in three European studies; DECIMAL trial (Decompressive Craniectomy in Malignant Middle Cerebral Artery Infarcts), in DESTINY trial (Decompressive Surgery for the Treatment of Malignant Infarction of the Middle Cerebral Artery) and in HAMLET (Hemicranietomy after Middle Cerebral Infarction with Life-threatening Edema Trial). Besides above mentioned trials two other randomized studies were done in past decade (Table 3).

| Author | Right MCA, n | Left MCA, n | Mean Age, y | Patients With Early Surgery, n (%) | Patients With Brainstem Signs, n (%) | Mean Time to Follow-Up, mo | Patients With Good Outcome, n (%) | Patients Died, n (%) |
|---|---|---|---|---|---|---|---|---|
| Carter et al | 14 | 0 | 49 | 5(36) | 14(100) | 12 | 8(57) | 3(21) |
| Walz et al | 10 | 8 | 50 | 9(50) | NA | 14 | 6(33) | 6(33) |
| Leonhardt et al | 26 | 0 | 50 | 11(42) | NA | 12 | 11(42) | 6(23) |
| Holtkamp et al | 9 | 3 | 65 | 4(33) | 0(0) | 7 | 1(8) | 4(33) |
| Delashaw et al | 9 | 0 | 57 | 3(33) | 7(78) | 15 | 4(44) | 1(11) |
| Rieke et al | 26 | 6 | 49 | 8(25) | 24(75) | 13 | 16(50) | 11(34) |
| Koh et al | 4 | 3 | 45 | NA | NA | 7 | 2(29) | 1(14) |
| Rengachary et al | 3 | 0 | 31 | 0 | 3(100) | 21 | 1(33) | 0(0) |
| Kalia and Yonas | 2 | 2 | 34 | 1(25) | 2(50) | 17 | 3(75) | 0(0) |
| Young et al | 1 | 0 | 59 | 0(0) | 1(100) | 9 | 0(0) | 0(0) |
| Ivamoto et al | 1 | 0 | 49 | 0 | 1(100) | 7 | 1(100) | 0(0) |
| Kondziolka et al | 3 | 1 | 42 | 2(50) | 4(100) | 20 | 4(100) | 0(0) |
| Gupta et al | 5 | 4 | 53 | 2(22) | 6(66) | 8 | 1(11) | 1(13) |

Table 2. Summary of Case series of the Decompressive Craniectomy (Gupta analysis, 2004)

DECIMAL and DESTINY were stopped in 2006 because of the benefit of the surgery on mortality, but primary clinical end point (benefit for the patient with mRS less or equal to 3) failed. (Jüttler et DESTINY Study Group, 2007; Vahedi et Decimal investigators, 2007) HAMLET study was finished in 2009 with the conclusion that there is no evidence that this operation improves the functional outcome when it is delayed for up to 96 hours after the stroke onset. (Hofmeijer et Hamlet investigators, 2009 )

In 2007 the results from the three European randomised controlled trials (DECIMAL, DESTINY, HAMLET) were pooled to obtain sufficient data to reliably estimate the effects of decompressive surgery not only on the reduction in mortality but also in order to increase the number of patients with a favourable outcome. As the favourable outcome was chosen mRS equal or less than 4 in spite the fact that in the most studies score mRankin <= 3 is accepted. Distribution of the modified Rankin score after 12 months between the group treated with and without decompressive surgery is shown in Table 4 .(Vahedi et al,2007) The favourable outcome defined in mRankin scale 0-4 has given rise to discussion again among neurologists and neurosurgeons. Many clinicians do not consider the state of the patient rated in mRankin scale 4 as a favourable outcome. But decompressive hemicraniectomy based on the above studies was recommended in strictly selected patients in the European Stroke Organization guidelines 2008. (European Stroke Organization (ESO), 2009)

| Authors | n | Design | Conclusions |
|---|---|---|---|
| Pooled analysis | 93 | Multicentre International RCT. 51 patiens | ´Good outcome´ defined as MRS ≤4 10/42 (24%) |
| DECIMAL, | | randomized to surgery along standard protocol/ | MRS < 4 at 1 year in medical group, 22/51 (43%) |
| DESTINY and | | technique,42 managed medically(Mean age | in surgical group |
| HAMLET | | 45.1)Main Inclusion criteria:age 18-60,>50% | Most patients randomized < 24 hours, Subgroup |
| (2007) | | MCA infarct on CT,<45 hours symptom onset. | analysis not possible due to insufficient numbers. |
| | | Exclusion criteria: Haemorrhage,MRS ≥ 2, | Largerst RCT to date |
| | | expectancy < 3 years | |
| HeadDDfirst | 26 | Multicentre RCT.Inclusion: MCA infarct with | Stopped early due to very large difference in in 21 day |
| | | clinical or radiological deterioration after 96 hours | mortality favouring surgical group. Publication |
| | | of onset.Age < 75 | pending |
| Mori et al. | 71 | retrospective analysis of massive hemispheric | 6/12 Mortality in medical group 71.4% |
| (2004) | | infarcts(volume > 200 cm3).Divided into 3 | Late DC 27.6 % at 6/12 |
| | | groups-21/71 medical management alone.50/71 | Early DC 19.1 % at 6/12 |
| | | underwent DC+Duroplasty subdivided into 21 | 6/12 outcome in suvivors revelead statistically |
| | | ´early´ DC and 29´late´ DC after clinical/ | significant improved GOS in early DC vs |
| | | radiological herniation | conservative. Little difference between late DC vs conservative. |

Table 3. Randomized controlled trials on DC for malignant MCA infarction (Kakar et al, 2009)

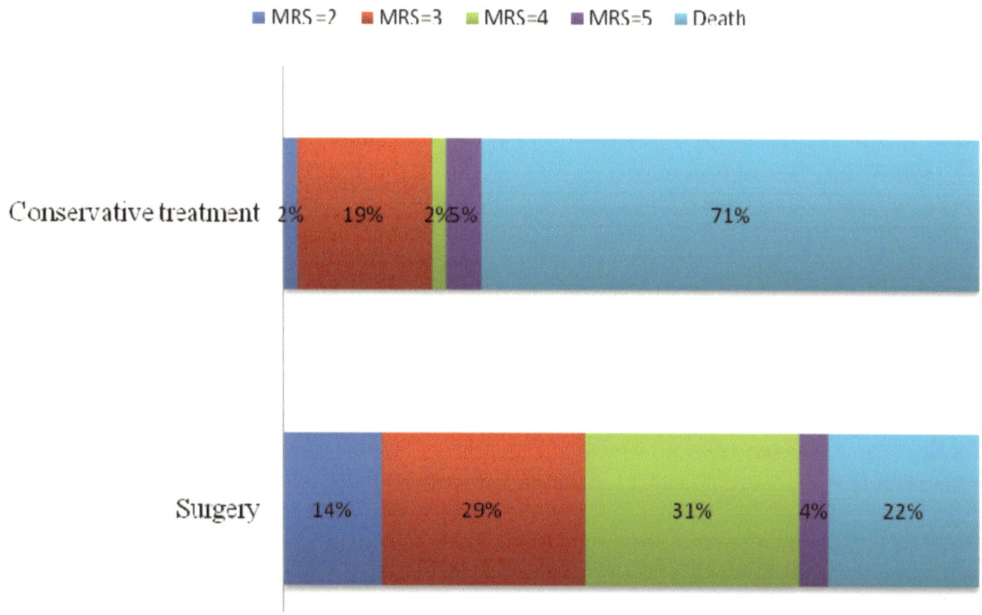


Table 4. Pooled analysis of DECIMAL, DESTINY, HAMLET, Distribution of the modified Rankin score after 12 months among the group treated with and without the decompressive surgery, (Vahedi et al,2007)

4.1.1.2 Patients selection

On the basis of the above mentioned pooled analysis, eligible criteria have been determined for carrying out the decompressive craniectomy(Table No 5).(Vahedi et al,2007; European Stroke Organization (ESO), 2009)

| Inclusion criteria | Main Exclusion criteria |
|---|---|
| age range 18-60 years | prestroke score on the MRS > =2 |
| ischemic infarction in the territory of the | coma with two dilated pupils |
| MCA with a score on the National Institutes of Health stroke scale (NIHSS) >15 | other serious illness |
| less than 45 hours from the symptoms onset to surgery | contralateral ischemia or other brain lession |
| decrease in the level of consciousness to a score 1 or greater on item 1a of the NIHSS | |
| CT evidence of at least 50% infraction in the MCA territory,or infarct (volume > 145 cm3 on diffusion-weighed MRI) | |

Table 5. Inclusion and Exclusion criteria of DC for MCA stroke

4.1.1.3 Timinig of procedures

One of the most important factors which decide about a good result in operated patients with malignant MCA infarction is the right timing of the operation. The timing is closely related to monitoring the intracranial pressure (ICP) increase, cerebral perfusion pressure (CPP) dynamics, also to radiologic monitoring of the development of the malignant edema as well as monitoring the clinical state of the patient. ICP and CPP measuring requires invasive approach. Nowadays there is guideline for ICP monitoring only for Traumatic Brain Injury management. (Adelson et al, 2003)

We use repeated CT examinations for monitoring progression of brain edema and midline shift. Besides noninvasive monitoring of the midline shift it is also possible to use noninvasive transcranial duplex colour coded sonography (TCCS) examination. Gerriets et al demonstrated that TCCS monitoring of midline shift is a useful tool in management of critically ill patients who cannot undergo repeated CT scans. (Gerriets et al, 2001) It must be pointed out that there are no exact radiologic indicative criteria for performing the DC.

Mori et al proved that the benefit of the operation is bigger even before the herniation of the brain tissue. In his study he divided patients with ischemia bigger than 200cm3 into 3 groups, he treated the first group conservatively, the second group was treated before the herniation of the brain tissue, and in the third group he carried out decompressive craniotomy but after herniation. In his work he proved a statistically significant benefit assessed after 6 months from the stroke in the Glasgow outcome scale (GCO) and also in the Barthels scale for the benefit of the patients who underwent the timely operation. (Mori et al, 2004) On the other hand, there are other studies which do not confirm the effect of timely " preventive " operations and these studies encourage clinicians to be more conservative and to wait for the time of developing the mass effect and midline shift. (Uhl et al, 2004; Rabinstein et al, 2006)

Bar et al demonstrated in his studies that the size of ischemia does not have any influence on the favourable outcome (mRankine 0-4) assessed 3 months after the operation. He also did not identify the timing as an important variable affecting the outcome but in his work only a few patients were indicated early and this masked the benefit of early versus late surgery. (Bar et al, 2011). In the pooled analysis (DECIMAL, DESTINY HAMLET) no difference was found between patients treated on the first and the second day. (Vahedi et al 2007) Hamlet demonstrates no benefit of late surgery between 48-96 hours from the stroke onset between groups of patients who were operated on and those who were not operated on. (Hofmeijer et al ,2009)

In conclusion on basis of the literature we believe that probably early decompressive surgery (that means before herniation and poor clinical status) is more beneficial than late timing. In our opinion "preventive surgery "up to 24 hours from the operation in patients with the whole middle cerebral artery territory stroke means prevention from irreversible demage of the brain tissue.

4.1.1.4 Utilization of decompressive surgery for malignant MCA infarction

The number of patients with malignant MCA ischemia who fulfilled the new indicative criteria for DC is not clear. Even the number of all patients who are indicated for DC is not clear. Hacke et al study, 1993, which is cited by the majority of authors, implies that the prevalence of patients with malignant ischemia is approximately 10% of all the patients who suffered the cerebral MCA ischemia. Unfortunately there is no known data of how many patients with malignant ischemic stroke undergo decompressive surgery generally. (Bar et al, 2011)

Bar et al analysed the retrospective occurrence of a malignant edema in all the patients with MCA ischemic stroke who were admitted in 2009 into the Comprehensive stroke centre in Ostrava, the Czech Republic. They identified that 22 (10%) out of 217 patients admitted for acute ischemic stroke in the anterior circulation had a malignant supratentorial infarction and five patients (2.3%) met the indication criteria for decompressive surgery. Seventeen patients did not meet the criteria because they were aged >60 years in all cases.(Bar et al 2011)

In spite of the clear guidelines from 2008, the utilization of decompressive surgery for stroke patients with malignant ischemia did not increase essentially. In the Czech republic the number of procedures increased from 39 in 2006 to 56 in 2009. We estimate that only about 10% of the patients who met the criteria underwent the surgery. (Bar et al 2011)

In the United States the rate of hemicranietomies increasing by 21% per year but the operation was done only in 426 patients during the period between 2005-2009. That means in fact only 0.072 % of the patients with an acute MCA ischemic stroke who were registered in the Premier database. (Adeyoe et al 2010) There are several factors explaining the poor utilization of decompressive surgery:

- the guideline are relatively new and they have not yet entered the consciousness of neuorologists and neurosurgeons.
- clinicians have not yet associated with the idea that the outcome mRankin=4 is favourable and therefore do not indicate the patients for surgery .
- doctors do not believe that patient with ischemia size 50% MCA territory on a CT or 145cm3 without any signs of an edema or without a mass effect and midline shift should be indicated for an operation. They do not believe that "preventive" surgery is useful for patient.

In conclusion it is necessary to state that in the period of the past 5 years there has been a rise in the number of patients who underwent the operation, unfortunately this number is insufficient not only for the prevalence of the malignant ischemia occurrence but also for the number of patients who fulfil the guidelines criteria for DC as well.

#### 4.1.2 Decompressive craniectomy for space occupying cerebellar ischemic infarction

Suboccipital Decompressive craniectomy with or without resection of necrotic cerebellar tissue is generally accepted among clinicians as an effective and lifesaving treatment strategy for cerebellar infarction. In spite of the lack of evidence based medicine this procedure is accepted more than craniectomy in malignant supratentorial infarction. ( Merenda & DeGeorgia 2010; Mathew et al ,1995; Racoet al, 2003) Doctors fear a rapid expansion of the cereberall forman magnum or cerebellar tentorial herniation which leads to the compression of the brainstem followed by death. Deterioration of consciousness and sixth nerve palsy are the first signs of brainstem compression. Mortality in this case has been estimated as high as 80% (Kakar et al, 2009; Ganapathy et al, 2003;Chen et al, 1992) Progressive deterioration of consciousness , decerebral fits and CT demonstration of mass effects strongly support performing decompressive surgery (with or without ventriculostomy for treatment of hypdrocephalus). The presence of the brainstem infarction has been associated with a poor outcome and the brainstem infarction has been analysed as the only independent predictive factor which has been associated with the poor clinical outcome. (Merenda & DeGeorgia 2010; Pfefferkorn et al, 2009; Chen et al, 1992) The other predictors, such as age, bilateral cerebellar infarction, and the time to surgery have not been significantly related to the poor outcome. (Pfefferkorn et al, 2009) Ventriculostomy and decompressive surgery are considered treatment of choice for space-occupying cerebellar infarctions (Class III, Level C).(European Stroke Organization (ESO),2009) But there are no randomized clinical trials which would prove this recommendation. (Adams et al, 2007) Currently we found no level I or II evidence to support of surgical treatment of space occupying cerebellar infarction. Therefore there is no optimal surgery strategy which would help choose patients with the highest benefit of the operation. The prognosis among survivors can be very good, even in patients who are comatose before the surgery. There is uncertainty of the prognostic value of age and preoperative Glasgow Coma Scale and large prospective case series is warranted.

### 4.1.3 Decompressive surgery for subarachnoid hemorrhage (SAH) and spontaneus intracerebral hemorhage (ICH)

Decompressive Craniectomy for SAH with elevated ICP remains controversial. We can notice that the intracranial pressure could escalate in both groups of patients with intracerebral haematoma; with the mass effect and also in patients with only subarachnoid hemorrhage where intracranial hypertension develops on the basis of the generalised brain swelling. In case of the delayed ischemic deficit, intracranial hypertension can occur between 5th and 15th day from the SAH onset. A number of recent studies have explored the role of craniectomy in the setting of aneurysmal subarachnoid hemorrhage associated with the large intracerebral hemorrhage (Schimer et al, 2008; Smith et al, 2002; Güresir et al, 2009). The patients indication, and the timing of the operation were discussed in past two decades. Schirmer et al showed that even in case of SAH without a large intracranial hematoma, DC led to a significant reduction in mortality. He reached a better outcome in an early DC (up to 48 hours) than in patients who undertook the decompression later. (Schimer et al, 2007) Nevertheless other authors have not confirmed these results and have not found any significant difference in the final outcome between the groups of patients with the elevated intracranial pressure who undertook the decompression and who were treated conservatively. (Buschmann et al, 2007; D'Ambrosio et al, 2005) There are no data nowadays for any kind of guidelines for performing DC in this indication. In our opinion DC for SAH with or without intracerebral hematoma should be considered only as an option of the treatment of the elevated intracranial pressure in a patient after SAH with or without intracerebral hematoma.

According to the only one randomized large study of the surgical treatment of ICH only in patients with lobar hemorrhage within 1 cm of the surface standard craniotomy may be considered(Class IIb). ( Steiner et al 2006) Decompressive craniectomy together with the ICH evacuation is supposed to be a life- saving procedure due to the decreasing ICP level. Some studies suggest that decompressive craniectomy and ICH evacuation might improve mortality in selected groups of patients. (Ma et al, 2010; Green et al 2010) Larger, randomized studies are needed to verify this recommendation.

#### 4.1.4 Decompressive craniectomy for traumatic brain Injury (TBI)

It is recognized and widely accepted, that uncontrolled intracranial hypertension is associated with worse ourcome after traumatic brain injury. There are several deterious mechanisms starting immediately after traumatic impact resulting in secondary brain injury. These mechanisms may cause disruption of cellular haemostasis that leads to vicious circle elevated ICP - cell death - more oedema - worse perfusion - further elevation of ICP. Decompressive craniectomy is believed to interrupt this circle by decreasing ICP, but it has to be done early a appropriately sized. Despite wide and frequent use, to date there is no class I evidence showing improved outcome following decompressive craniectomy after TBI. In past 15 years 4 publications of class II and 23 of class III with positive conclusions were published. (Kakar et al, 2009) The most promising study on this topic to be under way is the RESCUEicp comparing the efficacy of DC versus optimal medical management for refractory intracranial hypertension following TBI. (Hutchinson et RESCUEicp investigators, 2006)

Up to date there are no specific guidelines or protocols stating exactly when or in what circumstances DC is appropriate, but there are some recommendations:

- A Cochrane review (2006) recommended DC may be justified in some children with medically intractable ICP after head injury but concluded there was no evidence to support its routine use in adults. (Sahuquillo & Arikan, 2006)
- European Brain Injury Consortium recommend DC as an option for refractory intracranial hypertension in all ages. (Maas et al,1997)
- The North American Brain Trauma Foundation suggests DC may be the procedure of choice in the appropriate clinical context and also considering the use of DC in the first tier of TBI management. (Bullock et al, 2006)

Most definitions of decompressive craniectomy describe this procedure as an option for managing refractory intracranial hypertension. Attention is focused on ICP, that is measured and therapy is aimed to lower rised intracranial pressure. Animal models confirm that decompressive craniectomy improves cerebral compliance and reduces ICP. (Zweckberger et al 2003)

But there are opinions that intervention in situation of refractory IC hypertension is delayed, and as known from our daily practice, in many cases decompression under these circumstances is predetermined for failure. In other words, we are looking for warning signs, that would induce early effective therapy that would preserve excesive brain swelling and conus formation. Microdialysis as a functional measurment and MRI perfusion/diffusion imaging with prognosis of extent and localization of tissue at risk (penumbra) seem to be very promising and are still waiting for clear definition of their roles.

## 5. Key steps of decompressive craniectomy

Decompressive craniectomy describes the temporary removal of a portion of the skull for the relief of high intracranial pressure. This can be achieved by removal of the fronto-temporal-occipital bone over one or both cranial hemispheres or can involve a bifrontal craniectomy. (Schirmer et al , 2008) Most common unilateral hemicraniectomy is typicaly indicated for unilateral space occupaying lesion. The procedure is started typically with large question mark skin incision and then large craniectomy is performed. Jiang in his work describes standard size of craniectomy 15x12cm to be more effective compared to limited craniectomy (8x6cm) (Jiang et al,2005). The procedure aims to reduce compression of brain structures, especially brain stem by swollen brain. Techniques describing simple bone removal without dural opening are believed not to be sufficient. There is no universally stadardized performance of DC and techniques may vary according to institution traditions. Anyway it is widely accepted, that decompression must be spacious enough to avoid cerebral tissue squeezing against the edges of craniectomy. The size of craniectomy defect seems to be crucial. It is stressed to remove temporal squama to ensure temporal lobe decompression (to avoid uncal herniation). Another point of discussion is dural closeure. Some authors do not close dura at all, some use auto- or allogenous grafts to perform duraplasty to prevent CSF leak and make the preparation for cranioplasty easier. Most recent essential requirements for "standard surgical technique" were described in DC for TBI in ongoing study (RESCUEicp) as follows: (Hutchinson et al, 2006)

- Wide (≥12 cm in diameter) decompressive craniectomy (avoiding brain herniation, a. k. a. fungus cerebri).
- Opening the dura and leaving it open (with an option of duraplasty).
- Avoiding tight bandage or positioning patient head on the craniotomy side, after decompression.

It is also recommended, although not absolutely essential:

- For diffuse brain swelling to use a bifrontal decompressive craniectomy with bilateral U-shaped opening of the dura, based on the superior sagittal sinus and with ligation and division of the sinus and falx anteriorly for maximum decompression of the frontal regions. The frontal sinus, if inadvertently opened during craniectomy, should be cranialized (excision of posterior wall, stripping of mucosa and plugging of osteum with the pericranium and/or free muscle and/or tissue glue).
- For predominantly unilateral swelling with midline shift a–wide (≥12 cm in diameter) "trauma" craniectomy with temporal decompression on the side of the swelling.
- If it is not feasible to keep the existing ICP monitor in place during the operation, to replace the ICP monitor following craniectomy via separate burr hole / bolt, at least 3 cm away from the bony edge of craniectomy.
- Performing cranioplasty within 6 months following decompressive craniectomy.

## 6. Complications

The procedure itself seems to be relatively safe with low reported occurence of acute surgical complications. Morbidity and mortality are associated with late comlications secondary to surgical decompression. Many of these complications arise from normal pathophysiological alterations in cerebral compliance after removal of large piece of skull. Among well recognized complications are progression of haemorrhagic contusion, external cerebral herniation, subdural hygroma, infection, hydrocephalus, syndrome of trephined and epilepsy. Margules et al, 2010)

Yang et al. reported 50% complication rate after decompressiove craniectomy with 25,9% of patients who developed more than one complication. (Yang et al, 2008) There seems to be an association between the severity of the initial injury measured by the Glasgow Comas Scale, and the outcome of decompressive craniectomy. Yang et al in his work found patients with worse GCS score had higher complication rate and worse prognosis.

Herniation of swollen brain through craniectomy defect may significantly worsen patient´s prognosis, as it may lead to laceration of brain tissue and damage to cortical veins. Post-craniectomy brain oedema may be a consequence of hyperperfusion syndrome of decompressed brain. In Yang series brain herniation over bony edges has been reported in 27,8% of patients. This complication is more pronounced when small-sized craniectomy was performed. Techniques minimizing risk of herniation include suffitiently large craniectomy, augmentative duraplasty to limit cephalocele (this technique also limits postoperative hygroma formation) and insertion of "vascular cushions" formed by absorbable sponge adjacent to large draining veins to reduce risk of venostasis.

Nowadays with routine intraoperative antibiotic prophylaxis the risk of infection complications after decompressive craniectomy should not be more than 3-7%.Syndrome of the trephined (also known as sinking skin flap syndrome) appears weeks of months after creniectomy. (Stiver et al, 2009) Symptoms include headache, dizziness, irritability, concentration difficulties, memory problems and mood disturbancies. Sometimes also motor deficit may develop. The mechanism underlying this condition is probably transmission of atmospheric pressure over the brain tissue that impairs cortical brain perfusion. For this reason early cranioplasty is the treatment option.

## 7. Outcome

Early surgery - up to 24- 48 hours, age bellow 60 (and 50 years) and clinical status were identified as predictors of a favourable outcome after decompressive surgery in acute supratentorial stroke. (Vahedi et al, 2007; Bar et al 2011; Gupta et al, 2004) Unfortunately, radiologic criteria (infarction volume threshold and midline shift size) of a good clinical outcome have not yet been defined (Schimer et al, 2008). Only in patients where the ischemia is bigger than 145cm3 according to DWI MR which are made within 14 hours from the start of the stroke, there are potential candidates for malignant ischemia formation (Oppenheim et al, 2000). That means that patients with the MCA or MCA and Internal Carotid Artery (ICA) occlusion where early recanalisation has not been carried out and the brain ischemia in the region of the whole territory of the middle cerebral artery developed are potentially threatened by malignant edema. Patients with midline shift more than 4 mm according to transcranial color-coded sonography at 24 hours from stroke onset reached poor outcome (Gerriets et al, 2001). There is no evidence that patients with the dominance of infarction have a poorer favourable outcome than patients with nondominance supratentorial infarction. The dominance of infarction should not be evaluated as an exclusion criterion for selection of patients to DC. (Merenda & DeGeorgia, 2010)

Bar et al identified that the clinical status in NIHSS was significantly and independently associated with a poor outcome, which was confirmed in many studies. (Bar et all 2010, 2011;Vahedi et al 2007; Gupta et al , 2004) DC performed prior to the clinical signs of herniation is associated with a favourable clinical outcome.(Chen et al 2007, Oppenheim et al,2000) A weakness of the randomized trials is the lack of the data on older patients . These randomized studies were carried out in patients younger than 60 and therefore the DC for malignant supratentorial infarction is recommended only for this age group in the recent guidelines. There is also evidence that DC can be beneficial even in older patients. (Jüttler & Hacke, 2011)

We conclude that the most important positive predictors of favourable outcome after DC in acute supratentorial stroke are age , clinical status in NIHSS ,time to surgery up to 24 (48) hours. For other indications (space occupying cerebellar ischemic infarction, SAH, ICH and traumatic brain injury) the outcome predictors have not been determined yet.

## 8. Expert suggestion

The intracranial hypertension means a very serious complication of various diseases of the central nervous system. The conservative treatment of ICP such as the management of the airway, breathing and circulation (ABCs), osmotherapy, sedation, steroid, hyperventilation, and induced therapeutic hypothermia very often fails and mortality in conservatively treated patients reaches 80%. Decompressive craniectomy is a surgical therapeutic option for the treatment of a massive middle cerebral artery infarction, space occupying cerebellar infarction, lobar intracerebral hemorrhage, severe aneurysmal subarachnoid hemorrhage and traumatic brain injury. The strongest evidence of the effectiveness of the treatment is nowadays available in patients with a malignant suratentoriálním infarction. Decompressive craniectory should be performed within 48 hours from the ischemic stroke occurance in every patient younger than 60 with a severe deficit (NIHSS scale more than 15 points) and at least a minor consciousness deterioration (Class I, Level of evidence A). Decompressive craniectomy in other types of a stroke is still a controversial issue. It is the most accepted by doctors in cases of space-occupying cerebellar stroke where the guidelines for executing the performance of type Class II, level of evidence C are valid. In case of subarachnoid and intracerebral haemorrhages there are no particular guidelines and doctors approach this treatment based on their individual experience and decisions.

In traumatic brain injury decompressive craniectomy is believed to interrupt the vicious circle of secondary brain damage by decreasing ICP, but it has to be done early a appropriately sized. There is no class I evidence showing improved outcome following decompressive craniectomy after TBI to date. The most promising study on this topic to be under way is the RESCUEicp.

## 9. Explicative cases

### Case report 1. Supratentorial malignant ischemic stroke

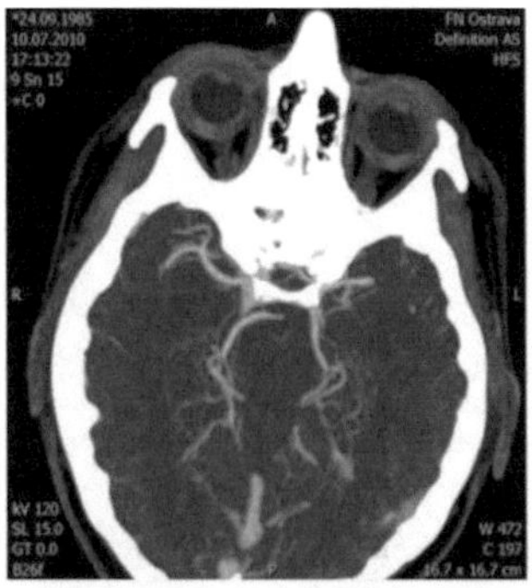

Fig.1

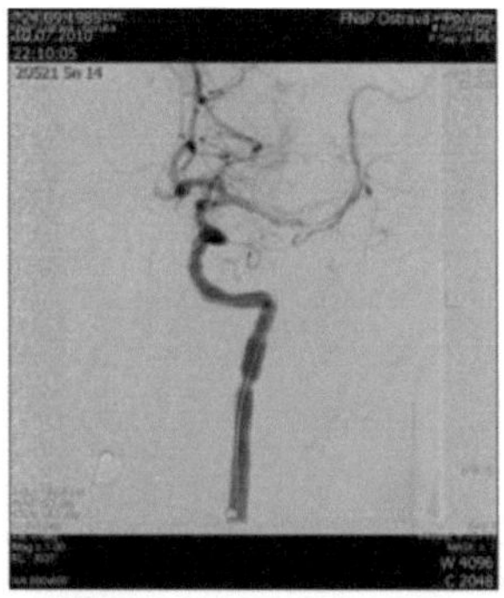

Fig.2

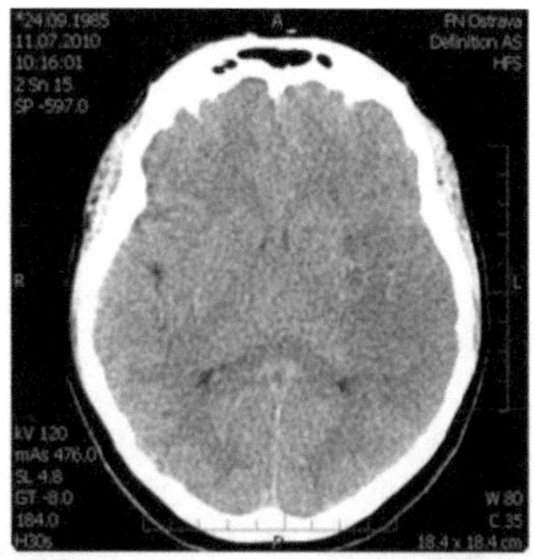

Fig3

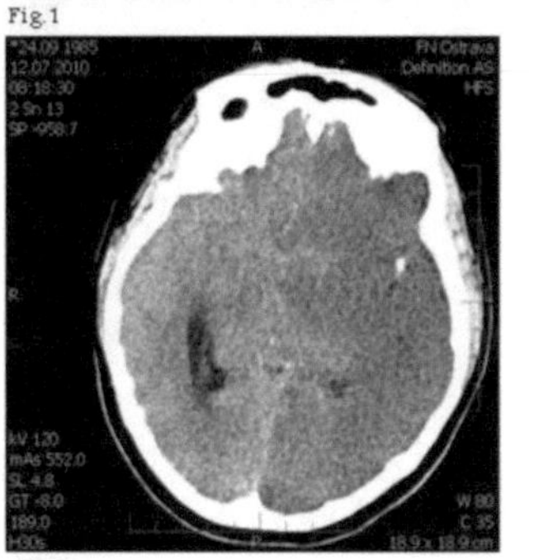

Fig4

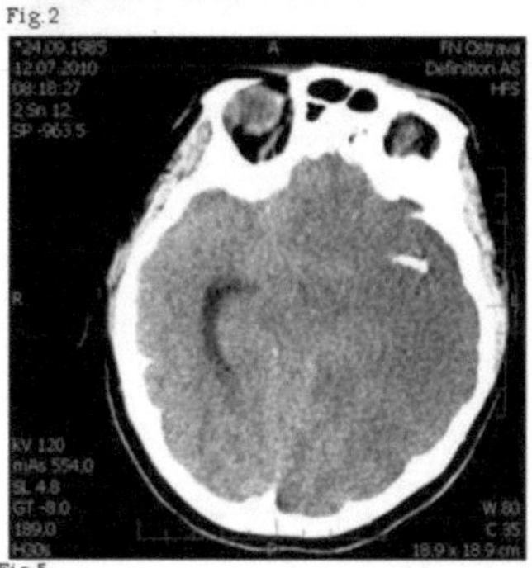

Fig5

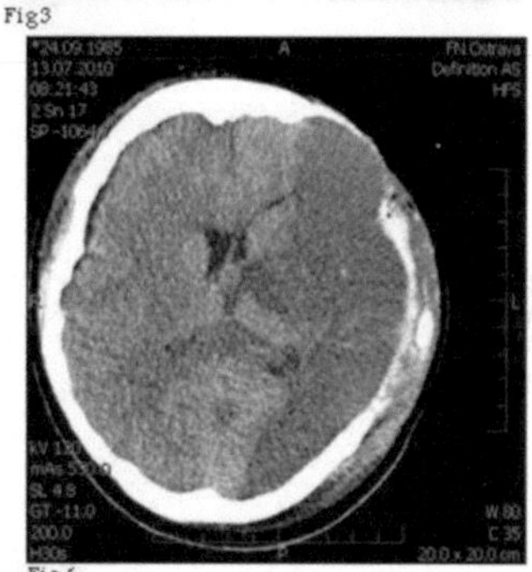

Fig6

Case report: Supratentorial malignant ischemic stroke. Female, 25 years old, was admitted to hospital for severe rightside hemiparesis, gaze palsy and aphasia. CT angiography ACM-M1 segment artery occlusion (fig 1) Mechanical recanalization (Wingspanstent) was done within 5th hours from the stroke onset with only partial recanalization. (Digital subraction on angiography – fig 2) The CT scan 24 hours after the stroke onset shows massive ischemia in MC A territory on the left side (fig 3). The CT scan just before surgery showed space occupying lesion, midline shift and tenitorial herniation (fig 4,5). The patient was operated on in 48 hours after the stroke. Decompressive craniectomy shows fig 6. She final outcome in 12 months time after the stroke is mRankin3, but cortical blindness is present. In our opinion, the patient was indicated to surgery too late and after tentoral herniation

## Case report 2. Space occupying cerebellar infarction

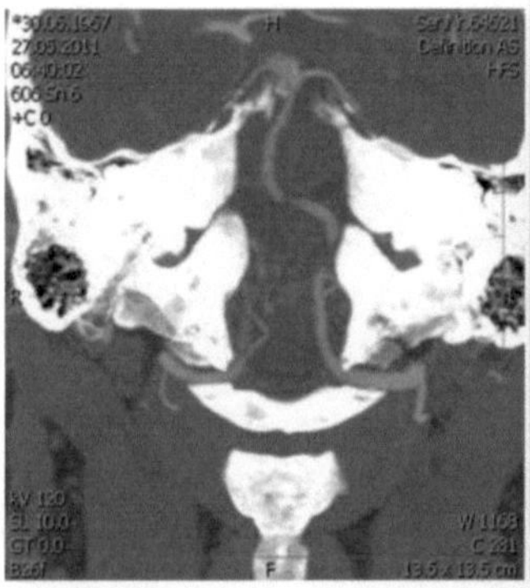

Fig.1

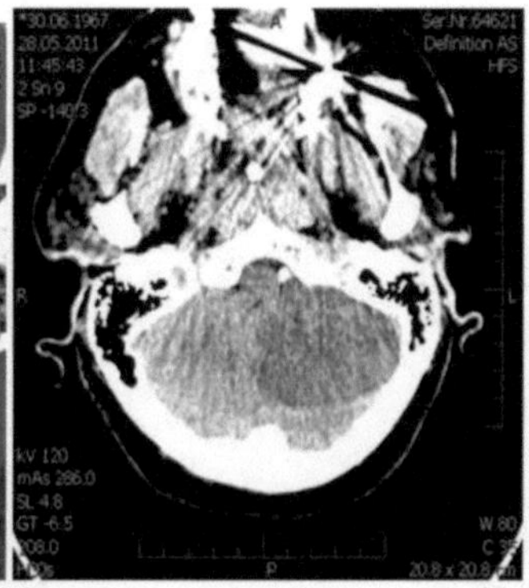

Fig2

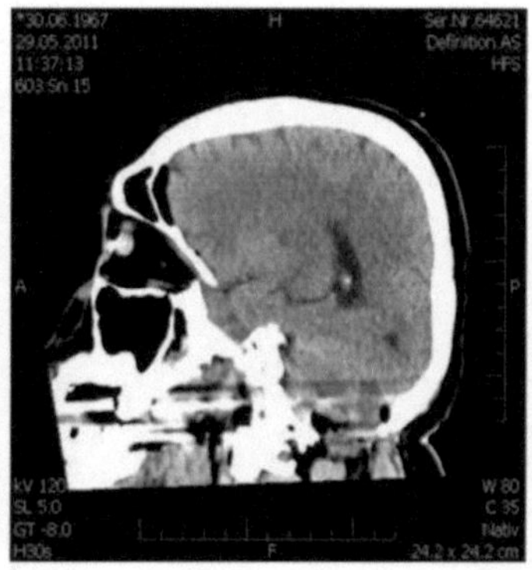

Fig3

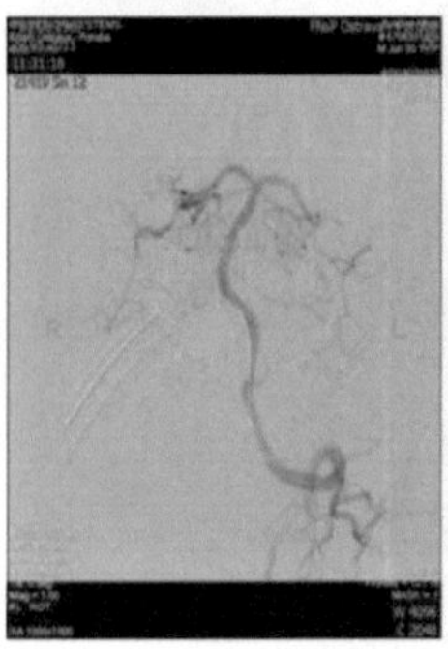

Fig4

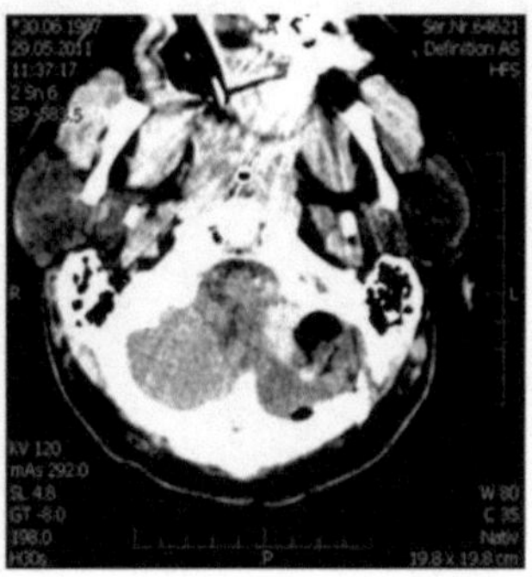

Fig.5

Case report: Space occupying cerebellar infarction. Male, 45 years old, was admitted to hospital for vertigo and desorientation. CT Angiography confirms occlusion of V4 segment of the right vertebral artery and the stenosis of V4 segment of the left vertebral artery (Fig 1). Mechanical recanalisation of the left vertebral artery was done within 5th hour, unfortunately iatrogenic occlusion of the left posterior inferior cerebellar artery (PICA) happened within the procedure (DSA, fig 4). This occlusion was followed by ischemia in PICA territory with the beginning expansion of the left cerebellar hemisphere and partial displacement of the 4th ventriculi (fig 2, 3). Suboccipital decompressive craniectomy with resection of necrotic tissue and duroplasy was done 72 hours after the stroke onsed (fig 5). The outcome in the modified Rankin score is 4 in three months after the stroke.

**Case report 3. Traumatic brain injury**

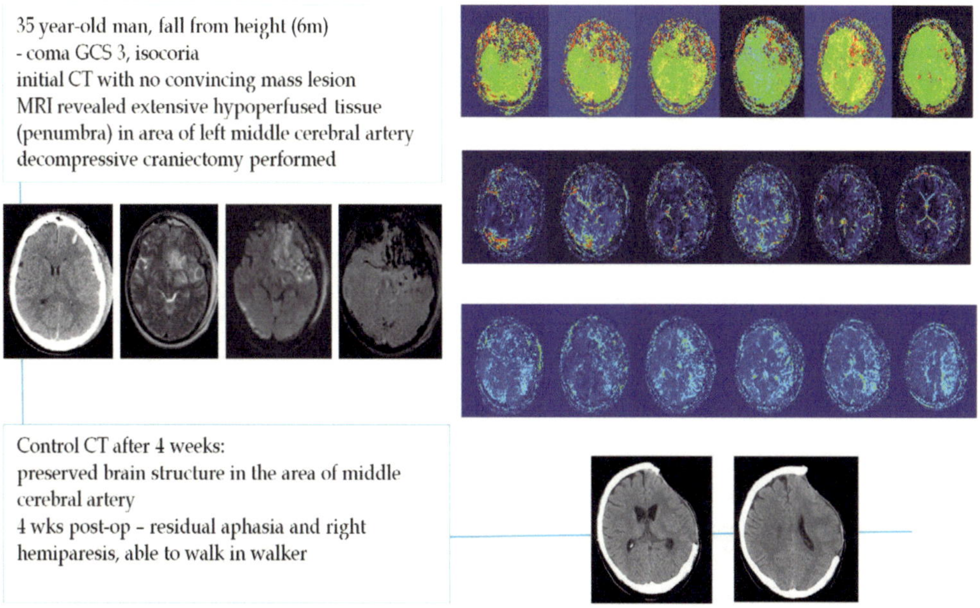


## 10. Conclusion

Decompressive craniectomy is widely used as the treatment of intractable intracranial hypertension in patients after severe traumatic brain injury and ischemic stroke. It is believed that sufficiently large and correctly performed craniectomy may significantly improve patients outcome. In our opinion „preventive decompressive surgery" up to 24 hours from stroke onset means prevention from irreversible damage of the brain tissue and can reduce disablity. But undisputably the most important factor that is still subject of discussion is the timing of such a radical surgical procedure, in order not only to reduce mortality but also to improve the quality of life of the patients.

In traumatic brain injury the timing of decompressive craniectomy seems to be crucial. Early selection of patients that would have benefit from decompression is chalenge for new diagnostic methods (brain tissue microdialysis and MRI perfusion/diffusion imaging).

## 11. References

Adams, H.P. Jr, del Zoppo, G., Alberts M. J. et al. (2007). Guidelines for the early management of adults with ischemic stroke: a guideline from the American Heart Association/American Stroke Association Stroke Council, Clinical Cardiology Council, Cardiovascular Radiology and Intervention Council, and the Atherosclerotic Peripheral Vascular Disease and Quality of Care Outcomes in Research Interdisciplinary Working Groups: The American Academy of Neurology affirms the value of this guideline as an educational tool for neurologists. *Circulation*, Vol. 115, No. 20, (May 2007), pp e478-534, ISSN 0009-7322

Adams, R.D., Victor, & M., Ropper, A.H. *Principles of Neurology*. 6th ed. New York, McGraw-Hill, 1997. Chap. 31. Intracranial neoplasms and paraneoplastic disorders, Figure 31-2 [Mass shifts associated with a parietal lobe tumor], pp 648, ISBN 0-07-067439-6

Adelson, P.D., Bratton, S.L., Carney, N.A. et al. (2003). Guidelines for theacute medical management of severe traumatic brain injury in infants, children, and adolescents: chapter 5. Indications forintracranial pressure monitoring in pediatric patients withsevere traumatic brain injury. *Pediatric Critical Care Medicine*, Vol. 4, 3-Suppl., (Jul 2003), pp S19-24, ISSN 1529-7535

Adeoye, O., Hornung, R., Khatri, P. et al. (2011). The rate of Hemicranietomy for Acute Ischemic Stroke is increasing in USA. *Journal of Stroke and Cerebrovascular Disease*. Vol. 20, No. 3, (May-Jun 2011), pp251-4, ISSN 10523057

Bamford, J., Sandercock, P., Dennis, M. et al. (1990). A prospective study of acute cerebrovascular disease in the community: the Oxfordshire Community Stroke Project--1981-86. 2. Incidence, case fatality rates and overall outcome at one year of cerebral infarction, primary intracerebral and subarachnoid haemorrhage. *Journal of neurology, neurosurgery, and psychiatry*, Vol. 53, No. 1, (Jan 1990), pp16-22 ISSN 0022-3050

Bar, M., Mikulik, R., Skoloudík. D. et al. (2011). Decompressive surgery for malignant supratentorial infarction remains underutilized after guideline publication. *Journal of Neurology*, DOI: 10.1007/s00415-011-6003-3, (Mar 2011 Epub ahead of print), ISSN 0340-5354

Bar, M., Mikulik, R., & Skoloudík, D., et al. (2010). Nationwide study of decompressive surgery for malignant supratentorial infarction in the Czech Republic: utilization and outcome predictors. *Journal of Neurosurgery*, Vol. 113, No. 4, (Oct 2010), pp 897-900, ISSN 0022-3085

Bullock, M.R., Chesnut, R., Ghajar, J., et al. (2006). Surgical management of traumatic parenchymal lesions. *Neurosurgery*, Vol. 58, No. 3 suppl., (Mar 2006), pp S25-46, ISSN 0148-396X

Buschmann, U., Yonekawa, Y., & Fortunati, M. (2007). Decompressive hemicraniectomy in patients with subarachnoid hemorrhage and intractable intracranial hypertension. *Acta neurochirurgica*, Vol. 149, No. 1, ( Jan 2007), pp 59-65, ISSN 0001-6268

D'Ambrosio, A. L., Sughrue, M.E., Yorgason, J.G., et al. (2005). Decompressive hemicraniectomy for poor-grade aneurysmal subarachnoid hemorrhage patients with associated intracerebral hemorrhage: clinical outcome and quality of life assessment. *Neurosurgery*, Vol. 56, No. 1, (2005), pp 12-9, ISSN 0148-396X

Dorfer, C., Frick, A., Knosp, E. et al. (2010). Decompressive hemicraniectomy after aneurysmal subarachnoid hemorrhage. *World Neurosurgery*, Vol. 74, No. 4-5, (Oct-Nov 2010), pp. 465-71, ISSN 1878-8750

Ganapathy, K., Girija, T., Rajaram, R. et al. (2003). Surgical management of massive cerebellar infarction. *Journal of clinical neuroscience*, Vol.10, No. 3, (May 2003), pp 362-4, ISSN 0967-5868

Gerriets, T., Stolz, E., König, S. et al. (2001). Sonographic monitoring of midline shift in space-occupying stroke: an early outcome predictor. *Stroke*, Vol. 32, No. 2, (Feb 2001), pp 442-7, ISSN 0039-2499

Güresir, E., Schuss, P., Vatter, H. et al. (2009). Decompressive craniectomy in subarachnoid hemorrhage. *Neurosurgical Focus*, Vol. 26, No. 6, (Jun 2009), pp E4, ISSN 1092-0684

Gupta, R., Connolly, E.S., Mayer, S. et al. (2004). Hemicraniectomy for massive middle cerebral artery territory infarction: a systematic review. *Stroke*, Vol.35, No. 2, (Feb 2004), pp 539-43, ISSN 0039-2499

Green, T.L., Newcommon, N., & Demchuk, A. (2010). Quality of life and caregiver outcomes following decompressive hemicraniectomy for severe stroke: a narrative literature review. *Canadian journal of neuroscience nursing*, Vol. 32, No. 2, (2010), pp 24-33, ISSN 1913-7176

Guidelines for Management of Ischaemic Stroke and Transient Ischaemic Attack 2008. (2009), In: *The European Stroke Organization (ESO) Executive Committee and the ESO Writing Committee.* (2009. 2011-02-08, Available from: <http://www.eso stroke.org/pdf/ESO%20Guidelines_update_Jan_2009.pdf>

Hacke, W., Schwab, S., Horn. M. et al.(1996). 'Malignant' middle cerebral artery territory infarction: clinical course and prognostic signs. *Archives of neurology*, Vol. 53, No. 4, (Apr 1996), pp 309-15, ISSN 0003-9942

Hofmeijer, J., van der Worp, H. B., & Kappelle, L. J.(2003). Treatment of space-occupying cerebral infarction. *Critical Care Medicine*, Vol. 31, No. 2, (Feb 2003), pp 617-25, ISSN 0090-3493

Hofmeijer, J., Kappelle, L. J., Algra, A. et al. (2009). Surgical decompression for space-occupying cerebral infarction (the Hemicraniectomy After Middle Cerebral Artery infarction with Life-threatening Edema Trial [HAMLET]): a multicentre, open, randomised trial. *Lancet neurology*, Vol. 8, No. 4, (Apr 2009), pp 326-33, ISSN 1474-4422

Huang, A.P., Tu, Y.K., Tsai, Y.H. et al. (2008). Decompressive craniectomy as the primary surgical intervention for hemorrhagic contusion. *Journal of Neurotrauma*, Vol. 25, No. 11, (Nov 2008), pp 1347-54, ISSN 0897-7151

Hutchinson, P.J., Corteen, E., Czosnyka, M. et al. (2006). Decompressive craniectomy in traumatic brain injury: the randomized multicenter RESCUEicp study. *Acta Neurochirurgica*, (2006), No. Suppl. 96, pp 17-20, ISSN 0065-1419

Chen, C.C., Cho, D.Y., & Tsai, S.C. (2007). Outcome and prognostic factors of decompressive hemicraniectomy in malignant middle cerebral artery infarction. *Journal of the Chinese Medical Association*, Vol. 70, No. 2, (Feb 2007), pp 56-60, ISSN 1726-4901

Chen, H.J., Lee, T.C., & Wei, C.P. (1992). Treatment of cerebellar infarction by decompressive suboccipital craniectomy. *Stroke*, Vol. 23, No. 7, (Jul 1992), pp 957-61, ISSN 0039-2499

Jiang, J.Y., Xu, W., & Li, W.P. (2005). Efficacy of standard trauma craniectomy for refractory intracranial hypertension with severe traumatic brain injury: a multicenter, prospective, randomized controlled study. *Journal of Neurotrauma*, Vol. 22, No. 6, (Jun 2005), pp 623-8, ISSN 0897-7151

Jüttler, E., Schellinger, P.D., & Aschoff, A. (2007). Clinical review: Therapy for refractory intracranial hypertension in ischaemic stroke. *Critical Care*, Vol. 11, No. 5, ( 2007), pp 231, ISSN 1364-8536

Jüttler, E., Schwab, S., Schmiedek, P. et al. (2007). Decompressive Surgery for the Treatment of Malignant Infarction of the Middle Cerebral Artery (DESTINY): a randomized, controlled trial. *Stroke*, Vol. 38, No. 9, (Sep 2007), pp 2518-25, ISSN 0039-2499

Jüttler, E., & Hacke, W. (2011). Early decompressive hemicraniectomy in older patients with nondominant hemispheric infarction improves outcome. *Stroke*, Vol. 42, No. 3, (Mar 2011), pp 843-4), ISSN 0039-2499

Kakar, V., Nagaria, J., & Kirkpatrick, P. J. (2009). The current status of decompressive craniectomy. *British Journal of Neurosurgery*, Vol. 23, No. 2, (Apr 2009), pp 147-57, ISSN 0268-8697

Ma, L., Liu, W.G., Sheng, H.S. et al. (2010). Decompressive craniectomy in addition to hematoma evacuation improves mortality of patients with spontaneous basal ganglia hemorrhage. *Journal of stroke and cerebrovascular diseases*, Vol. 19, No. 4, (2010), pp 294-8, ISSN 1052-3057

Margules, A. & Jallo, J. (2010) Complications of Decompressive Craniectomy. *JHN Journal*, Vol. 5, No. 1, (2010), pp.9-12.

Maas, A.I., Dearden, M., Teasdale, G.M., et al. (1997). EBIC-guidelines for management of severe head injury in adults. European Brain Injury Consortium. *Acta neurochirurgica*, Vol. 139, No. 4, (1997), pp 286-94, ISSN 0001-6268

Mathew, P., Teasdale, G., Bannan. A. et al. (1995). Neurosurgical management of cerebellar haematoma and infarct. *Journal of neurology, neurosurgery, and psychiatry*, Vol. 59, No. 3, (Sep 1995), pp 287-92, ISSN 0022-3050

Merenda, A., & DeGeorgia, M. (2010). Craniectomy for acute ischemic stroke: how to apply the data to the bedside. *Current opinion in neurology*, Vol. 23, No. 1, (Feb 2010), pp 53-8, ISSN 1350-7540

Mori, K., Nakao, Y., Yamamoto, T. et al. (2004) Early external decompressive craniectomy with duroplasty improves functional recovery in patients with massive hemispheric embolic infarction: timing and indication of decompressive surgery for malignant cerebral infarction. *Surgical neurology*, Vol. 62, No. 5, (Nov 2004), pp 420-9, discussion 429-30, ISSN 0090-3019

Morley, N.C., Berge, E., Cruz-Flores, S. et al. (2002). Surgical decompression for cerebral oedema in acute ischaemic stroke. *Cochrane database of systematic reviews* (Online), No.3, (2002), pp CD003435, ISSN 1469-493X

Oppenheim, C., Samson, Y., Manaï, R. et al. (2000). Prediction of malignant middle cerebral artery infarction by diffusion-weighted imaging. *Stroke*, Vol. 31, No. 9, (Sep 2000), pp 2175-81, ISSN 0039-2499

Pfefferkorn, T., Eppinger, U., & Linn, J. (2009). Long-term outcome after suboccipital decompressive craniectomy for malignant cerebellar infarction. *Stroke*, Vol. 40, No. 9, (Sep 2009), pp 3045-50, ISSN 0039-2499

Rabinstein, A.A., Mueller-Kronast, N., Maramattom, B.V. et al. ( 2006). Factors predicting prognosis after decompressive hemicraniectomy for hemispheric infarction. *Neurology*, Vol. 67, No. 5, (Sep 2006), pp 891-3, ISSN 0028-3878

Raco, A., Caroli, E., & Isidori, A. (2003). Management of acute cerebellar infarction: one institution's experience. *Neurosurgery*, Vol. 53, No. 5, (Nov 2003), pp 1061-5, ISSN 0148-396X

Sahuquillo, J., & Arikan, F. (2006). Decompressive craniectomy for the treatment of refractory high intracranial pressure in traumatic brain injury. *Cochrane database of systematic reviews* (Online), No. 1 (Jan 2006), pp CD003983, ISSN 1469-493X

Sankhyan, N., Vykunta Raju, K.N., Sharma, S. et al. (2010). Management of raised intracranial pressure. *Indian Journal of Pediatrics*, Vol. 77, No. 12, (Dec 2010), pp 1409-16, ISSN 0019-5456

Scarcella, G. (1956). Encephalomalacia simulating the clinical and radiological aspects of brain tumor; a report of 6 cases. *Journal of neurosurgery*, Vol. 13, No. 4, (Jul 1956), pp 278-92, ISSN 0022-3085

Servadei, F. (2011). Clinical value of decompressive craniectomy. *The New England journal of medicine*, Vol. 364, No.16, (Apr 2011), pp 1558-3, ISSN 0028-4793

Schirmerm, C.M., Ackil, A.A. Jr, & Malek, A.M. (2008). Decompressive Craniectomy. *Neurocritical Care*, Vol. 8, No. 3, (2008), pp 456-70, ISSN 1541-6933

Schirmer, C. M., Hoit, D. A., & Malek, A. M. (2007). Decompressive hemicraniectomy for the treatment of intractable intracranial hypertension after aneurysmal subarachnoid hemorrhage. *Stroke*, Vol. 38, No. 3, (Mar 2007), pp 987-92, ISSN 0039-2499

Smith, E.R., Carter, B.S., Ogilvy C.S. (2002). Proposed use of prophylactic decompressive craniectomy in poor-grade aneurysmal subarachnoid hemorrhage patients presenting with associated large sylvian hematomas. *Neurosurgery*, Vol. 51, No. 1, (Jul 2002), pp 117-24, ISSN 0148-396X

Steiner, T., Kaste, M., Forsting, M. et al. (2006). Recommendations for the management of intracranial haemorrhage - part I: spontaneous intracerebral haemorrhage. The European Stroke Initiative Writing Committee and the Writing Committee for the EUSI Executive Committee. *Cerebrovascular diseases*, Vol. 22, No. 4, (2006), pp 294-316, ISSN 1015-9770

Stiver, S.I. (2009). Complications of decompressive craniectomy for traumatic brain injury. *Neurosurgical Focus*, Vol. 26, no. 6, (Jun 2009), pp E7, ISSN 1092-0684

Uhl, E., Kreth, F.W., Elias, B. et al. (2004). Outcome and prognostic factors of hemicraniectomy for space occupying cerebral infarction. *Journal of neurology, neurosurgery, and psychiatry*, Vol. 75, No. 2, (Feb 2004), pp 270-4. ISSN 0022-3050

Vahedi, K., Hofmeijer, J., Juettler, E. et al. (2007). Early decompressive surgery in malignant infarction of the middle cerebral artery: a pooled analysis of three randomised controlled trials. *Lancet Neurology*, Vol. 6, No. 3, (Mar 2007), pp 215-22, ISSN 1474-4422

Vahedi, K., Vicaut, E., Mateo, J. et al. (2007). Sequential-design, multicenter, randomized, controlled trial of early decompressive craniectomy in malignant middle cerebral artery infarction (DECIMAL Trial). *Stroke*, Vol. 38, No. 9, (Sep 2007), pp 2506-17, ISSN 0039-2499

Zweckberger, K., Stoffel, M., Baethmann, A., et al. (2003). Effect of decompression craniotomy on increase of contusion volume and functional outcome after controlled cortical impact in mice. *Journal of neurotrauma,* Vol. 20, No. 12, (Dec 2003), pp 1307-14, ISSN 0897-7151

# 6

# Suboccipital Concentric Craniotomy as Variant for Posterior Cranial Fossa Surgery

Abraham Ibarra-de la Torre[1], Fernando Rueda-Franco[2] and Alfonso Marhx-Bracho[2]
*[1]Hospital Central Sur de Alta Especialidad, PEMEX and*
*[2]Instituto Nacional de Pediatría*
*Mexico*

## 1. Introduction

In the early development of neurosurgery, a common procedure was the posterior cranial fossa surgery exposition using craniectomy.

The approaches to the posterior fossa were directed largely via the occipital squama; with figure of some authors that proposed suboccipital craniectomy and/or craniotomy. The suboccipital concentric craniotomy it's a variant for posterior cranial fossa surgery which considers the principle of fronto-orbital approach, use the concentric craniotomy technique by Laligam N Sekhar, Fotios N Tzortzidis and Jair L Raso in 1997.

## 2. Alternative procedures

As told, in the early development of neurosurgery, the posterior cranial fossa surgery exposition using craniectomy and/or craniotomy was a common procedure and several authors had described this approach, including combined approaches. Including midline suboccipital craniotomy, superior or inferior, for lesions such tumors of the culmen, pineal tumors, medulloblastoma, cerebelar hemisphere astrocytoma, ependimoma of the IV ventricle, foramen magnum tumors, respectively. The lateral suboccipital craniotomy or paramedian and the lateral suboccipital retrosigmoid approach opening is placed entirely within the squamous portion (immediately inferior to transverse sinus and posteromedial to jugular bulb) out in a retromastoid fashion, the access it offers to the lateral surface of the cerebellar hemisphere is excellent. It is the flap that permits one to work effectively in the pontocerebelllar angle, the jugular foramen, or along the lateral surface of the medulla oblongata and pons. Neurinomas, meningiomas, epidermoids, dermoids, chordomas, chondromas, metastases, and cysts constitute the majority of tumors in this region. These techniques had risk of iatrogenic injury to venous sinuses and causing profuse venous bleeding or air emboli. We recently described the suboccipital concentric craniotomy as a variant for posterior cranial fossa surgery, as a variant that have advantage for minor risk of injuries on the venous sinuses, in midline or lateral suboccipital approaches. This paper is dedicated for the latest technique.

## 3. Indications and contraindications

Injuries of the posterior fossa are varied and different neurosurgical diseases. The indications in this case series were medulloblastoma 5 cases, midline suboccipital craniotomy; pineal germinoma 4 cases, using midline (superior) suboccipital craniotomy; pilocytic atrocytoma in 2 cases, one midline suboccipital craniotomy and the other lateral suboccipital craniotomy; each one case for arteriovenous malformation and aneurysm associated, cerebellar metastases, neurinoma, trigeminal neuralgia. We consider that the suboccipital concentric craniotomy may be used in the different neurosurgical lesions in the posterior fossa, including cerebellar, pineal and the pontocerebellar angle tumors, cerebellar metastasis, vascular lesions and vascular decompression in cranial nerves. This technique has application in children and/or adults. Without contraindications in these cases. Maybe using this craniotomy with combined approach for petroclival meningiomas, supra-infratentorial pre-sigmoid sinus avenue, such previous reports for Al-Mefty et al. and Samii and Ammirati, in 1988 or Miller et al, in 1993.

## 4. Preoperative planning

### 4.1 Imaging

Computed tomography (CT) or magnetic resonance Imaging (MRI) can establish the diagnosis (alone or together) of the posterior fossa lesion.

### 4.2 Preoperative preparation

Most of the patients diagnosed with a posterior fossa lesion can be stabilized by using steroids, this given 8 to 48 hours before tumor resection in hopes of reducing peritumoral edema and lowering ICP administer a histamine blockers as prophylactic are at the clinican's discretion; and cerebrospinal fluid diversion, for treat the hydrocephalus using external ventricular drain (EVD) or shunt insertion; the EVD inserted just before the craniotomy, during the same anesthetic; postoperatively, remove bloody, debris-laden cerebrospinal fluid and avoid the risk of acute postoperative hydrocephalus.

### 4.3 Position

The anesthetized patient is placed in the sitting position (the prone position, the venous oozing obscured the operative field), and the Mayfield three-point fixation device is used to fix the head and the neck slightly flexed forward, for midline approach and a midline linear skin incision (6-7 centimeters in lenght) begins 2-3cm above the level of the external occipital protuberance and extends as far as $C_{2-3}$. Dissection of the underlying soft tissue is completed. For the lateral suboccipital approach the skin incision begins approximately 3 cm above and slightly lateral to the external occipital protuberance and extends linearly down 6-8 cm toward the base of the occiput, but may vary. The transesophageal echography was use only in the cases of pineal tumors.

The position and size of major dural sinus were identified for using neuroimaging (see Fig. 2-J). In the midline superior suboccipital craniotomy, lesions such pineal tumor, we don't open the foramen magnum.

### 4.4 Anatomic landmarks in the posterior cranial fossa

The orientation for any neurosurgical approach begins with consideration of surface anatomic landmarks; the relationships of surface structures to the internal anatomy, and the proper placement of the bony opening (strategic or initial burr-hole). The transverse and sigmoid sinuses are the natural limits of these exposures, the knowledge of the cranial topography constitutes the main factor in the planning of these posterior approaches and reliable landmarks would therefore guide the surgeon in order to reduce the risk of iatrogenic injuries.

The inion and superior nuchal line, the sagittal, lamboid, occipitomastoid, and parietomastoid sutures are recognizable structures on the external cranial surface and their relationships with the transverse and sigmoid sinuses and torcular herophili or superior sagittal sinus; the asterion, the junction of the lamboid, parietomastoid, and occipitomastoid sutures, has been used in posterior fossa surgery to locate the transverse-sigmoid sinus transition complex.

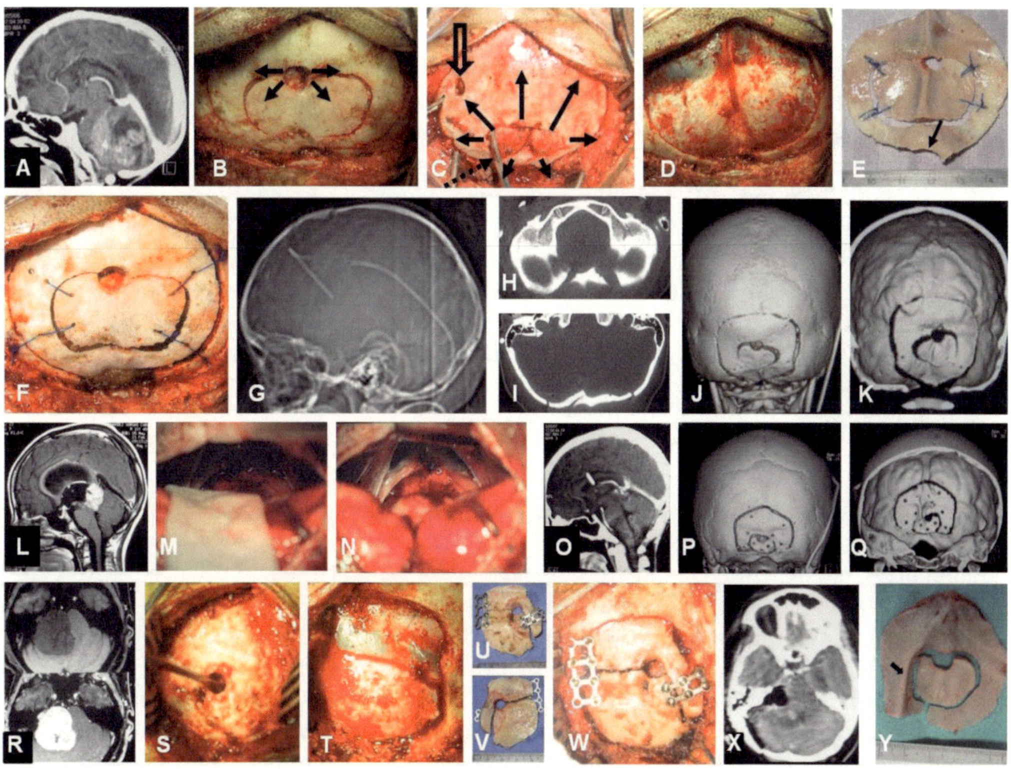


Fig. 1. Surgical technique. Cases 3 (*A,B, D* to *G*), 11 (*C*), 6 (*H* to *K*), 10 (*L* to *Q*), 16 (*R* to *X*) and 4 (*Y*); the patient with a medulloblastoma by cranial computed tomography (CT) (***A***) suboccipital concentric craniotomy, medial approach, initial burr-hole inferior to inion and epidural dissection (*arrows*) for initial craniotomy (***B***), follow with new epidural-venous sinus dissection (*black arrows*), look the venous sinus separating (*open arrow*) with use of dissector through the initial craniotomy (*dotted arrow*) (***C***), and cut the complete craniotomy (***D***) without venous sinus injury; internal cranial view of bone flap with foramen magnum opening (*arrow*) (***E***), fixed the bone flap (***F***), in neuroimaging using CT with reconstruction

suboccipital, (***G***), foramen magnum (***H***), occipital squama (***I***), tridimensional reconstruction (***J,K***). Suboccipital concentric craniotomy, medial approach, the patient with germinal tumor in pineal region, neuroimaging using magnetic resonance imaging (MRI) T1 weighted with gadolinium (***L***), infratentorial-supracerebellar approach with the tentorium *in situ* (***M***) and after retraction gentile (***N***); CT in the post-surgical (***O***) and tridimensional reconstruction without foramen magnum opening (***P,Q***). Suboccipital concentric craniotomy, lateral approach, the patient with right pontocerebellar angle neurinoma in MRI T-1 weighted simple and with gadolinium (***R***), and in the surgical approach the initial burr-hole inferior and medial to the asterion, dissector in the epidural level (***S***) and exposure de venous sinus – transverse sinus (TS) with junction to sigmoid sinus (SS) and right infra- and supratentorial dura mater (***T***), the bone flap with two craniotomies fixed to the cranium (***U-W***), CT post-surgical; and a case with bone "keel-like" projection intracranially, *arrow* (***Y***).

## 5. Key steps of the procedure

### 5.1 Surgical technique

Patient place in prone and/or sitting position, the Mayfield three-point fixation device is used to fix the head. Midline or lateral linear incision and dissection of the underlying soft tissue is completed. The bone flap of concentric craniotomy, using high velocity drill, in midline or lateral suboccipital craniotomy; initial burr hole inferior to inion, 1cm inferior and medial to asterion, for midline and lateral approach, respectively; and epidural dissection of internal occipital through the burr hole, cut a small-initial bone flap, after this, it´s necessary to make an epidural-venous sinuses dissection from internal occipital trying separating it, cut de bone flap for a complete approach requiring with preservation of venous sinuses. Dural open and microsurgical approach is made. Close dural and the two bone flap are fixed; follow with close standard form in the level muscular and skin (Fig. 1).

## 6. Postoperative care

For the first days after posterior fossa craniotomy, we must attend postoperative pain; intravenous morphine is the standard for analgesia in the intensive care unit. Synthetic opioids such as fentanyl are also available. Ketorolac and other nonsteroidal anti-inflammatory agent would avoid these probably for fear of their antiplatelet effects and increased risk of bleeding. Corticosteroids are given in constant doses in the postoperative, primarily dexamethasone (1-10 mg q6h), are frequently used postoperatively in neurosurgical patients. Complications of delayed wound healing, gastric ulceration, and infection should be monitored; as well as histamine blockers (ranitidine 50mg IV q8h, famotidine 20mg IV q12h) or proton pump inhibitor is reasonable in the immediate postoperative period. Patients receiving prolonged steroid therapy could considered for continued ulcer prophylaxis. Antibiotic prophylaxis for neurosurgical conditions has various antibiotic regimens such gentamicin with vancomycin, cefalozin, piperacillin, or oxacillin, first-generation cephalosporin for minor risk of infection.

We can use external ventricular derivation or shunt in which symptoms of hydrocephalus occur.

Risks of operation include wound infection, ventriculitis/meningitis, cerebrospinal fluid leak, cerebellar signs or the posterior fossa syndrome of mutism or death.

Postoperative scans to determine whether residual lesion and suboccipital anatomical reconstruction.

## 7. Complications

Using the suboccipital concentric craniotomy in these cases, we none had injuries and/or tear of venous sinuses, in the posterior cranial fossa surgery.

## 8. Outcome

We reviewed 17 consecutive patients, who underwent surgical resection for posterior cranial fossa lesions at the Departments of Neurosurgery, in the *Hospital Central Sur de Alta Especialidad, PEMEX* and the *InstitutoNacional de Pediatría*, from Mexico City, between March 2005 to February 2008. The charts with the clinical data (age, sex, preoperative symptoms and signs), pre- and postoperative imaging studies, and operative notes (extent of resection, surgical technique) were analyzed.

The seventeen patients who were treated with suboccipital concentric craniotomy and were reported previously, show important data: age from 2 to 64 years old, media 17.23; 9 were male and female 8; 14 children and 3 adults (Table 1).

The diagnosis of the neurosurgical lesions in the posterior fossa were 15 tumors (6 medulloblastomas, 4 pineal tumors, 3 pilocytic astrocytoma, 1 neurinoma, 1 metastasis.), 1 vascular lesion and 1 trigeminal neuralgia.

Additional data: the suboccipital concentric craniotomy shows the surface in the craniotomy measures in children for medial approach was of 37.3 $cm^2$ (range 22.5$cm^2$ to 47.5$cm^2$) and lateral approach 15.5$cm^2$ (range 14.0$cm^2$ to 17.1$cm^2$) and in the adults, for medial approach 32.5$cm^2$ and lateral approach 15.37$cm^2$ (range 10.5$cm^2$ to 20.25$cm^2$).

In these cases, we don´t have complications for neurosurgical procedure.

## 9. Expert suggestions

The suboccipital concentric craniotomies for posterior cranial fossa surgery, in the midline and/or lateral, permit access to several infratentorial lesions and with risk reduced for injuries to venous sinuses and avoid profuse bleeding and/or air embolism; useful the external landmarks for initial burr hole and follow the craniotomy.

Too necessary technical aspect, such in the 4 case, that presented a bone "keel-like" projection intracranially (see Fig. 1,Y). With the principle of suboccipital concentric craniotomy, for preservation of dural and/or venous sinuses, too have applications in other cases for incomplete resection as cerebellar abscess and edema (performed a previously craniectomy), for cerebellar hemangioblastoma and edema and/or for sagittal synostectomy in sagittal craniosynostosis (in a patient with multiple synostosis)(Fig. 2).

## 10. Explicative cases

Case 6. This 6 year old girl was admitted with headache, vomiting, asthenia, with early symptomatic management for gastrointestinal disease without improvement for one month.

| Case | Gender (♂/♀) age (years) | Clinical manifestations | Image | Diagnostics | Suboccipital concentric craniotomy | | | | | | Compli-cations. |
|---|---|---|---|---|---|---|---|---|---|---|---|
| | | | | | *Measure* (cm) | | | | *Surface* ($cm^2$) | | |
| | | | | | Middle | | Lateral | | | | |
| | | | | | Initial | Complete. | Initial | Complete | Initial | Complete | |
| 1 | ♀8 | ICH, CerSx. | CT | Medulloblastoma, HCF. | 3.0x3.5 | 4.5x6.0 | No. | No. | 10.5 | 27.0 | No. |
| 2 | ♀9 | ICH. | CT, MRI | Medulloblastoma, HCF. | 2.5x3.0 | 4.5x5.5 | No. | No | 7.5 | 24.7 | No. |
| 3 | ♂5 | ICH, CerSx. | CT | Medulloblastoma, HCF. | 2.2x3.5 | 5.2x6.2 | No. | No. | 7.7 | 32.2 | No. |
| 4 | ♂15 | ICH, ParinaudSx. | CT, MRI | Pineal germinoma ,HCF | 2.0x2.5 | 5.0x6.0 | No | No | 5.0 | 30.0 | No. |
| 5‡ | ♀9 | ICH, CerSx. | CT, MRI | Medulloblastoma. | No. | No. | 1.2x2.3 | 3.5x4.0 | 4.2 | 14.0 | No. |
| 6 | ♀6 | ICH. | CT, MRI | Medulloblastoma, HCF. | 2.5x3.0 | 6.6x7.2 | No. | No. | 7.5 | 47.5 | No. |
| 7≠ | ♂4 | Cephalea. | CT, MRI | AVM and aneurysm associate. | 2.0x3.2 | 4.6x5.8 | No. | No. | 6.4 | 26.7 | No. |
| 8 | ♂6 | ICH, CerSx. | CT, MRI | Medulloblstoma,HCF. | 1.4x2.0 | 4.9x5.4 | No. | No. | 2.8 | 26.5 | No. |
| 9 | ♂13 | ICH, ParinaudSx. | CT, MRI | Pineal germinoma, HCF | 1.8x2.8 | 4.5x5.0 | No. | No. | 5.0 | 22.5 | No. |
| 10 | ♂10 | ICH, ParinaudSx. | CT, MRI | Pineal germinoma, HCF | 1.7x2.6 | 4.7x5.8 | No. | No. | 4.4 | 27.3 | No. |
| 11 | ♀7 | ICH, CerSx. | CT, MRI | Pilocytic astrocytoma. | 1.9x3.5 | 6.1x7.4 | No. | No. | 6.6 | 45.1 | No. |
| 12 | ♂2 | ICH, CerSx. | CT, MRI | Pilocytic astrocytoma, HCF. | 1.8x3.3 | 5.5x6.5 | No. | No. | 5.9 | 35.7 | No. |
| 13 | ♂10 | ICH, ParinaudSx. | MRI | Pineal germinoma,HCF | 2.0x3.2 | 5.0x5.5 | No. | No. | 6.4 | 27.5 | No. |
| 14 | ♂7 | ICH, CerSx. | MRI | Pilocytic astrocytoma.¶ | No. | No. | 2.0x2.4 | 3.5x4.9 | 4.8 | 17.1 | No. |
| 15 | ♀59 | ICH, CerSx. | CT, MRI | Cerebellar metastasis | 4.0x3.0 | 6.5x5.4 | No. | No- | 12.0 | 32.5 | No. |
| 16 | ♀59 | ICH, CerSx. | CT, MRI | Neurinoma | No. | No. | 3.5x3.0 | 4.5x4.5 | 10.5 | 20.25 | No. |
| 17 | ♀64 | Facial pain. | MRI | Trigeminal neuralgia | No. | No. | 2.5x3.0 | 3.0x3.5 | 7.0 | 10.5 | No. |

CerSx: cerebelar syndrome (gait abnormality, ataxia, incoordination); HCF: hydrocephalus; ICH: Intracraneal hypertension (cephalea, irritability, nausea, vomiting, papilledema); CT: computed tomography; MRI: Magnetic resonante imaging; AVM: arteriovenous malfomation; ‡ lateral resection of craniotomy 3.5x1.0cm;≠ and cerebral diagnostic angiography; ¶ relapse, resection 5 years ago.

Table 1. Present the consecutive cases and results for use the suboccipital concentric craniotomy.

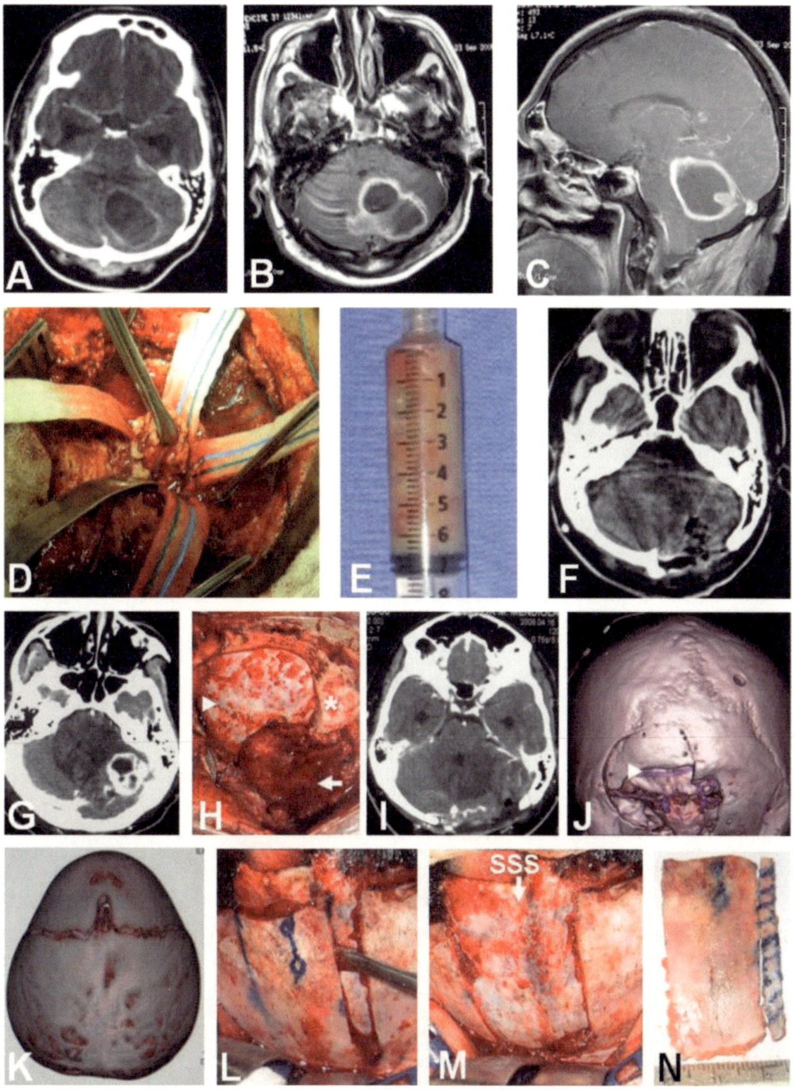


Fig. 2. Other applications with the principle of concentric craniotomy for preservation dural and/or venous sinuses. Such as a case of diabetic patient without take her hypoglycemic treatment, with cerebellar abscess and edema, posterior to drainage for sterotactic approach two weeks early, imaging CT and MRI, annular lesion and mass effect (***A***, ***B***, ***C***), intraoperative capsular resection (***D***), the pus (***E***), CT post/operative (***F***), in this patient performed shunt previously and craniectomy; too another case had before craniectomy and derivation ventricular external for hydrocephalus and hemangioblastoma (***G***), that performed re-operation see the cerebellum with congestion and herniated (*arrow*), preservation dural and transverse sinus (*arrowhead*) in the left side (***H***) total resection of tumor (I), duraplasty, concentric craniotomy and left transverse sinus (*arrow*) by CT tridimensional (***J***); and other patient with craniosynostosis for oxicephaly (***K***), with dissection dural and sagital superior sinus (SSS)with early craniotomy parasagital longitudinal (***L***), preservation of SSS (***M***) and sagittal synostectomy (N). *Inion.

Neurological examination revealed papilledema, horizontal nystagmus towards the left, incoordination and left brachial hypotonic (maneuver`s Stewart-Holmes positive). Imaging, in the CT and MRI with obstructive hydrocephalus and tumor in the posterior fossa in the medline probably rising on the cerebellar vermis and quadrigeminal cistern extensions. First was we installed a shunt, with improvement. The operation performed with the patient in the sitting position, midline incision and suboccipital "concentric" craniotomy, without dural tear and/or venous sinuses injuries, following tumor resection (see Fig. 1, *H* to *K*). Postoperative course, the patient with improvement and had anatomical suboccipital reconstruction.

Case 17.A 52 year old female with headache, staggering gait with vertigo for one month and lowering of the hearing. Neurological examination revealed papilledema, incoordination and adiadochokinesia on the right side. Imaging, TC and MRI, showed obstructive hydrocephaly and a vestibular schwannoma in the right cerebellopontine angle. Was need performed a shunt and the operation (see Fig. 1, *R* to *X*), with total resection for lateral suboccipital craniotomy using the "concentric" form, without dural and/or venous sinuses injury exposed. Postoperative course, the patient had right facial paralysis and hypoesthesia V1, V2; with anatomical suboccipital reconstruction.

## 11. Acknowledgments

To David Alejandro Díaz Méndez, M.C., and Gloria Angélica Díaz Méndez, M. D., Doria Díaz Ibarra, by preparing this manuscript.

## 12. References

A proposal for more informative abstracts of clinical articles.Ad Hoc Working Group for Critical Appraisal of the Medical Literature.*Ann Intern Med* 1987; 106:598-604.

Abolghassem S, Ulrich K. Osteoplastic lateral suboccipitalapproach for acoustic neuroma surgery, technical note.*Neurosurgery* 2000;48:229-231.

Al-Mefty O, Fox JL, Smith RR. Petrosal approach for petroclivalmeningiomas. *Neurosurgery* 1988; 22:510-517.

Avci E, Kocaogullar Y, Fossett D, Caputy A. Lateral posteriorfossa venous sinus relationships to surface landmarks. *Surg Neurol* 2003; 59: 392-7.

Bozbuga M, Boran BO, Sahinoglu K. Surface anatomy of theposterolateral cranium regarding the localization of the initialburr-hole for a retrosigmoid approach. *Neurosurg Rev* 2006;29:61-63.

Bucy PC. Exposure of the posterior or cerebellar fossa.*J Neurosurg*1966; 24: 820-832.

Critchley M.: Discussion on the differential diagnosis of lesions of the posterior fossa. *Proc R Soc Med* 1953; 46:719-738.

Dandy WE.The treatment of trigeminal neuralgia by the cerebellar route.*Ann Surg*1932; 96:787-795.

Day JD, Kellogg JX, Tschabitscher M, Fukushima T. Surfaceand superficial surgical anatomy of the posterolateral cranialbase, significance for surgical planning and approach. *Neurosurgery* 1996; 38: 1079-1084.

Day JD, Tschabitscher M. Anatomic position of the asterion. *Neurosurgery* 1998; 42: 198-199.

Gharabaghi A, Rosahi SK, Feigl GC, Liebig T, Mirzayan JM, Heckl S, Tatagiba M, Samii M. Image guided lateral suboccipital approach: part 1individualized landmarks for surgical planning. *Neurosurgery* 2008; 62:S18-S23.

Haynes RB, Murlow CD, Huth EJ, Altman DG, Gardner MJ. More informative abstracts revisited. *Ann Intern Med* 1990; 113:69-76.

Ibarra A, Aguilar R. Craneotomía suboccipital concéntrica como variante en cirugía de fosa posterior: nota técnica. *Arch Neurocien (Mex),* 2009; 14:206-210.

Ibarra A, Marhx A, Rueda F, Mora I. Craneotomía suboccipital concéntrica para cirugía craneal infratentorial: resultados quirúrgicos en una serie de 14 casos. *Arch Neurocien (Mex),* 2009; 14:151-156.

Ibarra A, Marhx A, Rueda F. Suboccipital concentric craniotomy as variant for posterior cranial fossa surgery: outcome in a case series (paper 90). Presented at the 38th Annual Meeting of the International Society for Pediatric Neurosurgery, Jeju, South Korea, October 31 to November 4, 2010. *Childs Nerv Syst* 2010; 26: 1435-1476.

Jannetta PJ. Hemifacial spasm.*In*: Samii M, Jannetta PJ (editors), *The cranial nerves, anatomy, pathology, pathophysiology, diagnosis, and treatment*. Springer-Verlag, Berlin, 1981.

Jannetta PJ. Vascular decompression in trigeminal neuralgia. In: Samii M, Jannetta PJ (editors), *The cranial nerves, anatomy, pathology, pathophysiology, diagnosis, and treatment*. Springer-Verlag, Berlin, 1981.

Kempe LG. *Operative neurosurgery, posterior fossa, spinal cord, and peripheral nerve disease.* Springer-Verlag, New York, 1970.

Lang J Jr, Samii A. Retrosigmoid approach to the posterior cranial fossa, an anatomical study. *Acta Neurochir (Wien)* 1991; 111: 147-153.

Lang J Jr, Samii A. Retrosigmoid approach to the posteriorcranial fossa, an anatomical study. *Acta Neurochir (Wien)* 1991;111:147-153.

Levy ML, Apuzzo ML.: Supracerebellarinfratentorial approaches to the pineal region. *In*: Rengachary SS, Wilkins RH (editors), *Neurosurgical operative atlas.* Vol. 4, Park Ridge, Illinois, American Association of Neurological Surgeons, 1995, pp. 29-36.

Marlin AE, Gaskill SJ.Cerebellar medulloblastoma.*In*:Rengachary SS, Wilkins RH (editors), *Neurosurgical operative atlas.*Vol. 1, Williams and Wilkins, Baltimore, *American Association of Neurological Surgeons* 1991, pp 176-83.

Miller CG, van Loveren HR, Keller JT, Pensak M, El-Kalliny M,Tew JM Jr. Transpetrosal approach: surgical anatomy andtechnique. *Neurosurgery* 1993; 33:461-469.

Ogilvy CS, Ojemann RG. Posterior fossa craniotomy for lesionsof the cerebellopontine angle.*J Neurosurg*1993; 78: 508-9. 19.

Page LK. The infratentorial-supracerebellar exposure of tumors in the pineal area. *Neurosurgery* 1977; 1: 36-40.

Poppen JL. *An atlas of neurosurgical techniques.*WB. Saunders, Philadelphia, 1960.

Raimondi AJ. *Pediatric neurosurgery, theoretical principles artof surgical techniques.* Springer-Verlag, New York. 1987.

Rhoton AL Jr. The posterior cranial fossa, microsurgical anatomy and surgical approaches.*Neurosurgery* 2000; 47:S5-S6.

Ribas GC, Rhoton AL Jr, Cruz OR, Peace D. Suboccipital burrholes and craniectomies. *Neurosurg Focus* 2005; 19: 1-12.

Samadiana M, Nazparvar B, Haddadian K, Rezaei O, Kormaee F. The anatomical relation between the superior sagittal sinus and the sagittal suture with surgical considerations. *Clin Neurol Neurosurg* 2011;113:89-91.

Samii M, Ammirati M. The combined supra-infratentorialpresigmoidsinus avenue to the petro-clival region.Surgicaltechnique and clinical applications. *Acta Neurochir (Wien)* 1988;95:6-12.

Sekhar LN, Tzortzidis F, Raso J. Fronto-orbital approach. *In*: Sekhar LN, De Oliveira E (editors), *Cranial microsurgery,approaches and techniques*, Thieme, New York, 1997: 54-60.

Stein BM. The infratentorialsupracerebellar approach to pineal lesions. *J Neurosurg*1971; 35: 197-202.

Stein BM. The infratentorial-supracerebellar exposure of tumors in the pineal area. *Neurosurgery* 1977; 1: 36-40.(Comment).

Tew JM, van Loveren HR. *Atlas of operative microneurosurgery*.W. B. Saunders Company, Philadelphia, 1994.

Tubbs RS, Loukas M, Shoja MM, Bellew MP, Cohen-Gadol AA. Surface landmarks for junction between the transverse and sigmoid sinuses: application of the "strategic" burr hole for suboccipital craniotomy. *Neurosurgery* 2009; 65:S37-S41.

Tubbs RS, Salter G, Elton S, Grabb PA, Oakes WJ. Sagittal suture as an external landmark for the superior sagittal sinus. *J Neurosurg* 2001; 94:985-987.

Tubbs RS, Salter G, Oakes WJ.Superficial surgical landmarksfor the transverse sinus and torcularherophili. *J Neurosurg* 2000; 93: 279-281.

Yasargil MG, Fox JL. The microsurgical approach to acousticneurinomas.*SurgNeurol*1974; 2: 393-8.

Yasargil MG. *Microneurosurgery*. Georg ThiemeVerlag,Stuttgart, 1984; (1):238-244.

Yasargil MG. *Microneurosurgery*.IVB, Georg ThiemeVerlag,Stuttgart, 1996.

7

# Diagnostic Evaluation of the Lesions of the Sellar and Parasellar Region

Roberto Attanasio[1], Renato Cozzi[2], Giovanni Lasio[3] and Regina Barbò[4]

[1]*Endocrinology, Galeazzi Institute, Milan*
[2]*Endocrinology, Niguarda Hospital, Milan*
[3]*Neurosurgery, Humanitas Institute, Milan*
[4]*Neuroradiology, Gavazzeni-Humanitas, Bergamo*
*Italy*

## 1. Introduction

The sellar and parasellar region is an anatomically complex area that represents a critical junction for important contiguous structures (Ruscalleda, 2005). While the sellar region has specific anatomical landmarks, the parasellar region is not clearly delineated. It includes, laterally, the dural walls of the cavernous sinus (Smith, 2005), and is in close relation with the basisphenoid and sphenoid sinus inferiorly, and superiorly with the suprasellar subarachnoid spaces (Ruscalleda, 2005). The nasopharynx and the temporal lobes are also closely related to the region (Smith, 2005). A wide range of neoplastic, inflammatory, infectious, developmental and vascular diseases may embroil vital structures in this region (Freda & Post, 1999). The most frequently involved are the brain parenchyma, meninges, the optic pathways and cranial oculomotor nerves (III, IV, VI) and the V1 and V2 branches of the trigeminal nerve, major blood vessels, hypothalamo-pituitary system, tuber cinereum, anterior third ventricle and bone compartments.

Data from cancer registries suggest that prevalence of primary central nervous system (CNS) tumors is 130–230 cases per 100,000 of the population (Davis et al., 2001). Lesions of the sellar and parasellar region are very common, accounting for 10–15% of intracranial masses based on surgical experience (Terada et al., 1995), and in 3-24% of unselected autopsies depending on the sections examined (Kovacs et al., 2001).

The malignant potential of these tumors may be defined according to the WHO classification of tumors of the CNS (Louis et al., 2007; Lloyd et al., 2004b):

- WHO grade I, i.e. tumors with low proliferative potential and possibility of cure following surgical resection;
- WHO grade II, i.e. infiltrative tumors with low mitotic activity that can recur and progress to higher grades of malignancy;
- WHO grade III, i.e. tumors with histological evidence of malignancy;
- WHO grade IV, i.e. mitotically active tumors with rapid evolution of disease.

A number of other non-neoplastic lesions, such as inflammatory, granulomatous, infectious and/or vascular pathologies can also involve the parasellar region. The different lesions are listed in table 1, according to an etiologic and anatomic classification, and systematically addressed in the following section. Classifications are created to accommodate a large spectrum of entities, from the typical and frequent to the unusual and exceptional, but they are never comprehensive enough to satisfactorily reflect the diversity of nature and the wide range and variety of human diseases (Kovacs et al., 2001).

Pituitary adenomas account for about 90% of lesions of the sellar and parasellar region according to different large surgical series: Freda & Post (Freda & Post, 1999) collected 1120 cases in 18 years in a single center, the German Registry of pituitary tumors (Saeger et al., 2007) collected 4122 cases in 10 years, Valassi et al. (Valassi et al., 2010) collected 1469 cases in 10 years in a single center. Thus in ~8-15% of cases, an etiology other than a pituitary adenoma is encountered: other tumors in 4.2-5.6%, malformative lesions in 2.9-5.2%, inflammatory lesions in 0.7-1.2% of cases (Freda & Post, 1999; Saeger et al., 2007; Valassi et al., 2010). In these series vascular lesions are of course underrepresented.

A recent radiological series, retrospectively evaluating 2598 MRIs performed over 11 years (Famini et al., 2011), showed that after exclusion of normal pituitaries (47%), non-adenomatous lesions accounted for 18% of observed lesions.

Sellar and parasellar masses occur with overlapping clinical and radiological features, ranging from asymptomatic incidental presentations to hormonal symptoms, or compressive local mass effects on nearby vital surrounding structures. The severity depends on the location, size and growth potential of the tumors (Famini et al., 2011; Glezer et al., 2008).

The most common symptom is represented by visual troubles (from minimal visual field defect to blindness) and headache that may be severely disabling. Several mechanisms have been proposed to explain headaches in patients harboring pituitary masses. Some are not related to the volume of the mass, such as distortion of the sellar diaphragm or irritation of the parasellar dura (Arafah et al., 2000; Levy et al., 2004).

Hypopituitarism and hyperprolactinemia (due to the lack of physiologic dopamine inhibition of PRL secretion) are common, whereas diabetes insipidus (DI) and cranial nerve palsies are atypical for adenomas but common for other lesions of the region (see below).

Hypothalamic localization may produce the diencephalic syndrome in children, manifesting as wasting, poor development and sexual immaturity, whereas disruption of appetite control can occur in adults, causing severe obesity or starvation.

A correct diagnosis of such lesions thus implicates a multidisciplinary approach, requiring detailed endocrine, neuroimaging, and ophthalmological studies. Correct diagnostic orientation is crucial in order to choose the proper treatment for each different case (Kaltsas et al., 2008). Histological confirmation is not necessary in formulating a management plan in most cases. It is indeed redundant (and may be even dangerous) when clinical, endocrine and/or radiological features are clear-cut. But what about the uncommon borderline situations? Samples for histological evaluation can be nowadays collected by mini-invasive image-guided techniques (Frighetto et al., 2003; Samandouras et al., 2005). The procedure should be reserved only to those cases when radiologic features are not clearcut, but risks and benefits of such procedures must be strongly considered.

| | | |
|---|---|---|
| **Tumors deriving from adeno-hypophyseal cells** | Pituitary adenoma<br>Pituitary carcinoma | |
| **Tumors deriving from neuro-hypophyseal cells** | Pituitocytoma<br>Granular cell tumor (choristoma) | |
| **Parasellar tumors** | **Malignant** | Glioma<br>Germ cell tumor<br>Primary lymphoma<br>Pituitary metastases<br>Supratentorial primitive neuroectodermal tumor<br>Ependymoblastoma |
| | **Potentially malignant (low-grade)** | Chordoma<br>Chondrosarcoma<br>Chondroma<br>Langerhans' cell histiocytosis<br>Hemangiopericytoma<br>Solitary fibrous tumors<br>Plasmacytoma |
| | **Usually benign** | Craniopharyngioma<br>Meningioma<br>Paraganglioma<br>Lipoma<br>Neurinoma/Schwannoma<br>Gangliocytoma |
| **Malformative lesions** | Rathke's cleft cyst<br>Epidermoid<br>Dermoid<br>Hamartoma<br>Empty sella<br>Arachnoid cyst | |
| **Granulomatous, infectious and inflammatory lesions** | Hypophysitis<br>Pituitary abscess<br>Pseudotumor<br>Tuberculosis<br>Mycoses<br>Sarcoidosis<br>Wegener's granulomatosis<br>Sphenoidal mucocele | |
| **Vascular lesions** | Aneurysm<br>Carotid-cavernous fistula<br>Cavernous sinus thrombosis | |

Table 1. Classification of sellar and parasellar lesions

## 2. From theory to practice

Patient 1 is a 55 year-old woman, complaining of headache and visual troubles for a few months. She had two pregnancies and is post-menopause since two years. Previous medical history is unremarkable, except for hypertension, treated with ACE-inhibitor since 5 years. Physical examination is negative, except for peripheral visual loss at confrontation.

Patient 2 is a 34 year-old woman, complaining of amenorrhea since 8 months. She had one uneventful pregnancy and lactated 3 years ago. Previous medical history is unremarkable. On physical examination she is slightly overweight.

Patient 3 is an 8 year-old male whose parents perceived growth arrest and worsening of school performance. After his pediatrician's evaluation showing GH deficiency, he performed MRI and was referred to neurosurgeon for a mass in the sellar region. The neurosurgeon requires an endocrine evaluation prior to the planned mass resection.

Patient 4 is a 45 year-old male, referred to the endocrinologist after finding a 7-mm lesion in the pituitary on MRI performed after a road accident.

## 3. Systematic of sellar and parasellar lesions

### 3.1 Lesions deriving from adeno-hypophyseal cells

#### 3.1.1 Pituitary hypertrophy/hyperplasia

First of all, it should be stressed that also physiological conditions can drive enlargement of the pituitary gland. Sex- and age-dependent variations in size and shape of the pituitary have been indeed reported (Chanson et al., 2001). Pituitary height in healthy subjects can be higher than 9 mm in 0.5%, simulating a pituitary lesion, mostly in adolescent girls (figure 1 a, b) but also in menopausal women (Tsunoda et al., 1997). Furthermore, reversible pituitary hyperplasia can be observed during pregnancy (Elster, 1991) as well as in pathological conditions such as long-term severe failure of target organs (hypothyroidism - Hutchins et al., 1990 -, hypoadrenalism – Clayton et al., 1977 -, hypogonadism - Kido et al., 1994) (figure 1 c, d) and CRH or GHRH hypersecretion (Asa et al., 1984; Sano et al. 1988). In such conditions the pituitary gland is homogeneously increased both on plain and contrast-enhanced images.

It is worth considering this diagnosis in the patients undergoing MRI for any reason, particularly in young females.

A biopsy is not necessary to diagnose such lesions. In the event tissue is examined in cases of GHRH or CRH hypersecretion, silver stains (Gomori, Gordon-Sweet, etc.) are needed in order to distinguish hyperplasia from adenoma. These techniques demonstrate the delicate reticulin fiber network, surrounding the acini. This acinar pattern is preserved in hyperplasia and disrupted in adenoma (Kovacs et al., 2001).

#### 3.1.2 Pituitary adenomas

*Classification and epidemiology*

Pituitary adenomas are defined as benign lesions arising in the anterior pituitary. They can be classified according to size (microadenomas and macroadenomas being, respectively, smaller and larger than a conventional 10-mm cut-off), extension (intrasellar and extrasellar, being, respectively, enclosed or not within sellar limits, irrespective of their size), and secretory status. Most adenomas are PRL-secreting, followed by clinically non-functioning (NFPA), GH-secreting, ACTH-secreting, and last by TSH-secreting ones.

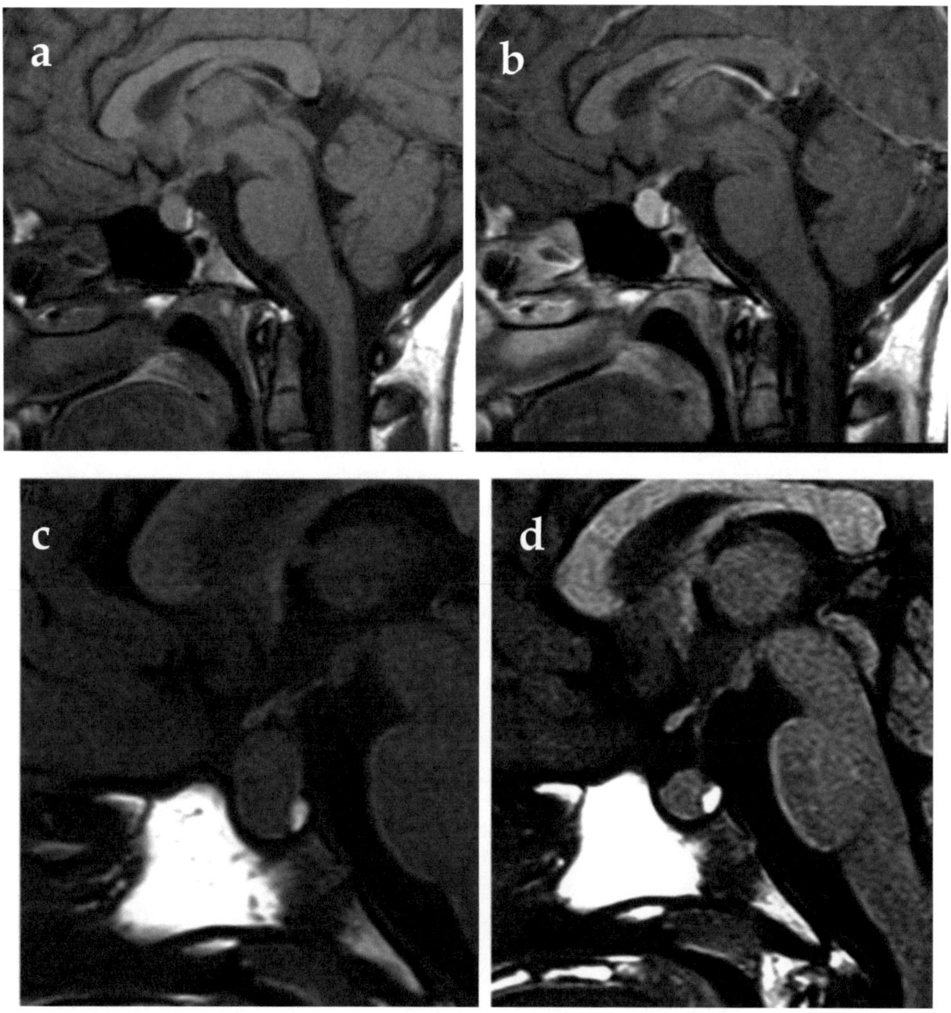


Fig. 1. a and b: adolescent girl (courtesy of P. Doneda, MD). T1 MRI shows diffuse enlargement of the pituitary gland, with convex superior margin and posterior pituitary "bright spot" (a), homogeneously enhancing (b). c and d: 8 yo girl, with primary hypothyroidism. MRI at diagnosis (c) shows enlarged, homogeneously enhancing pituitary gland with suprasellar extension; after replacement treatment with L-thyroxine pituitary size is reduced and normal (d).

Adenomas can be eventually classified as typical or atypical. The atypical adenoma is defined as an invasive tumor with elevated mitotic index, Ki-67 (MIB-1) proliferation index of 3% or more, and an extensive nuclear immuno-staining for p53 (Jaffrain-Rea et al., 2002; Turner & Wass, 1999.). The poorer prognosis of this adenoma is due to a higher degree of invasiveness, larger size, and accelerated growth that reduce the chances of radical removal. It accounts for less than 3% of pituitary tumors in the German Registry (Saeger et al., 2007) and differs from pituitary carcinoma (0.12% of cases in the German Registry) only in the lack of metastases (see below).

As for epidemiology, a pathological systematic review (Ezzat et al., 2004) combined the findings from seven autopsy series: among a total of 3375 autopsied pituitaries, the overall prevalence of adenomas was 14.4% and the most frequent were PRL-staining ones. Thereafter, in a single series of 3048 autopsy (Buurman & Saeger, 2006) a total of 334 adenomas in 316 pituitary glands were reported, only 22.7% being > 3 mm (3 macroadenomas).

The mean radiological prevalence of pituitary adenomas was 22.3%. In a combined analysis including both radiological and pathological data, the prevalence of unsuspected pituitary adenomas was 16.7% (Daly et al., 2009).

From the clinical point of view, it was recently indicated that prevalence of pituitary adenomas is 3–5 times higher than previously believed. In 2006 a cross-sectional study in a definite area of Belgium using an intensive case-finding approach involving all the general practitioners and relevant specialists, reported a mean prevalence of 94 cases per 100,000 (Daly et al., 2006). Once again the most frequent tumors were prolactinomas, accounting for 2/3 of cases. An international, multicenter study in Europe, South America and other sites with a total population of 862,000 found similar results (Daly et al., 2009).

*Clinics*

Macroadenomas can cause a common clinical picture, due to mass effect of expanding tumor impinging on neighbor structures: visual defects (from minimal visual field defect to typical hemianopsia to amaurosys), headache, and hypopituitarism. Giant adenomas can give rise to cavernous sinus syndrome with oculomotor nerve palsies or seizures (when expanding through cavernous sinus to temporal lobe), or DI. These latter manifestations are so rare that must prompt an accurate differential diagnosis with non-adenomatous lesions of the region.

Each secretory adenoma causes a typical hypersecretory syndrome:

- PRL-secreting adenomas produce amenorrhea and galactorrhea in women, loss of libido and hypogonadism in men, and secondary osteoporosis in both sexes (Colao, 2009);
- GH-secreting adenomas cause acromegaly (or giantism before puberty)(Melmed, 2006);
- ACTH-secreting adenomas are the main cause of Cushing's disease (Bertagna et al., 2009);
- TSH-secreting adenomas cause central hyperthyroidism (Beck-Peccoz et al., 2009).

All these entities, mostly Cushing's disease and acromegaly, are associated to increased morbidity and mortality, when untreated.

Although commonly defined as benign tumors, invasion of surrounding tissues can occur in half of pituitary adenomas (Bonneville et al., 2005; Meij et al., 2002), depending on size and subtype (in increasing order from the lowest rate in Cushing's disease, to intermediate in acromegaly, PRLomas, null cell, and plurihormonal adenomas, to the highest in Nelson's syndrome, and TSHomas).

*Imaging*

MRI is nowadays the gold standard for imaging pituitary gland and hypothalamic disorders.

The normal anterior pituitary has signal intensity similar to the white matter on T1 and T2, whereas a spontaneous hyperintensity on T1 images, the so-called bright spot, appears in the posterior pituitary of most patients (figure 2). It is related to the phospholipid membrane of the ADH-containing neuro-secretory granules in the posterior pituitary. The lack of bright spot is closely correlated with a loss of function of the neuro-hypophysis but nonspecific because it occurs also in 10-20% of normal subjects. With the administration of paramagnetic contrast agent, the pituitary and its stalk enhance or become brighter in signal intensity (Freda & Post, 1999).

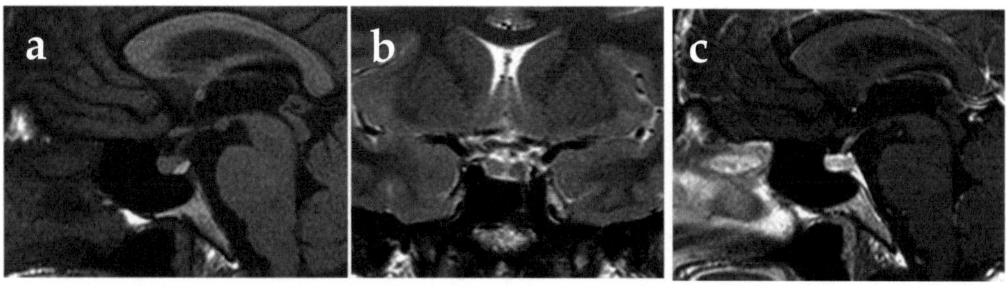


Fig. 2. Normal MRI of pituitary. Anterior pituitary has signal intensity similar to white matter on T1 (a) and T2 (b). The typical "bright spot" is shown in posterior pituitary gland. The pituitary and stalk enhance strongly (c).

Most microadenomas on precontrast T1-weighted images show abnormal low signal, whereas some may appear hyperintense due to internal bleeding (Rumboldt, 2005). On T2-weighted images microprolactinomas are usually hyperintense and GH-secreting adenomas are iso-hypointense (Bonneville et al., 2005)(figure 3). About 5% to 10% of microadenomas are detected exclusively on post-contrast images.

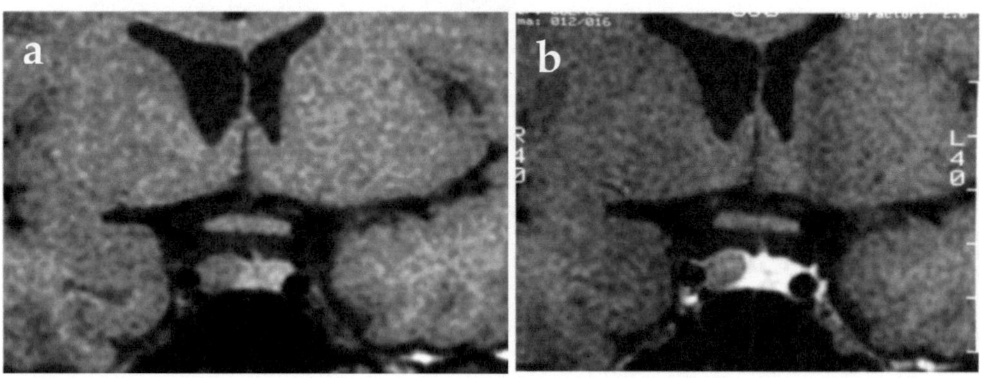


Fig. 3. Typical microadenoma: coronal MRI on T1 (a) shows a well-demarcated hypointense intrapituitary mass, < 10 mm in diameter, with contralateral stalk deviation. Contrast enhancement is slower into the microadenoma (b).

The peculiar vascularization of the adeno-hypophysis, supplied by a portal rather than an arterial circle, allows dynamic MR imaging. Using this technique, the normal gland enhances later than the pituitary stalk and cavernous sinuses. The tumors show delayed enhancement. Dynamic post-contrast imaging is thus a useful tool to increase the sensitivity of the exam (Bonneville et al., 1993). Indirect radiologic signs, like unilateral bulging of the superior pituitary margin and stalk deviation, may be helpful. Anyway, stalk deviation is a nonspecific sign, being observed even in normal subjects. Moreover, the deviation can be either contralateral or more rarely ipsilateral to the microadenoma (Ahmadi et al., 1990).

The finding of a focal pituitary lesion may be incidental (so-called incidentaloma, see below) and not related to any clinical picture (Teramoto et al., 1994).

Macroadenomas are occasionally heterogeneous on MRI. Cystic, necrotic, or hemorrhagic portions may appear as hyperintense areas (Rumboldt, 2005) (figure 4). Sometimes macroadenomas with suprasellar extension, due to constriction at the level of the diaphragm appear like a number 8 or a snowman. Further information provided by MRI is that bizarre and irregular shape usually points to PRLomas. Tumors that are iso-hypointense with the normal gland on T2-weighted sequences tend to be more fibrotic (Elster, 1993). Post-contrast images are acquired in order to visualize the normal pituitary tissue, strongly enhancing and displaced (laterally or posteriorly or superiorly) by the expanding mass, as well as the relationships with the optic pathways and cavernous sinus (Cottier et al., 2000; Knosp et al., 1993).

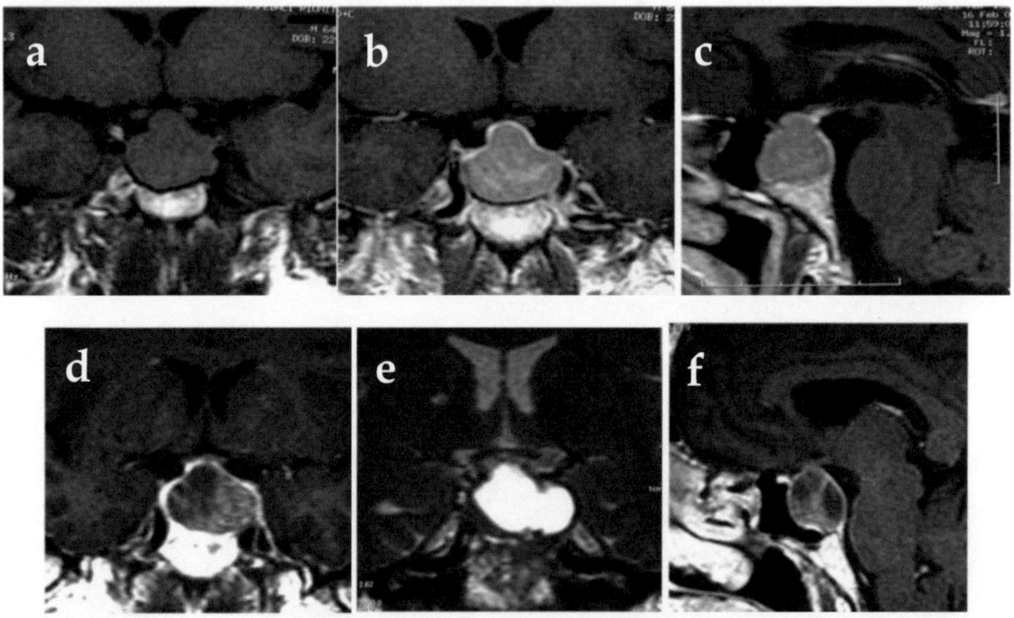


Fig. 4. a-c: Typical macroadenoma. Coronal (a and b, before and after contrast administration, respectively) and sagittal (c) MRIs show intra/suprasellar mass. The lesion looks like a "snowman" on morphology, is isointense with gray matter and enhances homogeneously. It compresses optic chiasm and left cavernous sinus without definite invasion. d-f: cystic macroadenoma in another patient. The lesion appears homogeneously hyperintense on T2 (e), moderately and heterogeneously enhancing (d and f).

*Pituitary incidentaloma*

Pituitary adenomas have been found at post-mortem examination in 10-15% of subjects without any clinical manifestation, regardless of age or gender. Very few were macroadenomas. It was thus hypothesized (Molitch, 2009) either that the growth from micro- to macroadenoma is an exceedingly uncommon event, or that a macroadenoma cannot miss clinical diagnosis, but more data are needed.

Due to the large availability of sophisticated imaging techniques an ever-growing amount of lesions in the pituitary region are incidentally found. MRI scans of subjects examined for reasons unrelated to pituitary disease (excluding thus scans performed for visual loss, or a clinical manifestation of hypopituitarism or hormone excess) have visualized silent pituitary tumors sized ≥ 3 mm in approximately 10% of them (Hall et al., 1994). Therefore there is an outbreak of so-called pituitary incidentalomas, in analogy to adrenal lesions. In this setting also macroadenomas can be encountered in 0.2-0.3% of normal subjects (Nammour et al., 1997; Vernooij et al., 2007; Yue et al., 1997).

What is the correct and cost-effective approach to this situation, both at diagnosis and during follow-up (Dekkers et al., 2008; King et al., 1997; Randall et al., 2010), considering that sensitivity and specificity of MRI were reported to be of 99% and 29%, respectively (Famini et al., 2011)?

To screen hypersecretory syndromes, even without a clear-cut clinical picture, is mandatory. The minimal panel to diagnose hypersecreting adenomas includes:

- PRL assay after thorough exclusion of physiological, i.e. pregnancy and stress, pharmacological (mostly anti-psychotic, anti-depressive, and gastroenteric drugs, acting as anti-dopaminergic) and pathological causes of secondary increase of plasma PRL levels (such as hypothyroidism, renal or liver failure, lung or kidney tumors) to rule out hyperprolactinemia;
- IGF-I levels to rule out acromegaly, when a reliable assay is available and main causes of spurious decrease, i.e. liver disease and malnutrition have been excluded;
- free thyroxine ($FT_4$) and TSH to rule out central hyperthyroidism;
- morning cortisol after overnight suppression test (or night salivary cortisol if available) to rule out Cushing's disease.

More formal evaluation can be required as a subsequent step, if first level assessment is uncertain.

- Whereas very high PRL levels (i.e. > 200 ng/mL) are diagnostic of PRLomas, lower levels may require further testing to distinguish between stalk compression (due to any mass in the region, inhibiting the physiologic dopamine inhibition of PRL secretion, with PRL levels seldom exceeding 100 ng/mL) and different clinical conditions. Serial PRL sampling will overcome stress, sample dilutions or PEG precipitation will rule out, respectively, hook effect (due to saturation of capture antibodies in presence of large amounts of antigen, as observed in very large PRL-secreting tumors) or macroprolactinemia (circulating macroaggregates of PRL without biological effect).
- GH assay during oral glucose load because the physiologic GH suppression is lost in GH-secreting tumors.

- One or more among the numerous available tests for diagnosing Cushing's disease.

To establish a diagnosis of hypopituitarism it is useful to perform assays of serum cortisol at 8 a.m., $FT_4$, and testosterone, to rule out hypoadrenalism, hypothyroidism, and male hypogonadism, respectively. To evaluate gonadal function in females, a history of regular menses in fertile age or FSH assay post-menopause is sufficient. Hypopituitarism can be partial or total and it generally occurs only in patients with macroadenoma (up to half of patients). Microadenomas usually do not cause disruption of normal pituitary function, even though it has been recently reported GH deficiency even in this setting (Yuen et al., 2008). Thus, all patients bearing a macroadenoma should be screened for hypopituitarism. It is commonly accepted that GH deficiency should be screened only in those patients candidate to ensuing GH substitutive treatment.

Obviously all hypersecreting tumors, whether clinically or incidentally diagnosed, should be appropriately treated with surgery or drugs, according to type of tumor and relative guidelines (Biller et al., 2008; Cozzi et al., 2009a; Melmed et al., 2011). This is not always the case for clinically non-functioning pituitary adenoma (NFPA). Whereas surgery is clearly indicated in macroadenomas impinging or near the optic pathways, unless absolute contraindications exist, the same is not true for the incidentally found microadenoma or macroadenoma. NFPAs are a very heterogeneous population from a biological and clinical point of view (Honegger et al., 2008), and some series with serial evaluation over many years clearly demonstrated that progressive growth is not the rule. It was observed only in 10% of microadenomas, while any change in size has been shown in the vast majority and even a reduction occurred in 6% (Dekkers et al., 2007; Karavitaki et al., 2007.).

In a meta-analysis, 8.2% of incidentalomas enlarged per year (1.7% of microincidentalomas) with a follow-up of 472 person-years (Fernandez-Balsells et al., 2011). Importantly, none of the patients with microincidentalomas developed new visual field defects requiring surgery. Watchful waiting can thus be considered a safe option (Freda et al., 2011). In microadenomas we suggest to perform the first MRI at 12 months, and the second after additional 18-24 months: if no growth is observed further monitoring can be safely withdrawn, unless new neuro-ophthalmological symptoms occur. In macroadenomas not undergoing surgery, we recommend visual assessment every 6 months; MRI should be performed at 6-month intervals for the first year, then yearly. Images must be always personally compared with the first one (and not only with the last): if no growth occurs and visual fields are intact, intervals between imaging can be progressively lengthened.

Unless clinical picture changes, it is useless to repeat screening of hypersecretions during follow-up. Yearly evaluation of basal serum cortisol, $FT_4$ and testosterone is warranted in macroadenomas, to timely start substitutive treatment(s) when necessary.

*Pituitary apoplexy*

An acute condition to be aware of is pituitary apoplexy. This may be a life-threatening clinical syndrome, characterized by sudden onset of headache, vomiting, visual impairment and decreased consciousness caused by the rapid expansion of sellar-suprasellar mass. It is usually the result of a hemorrhage or an infarction in a preexisting adenoma (most often a NFPA, but any type can be involved), and it has a rapid clinical progression (within hours or days) (Nawar et al., 2008).

Notably, in 60-80% of cases the adenoma was previously unknown. Pituitary tumor apoplexy occurs as the first manifestation of disease in a previously asymptomatic patient mainly in the fifth or sixth decade.

The apoplexy syndrome should be distinguished from two different situations: ischemic changes occurring in otherwise normal pituitary glands, after prolonged hypotensive episodes, generally in women after excessive postpartum bleeding (Sheehan's syndrome-Dash et al., 1993), and small hemorrhages frequently (up to 25% of cases) found in adenomas without any specific acute clinical picture. These are sometimes inappropriately defined as silent or subclinical pituitary tumor apoplexy. The term apoplexy is appropriate only when signs of compression of perisellar structures or meningeal irritation occur after hemorrhagic infarction of an adenoma (Arafah et al., 1997; Dubuisson et al., 2007; Nielsen et al., 2006; Onesti et al., 1990; Randeva et al., 1999; Sibal et al., 2004).

The reported incidence is near 2% (Bonicki et al., 1993; Nawar et al., 2008).

On a retrospective evaluation, a lot of events have been advocated as precipitating factors in at least 25-30% of patients (Biousse et al., 2001; Möller-Goede et al., 2011; Semple et al., 2007). Anticoagulant/antiaggregant therapy and coagulopathies, head trauma, hypotension or hypertension, previous irradiation, myocardial infarction, major surgery (in particular coronary artery bypass surgery), hemodialysis, angiography, spinal anesthesia, initiation or withdrawal of dopamine agonists, pregnancy and estrogen therapy, and dynamic testing of pituitary function have been reported. Gonadotrophin-releasing hormone, thyrotrophin-releasing hormone, corticotrophin-releasing hormone and insulin tolerance test have all been reportedly involved in apoplexy. Whenever the association with dynamic tests was described, it occurred within 2 hours in 83% and within 88 hours in all patients (Levy, 2003; Yoshino et al., 2007). This finding coupled to inefficiency in differential diagnosis and cost of testing prompted a drastic reduction in the overall use of such procedures in the last years and suggests that these procedures should be abandoned.

The earliest and most frequent symptom of pituitary tumor apoplexy is sudden and severe headache (75-100%), often accompanied by vegetative (nausea and vomiting) and neurological symptoms. Cranial nerve palsies, mainly diplopia, occur in 70% of patients; visual impairment, from visual field defects to decreased visual acuity up to blindness, occurs in nearly 75% of the cases.

Hypopituitarism is very common (near 80%) and may be life-threatening if unrecognized and untreated. In contrast to the common rule that ACTH-secreting cells are the most resistant to injuries of any kind, central hypoadrenalism is reported in up to 70% of the patients. DI is rare (8%) but may occur and be permanent. Low PRL levels indicate a poor prognosis for pituitary function recovery (Zayour et al., 2004). On the other hand, pituitary hypersecretion can be "cured" in patients surviving apoplexy (Glezer et al., 2008).

Blood in the tumor is characteristically appreciated on imaging according to time elapsed from bleeding. Within 3 hours from onset CT (performed without contrast administration) is superior to MR. A high-density or heterogeneous gland with or without evidence of subarachnoid hemorrhage can be visualized on the former, but no specific sign on the latter. With the progressive breakdown of oxyhemoglobin to deoxyhemoglobin after 3 hours from bleeding and owing to the paramagnetic properties of intracellular or extracellular methemoglobin, apoplectic pituitary appears isointense on T1-weighted images and very hypointense on T2-weighted images (figure 5). Thereafter there is focal hyperintensity on T1-weighted images, and focal hyper- or hypointensity on T2-weighted images. Areas of old bleeding appear cystic on CT and often hypointense on T1-weighted MRI due to increased proton density (Piotin et al., 1999). Late follow up usually shows a decrease in tumor volume.

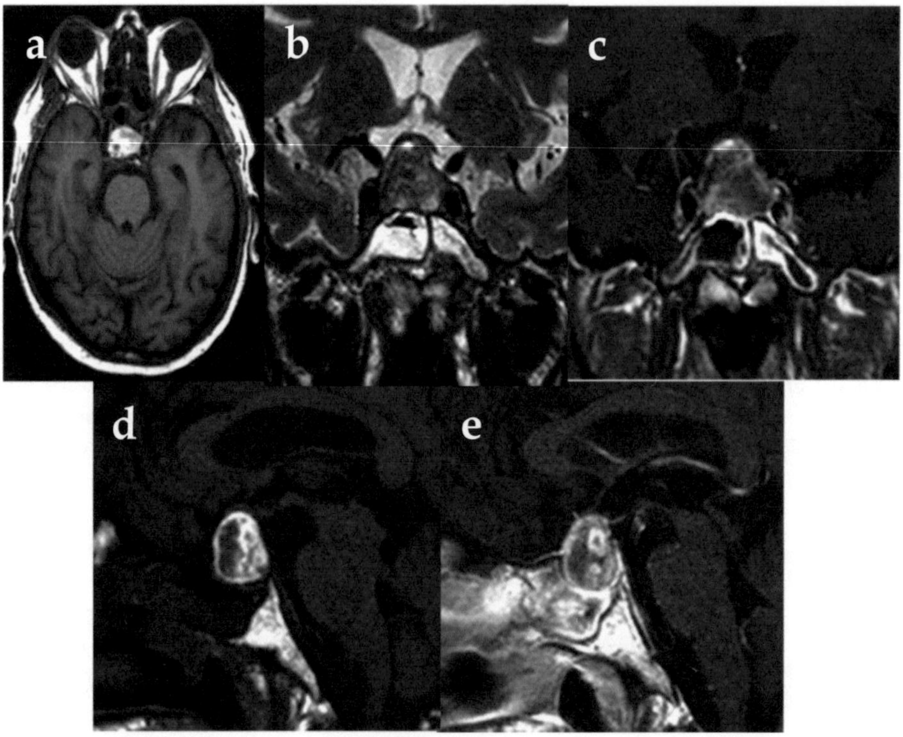


Fig. 5. Hemorrhagic pituitary apoplexy (MR performed 6 hours after the onset of clinical picture). Axial and sagittal T1 (a and d) show confluent hyperintensity in enlarged gland, with moderate, rim enhancement. On coronal T2 (b) the intra and suprasellar mass appears hypointense. Optic chiasm is strained (c and e).

According to recent British Guidelines (Rajasekaran et al., 2011), a high degree of clinical suspicion is needed to diagnose pituitary apoplexy. All patients presenting with acute severe headache with or without neuro-ophthalmic signs, should be submitted to urgent neuroradiological imaging. Patients should undertake visual fields assessment as soon as possible when clinically stable, and be administered iv steroids after baseline endocrine function tests (serum cortisol and $FT_4$) if hemodynamically unstable. Urgent referral to a neurosurgeon is mandatory when visual deterioration is present. Emergency surgery is usually indicated in these cases.

### 3.1.3 Pituitary carcinoma

Most pituitary tumors are noninvasive adenomas with local expansion along the lines of minor resistance. Near half can become locally invasive infiltrating surrounding tissues (dura and bone) by radiologic or pathologic criteria (Meij et al., 2002), and some are defined "atypical", according to a proliferative index higher than 3% in pathology sections. The proliferative index (Ki67/MIB-1) has no useful clinical relevance, in our experience, and no particular follow-up is needed in these cases.

Pituitary carcinoma is a rare entity (< 0.5% of pituitary adenomas) whose definition until now relies upon the presence of metastases (Kaltsas et al., 2005). It must be stressed that this definition is far from be satisfying from a clinical (and logical) point of view. Very aggressive tumors, requiring multiple resections by skilled operators and adjuvant radio and chemotherapy cannot be labeled carcinomas owing to the lack of metastases. Metastases are sometimes found in patients whose tumor has the same proliferative index, mitoses, hypercellularity, nuclear pleomorphism, necrosis, hemorrhage, etc. of "normal" adenomas (Kovacs et al., 2001).

Current working consensus to diagnose pituitary carcinoma requires fulfillment of all the following criteria (Lloyd et al., 2004a):

- histologic diagnosis of primary pituitary tumor;
- presence of metastases without any continuity with primary pituitary tumor;
- strict correspondence or at least similarity in cytohistologic features and biomolecular markers between metastases and primary pituitary tumor;
- exclusion of any possible alternative primary tumor.

The great majority of pituitary carcinomas are associated with excessive hormonal secretion (mostly ACTH or PRL, but any type was reported), with progressive loss of hypersecretion heralding dedifferentiation. A variable latency period (mean 7 years, Kaltsas et al., 2005) elapses between the clinical onset of what is initially diagnosed as an aggressive pituitary macroadenoma and the appearance of metastases. Thereafter the mean survival is less than 4 years, even though a wide variation is described.

Metastases can localize in the brain and spine (40%, through invasion into the subarachnoid space), can be systemic (47%, through hematogenous or lymphatic dissemination, common sites being liver and bone) or can be found at both locations (13%) (Kaltsas et al., 2005).

### 3.2 Lesions deriving from neuro-hypophyseal cells

#### 3.2.1 Pituitocytoma

Pituicytes are specialized glial cells lodged in the stalk and posterior pituitary. They can transform in pituitocytoma, a rare low-grade neuro-hypophyseal glial tumor, also known as pituitary astrocytoma, histologically distinct from pilocytic astrocytomas (Brat et al., 2000; Huang & Castillo 2005; Katsuta et al., 2003).

Pituicytomas usually occur in young to middle-aged women; they are ubiquitarious in the hypothalamic-pituitary axis and can be entirely intrasellar or suprasellar or involve both compartments. Clinical presentation is similar to that of other regional masses: headache and hypopituitarism are the most common trouble. Despite the neuro-hypophyseal origin, DI is not common.

Imaging does not enable differentiation from other neuro-hypophyseal tumors and the diagnosis is histologic. MRI shows a solid, demarcated, enhancing sellar or suprasellar mass, usually isointense to gray matter on T1 and hyperintense on T2, occasionally displacing anteriorly the normally enhancing adeno-hypophysis (figure 6).

Although histologically benign, the location and high vascularization can make radical resection difficult (Glezer et al., 2008; Kowalski et al., 2004).

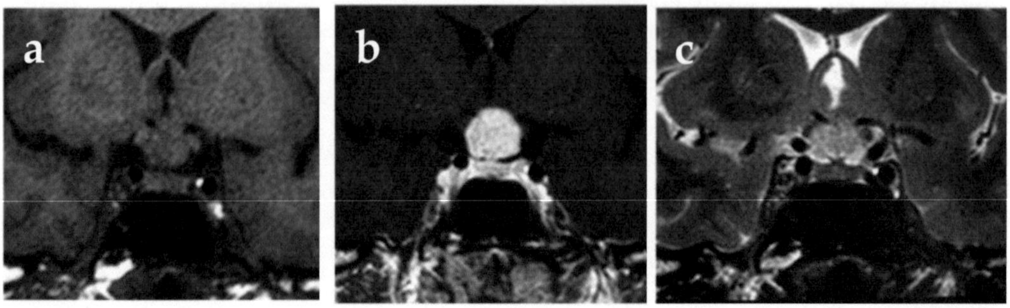


Fig. 6. Pituitocytoma in a young man complaining headache, decreased libido, and diabetes insipidus. MRI depicts a suprasellar, nodular mass, arising from pituitary stalk, isointense on T1 and T2 (a and c, respectively), strongly enhancing (b), like meningioma, compressing the optic chiasm.

### 3.2.2 Granular cell tumor

They are the most common (found in up to 17% of non selected adult autopsies) primary tumor originating from either the neuro-hypophysis or infundibulum, also referred to as choristomas, myoblastomas, and infundibulomas (Freda & Post, 1999; Huang & Castillo, 2005; Kaltsas et al., 2008).

Granular cell tumors are benign tumors, arising from granular cell-type pituicytes (Cohen-Gadol et al., 2003). They are usually asymptomatic, even though they can present, mainly in the fifth decade, with symptoms related to size and mass effect. Headache is common, 90% of symptomatic patients have visual complaints, and 50% have hypopituitarism or hyperprolactinemia. In spite of their origin from the infundibulum and/or posterior lobe, they are not typically associated with DI.

Most symptomatic patients have intra and suprasellar tumors, but in 11% tumor is purely intrasellar. The imaging appearance is nonspecific (Bubl et al., 2001; Iglesias et al., 2000). They appear isointense to gray matter on both T1- and T2-weighted sequences, with intense enhancement reflecting high vascularity. Calcifications may be present, as well as the loss of the so-called bright spot.

Surgical treatment for symptomatic granular cell tumors is indicated.

## 3.3 Malignant parasellar tumors

### 3.3.1 Glioma

Gliomas may arise in the hypothalamus and optic pathways.

Optic nerve gliomas are rare tumors accounting for 3.5% of intracranial tumors in children and 1% of intracranial tumors in adults, in whom they have a malignant behavior (Black & Pikul 1999; Freda & Post, 1999; Guillamo et al., 2001; Kaltsas et al., 2008; Kitange et al., 2003).

The **childhood variety**, occurring within the first decade of life, is typically pilocytic astrocytoma (WHO grade I), a benign and slow-growing lesion. The tumor usually grows infiltrating the chiasm and optic nerves. About 30% of patients with optic pathway gliomas have neurofibromatosis type 1 (NF-1), while about one third of patients with NF-1 will develop multicentric optic pathway gliomas, low-grade brain stem gliomas and basal ganglia non-neoplastic hamartomas (Kornreich et al., 2001). The most frequent presenting symptoms in children are loss of vision, headaches, and proptosis. Often, the visual loss remains unrecognized until the tumor is advanced. Imaging shows a hypointense lesion on T1 sequences with contrast enhancement, in the chiasm or optic nerve. The best therapy for optic gliomas confined in one optic nerve is surgery. Surgery plus radio and chemotherapy are an option in all the other cases, but a rule does not exist at the moment.

The **young adult type** of gliomas can develop in the brainstem and extend into the parasellar region. Diffuse intrinsic low-grade glioma (WHO grade II) is the most prominent type, whereas purely malignant brainstem glioma (WHO grades III–IV) occurs in 31% of cases. The initial presentation is often monocular blurring of vision and retrobulbar pain, which may progress rapidly to blindness (Glezer et al., 2008). The pattern of field defects is extremely variable and nonspecific. Presentation of an optic nerve glioma as an intrasellar cystic mass is exceedingly rare. On MR imaging, these lesions can usually be localized into the optic chiasm. The sella is normal in most patients. Typically, they are isointense to hypointense on T1-weighted images and hyperintense on T2-weighted images, with infiltration along the optic nerves and optic tracts, homogeneously enhancing. Radiotherapy is probably the best palliative therapy.

**Hypothalamic gliomas** present almost always in early life, with disruption of hypothalamic function, failure to gain weight, DI, and visual loss with optic atrophy. On MR imaging, these tumors do not spread along the optic nerves but rather are large masses in the suprasellar region, more invasive into the hypothalamus, infiltrating the brain and the third ventricle. Hypothalamic gliomas are hypo to isointense on T1-weighted images and isointense to hyperintense on T2-weighted images, homogeneously enhancing (figure 7). The tumor may extend into the suprasellar cistern or the surrounding brain parenchyma, usually without necrosis, hemorrhage or calcification. They may encase the vessels of the circle of Willis, and hydrocephalus is common (Smith, 2005).

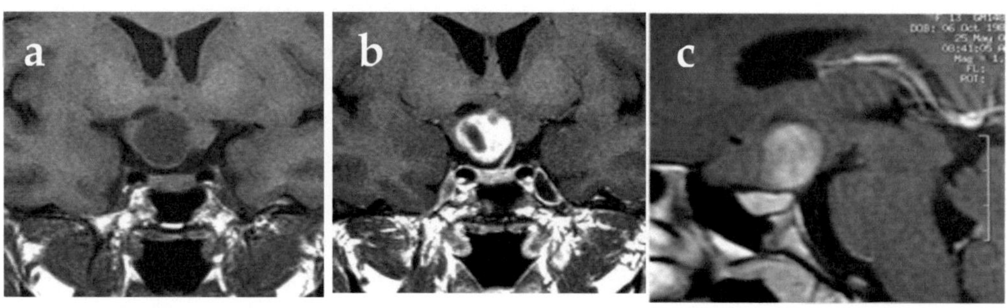


Fig. 7. Hypothalamic glioma in a 10 yo girl with NF1, complaining sight loss, without endocrine disturbances. Coronal and sagittal MRIs reveal an infiltrating hypothalamic mass involving the optic chiasm, isointense to the brain, with nodular and cystic components. The nodular portion enhances brightly and dislocates the pituitary stalk to the left.

Diagnosis can be accomplished by stereotactic or open biopsy.

Optic pathway gliomas are generally very slow growing tumors, while tumors around the chiasm/hypothalamus can be more aggressive (5-year survival 50%).

The best therapeutic approach is uncertain: watchful waiting, surgery, glucocorticoids and irradiation, and chemotherapy with temozolomide and/or other agents have been proposed with variable degree of success.

### 3.3.2 Germ cell tumors

Intracranial germ cell tumors are rare malignant tumors, representing 0.1-2% of all primary brain neoplasms. They are tumors of the suprasellar region arising from totipotent germ cells that fail to migrate to the genital crest during embryonic life. They are subdivided into germinomas (two thirds of the intracranial ones), teratomas, embryonal cell carcinoma, choriocarcinoma, endodermal sinus (yolk sac) tumors, and mixed germ cell tumors (Huang & Castillo 2005).

Their usual localization is in the midline, most frequently at the pineal gland region (80%). Three patterns are described: germinomas of the ventral hypothalamus associated with germinoma in the pineal region; germinomas in the anterior third ventricle that can involve the pituitary fossa as an extension; and intrasellar germinoma mimicking an intrasellar adenoma (Packer et al., 2000). All these can spread to involve the chiasm and optic nerves and may disrupt pituitary function.

Germinomas have a peak incidence in children and adolescents. Pineal localization is more frequent in males and supra and intrasellar one is more frequent in females.

Patients most commonly present with endocrine abnormalities: DI is the most common symptom (80%). It is worth noting that DI may persist for years before a diagnosis is made. Other manifestations include hypopituitarism in children and adolescents and hypogonadism in adults. Hyperprolactinemia and precocious puberty have been observed. Large tumors and primarily suprasellar tumors may present with visual field defects or optic atrophy, oculomotor palsies or hydrocephalus, and signs of increased intracranial pressure (Freda & Post, 1999; Glezer et al., 2008; Janmohamed et al., 2002; Kaltsas et al., 2008).

Diagnosis is established by histology but a subgroup can be diagnosed on the basis of elevation of specific tumor markers (Calaminus et al., 2005), or typical radiological features. Alpha-fetoprotein and chorionic gonadotrophin can be detected in the serum and/or cerebro-spinal fluid (CSF), and they are a pathognomonic sign of yolk sac tumors and choriocarcinomas, respectively (Calaminus et al., 2005; Matsutani et al., 1997).

CT scanning depicts isodense or hyperdense masses, sometimes multicentric, which enhance markedly. The concomitant presence of similar lesions in the suprasellar and pineal region is diagnostic (Freda & Post, 1999; Glezer et al., 2008; Kaltsas et al., 2008; Smith, 2005).

On MRI the lack of the posterior bright spot is an early but unspecific sign. It can be followed by swelling of the stalk and subsequent mass formation, which may displace anteriorly the enhancing pituitary gland (figure 8). At last a germinoma can appear as an enhancing solid homogenous mass with well defined margins, that appears isointense to gray matter on T1-weighted images and isointense-slightly hyperintense on T2-weighted images, displacing anteriorly the adeno-hypophysis with or without suprasellar extension (Rennert & Doerfler, 2007). Cystic changes, hemorrhage, or calcification are rarely observed (Freda & Post, 1999; Glezer et al., 2008; Kaltsas et al., 2008; Rennert & Doerfler, 2007; Smith, 2005; Sumida et al., 1995).

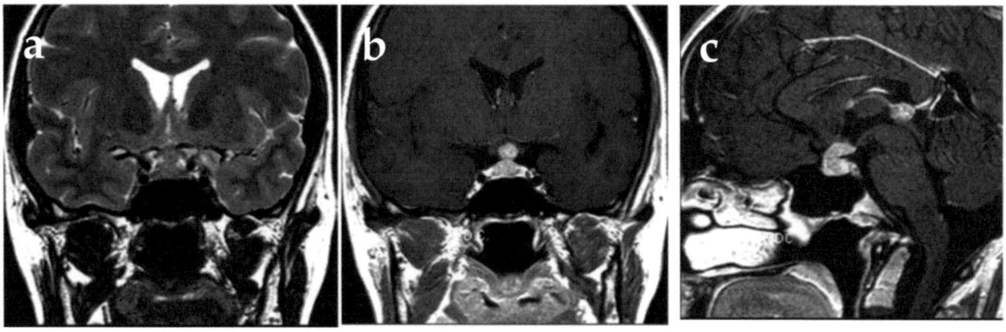


Fig. 8. Germinoma in a young boy with diabetes insipidus at presentation. Coronal MR shows a sellar and suprasellar lesion, isointense on T2 and homogeneously enhancing. Sagittal MRI (c) depicts a synchronous lesion in the pineal region, that "engulfs" the pineal gland.

Teratoma appears in imaging as a well-delineated mixed cyst with fat and calcification. This tumor can undergo ossification, teeth formation, or malignant transformation (Glezer et al., 2008).

Histological confirmation on a sample obtained using stereotactic or neuroendoscopic biopsy is the 'gold standard' diagnostic method. It will show a granulomatous infiltrate around germ cells. Biopsy can be avoided if clear-cut results have been obtained by imaging and biochemical markers (Calaminus et al., 2005).

Direct surgery is rarely indicated and ventricular shunting may be the only surgical procedure required (Janmohamed et al., 2002). Germinomas usually respond well to chemotherapy and radiotherapy.

### 3.3.3 Primary parasellar lymphoma

Primary CNS lymphoma is defined as a lymphoma limited to the cranio-spinal axis without systemic disease. Most originate from B-cell. They are distinct from systemic lymphomas that secondarily metastasize to the CNS (an event reported in about 30% of patients), and account for 1-2% of non-Hodgkin lymphomas and for about 3% of all intracranial neoplasms (Giustina et al., 2001). Primary localization at the pituitary is extremely rare (less than 1% in patients undergoing trans-sphenoidal surgery - TSS - for a sellar mass) (Freda & Post 1999, Moshkin et al., 2009). They were initially described in immunocompromised patients, but recently they have been documented even in immunocompetent patients (Giustina et al., 2001).

Peak incidence is between the 6th and 7th decade in non immune-depressed subjects and earlier in the immune-depressed ones, with a male preponderance (Pels et al., 2000).

Systemic symptoms, such as fever of unknown origin, are uncommon at presentation (22%), whereas local compressive symptoms are more frequent (headache, diplopia, and visual field defects in 56%, 39%, and 28%, respectively), as well as hypopituitarism (72%) and DI (39%) (Liu et al., 2007).

Lymphomas usually appear iso- or hyperdense on CT scanning, whereas appearance may be different on MRI based on whether patients have normal or suppressed immunity (Erdag et al., 2001; Huang & Castillo 2005; Johnson et al., 1997). Imaging of a sellar localization is largely nonspecific with diffuse enlargement of the pituitary (94%), suprasellar extension (44%), cavernous sinus extension (39%) and stalk thickening (22%). Most cases appear isointense on T1-weighted sequences, homogeneously or heterogeneously enhancing, usually without calcifications and hemorrhages, but isointense to hypointense relative to gray matter on T2-weighted imaging (Buhring et al., 2001).

The diagnosis of primary lymphoma is established histologically by stereotactic biopsy, but noninvasive tests can now be used with confidence, such as SPECT or PET or rather identification of EBV DNA in the CSF that is sensitive and usually unique for this disease (Castagna et al., 1997).

Treatment options include surgery, chemotherapy and radiotherapy (Glezer et al. 2008).

### 3.3.4 Metastases to the sellar and parasellar region

Metastases to this region are rare, less than 1% of patients undergoing TSS for sellar/parasellar lesions (Komninos et al., 2004). Autoptic series reported involvement of the region in up to one quarter of patients with intracranial dissemination. Furthermore, metastases have been diagnosed more and more frequently in recent years, owing to amelioration of imaging techniques, as well as improved survival in oncologic patients.

Even though metastases are usually part of a generalized spread in elderly patients without sex predominance, they can occur in young patients too, and occasionally are the first manifestation of an occult cancer or the only site of metastasis.

The most common primary tumors are breast and lung cancer, in females and males, respectively, accounting for two-third of reported cases, but any neoplasm can spread to the pituitary region and the primary tumor remains undetected in approximately 3% of cases despite intensive investigation.

Metastatic cells can spread to the sellar region via different ways: through the portal vessels, through the suprasellar cistern, by extension from the skull base, and directly through arterial blood circulation.

DI is the most frequent symptom at presentation, reported in 28% to 70% of patients (up to 100% in some series). It may be the initial manifestation of the malignancy. Anatomical reasons account for this pattern: the posterior lobe is directly supplied by arterial vessels and has a larger area of contact with the adjacent dura, in contrast with the anterior lobe supplied by the portal system. DI may occasionally be transient or intermittent, because regeneration of neuro-hypophyseal fibers may occur. In addition it can be masked by concomitant central hypoadrenalism until corticosteroid treatment is started (Freda & Post, 1999; Kaltsas et al., 2008).

Hypopituitarism is less frequent, both for the above described anatomical reasons and because it can be clinically masked by nonspecific symptoms (weakness, vomiting, weight loss) attributed to neoplasm. Cranial nerve palsies (mostly of the 6th nerve) may be found in 12-43% of patients.

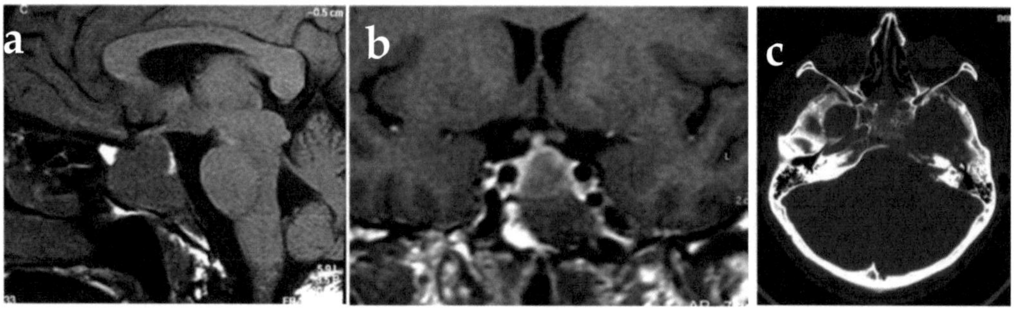


Fig. 9. Metastases in a 56 yo woman with breast cancer. Sagittal and coronal MRI reveals an intra and suprasellar solid mass, infiltrating the clivus and sphenoid sinus. The lesion is moderately hipointense on T1 and heterogeneously enhancing. Axial CT-bone (c) demonstrates a large erosion of the central skull base.

It is worth noting that the majority of metastases to the pituitary are clinically silent and even when symptomatic, cannot be reliably distinguished from primary sellar tumors on the basis of clinical and radiographic presentation. They often may mimic a pituitary adenoma or a variety of sellar area lesions, benign or malignant, especially when clinical evidence of primary malignancy is absent. Besides, even in patients with known malignancy, a sellar lesion is not always a metastasis; a benign lesion, like a pituitary adenoma, can be present and trigger clinical troubles in 1.8–16% of patients with known malignancy. It is thus essential a correct diagnosis, to appropriately plan the following therapeutic steps.

CT usually shows a hyperdense or isodense mass, homogeneously or inhomogeneously enhancing (if cystic degeneration, hemorrhage, or necrosis exists).

On MRI, pituitary metastatic lesions appear as enhancing isointense or hypointense sellar/suprasellar mass on T1, and usually hyperintense on T2. The mass may sometimes overrun the sellar diaphragm (so-called dumbbell-shape best seen on sagittal images), in contrast to adenomas, which usually upward displace the diaphragm (figure 9). Bone erosions, as well as the loss of posterior pituitary bright spot and stalk thickening, are nonspecific findings (Freda & Post, 1999; Kaltsas et al., 2008).

Lumbar puncture may be essential, pointing to malignancy in cases in which a meningeal spread is present.

Most of the times in absence of a primary and/or other metastatic lesions, diagnosis relies on histology. Immunohistochemical analysis is mandatory because local infiltration and cytological features such as nuclear pleomorphism, multinucleate cells and mitotic figures cannot reliably distinguish between malignancy and adenomas.

As a trans-sphenoidal approach is needed to gain a histological diagnosis in all sellar-suprasellar masses, resection, as radical as possible, should be undertaken. An extended approach is needed in almost every case. Adjuvant treatments by radiation and chemotherapy should be individually tailored, with adequate hormonal substitution.

The overall prognosis is poor, owing to the aggressiveness of the primary neoplasm, with a median survival of less than 2 years (Laigle-Donadey et al., 2005).

### 3.4 Potentially malignant parasellar tumors (low-grade malignant tumors)

#### 3.4.1 Tumors of cartilaginous origin

Approximately 10% of non-pituitary parasellar lesions are cartilaginous (chordomas, chondromas and chondrosarcomas) originating from the primitive notochord in the skull base (Kaltsas et al., 2008). They are located within the clivus in nearly 40% of cases or elsewhere within the sellar or parasellar region.

**Chordomas** are rare (1% of all malignant bone tumors and 0.1-0.2% of all intracranial neoplasms), locally invasive slow-growing tumors of the midline, most commonly arising around the ends of the notochord, within the sacrum and clivus. In 35% of cases they arise in skull base around the spheno-occipital synchondrosis, and rarely within the sella, in which case they are difficult to distinguish from pituitary macroadenomas (Thodou et al., 2000). They can occur in adults of all ages, mostly between 30 and 50 years.

Symptoms depend on the direction of tumor growth, usually posterior with extension into the prepontine cistern (Rennert & Doerfler, 2007). The most common presenting symptoms are headache (occurring early in a third of patients) and visual complaints, mainly diplopia due to typically asymmetric involvement of the sixth, third, or fourth cranial nerve. Field defects, when present, are similar to those seen with pituitary adenoma. Chordomas can reach considerable size at the time of diagnosis and patients may develop neck pain and nasopharyngeal obstruction (Rennert & Doerfler, 2007). Endocrine dysfunction is unusual, but hypopituitarism or mild hyperprolactinemia may occur. Less common presentations include dizziness, tinnitus, facial sensory deficits, ataxia, and hemiparesis.

Chordomas can be quite aggressive, causing local infiltration and extensive bone destruction in the skull base; in addition, they relapse and may progress to malignant transformation (Erdem et al., 2003; Gehanne et al., 2005).

CT scan of patients with clival chordoma shows a bone destroying mass, with frequent intra-tumoral calcifications (50%). MRI shows a destructive invasive lesion in the clivus, isointense to gray matter on T1, heterogeneously hyperintense on T2, heterogeneously enhancing with honeycomb-like internal septations, with involvement of the neural and vascular structures (Korten et al., 1998)(figure 10). Occasionally, cyst-like hypodense centers secondary to necrosis can be found (Erdem et al., 2003; Gehanne et al., 2005; Rennert & Doerfler 2007). In some cases, the normal pituitary gland can be distinguished from the tumor, a helpful finding to differentiate chordomas from invasive pituitary adenomas, which can likewise produce extensive bone destruction, even though usually causing sellar ballooning rather than destruction (Glezer et al., 2008).

**Chondroma** is another bone destructing, nodular/lobular tumor, arising from cartilaginous remnants in the area of the foramen lacerum, that undergo mucinous, cystic regression and calcification. Imaging findings are similar to those in chordoma (Rennert & Doerfler, 2007).

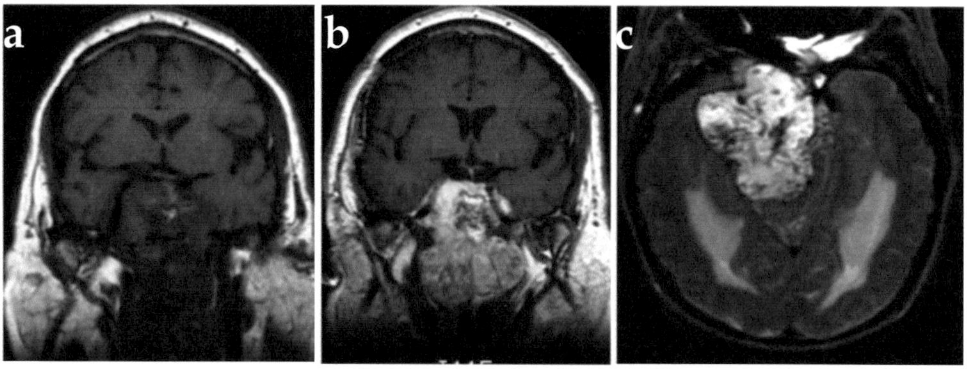


Fig. 10. Clival chordoma. Coronal T1 MR (a) reveals an invasive central skull base mass, infiltrating clivus and basisphenoid, sella, right cavernous sinus, and nasopharynx. The lesion is strongly and heterogeneously enhancing (b). On axial T2 (c) the signal is characteristically heterogeneously hyperintense.

**Chondrosarcoma** (Korten et al., 1998; Meyers et al., 1992) is a malignant tumor (WHO grades II–III), arising off the midline, at the petro-clival junction also associated with extensive bone destruction and compression on adjacent structures.

Chondromas and chondrosarcomas are centered along the lateral margin of clivus in petro-occipital fissure and display chondroid calcifications in more than half of cases.

An immunohistochemical distinction can be made as all these tumors are positive for S-100 protein but chondrosarcomas are negative for cytokeratin markers and epithelial membrane antigens (Kaltsas et al., 2008).

Surgery is the treatment of choice for all these tumors, but radical resection is usually not possible due to bone invasiveness (Glezer et al., 2008). RT adjuvant therapy is mandatory. Proton Beam therapy has shown the best results in chordomas, but in general the prognosis of these tumors remains poor on the long term.

### 3.4.2 Langerhans' cell histiocytosis

Langerhans' cell histiocytosis (LCH) or class I histiocytosis is a rare multisystem disorder. In the traditional classifications of parasellar tumors it is frequently described among the granulomatous disorders. Since it was discovered to be stemmed from the clonal proliferation of specific dendritic cells belonging to the monocyte-macrophage system, called Langerhans' cells, it is to be regarded as a genuine neoplastic disease.

Proliferation of histiocytes forms granulomas that infiltrate and destroy many sites, such as bone, lung, skin, hypothalamic-pituitary axis, and, less frequently, liver, spleen, lymph nodes, and bone marrow (Kaltsas et al., 2000).

The incidence is 3-4 cases per million per year in children younger than 15 years (only 1/3 of the cases are reported in adults), with males being 2 times more frequently affected than females (Glezer et al., 2008).

The disease has a particular tropism for the hypothalamo-pituitary system. DI affects half of the patients. Often it is the presenting sign and may even remain the unique feature of the disease. In childhood, LCH is the second most common cause of DI; consequently, this diagnosis should be actively pursued in childhood-onset DI (Prosch et al., 2006). Hypothalamic or stalk involvement can result in growth failure, frequent in children, or visual impairment. Bones may commonly appear as punched out, in particular skull, mandible, or long bones (Grois et al., 2004; Horn et al., 2006; Kaltsas et al., 2000; Makras et al., 2007).

On MRI there is no specific sign but in all patients with DI the 'bright spot' of the posterior pituitary is lost. In addition a suprasellar mass, hypothalamic lesions, and a thickened stalk (> 3.5 mm) are common findings (Kaltsas et al., 2000). They appear hypointense or isointense on T1 and hyperintense on T2, and enhance brightly with contrast (Lury et al., 2005)(figure 11).

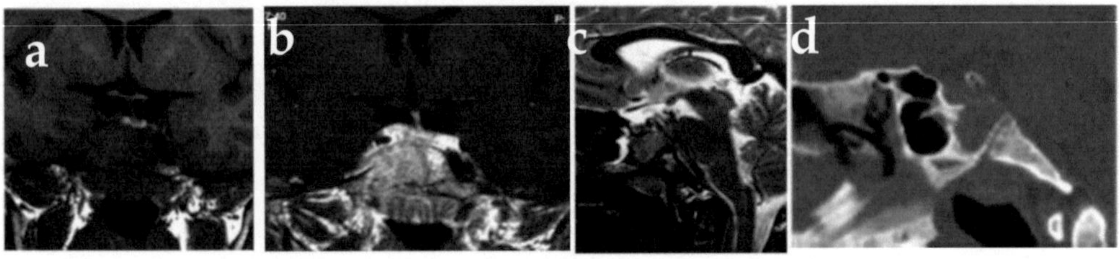


Fig. 11. Young female with known Langerhans' cell histiocytosis. MR shows a lesion in the basisphenoid, infiltrating the sella and nasopharynx, isointense on T1 (a) and slightly hiperintense on T2 (c). Sagittal CT-bone (d) demonstrates clivus and sellar erosion.

To achieve an early and accurate diagnosis is important due to the high mortality rate (20%) and permanent consequences (50%) associated to multisystem disease (Makras et al., 2007). The diagnosis may be established on the basis of symptoms, imaging, and biopsy of involved sites (Glezer et al., 2008; Kaltsas et al., 2000.), with immunohistochemical characterization of Langerhans' cells (S-100 protein, a CD1a antigen). Pituitary stalk biopsy is not routinely recommended in small lesions (< 7 mm).

Due to the systemic nature of the disease, chemotherapy is indicated, with possible radiotherapy on the parasellar region (Makras et al., 2007).

#### 3.4.3 Other tumors

Case reports described a lot of other tumors arising in the parasellar region: hemangioblastomas (Rumboldt et al., 2003), hemangiopericytomas (Jalali et al., 2008), fibrosarcomas (Lopes et al., 1998), rhabdomyosarcomas of the sphenoid sinus (Jalalah et al., 1987), solitary fibrous tumors (Furlanetto et al., 2009), esthesioneuroblastomas (Sajko et al., 2005), pituitary blastomas (Scheithauer et al., 2008), supratentorial primitive neuroectodermal tumors (Ohba et al., 2008), ependymomas (Mukhida et al., 2006), plasmacytomas (Sinnott et al., 2006), melanocytic tumors (Rousseau et al., 2005), and epidermoid carcinomas (personal observation).

### 3.5 Benign parasellar tumors

#### 3.5.1 Craniopharyngioma (Karavitaki et al., 2006, 2009)

Craniopharyngiomas are uncommon tumors (incidence is 0.13 per 100,000 person-years). They account for 2-5% of all primary intracranial neoplasms. There is no gender difference.

A bimodal age distribution is known, with peaks in children (5-14 years, 5.6-15% of intracranial tumors in children, 10-20 times more common than adenomas) and in older adults (50-74 years) (Karavitaki et al., 2005), but they may be detected at any age (Bailey et al., 1990). Nearly two thirds occur before the age of 20 years.

Craniopharyngiomas are grade I tumors, according to the WHO classification, but in spite of a benign histological appearance, their aggressive behavior with infiltrative tendency into critical parasellar structures heralds a significant surgical morbidity and mortality (Karavitaki et al., 2006). Malignant transformation, even if exceedingly rare (possibly triggered by previous irradiation) has been reported (Kristopaitis et al., 2000; Nelson et al., 1988). Craniopharyngiomas are derived from squamous cell rests in the remnant of Rathke's pouch between the adeno-hypophysis and neuro-hypophysis and can develop anywhere along the path of the craniopharyngeal duct, from the nasopharynx to the third ventricle. The majority (95%) is located in the sellar/parasellar region with a suprasellar component (purely suprasellar in 20-41%, both supra- and intrasellar in 53-75%), but also entirely intrasellar tumors can occur (Karavitaki et al., 2005; Van Effenterre & Boch, 2002).

Craniopharyngiomas are typically described as tumors with a lobular shape (Fahlbusch et al., 1999). Their consistency is purely or predominantly cystic in 46-64%, purely or predominantly solid in 18-39% and mixed in 8-36%. Calcifications are present in 45-57% (in 78-100% of children) with a pattern varying from solid lumps to popcorn-like foci or less commonly, to an eggshell pattern lining the cyst wall. Two pathological varieties are classically described - the adamantinomatous and the papillary - with occasional mixed forms (Zhang et al., 2002).

The adamantinomatous type is the most common, mainly affecting children and adolescents, even though it may occur at any age. There are solid and cystic components, necrotic debris, fibrous tissue, and calcifications. The cysts may be multiloculated, with a typical macroscopic appearance of machinery oil. Tumor margins are irregular, often intermingled with the surrounding brain tissue and the vascular structures. Three layers of cells are histologically visualized: a basal layer of palisading cells resembling the basal cells of the epidermis, an intermediate layer constituted by loose aggregates of stellate cells, and a top layer lining the cyst lumen with flattened and keratinized squamous cells, desquamating to form nodules of 'wet' keratin. These are heavily calcified and appear grossly as white speckles, capable of eliciting an inflammatory and foreign-body giant cell reaction.

The papillary type is typical of adults. It is usually better defined with respect to brain tissue, calcifications are rare and the cyst content is viscous. The histological examination shows rare mature squamous epithelial cells forming pseudopapillae and an anastomosing fibrovascular stroma.

Investigators have argued that papillary and adamantinomatous subtypes may represent two distinct entities located at the opposite ends of a pathological continuum (Zada et al., 2010).

The most common clinical presentations are, as usual for lesions in this area, DI, headache, nausea/vomiting, cranial nerve palsies, visual troubles and endocrine manifestations. Growth failure or delayed sexual development are described in 93% and 20% of children respectively, GH deficiency in 35-95% of the evaluated patients, FSH/LH deficiency in 38-82%, ACTH deficiency in 21-62%, TSH deficiency in 21-42%, and DI in 6-38%. The visual and endocrine abnormalities are frequently unrecognized initially (time elapsed between the onset of symptoms and diagnosis reportedly ranges between 1 week and 31 years), mostly in children that do not realize visual deficiency and increased thirst. As a result, these tumors can become large and cause liquoral obstruction and signs of increased intracranial pressure before the diagnosis is made. Hydrocephalus is observed indeed in up to 38% of cases and it is a more common finding in children (Karavitaki et al., 2005). Many patients suffer from chronic obesity even before surgery, secondary to hypothalamic dysfunction (Honegger et al., 1999; Karavitaki et al., 2006).

On CT, the cystic lesions are non-enhancing areas of low attenuation. The contrast medium enhances any solid portion, as well as the cyst capsule. Calcification is evident in 60% of tumors and it's more common in pediatric cases and in the adamantinomatous subtypes (Karavitaki et al., 2006. Sartoretti-Schefer et al., 1997).

The MR appearance of craniopharyngiomas depends on the proportion of the solid and cystic components, the content of the cyst(s), and the amount of calcification (Huang & Castillo 2005)(figure 12). The solid portions of the tumor appear as iso- or hypointense relative to the brain on pre-contrast T1-weighted images, but can also have a mottled appearance owing to calcific regions; they are usually of mixed hypo- or hyperintensity on T2-weighted sequences, and heterogeneously enhance following Gd administration (Choi et al., 2007; Hald et al., 1994). Large calcifications may be visualized as nodular or curvilinear areas of low signal on both T1- and T2 (Curran & O'Connor, 2005; Smith, 2005), and are more evident on CT. The cystic components are hyperintense on T1 with a thin peripheral contrast-enhancing rim, and have high or mixed intensity on T2 images (Sartoretti-Schefer et al., 1997). Fluid debris levels can be seen within the cysts. Protein, cholesterol and methemoglobin may cause high signal on T1, while very concentrated protein and various blood products may be associated with low T2-weighted signal (Sartoretti-Schefer et al., 1997). Whenever a craniopharyngioma is suspected, CT and MRI should both be acquired because the combination of these two exams is able to establish a firm diagnosis in almost every case.

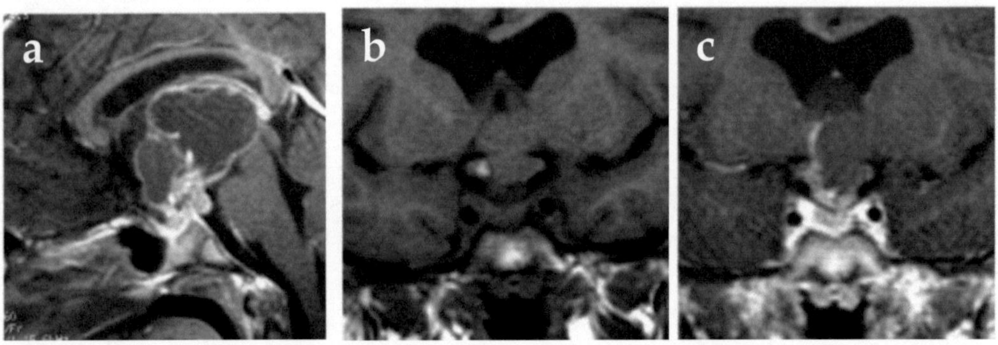


Fig. 12. Craniopharyngioma in a 10 yo girl. MRI on T1 shows a suprasellar, heterogeneous mass, with a small intrasellar component; solid portions and cystic walls enhance heterogeneously, with nodular and rim components (c).

Craniopharyngioma increases mortality (10-year survival rate is 83-92.7% overall and 29-70% in childhood), due to direct tumor effect on critical intracranial structures, surgery associated effects (among the others severe dehydration due to adipsic syndrome with likely complications), hypopituitarism, and increased cardio-cerebrovascular and respiratory mortality (Bülow et al., 1998; Müller, 2011).

It is often associated to severely impaired quality of life (Dekkers, 2006).

Up to now surgery is the only valid therapeutic option, with the goal of total removal at first operation, thus preventing recurrences, which are very difficult to remove completely at repeated surgery. In recent years the application of a trans-nasosphenoidal extended endoscopic approach in these cases has shown to be more effective and less harmful for the surrounding nervous structures than traditional craniotomic approaches. It is a matter of debate if surgery has to be necessarily performed in patients without neuro-ophthalmologic signs or symptoms. Radiosurgery can be a valuable option in case of residual tumor after an operation (Suh & Gupta, 2006). If large cystic portions cannot be resected, it has been reported that instillation of radioisotopes or bleomycin may provide benefits (Karavitaki et al., 2006). Systemic chemotherapy and interferon have been proposed in recurrent tumors and those that have undergone malignant transformation (Karavitaki et al., 2006). Recurrences usually develop within 4 years, occasionally with aggressive growth, even though longer delays have been described (up to 26 years).

### 3.5.2 Meningioma

Meningiomas are benign, slow-growing tumors arising from arachnoid cells. They can be localized in the sellar/suprasellar region and can reach considerable size at the time of diagnosis.

They are the most common non-glial primary brain tumor, accounting for 20% of all intracranial neoplasms, with an annual incidence of 6 per 100,000. Peak incidence is around 60-70 years and they are 2 times more common in females (Bondy & Ligon, 1996).

There is a strong association between meningiomas, neurofibromatosis (multiple tumors) and previous exposure to ionizing radiation (Hartmann et al., 2006).

According to the current WHO classification, around 90% are grade I tumors, 5-7% are atypical meningiomas (grade II) and 1-3% are anaplastic variants (grade III) (Hartmann et al., 2006; Whittle et al., 2004). Any type of meningioma, however, is able to assume a malignant behavior, although very rarely (Ko et al., 2007).

Meningiomas can arise from any part of the dura, most commonly at sites of dural reflections, at the skull vault, and from the skull base (Smith, 2005; Whittle et al., 2004). In 15-30% of cases, meningiomas may arise from the parasellar region (tuberculum sella, cavernous sinus, planum sphenoidale, diaphragma sellae, clinoid process). They represent the most common tumor of the region after pituitary adenomas; rarely, they grow entirely within the sella, arising from the undersurface of the diaphragma sella or from the dorsum sellae, but even from the floor or walls of the sella (Huang & Castillo, 2005).

Intra-suprasellar meningiomas may mimic NFPAs, with headache (both frontal and orbital), visual troubles, and endocrine abnormalities (hypopituitarism or hyperprolactinemia). Visual loss is the most common symptom, even without endocrine dysfunction, but intrasellar meningioma mimicking pituitary apoplexy was reported (Orakdogeny et al., 2004). The visual loss may begin with monocular blurring and then progresses to bilateral loss of vision. Different visual field defects have been reportedly associated to meningiomas: from deficits of either central or peripheral visual fields up to an asymmetric variant of bitemporal hemianopsia. Visual loss is gradual rather than abrupt. Optic atrophy is often observed but without pain on eye movement, in contrast to retrobulbar neuritis. Extraocular muscle palsies may occur. Meningiomas have been reported to increase in size during pregnancy and to become symptomatic (Freda & Post, 1999).

Imaging features of meningiomas are frequently characteristic and permit to distinguish them from other parasellar tumors (Smith, 2005). On CT meningiomas appear as a hyperdense lesion with well-defined margins, uniformly enhancing, arising from the dura with an extensive attachment. They can fill and expand the cavernous sinus; hyperostosis (thickening and sclerosis) of the contiguous bone can be present (Smith, 2005). Dense calcification is suggestive of meningiomas, in particular at the tuberculum sella (Glezer et al., 2008).

On MR meningiomas are typically isointense on T1 and T2, enhancing homogeneously and brightly, with occasional areas of diffuse calcification. Forty per cent are hyperintense on T2 (Karavitaki et al., 2009). Less commonly, they may have cystic or fat areas (Smith, 2005). The dural tail, a linear enhancing thickening of the dura in continuity with convexity extending away from the lesion, is not specific to meningioma (Guermazi et al., 2005). The sella is usually normal in size and the pituitary gland can be distinctly visualized. When a meningioma invades the cavernous sinus, the carotid artery lumen can be reduced more than with other tumors (Young et al., 1988) (figure 13).

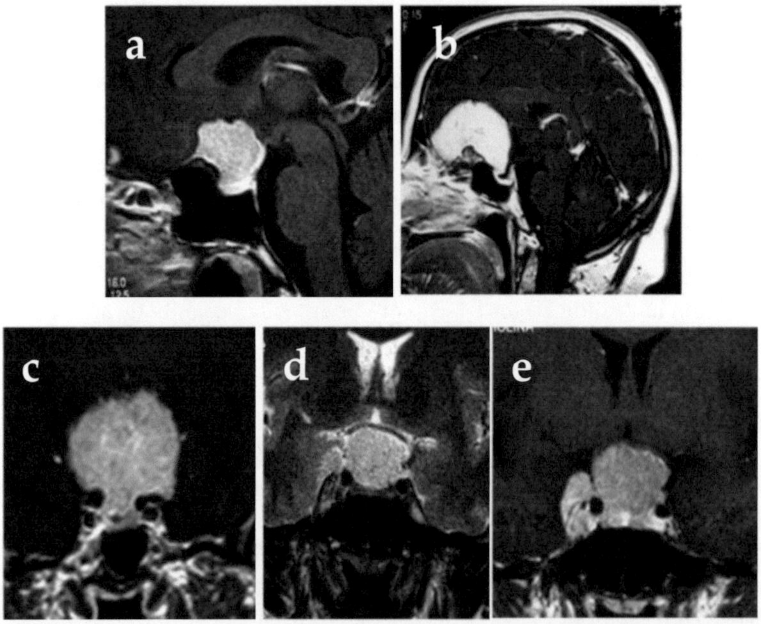


Fig. 13. Meningiomas. Coronal and sagittal contrast-enhanced MRIs show dural-based, mostly homogeneously enhancing mass. Planum sphenoidal meningiomas can completely (a) or partially (b) invade sella, compressing pituitary gland. Note typical hyperostosis and dural "tail". Diaphragma sellae meningiomas (c) can invade suprasellar cistern, compressing optic chiasm and lightly down-pushing normal pituitary gland (best seen on coronal T2, d), or they can overrun sella and cavernous sinus (e).

These lesions can remain stable for a long time and therefore can be safely followed-up only by serial imaging, but in the presence of symptomatic or growing lesions surgery is the treatment of choice. Most of these tumors are approached by a trans-cranial approach; in recent years, however, trans-sphenoidal extended endoscopic approaches have gained momentum (Cappabianca et al., 1999). A strong debate is underway among neurosurgeons about the approach to be preferred. Although benign, meningiomas can be locally aggressive, even with encasement and, ultimately, occlusion of an internal carotid artery. Furthermore they can recur after incomplete resection: in 7–20% of grade I tumors, in 39–40% and 50–78% of atypical and anaplastic tumors, respectively (Ko et al., 2007). Malignant histology is associated with a poor prognosis (survival less than 2 years) (Hartmann et al., 2006).

Also radiosurgery is used either as primary treatment of small (up to 3 cm diameter) tumors or for the treatment of residual disease or initial recurrence after surgery (Freda & Post, 1999). Nowadays it can be considered the choice treatment to prevent growing of small asymptomatic tumors. After the advent of the MRI, asymptomatic tumors are very frequently detected, thus posing a problem of treatment.

Due the presence of specific receptors in the tumor (Arena et al.), radiometabolic treatment with somatostatin analogs is under evaluation (Bartolomei et al., 2009).

Replacement treatment with estroprogestinic drugs in young females presenting with iatrogenic amenorrhea after radiosurgery is also a matter of debate due to the presence of estrogen and progesterone receptors on tumoral cells (Pravdenkova et al., 2006).

### 3.5.3 Paraganglioma (Naggara et al., 2005)

Paragangliomas (or glomangiomas) are rare benign encapsulated neoplasms (WHO grade I), arising in specialized neural crest cells associated with autonomic ganglia, and demonstrated in the pituitary also (Boari et al., 2006). Five percent of CNS paragangliomas produce metastasis (Boari et al., 2006). The presenting symptoms are nonspecific (mass effects and hypopituitarism).

MR images reveal a highly vascularized lesion, with characteristic "salt and pepper" appearance on T1. Salt corresponds to high signal areas in the tumor parenchyma secondary to subacute hemorrhage, whereas pepper zones are low signal foci from high-velocity flow voids. Bone-only CT can depict a wormhole pattern of sellar walls. CT, MRI and angiography (in order to search for other possible localizations of a multicentric tumor) are all required before surgical resection of this highly vascularized tumor.

### 3.5.4 Lipoma

Lipomas are benign fatty tumors (Smith, 2005) that may occur even in the sellar region, as lesions adherent to the surface of the infundibulum, floor of the third ventricle or adjacent cranial nerves. They are usually discovered incidentally but rarely may enlarge. On CT and MRI they appear as well delimitated, homogeneous not enhancing lesions, with possible rim calcification, that disappear on fat-suppressed sequences (Kurt et al., 2002; Smith, 2005)(figure 14). There is no indication to a treatment whatsoever.

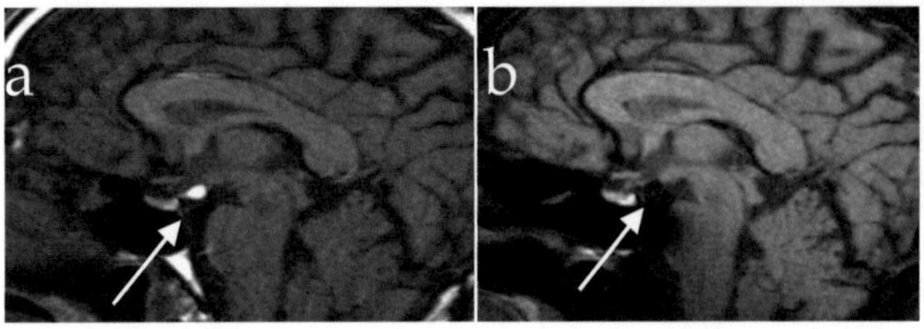


Fig. 14. Lipoma at the tuber cinereum, appearing as an ovoid hyperintense lesion on T1 (a) and disappearing on T1 fat-saturating sequence (b).

### 3.5.5 Schwannoma/neurinoma

These slow-growing tumors (WHO grade I) develop from the Schwann cells of sensory nerve sheaths. They are very rare in the parasellar region, usually arising from the first or second trigeminal branch or from oculomotor nerves (Rennert & Doerfler, 2007; Sarma et al., 2002). Schwannomas (associated in 60% with neurofibromatosis 2) can cause bone remodeling of the lateral portion of the sella or the apex of the petrous bone (Rennert & Doerfler, 2007). Symptoms depend on trigeminal involvement. They can rarely undergo malignant change. On CT and MRI, they appear as a parasellar mass that is isodense on CT, hypointense on T1 and usually hyperintense on T2 with intense homogenous contrast enhancement (Freda & Post, 1999; Rennert & Doerfler, 2007). Surgery and or radiosurgery are generally indicated.

### 3.5.6 Gangliocytoma

Ganglion cell tumors or gangliocytomas are rare benign tumors that may originate in the pituitary or elsewhere in the sellar and suprasellar regions. They may consist of purely neuronal or more frequently mixed adenomatous and neuronal tissue (Geddes et al., 2000). These tumors occur in adults and are more common in females. Approximately 75% of patients with pituitary gangliocytomas demonstrate pituitary hormone hypersecretion due to overproduction of hypothalamic releasing-hormones, either GHRH with consequent hypersecretion of GH and acromegaly or, more rarely, CRH causing Cushing's disease. Local mass effect can also occur. On MR imaging, these lesions may not be distinguishable from pituitary macroadenomas and appear as an enhancing sellar and suprasellar mass (Freda & Post, 1999).

## 3.6 Malformative lesions

### 3.6.1 Rathke's cleft cyst

Rathke's cleft cysts (RCCs) are non neoplastic cysts arising along the craniopharyngeal duct from remnants of squamous epithelium of Rathke's pouch, when there is incomplete obliteration of the central embryonic cleft separating the anterior lobe of the pituitary from the pars intermedia (Byun et al., 2000).

RCCs consist of a single layer of cuboidal or columnar epithelial cells with mucoid, cellular or serous components in the cyst fluid (Spampinato & Castillo, 2005).

They are often discovered incidentally and have been identified in up to 22% of the population according to routine examination of autopsy specimens. The peak age at the time of clinical presentation is generally 40-50 years, and they have a female to male ratio of 2:1 (Freda & Post, 1999).

RCCs can remain small, intrasellar, between the anterior and posterior pituitary lobes or anterior to the pituitary stalk, but 60% have some suprasellar extension, whereas the entirely suprasellar cases are rare (Billeci et al., 2005; Freda & Post, 1999; Mukherjee et al., 1997). Rarely, they may be associated with pituitary adenomas. RCCs range in size from a few millimeters to very large, in excess of 4.5 cm.

RCCs may become symptomatic in a minority (only 5-9% of all surgically resected sellar lesions, Aho et al., 2005; Kim et al., 2004), owing to slow cyst growth (due to an imbalance between secretion and reabsorption of cyst content) and/or more rarely intracystic bleeding or infection, leading to symptoms similar to those associated with adenomas (Isono et al., 2001; Billeci et al., 2005; Kim et al., 2004; Spampinato & Castillo, 2005). Less frequently, RCCs can present with aseptic meningitis, abscess, lymphocytic hypophysitis, or intracystic hemorrhage and apoplexy (Kim et al., 2004). RCCs can also cause symptoms in children, potentially resulting in somatic and/or sexual retardation (Zada et al., 2010).

On CT scanning, the cyst density ranges from hypodense, to isodense or to mixed (Billeci et al., 2005), without enhancement. Wall calcification is uncommon (Huang & Castillo, 2005). The lack of calcification is important to differentiate RCCs from craniopharyngiomas (Glezer et al., 2008).

On MRI, RCCs often appear as well circumscribed, centrally located spherical or ovoid, non-calcified cyst lesions of the sellar region (figure 15). The majority of these smooth contoured cysts are unilobar with a diameter ranging between 5-40 mm (Kim et al., 2004; Nishioka et al., 2006; Shin et al., 1999). The center of the lesion is often located in the region of the pars intermedia between the anterior and posterior pituitary gland. The normal pituitary gland may be displaced in any direction by a RCC, including circumferentially if the cyst arises in and remains encased within the gland. After the administration of Gd a thin peripheral rim of enhancement may be seen in a small number of cases and has been attributed to squamous metaplasia, inflammation or deposition of hemosiderin or cholesterol crystals in the cyst wall (Kim et al., 2004). Rim enhancement may be also present when a circumscribed area of pituitary tissue is present peripheral to the cyst.

MR signal intensity of cyst fluid never enhances after contrast administration (Byun et al., 2000), but basal signal demonstrates high variability on T1- and T2-weighted sequences: on T1 images, approximately half are hyperintense and half hypointense, whereas on T2 images, 70% are hyperintense and 30% iso- or hypointense (Billeci et al., 2005). Signal intensity correlates with the heterogeneous nature of the cystic content, which ranges from serous to mucinous (Tominaga et al., 2003). Although most RCCs display a homogeneous signal intensity, up to 40% contain a waxy intracystic nodule, presenting with lower T2 and higher T1 signal intensity than the rest of the cyst, composed of protein and cellular debris that typically fails to enhance following contrast administration and is virtually pathognomonic for the RCC (Byun et al., 2000). Sometimes differentiation from acute hemorrhage can be difficult.

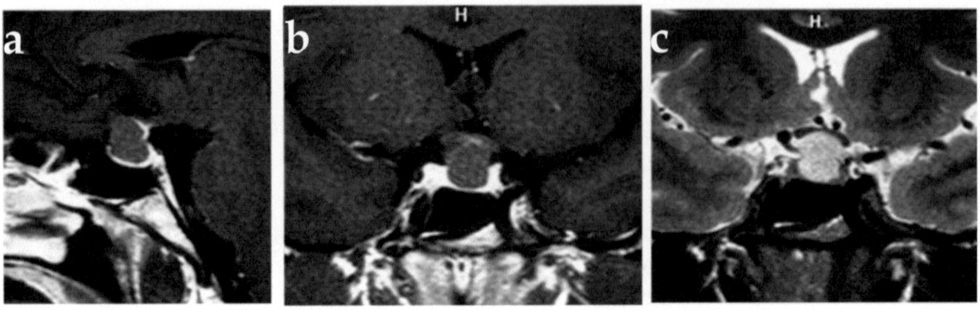


Fig. 15. Rathke's cleft cyst. MRI shows a well-delineated, lobulated, non-enhancing intra and suprasellar cyst, compressing normal pituitary gland and optic chiasm. The lesion is fairly isointense to CSF.

The symptomatic cases are managed by surgery (mostly TSS). A preoperative correct diagnosis is very important for surgical planning because the treatment of symptomatic RCCs differs from that of other sellar masses and usually consists of drainage of the cyst with or without resection of the cystic wall (Freda & Post, 1999; Mukherjee et al. 1997). The endocrine outcome following surgery remains poor, as the reversal of pituitary deficits is not common (Billeci et al., 2005).

### 3.6.2 Epidermoid and dermoid

These are benign tumors (WHO grade I), accounting for less than 2% of all intracranial tumors. They arise as a result of incomplete separation of the neuroectoderm from cutaneous ectoderm, with inclusion of epithelial elements during neural tube closure. They occur in the cerebellopontine angle, pineal region, middle cranial fossa, as well as in the suprasellar region (Kaltsas et al., 2008).

The clinical presentation may be due to local mass effect, but irritative symptoms are more frequent (Freda & Post, 1999).

**Epidermoid** tumors can occur anywhere in the intracranial cavity, but often arise away from the midline in the sellar and parasellar region (Tatagiba et al., 2000). The cyst contains a white cheesy material (keratin) within a thin capsule, lined with squamous epithelium, kerato-hyaline granule layers, and stratifications of "dry" keratin, but without hair follicles or sweat glands. Epidermoids usually present clinically in the 4th and 5th decades, when the cyst has grown by the accumulation of desquamated epithelial cells and exerts mass effect on adjacent structures (Gelabert-Gonzalez, 1998; Harrison et al., 1994). Some reports have also described an uncommon clinical presentation mimicking that of pituitary apoplexy. The cyst content can be caustic to the surrounding tissue, often resulting in hypophysitis, meningitis, or neurological deficits (Zada et al., 2010). The desquamated debris, which contains dead cells, keratin, and cholesterol crystals, appears almost identical to CSF on CT scans, and on T1- and T2-weighted MR images with no enhancement after contrast (Spampinato & Castillo, 2005).

Intracranial **dermoids** present earlier than epidermoids, in the 20-30-year age range, with a male predominance (Gelabert-Gonzalez, 1998; Harrison et al., 1994). They are also lined with squamous epithelium, but beyond desquamated epithelium the cysts contain sebaceous material, and, sometimes, dermal appendages, including hair follicles, teeth, and sweat and sebaceous glands. Unlike epidermoids, dermoids most commonly arise in the midline, usually in the posterior fossa or suprasellar area. Dermoids may break with leakage of tumor contents along the subarachnoid spaces, resulting in recurrent aseptic meningitis that may be a clue to the diagnosis (Smith, 2005). On imaging studies, dermoids are typically not enhancing midline well-circumscribed heterogeneous lesions, that appear hypodense on CT scanning, and heterogeneous and bright on T1-weighted images, owing to fat signal within the tumor, and heterogeneously hyperintense in T2-weighted images (Civit et al., 1999; Freda & Post, 1999; Rennert & Doerfler, 2007; Smith, 2005; Spampinato & Castillo, 2005.). Resection is the choice treatment.

Standard MR imaging cannot be reliably used in all cases to definitively establish a diagnosis of epidermoid or dermoid tumors, on account of their nonspecific features. Diffusion-weighted images can be helpful, typically showing a markedly restricted water diffusion in both (Rennert & Doerfler, 2007). Excision remains the most effective modality of treatment. Radical resection, however, is possible in less than half of cases, due to tight adhesion between the capsule of the lesion and key vascular and nervous structures. Symptomatic regrowth is reported in a quarter of patients.

### 3.6.3 Hamartoma

Hypothalamic hamartoma is a congenital malformation of neuronal origin characterized by disorganized, ectopic foci of gray matter, most frequently arising near the mammillary bodies or tuber cinereum. It is not a true neoplasm, but may increase in size slowly over time (Rennert & Doerfler, 2007). Hypothalamic hamartomas can be classified as parahypothalamic, arising from the floor of the third ventricle, sometimes pedunculated, with minimal or no displacement of the third ventricle, and intrahypothalamic, involving the hypothalamus or surrounded by hypothalamic tissue, with distortion of the third ventricle (Spampinato & Castillo, 2005).

Hamartomas mostly affect children and owing to their small size (usually < 1-2 cm) they produce few symptoms of mass effect (Freeman et al., 2004). Hamartomas usually present with partial and later generalized seizures and mental retardation with speech and behavioral abnormalities. Seizures originate from mechanical compression of the mammillary body and/or abnormal neuronal connections between the hypothalamus and the limbic system (Spampinato & Castillo, 2005). Rarely, but characteristically, the seizures may take the form of spasmodic laughter, so called gelastic seizures (Striano et al., 2005). The parahypothalamic type is typically associated with isosexual precocious puberty, present also in half of the intrahypothalamic type (Debeneix et al., 2001). Precocious puberty may be due to an abnormal secretion of LHRH by the hamartomas (GNRH1 neurons have been demonstrated in the tumor) or to aberrant stimulation by the hamartomas of LHRH-producing hypothalamic neurons (Judge et al., 1977). Occasional asymptomatic cases have been described.

On MRI, the characteristic appearance of hamartoma is a pedunculated, round, non-enhancing mass arising between the pituitary stalk and the mammillary bodies, best seen in coronal and sagittal images, isointense to gray matter on T1-weighted images and isointense or slightly hyperintense on T2-weighted images or FLAIR (Rennert & Doerfler, 2007; Smith, 2005; Spampinato & Castillo, 2005) (figure 16).

There is usually no indication to surgical resection. The only treatment is aimed to control precocious puberty or seizures.

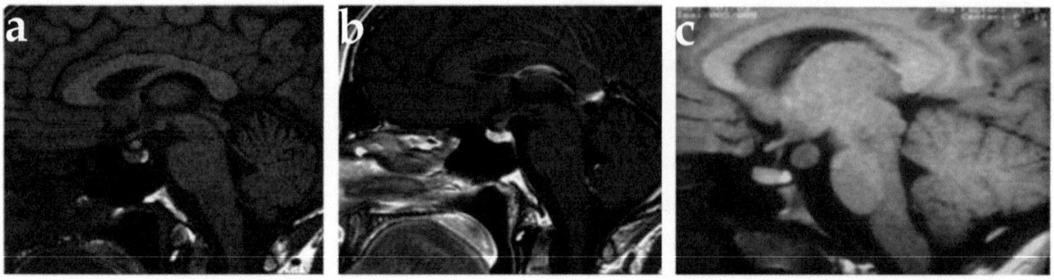


Fig. 16. Hamartomas. MRI on T1 shows a well delineated, nodular, not enhancing mass, isointense to the gray matter lesions, close to the pituitary stalk (a and b) or to the tuber cinereum (c). The pituitary gland appears normal and the "bright spot" in posterior pituitary gland is present.

### 3.6.4 Arachnoid cyst

Arachnoid cysts, arising from herniation of an arachnoid diverticulum through an incomplete diaphragma sellae, may be suprasellar or intrasellar. While the formers usually present in children with symptoms due to local mass effect, the latters are regarded as acquired and may become symptomatic later in life (Rennert & Doerfler, 2007).

Clinical symptoms may include increased intracranial pressure up to hydrocephalus, hormone deficiency, gait disturbance and visual impairment.

On MRI, arachnoid cysts appear as smooth, contoured, well-marginated lesions that are isointense to CSF on all sequences. Calcifications are absent, and these cysts do not exhibit central or rim enhancement with contrast. Although usually indistinguishable from RCCs, they typically displace anteriorly the adeno-hypophysis and posteriorly the infundibulum (Freda & Post, 1999; Nomura et al., 1996.). If needed, surgical treatment (either fenestration or derivation of the cyst) is the only therapeutic option.

### 3.6.5 Pars intermedia cyst

The pars intermedia is rudimentary in humans after fetal life. One or more small cysts (usually < 3 mm), regarded as embryological remnants of the Rathke's cleft, can be seen microscopically in pituitary specimens, coated by a single layer of cuboidal or columnar epithelium and filled with proteinaceous fluid or cellular debris. Occasionally, they can enlarge and become detectable on imaging within the pituitary gland (Spampinato & Castillo, 2005). No treatment is usually necessary.

### 3.6.6 Empty sella syndrome

Empty sella (ES) is defined as a herniation of the subarachnoid space into the sella turcica, associated with stretching of the pituitary stalk and flattening of the pituitary gland against the sellar floor (Giustina et al., 2010).

ES has been classified as either primary (attributed to congenital incomplete formation of the sellar diaphragm and/or increase in intracranial pressure, either unremitting or intermittent) or secondary to any cause, mainly necrosis of pituitary adenoma.

ES is a frequent finding, observed in up one third of subjects either at post-mortem examination or on in vivo imaging, mainly in obese females (De Marinis et al., 2005).

Primary ES may be an incidental radiologic finding. It has been variably associated to different clinical conditions (headache, obesity, hypertension, menstrual disturbances, and endocrine dysfunctions), even though a selection bias cannot be ruled out and a causal relation is far from being demonstrated. Compression of the pituitary gland and stretching of the pituitary stalk may sometimes trigger mild hyperprolactinemia (10-12%) and/or various degrees of hypopituitarism (mostly GH deficiency). DI and panhypopituitarism are very rare (Del Monte et al., 2006). On the other hand ES has been reportedly associated with active Cushing's disease (16%) or acromegaly (5%). Hypopituitarism and visual abnormalities are more frequent in children (where ES is less frequent) than in adults, regardless of the size of residual pituitary gland (Yamada et al., 2005). In this setting it was reported a strong association with defects in specific genes controlling the hypothalamo-pituitary development during fetal life (Naing & Frohman, 2007). CSF rhinorrhea is very uncommon.

On imaging (figure 17) ES can be conventionally classified as complete or partial, when less than half of the sellar cavity is occupied by CSF and pituitary thickness is still > 2 mm (De Marinis et al., 2005). Sellar size in primary ES may be normal or enlarged with symmetrical ballooning, usually without lateral displacing of the pituitary stalk, features allowing the differential diagnosis with secondary ES in which the dorsum sellae is usually posteriorly displaced. The radiological and clinical findings of primary ES generally remain constant over time (De Marinis et al., 2005). Surgical treatment is generally not necessary except when clear-cut campimetric or visual defects are present.

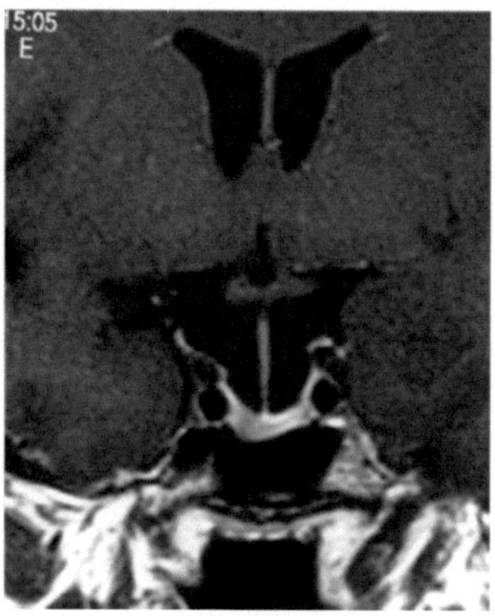


Fig. 17. Empty sella. Contrast-enhanced T1 MRI demonstrates CSF-arachnoid spaces protruding inferiorly through diaphragma sellae, compressing pituitary gland, enlarging sella without eroding sellar floor. The stalk is thin and centrally located.

### 3.7 Granulomatous, infectious and inflammatory lesions

#### 3.7.1 Hypophysitis

Primary hypophysitis is isolated to the gland, whereas secondary hypophysitis is usually associated with an underlying systemic disorder (Lury et al., 2005)(table 2).

| | | |
|---|---|---|
| **Primary** | Lymphocytic autoimmune<br>Granulomatous<br>Xanthomatous | |
| **Secondary** | Infectious | Tubercular<br>Bacterial<br>Fungal<br>Viral |
| | Non infectious | Wegener's<br>Sarcoidosis<br>Crohn's<br>Takayasu's<br>Ruptured cyst |

Table 2. Classification of hypophysitis (modified from Lury et al., 2005)

**Lymphocytic hypophysitis** is an autoimmune disorder frequently (20-25%) associated with other autoimmune diseases, most commonly autoimmune thyroiditis (about 75%), but also adrenalitis, ovarian failure, atrophic gastritis, pernicious anemia, or systemic lupus erythematosus.

It occurs mostly in women, and in 60% to 70% of cases it presents in the last two trimesters of pregnancy or until 6 months after delivery (Caturegli et al., 2005).

Headache and visual disturbances due to compression of adjacent structures are the most common (56-70%), and usually the initial, complaints. Other common symptoms are due to partial or complete deficiency of anterior pituitary hormones (66–97%). Secretion of ACTH is the most frequently affected, reported in 60–65% of cases (Rivera, 2006). In order of frequency, secretion of TSH (47%), gonadotropins (42.2%), and GH (36.7%) are then impaired. PRL may be increased (38%) or decreased (33.7%), with inability to lactate. It is worth underlining that hypopituitarism often appears disproportionate to the extent of changes on pituitary MRI, especially when compared with what usually happens in pituitary adenomas. DI (50%) corresponds well to pituitary stalk thickening on MRI and can be attributed either to direct immune destruction or to compression of the posterior lobe and infundibular stem (PRL levels are increased in the latter case) (Gutenberg et al., 2006). Occasionally presentation can resemble apoplexy (Dan et al., 2002).

The typical (95% of cases) MRI findings of lymphocytic hypophysitis include a symmetric enlargement of a homogeneous pituitary gland, a thickened stalk (rarely displaced, with a greater diameter > 3.5 mm at the level of the median eminence, and loss of the normal smooth tapering), a non specific loss of bright spot, and an usually intact sellar floor (Gutenberg et al., 2006, Lury et al., 2005)(figure 18). The lesion is contrast enhancing (70%)(Heinze & Bercu, 1997), often with suprasellar extension (62–75%) in some cases into the hypothalamus (Freda & Post, 1999). A triangular enhancement of the anterior pituitary (reflecting extension of the process towards the pituitary stalk) along with enhancement of the diaphragma sellae (possibly reflecting inflammation by contiguity), although described in a few cases only, and a tongue-like extension towards the hypothalamus (Honegger et al., 1997) seem to be particularly specific of lymphocytic hypophysitis. A ring-like enhancement is consistent with central necrosis (Rivera, 2006), a feature that may account for some cases of sterile pituitary abscesses (see below) in which no species are cultured and only inflammation is seen (Perez-Nunez et al., 2005). Dynamic MRI documented a hypothalamic-pituitary vasculopathy in some cases (Sato et al., 1998), showing delayed enhancement of the whole pituitary and doubling of peak time of posterior pituitary enhancement.

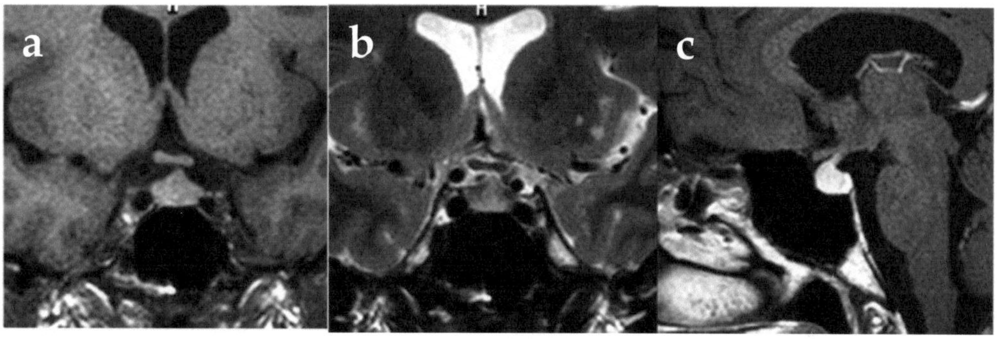


Fig. 18. Lymphocytic hypophysitis in a young female a few weeks after delivery. MRI on coronal (a) and sagittal (c) T1 shows an enlarged, uniformly enhancing pituitary gland and infundibulum. On coronal T2 (b) the characteristic central, triangular signal hyperintensity is shown.

Although the autoimmune nature of lymphocytic hypophysitis is well established, the pathogenic autoantigens targeted in this disease remain to be identified (Caturegli et al., 2005). PRL cell autoantibodies were the first to be detected, followed by antibodies to other pituitary hormone-producing cells (often, however, with low sensitivity and specificity) (Carpinteri et al., 2009). The role of anti-pituitary antibodies in this disease has yet to be clarified (Bellastella et al., 2003). Currently, a reliable serologic test based on implicated autoantibodies is not yet available for routine diagnostic purposes (Caturegli, 2007). Consequently, a diagnosis of lymphocytic hypophysitis can only be achieved with certainty by histological examination of the pituitary gland. Anyway, at present, approximately 40% of patients undergo surgery for a presumptive diagnosis of pituitary adenoma (Gutenberg et al., 2009). A diffuse polyclonal lymphocytic infiltration with predominance of T cells, particularly CD4 cells, is characteristic. Scattered plasma cells, a few eosinophils, edema, and fibrosis replacing pituitary acini are also commonly present. Electron microscopy has shown interdigitation of inflammatory cells with pituicytes and the presence of lysosomal bodies and oncocytic changes in some pituitary cells (Rivera, 2006).

The natural history of lymphocytic hypophysitis is thought to progress from inflammation (with enlargement of the gland corresponding to the period of mass-effect symptoms and often, subclinical hormone deficits) to fibrosis and subsequent tissue destruction and atrophy associated with permanent hypopituitarism, which can later present as an ES in imaging studies (Bellastella et al., 2003). In some cases the course of the disease can be rather insidious, and relapsing remitting cases have been reported (Matta et al., 2002). The inflammatory process can also be self-limited, spontaneously or with conservative corticosteroid and hormone replacement therapy, and radiological follow-up can show regression of the sellar mass in about 2 years. However, complete or partial DI may be permanent, probably because of neuronal destruction (Caturegli et al., 2005; Rivera, 2006).

Idiopathic **granulomatous hypophysitis**, a rare chronic inflammatory condition, is distinct from secondary granulomatous hypophysitis associated with systemic disorders (Caturegli et al., 2005). It is not yet definitely established whether lymphocytic and idiopathic granulomatous hypophysitis are different diseases or opposite ends of the spectrum of the same disease, with fibrosis representing the end stage of the inflammatory process (Flanagan et al., 2002). Granulomatous hypophysitis however lacks the key epidemiological features that are present in lymphocytic hypophysitis, such as the female preponderance, the occasional spontaneous resolution, the association with pregnancy and other autoimmune diseases (Caturegli et al., 2005; Cheung et al., 2001).

Granulomatous hypophysitis usually occurs in older patients and is characterized histologically by multinucleated giant cells, epithelioid histiocytes and true granulomas (Rivera, 2006).

Clinical presentation consists of headache, visual disturbances, nausea, vomiting, DI, and hyperprolactinemia, and pituitary function is severely impaired (Caturegli et al., 2005; Cheung et al., 2001).

The striking CT features are an intrasellar mass with cystic areas and ring enhancement. On MRI, the diffusely enlarged gland is usually isointense to gray matter on T1-weighted images (but also hyperintense due to hemorrhage) and heterogeneous on T2 sequences, with abnormal thickening of the infundibulum. Contrast enhancement is frequently homogeneous, occasionally extending to the optic chiasm, but cystic areas with ring enhancement may be seen. Findings suggesting inflammation, such as linear enhancement of the dura, sphenoid mucosal thickening, and adjacent bone marrow abnormality, may be also observed. These findings are nonspecific and indistinguishable from those caused by other neoplastic or inflammatory pituitary processes (Lury et al., 2005).

**Xanthomatous hypophysitis** is rare and can be considered an inflammatory response to ruptured cysts components (Glezer et al., 2008; Roncaroli et al., 2004). Cystic-like areas of liquefaction, infiltrated by lipid-rich foamy histiocytes and lymphocytes, are present in the pituitary gland (Caturegli et al., 2005).

Immunosuppression with high-dose glucocorticoids or other drugs, such as azathioprine, methotrexate and cyclosporin, have been reported effective in reducing pituitary mass, and improving pituitary function and DI (Rivera, 2006).

### 3.7.2 Tuberculosis

Pituitary tuberculosis is rare. It may present with meningitis, a dense plaque-like exudate mostly at the base of the brain, involving the sellar and parasellar region, or as a tuberculoma (suprasellar or intrasellar). Signs of mass lesion, and possible impairment of hypothalamic or pituitary function and involvement of the optic chiasm may be present (Domingues et al., 2002; Freda & Post, 1999).

Although most patients with hypothalamic-pituitary tuberculosis have signs of active tuberculosis elsewhere, this is not invariably true. As a result, the diagnosis of a tuberculoma in the region may, in some cases, be made only histologically after TSS (Freda & Post, 1999).

Imaging studies show involvement of pituitary fossa, along with thickening of the pituitary stalk. Simultaneous involvement of the clivus may be an additional unspecific feature. MRI shows a hypointense pituitary mass on T2, with or without an absent posterior pituitary bright signal. Tubercular pituitary abscesses appear isointense to hypointense on T1 (occasionally hyperintense owing to high protein/lipid content) and hyperintense on T2. Tuberculomas show strong enhancement with contrast and are often accompanied by thickening and enhancement of the stalk and dura. These signal characteristics are nonspecific and overlap those of pituitary adenomas. Tubercular abscesses may show peripheral contrast enhancement and adjacent meningeal enhancement on contrast-enhanced MR (Lury et al., 2005).

### 3.7.3 Other infections

Fungal (Histoplasma, Coccidioides, Cryptococcus, Candida, and Aspergillus), parasitic (Cysticercus) and opportunistic (Toxoplasma, Pneumocystis Carinii, Mucor) infections may rarely develop in the sellar region, particularly in immunocompromised patients, and may simulate a pituitary adenoma (Freda & Post, 1999).

**Aspergillosis** is a mycotic disease of paranasal sinuses, frequently extending into the orbital region, or invading the skull base. The organism has a typical tropism for vascular intima-media layer, thus enabling hematogenous spreading to basal nuclei, occasionally until hemorrhagic vasculitis. The invasive forms are usually observed in immunocompromised patients (Pinzer et al., 2006). Aspergillosis of the sphenoid sinus extending into the sellar region and simulating a pituitary tumor is extremely rare, but it was reported even in immunocompetent patients. Imaging studies show lesions moderately hyperintense on T1, hypointense on T2 and brightly enhancing. The diagnosis can be achieved only as a result of surgical exploration of the invaded areas (Carpinteri et al., 2009).

Another rare fungal infection to be considered when evaluating patients with a pituitary mass and ophthalmoplegia is **coccidioidomycosis**, where unilateral ophthalmoplegia may acutely appear and radiological studies show a mass lesion involving the pituitary gland and cavernous sinus (Scanarini et al., 1991).

### 3.7.4 Sarcoidosis

Sarcoidosis involves the CNS in 5-15% of patients with this disease. Neurosarcoidosis is usually associated with systemic sarcoidosis: only 5% of cases have no disease elsewhere. In rare cases neurosarcoidosis is the initial or only sign of the disease (Freda & Post, 1999).

Neurosarcoidosis has a predilection for the hypothalamic-pituitary region and therefore DI and headache are common, hyperprolactinemia and cranial neuropathy may be present.

On MR imaging, the intraparenchymal, meningeal, or sellar lesions of sarcoidosis appear isointense on T1 and variable on T2, and are contrast-enhancing. The stalk may be thickened and also enhancing. Very rarely a cystic appearance has been reported. Leptomeningeal involvement in the region of the hypothalamus and pituitary infundibulum may be seen as an isolated finding or associated with involvement of the basilar leptomeninges (Lury et al., 2004).

When neurosarcoidosis is suspected, CSF examination is indicated, evaluating angiotensin-converting enzyme, and cytology. In some patients, the diagnosis is made only by biopsy of the granulomatous lesion (Glezer et al., 2008).

Corticosteroids are the therapy of choice, but various adjuvant immunosuppressant drugs have been reportedly employed (Glezer et al., 2008).

### 3.7.5 Other systemic diseases

Pituitary granulomatous involvement has been described in isolated case reports with other systemic diseases (Carpinteri et al., 2009):

- Wegener's granulomatosis, with central DI usually occurring after pulmonary or kidney lesions in less than 1% of affected subjects (Goyal et al., 2000);
- Erdheim-Chester disease, with DI, hypopituitarism and hyperprolactinemia, cerebellar syndromes, orbital lesions, and extra-axial masses involving the dura (Kovacs et al., 2004);
- Crohn's disease, with hypopituitarism, progressive bitemporal haemianopsia and intrasellar mass (de Bruin et al., 1991);
- Takayasu's disease, with pituitary mass, hypopituitarism and DI (Toth et al., 1996);
- Cogan's syndrome, with pituitary enlargement, DI and secondary hypothyroidism (Kanatani et al., 1991).

### 3.7.6 Pituitary abscess

Pituitary abscess is a rare potentially life-threatening disease, occurring in all age groups, estimated to account for less than 1% of clinically apparent pituitary disease and 0.27% of pituitary surgeries (Famini et al., 2011; Vates et al., 2001).

In most cases, it develops from direct extension of an adjacent infection (sphenoid sinus meningitis, contaminated CSF fistula or very rarely cavernous sinus thrombophlebitis) or is caused by hematogenous seeding. The infection source cannot occasionally be identified (Glezer et al., 2008).

Abscess can be primary (in two thirds of the cases), occurring in a previously normal pituitary, or secondary, arising in glands that harbor a pre-existing lesion (adenoma, craniopharyngioma or RCC). Other risk factors include an underlying immunocompromised condition, previous pituitary surgery, CSF rhinorrhea with recurrent meningitis and irradiation of the pituitary gland (Freda & Post, 1999; Liu et al., 2011).

Isolated organisms are typically gram-positive cocci; fungi, such as Aspergillus, Cryptococcus or Candida Albicans, and other organisms (Mycobacterium Tuberculosis, Toxoplasma, Clostridium Difficile, Staphylococcus or Pseudomonas) have been reported as well (Famini et al., 2011; Freda & Post, 1999; Glezer et al., 2008; Liu et al., 2011). In at least half of cases pituitary abscesses are reported to be sterile.

Fever, meningism and leukocytosis have been reported in one third of cases only, in spite of the presence of meningitis along with the abscess in approximately 60% of patients. Most patients present with a chronic and indolent course with few infective manifestations, thus mimicking a pituitary tumor (Glezer et al., 2008). DI and headache are the most common presenting complaint (70%) (Fuyi et al., 2010), and over half of the patients complain of visual disturbances. Most patients (85%) have partial or total hypopituitarism (including PRL deficiency). In a recently reported series (Fuyi et al., 2010) the median time between the onset of symptoms and diagnosis was 6 months. Mortality can reach 30% to 50% of cases when it is complicated by meningitis (Glezer et al., 2008).

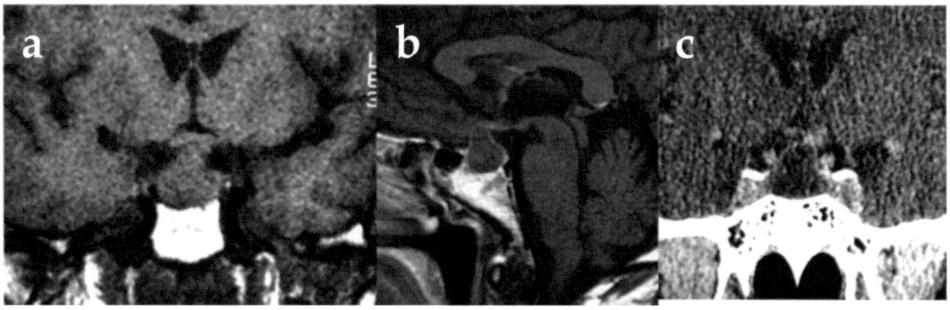


Fig. 19. Pituitary abscess in a patient with staphylococcal sepsis. Coronal T1 (a) and sagittal T1 enhanced (b) MRI shows an intra/suprasellar cystic lesion, isointense to the brain, with thin regular rim enhancement. Coronal CT after contrast (c) depicts a homogeneously hypodense lesion, with rim enhancement, sparing cavernous sinus. Note non pneumatized sphenoidal sinus.

The typical MR features of an abscess are the presence of a round cystic or partially cystic sellar mass that appears as hypo- or isointense on T1 and hyper- or isointense on T2, with an enhanced rim after Gd injection and a central cavity that is isointense to the brain (Freda & Post, 1999; Glezer et al., 2008; Rennert & Doerfler, 2007)(figure 19). The sella may be enlarged and, occasionally, extensively eroded.

Surgical resection and appropriate long-term antibiotic coverage is the choice treatment. Abscesses may recur requiring further surgery.

### 3.7.7 Sphenoid sinus mucocele

Primary mucocele is a congenital mucous retention cyst expansion, whereas the commoner secondary mucocele results from a chronic obstruction of the sinus that leads to accumulation and dehydration of secretions. Predisposing factors are inflammatory conditions, tumors, trauma, and previous surgery in the sphenoid sinus.

There is no specific age preponderance.

Mucocele can rarely extend to the pituitary fossa, parasellar and suprasellar regions, nasopharynx, orbits, clivus, or ethmoid air cells. A cystic accumulation of secretions expands and erodes the sinus walls, eventually compressing surrounding structures such as the cavernous sinus, the pituitary gland, the cranial nerves I through VI, and the carotid arteries. Sphenoid mucoceles usually evolve over a long period, often years, with nonspecific, usually severe, headaches and atypical facial pain with paresthesias secondary to trigeminal nerve irritation. Visual loss owing to direct nerve compression by the mass or from scarring caused by an inflammatory reaction is usually slowly progressive but may be suddenly worsened by vascular compromise of the optic nerve. Optic neuropathy is most often unilateral, and visual field deficits are typically absent. Exophthalmos is present in about half of patients. Diplopia due to dysfunction of the third and, less often, the fourth cranial nerves is common (Freda & Post, 1999). Hypopituitarism is less common.

On CT, a non-destructive mass causing a thinning and bulging of the bone sinus walls may be seen, and the sellar contents can mimic a para- or suprasellar mass.

MRI appearance is variable. Expansion of the sphenoid sinus, usually with intact but occasionally eroded walls, and prominent opacification of its content is present in most patients, most often with a high signal on T2 images and, because of its high protein content, a homogeneously hyperintense T1 signal. After contrast administration it appears a thin regular rim of enhancement (Akan et al., 2004; Glezer et al., 2008; Rennert & Doerfler, 2007) (figure 20).

Surgical drainage is indicated only when the lesion is highly symptomatic or erosive of bone.

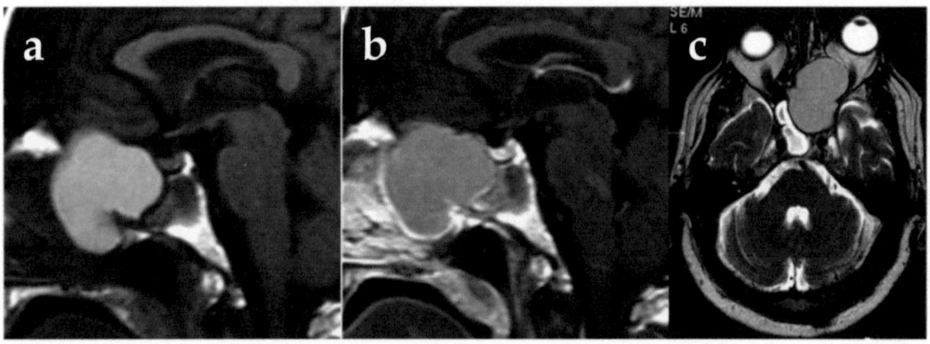


Fig. 20. Mucocele. Sagittal T1 (a) and axial T2 (c) MR show a cystic mass, filling and enlarging the left sphenoid sinus recess. The lesion appears homogeneously hyperintense on T1 (a) with rim enhancement (b). Chronic sinusitis is evident in the right sphenoidal recess.

### 3.8 Vascular lesions

#### 3.8.1 Aneurysm

Aneurysms of the sellar region account for approximately 10% of all cerebral aneurysms. They usually originate from the cavernous, infraclinoid, or supraclinoid internal carotid arteries, but also from the anterior or posterior communicating arteries, or the ophthalmic arteries. Aneurysms in the parasellar and suprasellar region may sometimes reach great dimensions and compress the optic nerve, chiasm, or both and produce signs of visual loss. They may also extend into the sella, causing direct pituitary compression and thus modest hyperprolactinemia and hypopituitarism (Freda & Post, 1999).

Intrasellar aneurysm can mimic other parenchymal masses and imaging is essential to distinguish among the different disorders before surgery. If within the sella, aneurysms are usually eccentrically located. Their appearance is mostly affected by the amount of calcification and thrombosis present within the aneurysm. Asymmetric enlargement and destruction of the sella turcica may occur in association with a giant aneurysm. CT cannot reliably distinguish an aneurysm from other pituitary lesion, but very intense, homogeneous blush with contrast may suggest an aneurysm (Rennert & Doerfler, 2007). On conventional spin-echo MRI, the aneurysm is contiguous to vessels, has well-defined margins, and appears heterogeneous (Glezer et al., 2008). Aneurysmatic sack may appear as a flow void or alternatively as a brightly enhancing spot corresponding to residual true lumen, according to vascular flow velocity. There may be variable amount of thrombosed lumen, which may contain crescent or ring shaped layers of different aged blood products or fibrosis, appearing heterogeneous on T1 and mostly hypointense on T2. There may be rings or arcs of calcification, especially at the periphery. A rim of calcification in the wall is characteristic but may resemble a craniopharyngioma.

There have been many case reports of aneurysms associated with pituitary adenomas (Smith, 2005). In any case, if an aneurism is suspected, angiography should be immediately performed. Angio-CT, angio-MRI or digital subtraction angiography are all suitable. The last is the gold standard because it allows concomitant treatment by embolization if needed.

### 3.8.2 Cavernous sinus thrombosis

Thrombosis of the cavernous sinus is a very rare condition, often secondary to iatrogenic or septic etiologies. On MRI and CT, enlargement of the cavernous sinus with internal filling defects and incomplete enhancement of the sinus may be noted. MRI shows high signal thrombus within the cavernous sinus. Additionally, periorbital edema, exophthalmos or dilatation of the superior ophthalmic vein can occur (Rennert & Doerfler, 2007).

### 3.9 Collision lesions

Collision tumors represent two morphologically different tumors attached to each other. Extending this definition, collision lesions refer to histologically different pathological conditions found in combination and may include neoplastic, vascular, congenital, or infectious/inflammatory lesions. The presence of a collision sellar lesion represents a very uncommon event. Most include a pituitary adenoma coexisting with a second lesion like a craniopharyngioma, arachnoid cyst, epidermoid cyst, lymphocytic or granulomatous hypophysitis, as well as sarcoidosis within a pituitary adenoma and metastatic carcinoma to a pituitary adenoma (Koutoroisiu et al., 2010)(figure 21).

Multiple pituitary adenomas are rarely encountered in patients undergoing pituitary surgery. In a large surgical cohort of more than 3,000 resected pituitary adenomas the percentage of double adenomas was 0.37% (Kontogeorgos et al., 1992). The same authors in the largest ever-reported autopsy study of more than 9,300 pituitary glands, identified 20 cases of multiple adenomas (Kontogeorgos et al., 1991).

Double pituitary adenomas can be divided into contiguous and clearly separated double tumors. Most contiguous tumors are surgically removed as one tumor and the co-existence of different adenoma types is established by immunohistochemical and electron microscopic examination of the surgical specimen (Kim et al., 2004). The most common hormone-active adenoma identified in surgical series of double adenomas is GH-secreting, but also ACTHomas are reported.

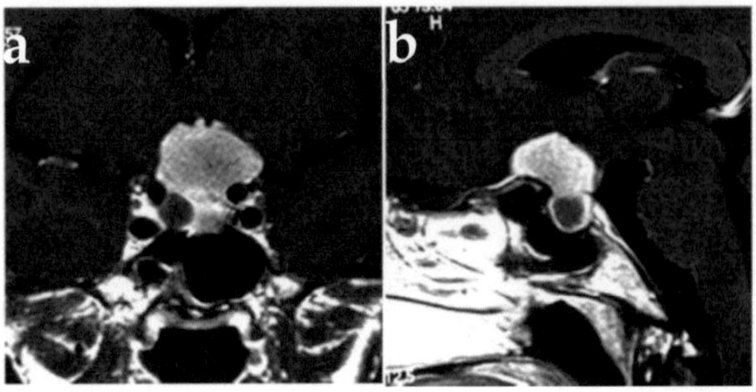


Fig. 21. T1 enhanced MR shows an intrasellar nodular, relatively hypointense, right lesion, characteristic for a pituitary microadenoma, close to a suprasellar mass, with features of diaphragma sellae meningioma.

## 4. Differential diagnosis

The differential diagnosis among the various neoplastic and non-neoplastic processes potentially involving the parasellar region is critical in the work-up of patients. It should always be performed jointly by the neurosurgeon, the endocrinologist and the neuroradiologist. The neuroradiological finding of a sellar mass may not always mean the presence of a pituitary adenoma, even though these are the great majority, and the correct screening among alternative diagnoses is crucial for an appropriate therapeutic planning. Some neoplasms should indeed not undergo surgery, unless requiring urgent decompression. A correct preoperative diagnosis allows to select the necessary treatment and eventually the correct surgical approach (trans-cranial vs. trans-sphenoidal) and strategy. Combining epidemiological, clinical and imaging data will allow progressively focusing of diagnosis.

### 4.1 Clinical data

Headache and hormone dysfunction are not always helpful in the differential diagnosis of a sellar suprasellar lesion (Valassi et al., 2010), unless hypersecretory syndrome occurs. The neuro-ophthalmological examination is the basic investigation that allows to raise suspicion of a lesion, but it is of no practical value to establish a diagnosis of nature of a para-suprasellar lesion.

Some classical campimetric defects are related to the location of a given lesion and its relationships with the visual apparatus (Freda & Post, 1999):

- Lesions extending over the sella, such as adenomas and RCCs, produce the typical bitemporal hemianopsia due to chiasmal compression from below;
- Lesions arising in the suprasellar area, such as meningiomas, can present with bitemporal field cuts of the classic superior chiasmal compression variety;
- Lesions anterior to the chiasm, such as meningiomas of the optic nerve sheath, can produce unilateral visual loss;
- Lesions compressing the visual system more posteriorly along the optic tract, such as meningiomas or aneurysms, provoke homonymous hemianopsia.

DI at presentation is highly atypical for pituitary adenomas, occurring in 0.01-3% vs. 11% of non-adenomatous lesions according to a recent overview (Famini et al., 2011). In our personal experience DI is associated to pituitary adenomas mainly when apoplexy occurs. DI should always lead to consider alternative diagnoses. Craniopharyngioma, metastases, and sarcoidosis are the most frequent. Vasopressin deficiency may be partial or transient because of spontaneous regeneration (Freda & Post, 1999). DI may apparently improve in some patients when hypoadrenalism develops.

The acute onset of cranial neuropathy often accompanies pituitary apoplexy, but the presence of ophtalmoplegia at presentation of a sellar/parasellar mass is suggestive of alternative etiologies (Freda & Post, 1999).

Hypothalamic dysfunctions may be observed in large tumors (exceptionally rare in adenomas) leading to poor development and sexual immaturity in children and disruption of the control of appetite in adults (Freda & Post, 1999).

### 4.2 Imaging data

Intratumoral calcifications are observed mainly in craniopharyngiomas, but also in meningiomas, teratomas, gliomas, cartilagineous tumors, and even in aneurysms and pituitary adenomas (Freda & Post, 1999).

Cartilagineous tumors and metastases typically destroy the bone of the skull base.

An enlarged pituitary stalk can be found in different diseases (hypophysitis, germinoma, lymphoma, tuberculosis, sarcoidosis, or LCH) (Gutenberg et al., 2009).

Neoplasms in the clival region include chordoma, chondrosarcoma, hemangiopericytoma, meningioma, lymphoma, plasmocytoma, paraganglioma, and metastasis (Rennert & Doerfler, 2007).

Location (midline vs. not midline) and consistence (mostly solid vs. cystic) of the lesion are among the key imaging data to consider (table 3).

| | **Midline** | **Away from midline** |
|---|---|---|
| **Solid** | Adenoma<br>Hypophysitis<br>Germinoma<br>Lymphoma<br>Chordoma<br>Metastases | Meningioma<br>Chondroma<br>Schwannoma<br>Glioma<br>LCH<br>(Metastases) |
| **Cystic** | Craniopharyngioma<br>RCC<br>Arachnoid cyst<br>Abscess | (Abscess)<br>Mycoses |

Table 3. Classification of lesions according to consistence and location

Tables 4 and 5 show synoptically key features of the different parasellar lesions (data are derived from the following references: Carpinteri et al., 2009; Famini et al., 2011; Freda & Post, 1999; Glezer et al., 2008; Huang & Castillo, 2005; Kaltsas et al., 2008; Karavitaki et al., 2006; Lury, 2005; Rennert & Doerfler, 2007; Ruscalleda, 2005; Smith, 2005; Spampinato & Castillo 2005).

| Lesion | Midline | Location | Age | Sex | DI* | Hypopit° | HypoPRL§ | CN palsies# |
|---|---|---|---|---|---|---|---|---|
| **NFPA** | yes | centered on sella | most > 40 yrs | | very rare | possible | no | rare |
| **Pituitary apoplexy** | yes | centered on sella | 30-50 yrs | | rare | frequent | yes | frequent |
| **Pituitary carcinoma** | yes | not different from adenoma except for metastases | | | | | | |
| **Pituitocytoma** | yes | intrasellar and/or suprasellar or stalk | young & middle aged | F | rare | frequent | | |
| **Choristoma** | yes | intrasellar and suprasellar | 40-50 yrs | | rare | common | | |
| **Germ cell tumor** | yes | suprasellar (+ pineal) or intrasellar | children and adolescents | | frequent | frequent | | common |
| **Lymphoma** | yes | intrasellar or suprasellar, cavernous sinus | 50-70 yrs | M | common | frequent | | |
| **Chordoma** | yes | clivus | 30-50 yrs | | | uncommon | | frequent |
| **Gangliocytoma** | yes | intrasellar and suprasellar | adult | F | | no (hyper$^+$) | | |
| **Metastases** | yes/not | intrasellar and/or suprasellar or stalk | usually elderly | | frequent | common | | common |
| **Hypophysitis** | yes | intrasellar and stalk | near pregnancy if lymphocytic, elderly if granulomatous | | common | frequent | possible | rare |
| **Hamartoma** | yes | parasellar or intrahypothalamic, tuber cinereum | childhood | | | | | |
| **Craniopharyngioma** | yes | suprasellar and/or intrasellar | 5-14 yrs and 50-74 yrs | | frequent | common | | possible |
| **Rathke's cleft cyst** | yes | intrasellar (and suprasellar) | 40-50 yrs | F | rare | possible | | |
| **Dermoid** | yes | suprasellar (posterior fossa) | 20-30 yrs | | | | | |
| **Abscess** | yes | intrasellar | | | frequent | frequent | yes | |
| **Arachnoid cyst** | yes | suprasellar | childhood | | | common | | |
| **Mucocele** | yes | sphenoid sinus extending in parasellar and suprasellar, nasopharynx, orbits, clivus, or ethmoid | | | | uncommon | | common |
| **Glioma** | no | optic nerve/hypothalamus | childhood or young adult/ hypothalamic in early life | | | | | |
| **Langerhans' cell hystiocytosis** | no | hypothalamus | < 15 yrs in 2/3 | M | frequent | common | | |
| **Meningioma** | no | dura at any site | 50-70 yrs | F | | common | | infrequent |
| **Tuberculoma** | no | intrasellar or suprasellar (paranasal sinuses, clivus) | | | | | | |
| **Chondrosarcoma** | no | petro-occipital fissure | | | | | | |
| **Schwannoma** | no | cavernous sinus | | | | | | |
| **Epidermoid** | no | intrasellar and parasellar | 30-50 yrs | | | | | |
| **Aneurysm** | no | cavernous sinus | | | | possible | | |
| **Lipoma** | yes | surface of the infundibulum, floor of the 3$^{rd}$ ventricle or adjacent cranial nerves | | | | | | |
| **Sarcoidosis** | yes | suprasellar | | | common | | | possible |

* Diabetes insipidus; ° Hypopituitarism; § PRL deficiency; # Cranial nerve palsies; $^+$ Hypersecretions

Table 4. Clinical aspects of the different parasellar lesions

| Lesion | Consistency | CT | CT contrast enhancement | Calcification | T1-weighed | T2-weighed | MR contrast enhancement | Notes |
|---|---|---|---|---|---|---|---|---|
| **NFPA** | solid (cystic) | isodense | moderate | rare | isointense (hyperintense with level if hemorrhagic) | isointense (hypointense if fibrotic) | heterogeneous, normal pituitary usually displaced laterally or upwards | nodular expansion towards suprasellar cisterns |
| **Pituitary apoplexy** | solid (mixed) | possible SAH, hyperdense | minimal or no | no | acute: hypointense (ischemic); isointense then hyperintense (hemorrhagic) | acute: hyperintense (ischemic); iso- hypointense (hemorrhagic) | rim | DWI: restricted diffusion |
| **Pituitary carcinoma** | not different from adenoma except for metastases | | | | | | | |
| **Pituitocytoma** | solid | hyperdense | strong | rare | isointense to hypointense | hypointense to isointense | strong, homogeneous | |
| **Choristoma** | solid | hyperdense | strong | possible | isointense | isointense | yes | |
| **Germ cell tumor** | solid (teratoma mixed) | isodense or hyperdense | strong | frequent in teratoma | Isointense or hyperintense | isointense/ hypointense | strong | precocious puberty (alfaFP, hCG) DWI: restricted diffusion |
| **Lymphoma** | solid | isodense or hyperdense | strong | no | isointense or slightly hypointense | isointense or slightly hypointense | yes | DWI: restricted diffusion |
| **Chordoma** | solid | bone destruction; iso to hyperdense | heterogeneous | common, diffuse | isointense to hypointense with septations and necrosis | hyperintense | heterogeneous | |
| **Gangliocytoma** | solid | isodense | moderate | rare | as macroadenomas | as macroadenoma | yes | acromegaly, Cushing's |
| **Metastases** | solid | hyperdense or isodense or hypodense | yes | rare | hypointense to hyperintense | hyperintense | yes | dumbbell |
| **Lymphocytic hypophysitis** | solid | hypodense | yes | no | hypointense | hyperintense | yes | symmetric enlargement, thickened stalk |
| **Granulomatous hypophysitis** | solid and cystic | hypodense to isodense | ring | no | isointense (hyperintense if blood) | heterogeneous | homogeneous, ring in cystic areas | thickened stalk |
| **Hamartoma** | solid | isodense | no | no | pedunculated isointense | isointense or slightly hyperintense | no | precocious puberty, seizures |
| **Cranio-pharyngioma** | cystic (solid) | heterogeneous | yes (solid portions) | frequent, nodular o curvilinear | solid: isointense or hypointense or mottled; cystic: hyperintense without levels | solid: hypointense or hyperintense; cystic: hyperintense or hypointense | strong in cyst walls, heterogeneous in nodular portions | normal pituitary usually displaced downwards, rare expansion in cavernous sinus |
| **Rathke's cleft cyst** | cystic | hypodense, isodense, mixed | no | uncommon | hypointense rarely iso-hyperintense | hyperintense (isointense), with small hypointense nodules | rim only if inflammatory, normal pituitary usually displaced downwards | meningitis |
| **Dermoid** | cystic | hypo-isodense | no | focal | hyperintense, heterogeneous | hyperintense | no | meningitis |

| Lesion | Consistency | CT | CT contrast enhancement | Calcification | T1-weighed | T2-weighed | MR contrast enhancement | Notes |
|---|---|---|---|---|---|---|---|---|
| **Abscess** | cystic | hypodense, sellar enlargement and erosion | rim | no | hypointense or isointense | hyperintense or isointense | rim (thick wall) | |
| **Arachnoid cyst** | cystic | hypodense | no | no | isointense to CSF | isointense to CSF | no | |
| **Mucocele** | cystic | hypodense to isodense, thinning and bulging of the bone sinus walls | rim | no | hyperintense | hyperintense | rim | facial pain and paresthesias |
| **Glioma** | solid | hypodense-isodense | variable | rare | hypointense; young adult isointense or hypointense; hypothalamic hypointense-isointense | hyperintense; hypothalamic iso-hyperintense | variable | proptosis, NF |
| **Langerhans' cell hystiocytosis** | solid | isodense | yes | no | isointense | hyperintense | bright, homogeneous of stalk | thickened stalk |
| **Meningioma** | solid | isodense or slightly hyperdense, hyperostosis | homogeneous, strong | common | isointense, very homogeneous | isointense (hyperintense or hypointense) | strong | carotid narrowing, normal pituitary usually displaced downwards, NF, ionizing radiation, increase during pregnancy |
| **Tuberculoma** | solid | isodense | yes | rare | isointense | hypointense | yes | thickened stalk |
| **Chondro-sarcoma** | solid | isodense to hyperdense, bone destruction | variable | yes | isointense to hypointense | hyperintense | heterogeneous | |
| **Schwannoma** | solid | isodense | yes | no | hypointense | hyperintense | intense, homogeneous | |
| **Epidermoid** | cystic | as CSF | no | no | as CSF | as CSF | no | DWI: restricted diffusion |
| **Aneurysm** | mixed | isodense to hyperdense | intense homogeneous blush | rim | mixed, hypointense | mixed, hypointense | bright, homogeneous | flow void |
| **Lipoma** | solid | hypodense | no | rim | hyperintense | hypointense | no | disappear with fat suppression |
| **Sarcoidosis** | solid | isodense to hyperdense | yes | no | isointense | isointense to hypointense | yes | thickened stalk |

SAH = subarachnoid hemorrhage; DWI: diffusion weighed images; NF = neurofibromatosis

Table 5. Imaging of the different parasellar lesions: for each lesion the most common picture is reported

### 4.2.1 Solid lesions

Sellar enlargement is typical but not exclusive of macroadenomas because it can occur in half of non-adenomatous masses of the region, such as meningiomas, craniopharyngiomas, empty sella, and RCCs. Therefore, only the lack of sellar enlargement is helpful in diagnosis, pointing to a non-pituitary lesion (Freda & Post, 1999).

Bone erosion or invasion is not particularly helpful in the differential diagnosis because it can be seen with adenomas, chordomas, intracavernous aneurysms, meningiomas of the middle fossa, RCCs, arachnoid diverticula, and elevated intracranial pressure from any source (Freda & Post, 1999).

The sudden onset of severe headache and ophthalmoplegia should always raise the suspicion of pituitary apoplexy. Since the presence of a pre-existing pituitary tumor is mostly unknown, diagnostic difficulties and delays can result in significant morbidity and rarely mortality. The diagnosis can often be difficult because patients may present in different clinical facilities, without immediate access to a skilled neuroradiologist. Clinical characteristics are not of help most of the times. On imaging CT and MRI will demonstrate an intrasellar mass and signs of bleeding or ischemia. Attention must be paid to the reported concomitant occurrence of pituitary adenomas and cerebral aneurysms (in 7%), requiring angiography. It must be pointed out that neuroradiology (CT scan and then MRI) is nowadays mandatory in every emergency case. Clinical data are of very little relevance in this setting.

**NFPA vs. hypophysitis**

On MRI lymphocytic hypophysitis appears as a symmetric enlargement of a homogeneous pituitary gland, with thickened but rarely displaced stalk and an intact sellar floor (Gutenberg et al., 2006; Lury, 2005), whereas macroadenomas are heterogeneous, frequently asymmetric lesions growing toward the suprasellar cistern and cavernous sinus, often displacing an intact stalk, depressing or eroding the sellar floor (Gutenberg et al., 2009; Lury, 2005). Intense and homogenous enhancement of the anterior pituitary, similar to that of the cavernous sinuses, is suggestive of hypophysitis.

It was suggested that hypophysitis should be suspected in a patient with pituitary dysfunction whenever there is the coexistence of 3 or more of the 9 following items (Rivera, 2006):

- young age;
- women presenting during the peripartum period;
- acute onset of headache with ophthalmoplegia, visual field defects, nausea or vomiting (present also in pituitary apoplexy where presentation is more catastrophic and imaging shows bleeding or ischemia);
- acute onset of DI with headache and mass-effect symptoms (present also in sarcoidosis and LCH, with a more insidious presentation);
- characteristic MRI findings;
- isolated, early or disproportionate impairment of ACTH secretion (usually the last hormone to be affected in patients with pituitary adenomas) and in general, disproportionate involvement of pituitary function for the magnitude of the changes on MRI;

- presence of other autoimmune conditions and/or autoantibodies;
- lymphomonocytic pleocytosis in the CSF, without clinical meningitis and antiviral antibodies;
- presence of circulating antipituitary antibodies, where available.

Recently a case-control study was performed on 402 lesions (histological diagnosis was NFPA and autoimmune hypophysitis in 304 and 98, respectively) evaluating the predictive value of different features before surgery (Gutenberg et al., 2009). Authors concluded that no single radiologic sign had sufficient accuracy to distinguish with certainty hypophysitis from pituitary adenomas. In a multiple logistic regression model, however, some features contributed significantly to the correct classification of lesions: relation to pregnancy, pituitary symmetry, stalk size, signal intensity and homogeneity after contrast supported the diagnosis of hypophysitis, whereas greater pituitary mass volume and mucosal swelling in the sphenoid sinus supported the diagnosis of adenoma.

**NFPA vs. meningioma**

Meningiomas grow typically in the suprasellar space, with obtuse margins at the edge. In the vast majority of cases pituitary function is normal, the sella is not invaded and a normal pituitary is easily recognizable even in the rare instance of sellar invasion.

If cavernous sinus is invaded, meningiomas tend to narrow the carotid artery lumen more than any other tumors (Young et al., 1988).

The so-called dural tail, previously regarded as pathognomonic of a meningioma, is now considered nonspecific, because it can be seen in association with adenoma, metastases, lymphoma, and lymphocytic hypophysitis (even though DI is frequent in these last 3 cases and not in meningiomas). This asymmetric tentorial enhancement is thought to be caused by venous congestion due to compression or invasion of the ipsilateral cavernous sinus rather than to meningeal inflammation or tumor invasion (Guermazi et al., 2005; Nakasu et al., 2001; Rumboldt, 2005)(figure 22).

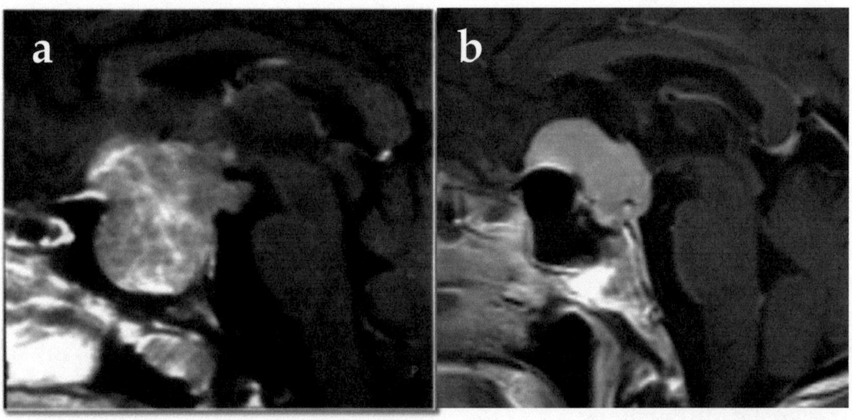


Fig. 22. Macroadenoma vs. meningioma (a vs. b): the former causes sellar enlargement and erodes sellar floor, the latter arising from planum sphenoidale, invades the sella that appears normal in size, and enhances strongly and homogeneously. In both cases dural tail is apparent.

Purely intrasellar meningiomas are extremely rare. They can be extremely difficult to distinguish from adenomas (Cappabianca et al., 1999). MRI is not different either on basal T1 or T2. However, post-contrast enhancement is marked, rapid and homogeneous in more than 90% of meningiomas, whereas adenomas generally enhance less intensely and more heterogeneously, with a longer time-to-peak enhancement on dynamic imaging (Huang & Castillo, 2005). Other features pointing to a meningioma (when present) are liquor cleft between the tumor and the gland, hyperostosis of the floor of the sella or adjacent bone structures, flow voids and prominent vessels, and calcifications (Huang & Castillo, 2005).

**NFPA vs. metastasis**

No radiological sign can accurately discriminate between the two conditions, even though bone lytic reactions usually accompany the latter (Komninos et al., 2004).

**NFPA vs. chordoma**

Posterior location, bone destruction with honeycomb aspect, and calcification as well as MR signal characteristics usually point to chordoma (Glezer et al., 2008).

**NFPA vs. solid craniopharyngioma**

Calcifications at CT are usually present in craniopharyngiomas. The apparent diffusion coefficient of craniopharyngiomas is higher than that of adenomas on average (Yamasaki et al., 2005; Zada et al., 2010).

**Meningioma vs. solid craniopharyngioma**

On T2-weighed images meningiomas typically appear isointense, whereas craniopharyngiomas (and RCCs) typically look hyperintense (Freda & Post, 1999).

**Meningioma vs. neurinoma**

Patients with neurinoma usually complain of 5$^{th}$ nerve pain or numbness and deficit is usually present at the neurological examination. Schwannomas follow the expected course of a cranial nerve or its branches, occasionally enlarging the cranial nerve outlet foramen in the skull base, such as the foramen ovale or rotundum (Smith, 2005). Furthermore, on dynamic contrast enhancing MRI sequences meningiomas usually show early enhancement, while neurinomas present gradual but brighter enhancement (Rennert et al., 2007).

**Lipoma vs. other tumors**

Lipomas can be distinguished from other lesions, similarly bright on precontrast T1-weighted images (such as hemorrhagic or proteinaceous lesions), by using suppressing fat sequences, which obtain their disappearance (Smith, 2005).

Fat containing dermoids and teratomas are less homogenous than lipomas.

**Hamartoma vs. other tumors**

Tuber cinereum hamartoma can be differentiated from other pathologies in this region (gliomas, LCH, and germ cell tumors) by clinical presentation, absence of contrast enhancement, and unchanging appearance on follow-up without growth or invasion (Spampinato & Castillo, 2005).

### 4.2.2 Cystic lesions

The spectrum of cystic pathologies occurring in the sellar region includes craniopharyngiomas, RCCs, arachnoid cysts, cystic pituitary adenomas, epidermoid cysts, dermoid cysts, and several others (Laws, 2008). A firm diagnosis is easily reached in most cases, while in others a diagnosis can be established only at surgery, when it is clinically indicated (Harrison et al., 1994; Zada et al., 2010).

**Cysts vs. ES**

Arachnoid cysts or RCCs may simulate ES, but in the latter the pituitary stalk remains usually in the median position and can be visualized down to the sellar floor (Giustina et al., 2010).

**Cystic NFPA vs. RCC**

Both intrasellar and suprasellar cysts can produce signs and symptoms similar to those of adenomas, such as visual impairment or hypopituitarism (Freda & Post, 1999).

Presence of a fluid-fluid level on sagittal or axial images is highly indicative of adenomas, representing intratumoral degeneration and hemorrhage, which almost never occur in cysts (Rumboldt, 2005).

RCCs are located in the center of the gland, have complete absence of contrast enhancement, and may contain characteristic nodules of low T2 signal or be completely hypointense on T2-weighted images (Byun et al., 2000).

**Cystic NFPA vs. craniopharyngioma**

Cystic pituitary adenomas are located within the anterior pituitary lobe, are surrounded by normal pituitary tissue, and the cyst wall consists of enhancing tumor tissue. Cystic craniopharyngiomas are more commonly suprasellar and located superior to the pituitary gland and show enhancing solid components and calcifications (Spampinato & Castillo, 2005).

**Cystic NFPA vs. abscess**

In contrast to adenomas, abscesses typically show ring enhancement and high signal intensities on diffusion weighted (DW) images together with a reduction in the apparent diffusion coefficient (ADC), whereas necrotic tumors display a hypointensity on DW images and higher ADC values (Takao et al., 2006). Furthermore, meningeal enhancement due to concurrent meningitis may be observed in pituitary abscess (Vates et al., 2001).

**RCC vs. cystic craniopharyngioma**

Presenting clinical features are not reliable in this differentiation.

The two lesions can be classically distinguished on MRI: craniopharyngiomas typically show prominent cystic components and calcifications, may be multilobulated or with an irregular shape or rim enhancement, with heterogeneous T1 signal demonstrating heterogeneous or strong homogeneous enhancement as well as solid enhancing nodules in the cyst; RCCs are typically small, round, purely cystic lesions lacking calcification with homogenous hypointense T1 signal intensity and midline anterior infundibular displacement (Famini et al., 2011). RCC may however have a variable imaging appearance depending on the nature of the cyst contents, making the differential diagnosis challenging in some cases.

Imaging parameters that can be used to support a diagnosis of craniopharyngioma over RCC include: presence of calcification, greater tumor diameter (> 2 cm), suprasellar location with superior tumor lobulation, and compression of the third ventricle (Choi et al., 2007). Radiological parameters supporting a diagnosis of RCC are an ovoid shape, small cyst volume, and thin or no cyst wall enhancement.

Suprasellar calcification in a child is highly suggestive of the diagnosis of craniopharyngioma. Although the presence of calcifications may be helpful in the differential diagnosis, it is not specific. On CT scanning 42–87% of craniopharyngiomas exhibited calcification, compared with only 0–13% of RCCs. It is important to note, however, that several cases of RCCs have been reported to occur with ossification and no evidence of neoplastic features, and that the presence of calcium is not necessarily pathognomonic for craniopharyngiomas (Zada et al., 2010).

**RCC vs. arachnoid cyst**

Arachnoid cyst typically contains CSF, while the content of RCC (and its imaging characteristics) is variable. RCC exhibits some degree of rim enhancement, as opposed to minimal or no enhancement in arachnoid cyst (Valassi et al., 2010).

**Epidermoid cyst vs. arachnoid cyst**

Neither epidermoids nor arachnoid cysts enhance but epidermoids are usually bright on FLAIR and DW images, while the arachnoid cyst is dark on both sequences. Furthermore, epidermoids tend to insinuate between vessels and other adjacent structures, while arachnoid cysts displace them (Spampinato & Castillo, 2005).

## 5. Back to clinics

### 5.1 Patient 1

The 55 yo woman with headache and visual troubles needs a careful ophthalmologic, neuroradiological and endocrine evaluation. Initially, visual troubles must be better defined by performing a complete examination, including formal visual field testing. Bitemporal hemianopsia is shown together with previously unknown decreased left visual acuity. MRI shows a solid mass isointense on T1, hyperintense on T2, heterogeneously enhancing after Gd administration. The lesion enlarges the sella, extends in the suprasellar region impinging on the optic chiasm, while apparently sparing the cavernous sinuses. The patient denies polydipsia and polyuria. No clinical sign of hypersecretion is present. Screening of hypersecretions is negative: PRL is 88 ng/mL (no change after serum dilution 1:10 to rule out hook effect), IGF-I is 120 ng/mL (that is normal for her age range), and morning cortisol is normally suppressed after overnight dexamethasone suppression test (0.5 μg/dL). Screening of hypopituitarism is negative as well: morning cortisol, $FT_4$, and FSH are 10 μg/dL, 1 ng/dl, and 45 U/L, respectively. All data (epidemiologic, clinical, endocrine and imaging) thus point to a diagnosis of NFPA. The patient is operated on by a trans-sphenoidal endoscopic approach, without perioperative steroid coverage (Cozzi et al., 2009b). Headache disappears and visual field normalizes. Histological evaluation confirms pituitary adenoma. Immunohistochemistry is negative for pituitary hormones, and Ki67 is 0.5%. Post-operative course is uneventful. At 4 months, a radical resection is shown on MRI, as well as normalization of visual acuity and visual fields; morning cortisol and $FT_4$ are 12 μg/dL and 1.1 ng/dL, respectively. Follow-up is scheduled with yearly evaluation of MRI for 3 years, thereafter progressively lengthening intervals.

### 5.2 Patient 2

In the 34 yo woman with amenorrhea since 8 months work-up must start from endocrine evaluation. PRL is 850 ng/mL. This value is diagnostic of prolactinoma, because no other disease is associated to such high values. It is useful to evaluate IGF-I levels, to rule out a concomitant GH hypersecretion (210 ng/mL, that is normal for her age range), and pituitary function to screen for hypopituitarism. Morning cortisol and $FT_4$ are within normal limits (13 μg/dL and 1.2 ng/dL, respectively), whereas estradiol, LH and FSH are low as expected (40 pg/mL, 0.7 U/L, and 3.5 U/L, respectively). Visual field examination shows superolateral bilateral quadrantopsia and MRI demonstrates a large mass, hypointense on T1, hyperintense on T2, heterogeneously enhancing after Gd administration due to multiple cysts, with irregular extrasellar extension up to optic chiasm, and in the sphenoid and cavernous sinuses. Macroprolactinoma is the only clinical situation where neurosurgery is not the first line therapeutic option in spite of visual pathways compression. Cabergoline, a selective dopamine agonist drug, is started at 0.25 mg/week at at bedtime, obtaining visual field normalization within one week. Follow-up is scheduled with clinical and PRL evaluation monthly for the first 3 months, at 3-month intervals in the first year, and at 6-month intervals in the following two years. PRL levels progressively decrease until normalization in 6 months, with menses restoration. After the first control at 3 months, MRI should be repeated at 6 and 12 months. If there is progressive shrinkage (in this patient it is substantial), successive controls can be performed yearly or even at more prolonged intervals, provided that PRL levels are still suppressed.

### 5.3 Patient 3

The 8 yo boy with growth arrest and mass in the sellar region needs a thorough evaluation. On physical examination height is at the $25^{th}$ centile (genetic target over $50^{th}$), weight at the $75^{th}$ centile, puberty at Tanner stage I. Adenoma is not the most frequent diagnosis in this age group, nonetheless the screening for prolactinoma and Cushing's disease (even though macroadenoma would be exceptionally rare) is warranted. PRL is 60 ng/mL and morning cortisol is normally suppressed after overnight dexamethasone suppression test (basal 9 μg/dL, after dexamethasone 0.8 μg/dL). Beyond growth arrest and worsening of school results, weight increase and excessive thirst are reported. Serum sodium is 148 mEq/L and glucose 65 mg/dL. Thyroid function is slightly impaired ($FT_4$ 0.7 ng/dL, with normal values 0.8-2.2). On the basis of history and sodium values, partial central DI is diagnosed and desmopressin is started. On MRI a heterogeneous intra and suprasellar mass is observed, with mottled appearance on T1, heterogeneously hyperintense on T2. Multicystic appearance is evident after Gd administration, with rim enhancement. CT scan shows multiple calcifications. Epidemiologic, clinical and radiological data point to craniopharyngioma. The patient undergoes neurosurgery by trans-sphenoidal approach. Post-operatively, DI worsens and panhypopituitarism develops, requiring full substitutive treatment with desmopressin, hydrocortisone and thyroxine. Follow-up is scheduled with MRI, to evaluate the radicality of resection. Metabolic and weight control is of particular concern. GH treatment is started. Puberty induction will be postponed until attainment of satisfactory height for the genetic target.

### 5.4 Patient 4

In the 45 yo male with the incidental finding of microlesion in the pituitary, the first task is screening of hypersecretory syndromes. PRL is 13 ng/mL, IGF-I 150 ng/mL, $FT_4$ 1 ng/dL, TSH 1 mU/L, and morning cortisol after overnight dexamethasone suppression test 1 μg/dL (all within normal limits). The 7-mm lesion is located in the left inferior portion of the gland, is hypointense on T1, hyperintense on T2, and moderately enhancing. All data point to a non-functioning microadenoma. On the basis of clinics (non functioning), size (micro) and location (far from critical structure), watchful waiting is an appropriate choice. MRI control is scheduled at 12 and 24 months, without any hormonal control. Size is unchanged and the patient is reassured about the lack of evolutivity of the lesion. There is disagreement between the neurosurgeon and the endocrinologist about further follow-up: it is to be prolonged life-long for the former (with MRI at 2-year intervals), and it is redundant for the latter.

## 6. Expert suggestions and conclusions

A few key-points are to be kept in mind.

- Most lesions are pituitary adenomas but alternative diagnoses must always be considered.
- A screening of hypersecretory syndromes and hormonal deficiencies is mandatory. This can be accomplished by a few focused hormonal assays.
- In diagnostic reasoning, consider epidemiological factors.
- Take always into account comorbidities: a hypothalamic-pituitary lesion can be a local manifestation of a systemic disease.
- Imaging must be critically reviewed together with the radiologist.
- Don't miss red flags even though virtually nothing is pathognomonic.

The flow-chart in figure 23 is a simple but not exhaustive guide to diagnostic reasoning.

A plausible diagnosis is possible in many cases of parasellar lesions on the basis of epidemiological, clinical and neuradiological data. This involves a multidisciplinary collaborative effort among the endocrinologist, the neuroradiologist, and the neurosurgeon. Skilled individuals in an organized team, the pituitary unit, better perform this task. In cases of doubt, a histological diagnosis may still be required for a correct diagnosis and to allow appropriate treatment planning. Although most parasellar tumors are slow growing and benign, it is important to identify on the basis of clinical context, laboratory data, and serial imaging those which exert a strong malignant potential or are malignant. Treatment as well involves a joint effort requiring the collaboration of different specialists: the neurosurgeon, the endocrinologist, and the radiotherapist, with the neuro-oncologist and the nuclear physician entering as a second-line in a few cases.

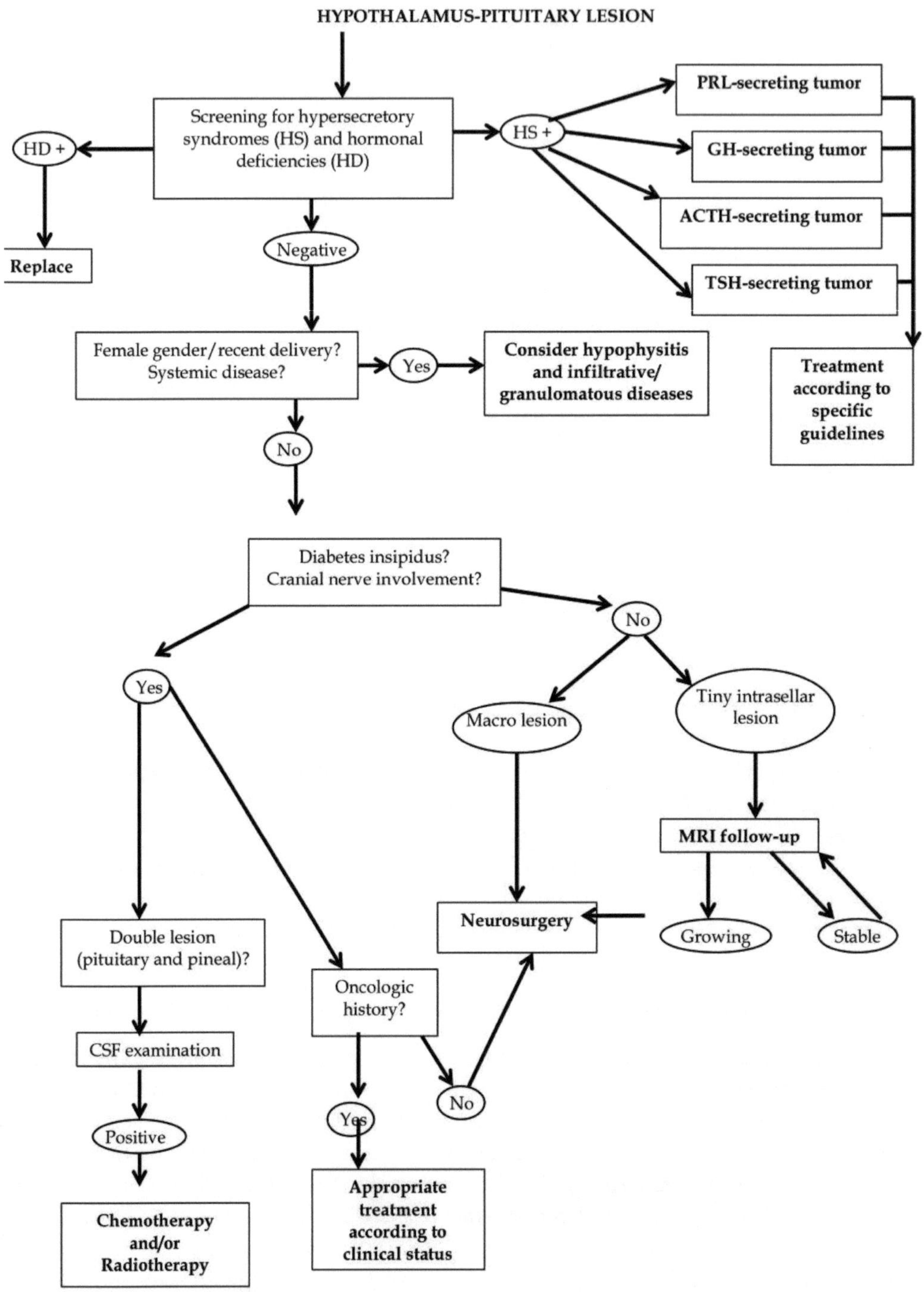


Fig. 23. Flow-chart for diagnosis

## 7. References

Arena S, Barbieri F, Thellung S, Pirani P, Corsaro A, Villa V, Dadati P, Dorcaratto A, Lapertosa G, Ravetti JL, Spaziante R, Schettini G, & Florio T. (2004). Expression of somatostatin receptor mRNA in human meningiomas and their implication in in vitro antiproliferative activity. *Journal of Neurooncology,* Vol. 66, pp. 155-166.

Ahmadi H, Larsson EM, & Jinkins JR. (1990). Normal pituitary gland: coronal MR imaging of infundibular tilt. *Radiology,* Vol. 177, pp. 389-392.

Aho CJ, Liu C, Zelman V, Couldwell WT, & Weiss MH. (2005). Surgical outcomes in 118 patients with Rathke cleft cysts. *Journal of Neurosurgery,* Vol. 102, pp. 189-193.

Akan H, Cihan B, & Celenk C. (2004). Sphenoid sinus mucocele causing third nerve paralysis: CT and MR findings. *Dentomaxillofacial Radiology,* Vol. 33, pp. 342-4.

Arafah BM, Ybarra J, Tarr RW, Madhun ZT, & Selman WR. (1997). Pituitary tumor apoplexy: pathophysiology, clinical manifestations and management. *Journal of Intensive Care Medicine,* Vol. 12, pp. 123-134.

Arafah BM, Prunty D, Ybarra J, Hlavin ML, & Selman WR. (2000). The dominant role of increased intrasellar pressure in the pathogenesis of hypopituitarism, hyperprolactinemia, and headaches in patients with pituitary adenomas. *Journal of Clinical Endocrinology and Metabolism,* Vol. 85, pp. 1789-1793.

Asa SL, Kovacs K, Tindall GT, Barrow DL, Horvath E, & Vecsei P. (1984). Cushing's disease associated with an intrasellar gangliocytoma producing corticotrophin-releasing factor. *Annals of Internal Medicine,* Vol. 101, pp. 789-793.

Bailey W, Freidenberg GR, James HE, Hesselink JR, & Jones KL. (1990). Prenatal diagnosis of a craniopharyngioma using ultrasonography and magnetic resonance imaging. *Prenatal Diagnosis,* Vol. 10, pp. 623-629.

Bartolomei M, Bodei L, De Cicco C, Grana CM, Cremonesi M, Botteri E, Baio SM, Aricò D, Sansovini M, & Paganelli G. (2009). Peptide receptor radionuclide therapy with (90)Y-DOTATOC in recurrent meningioma. European *Journal of Nuclear Medicine and Molecular Imaging,* Vol. 36, pp. 1407-1416.

Beck-Peccoz P, Persani L, Mannavola D, & Campi I. (2009). Pituitary tumours: TSH-secreting adenomas. *Best Practice and Research in Clinical Endocrinology and Metabolism,* Vol. 23, pp. 597-606.

Bellastella A, Bizzarro A, Coronella C, Bellastella G, Agostino SA, De Bellis A. (2003). Lymphocytic hypophysitis: a rare or underestimated disease? *European Journal of Endocrinology,* Vol. 149, No. 5, pp. 363-376.

Bertagna X, Guignat L, Groussin L, & Bertherat J. (2009). Cushing's disease. *Best Practice and Research in Clinical Endocrinology and Metabolism,* Vol. 23, pp. 607-623.

Billeci D, Marton E, Tripodi M, Orvieto E, & Longatti P. (2005). Symptomatic Rathke's cleft cysts: a radiological, surgical and pathological review. *Pituitary,* Vol. 7: pp. 131-137.

Biller BMK, Grossman AB, Stewart PM. Melmed S, Bertagna X, Bertherat J, Buchfelder M, Colao A, Hermus AR, Hofland L, Klibanski A, Lacroix A, Lindsay JR, Newell-Price J, Nieman L, Petersenn S, Sonino N, Stalla GK, Swearingen B, Vance ML, Wass JAH, & Boscaro M. (2008). Treatment of Adrenocorticotropin-Dependent Cushing's Syndrome: A Consensus Statement. *Journal of Clinical Endocrinology and Metabolism,* Vol. 93, No. 7: pp. 2454-2462.

Biousse V, Newman NJ, & Oyesiku NM. (2001). Precipitating factors in pituitary apoplexy. *Journal of Neurology, Neurosurgery and Psychiatry*, Vol. 71, pp. 542-545.

Black KL, & Pikul BK. (1999). Gliomas-past, present, and future. *Clinical Neurosurgery*, Vol. 45, pp. 160–163.

Boari N, Losa M, Mortini P, Snider S, Terreni MR, & Giovanelli M. (2006). Intrasellar paraganglioma: a case report and review of the literature. *Acta Neurochirurgica*, Vol. 148, pp. 1311–1314.

Bondy M, & Ligon BL. (1996). Epidemiology and etiology of intracranial meningiomas: a review. *Journal of Neurooncology*, Vol. 29, No. 3, pp. 197-205.

Bonicki W, Kasperlik-Zaluska A, Koszewski W, Zgliczynski W, & Wislawski J. (1993). Pituitary apoplexy: endocrine, surgical and oncological emergency. Incidence, clinical course and treatment with reference to 799 cases of pituitary adenomas. *Acta Neurochirurgica (Wien)*, Vol. 120: pp. 118-122.

Bonneville J-F, Cattin F, Gorczyca W, & Hardy J. (1993). Pituitary microadenomas: early enhancement with dynamic CT-implications of arterial blood supply and potential importance. *Radiology*, Vol. 187, pp. 857-861.

Bonneville J-F, Bonneville F, & Cattin F. (2005). Magnetic resonance imaging of pituitary adenomas. *European Radiology*, Vol. 15, pp. 543-548.

Brat DJ, Scheithauer BW, Staugaitis SM, Holtzman RNN, Morgello S, & Burger PC. (2000). Pituicytoma: a distinctive low-grade glioma of the neurohypophysis. *American Journal of Surgical Pathology*, Vol. 24, No. 3, pp. 362-368.

Bubl R, Hugo HH, Hempelmann RG, Barth H, & Mehdorn HM. (2001). Granular-cell tumour: a rare suprasellar mass. *Neuroradiology*, Vol. 43, No. 4, pp. 309-312.

Buhring U, Herrlinger U, Krings T, Thiex R, Weller M, & Kuker W. (2001). MRI features of primary central nervous system lymphomas at presentation. *Neurology*, Vol. 57, pp. 393–396.

Bülow B, Attewell R, Hagmar L, Malmström P, Nordström CH, & Erfurth EM. (1998). Postoperative prognosis in craniopharyngioma with respect to cardiovascular mortality, survival, and tumour recurrence. *Journal of Clinical Endocrinology and Metabolism*, Vol. 83, pp. 3897–3904.

Buurman H, & Saeger W. (2006). Subclinical adenomas in postmortem pituitaries: classification and correlations to clinical data. *European Journal of Endocrinology*, Vol. 154, No. 5, pp. 753–758.

Byun WM, Kim OL, & Kim D. (2000). MR imaging findings of Rathke's cleft cysts: significance of intracystic nodules. AJNR *American Journal of Neuroradiology*, Vol. 21, pp. 485-488.

Calaminus G, Bamberg M, Harms D, Jurgens H, Kortmann RD, Sorensen N, Wiestler OD, & Gobel U. (2005) AFP/beta-HCG secreting CNS germ cell tumors: long-term outcome with respect to initial symptoms and primary tumor resection. Results of the cooperative trial MAKEI 89. *Neuropediatrics*, Vol. 36, pp. 71–77.

Cappabianca P, Cirillo S, Alfieri A, D'Amico A, Maiuri F, Mariniello G, Caranci F, & de Divitiis E. (1999). Pituitary macroadenoma and diaphragma sellae meningioma: differential diagnosis on MRI. *Neuroradiology*, Vol. 41, No. 1, pp. 22-26.

Carpinteri R, Patelli I, Casanueva FF, & Giustina A. (2009). Inflammatory and granulomatous expansive lesions of the pituitary. *Best Practice & Research Clinical Endocrinology & Metabolism,* Vol. 23, pp 639–650.

Castagna A, Cinque P, d'Amico A, Messa C, Fazio F, & Lazzarin A. (1997). Evaluation of contrast-enhancing brain lesions in AIDS patients by means of Epstein-Barr virus detection in cerebrospinal fluid and 201 thallium single photon emission tomography. *AIDS,* Vol. 11, pp. 1522–1523.

Caturegli P, Newschaffer C, Olivi A, Pomper MG, Burger PC, &Rose NR. (2005). Autoimmune hypophysitis. *Endocrine Reviews,* Vol. 26, No. 5, pp. 599–614.

Caturegli P. (2007). Autoimmune hypophysitis: an underestimated disease in search of its autoantigen(s). *Journal of Clinical Endocrinology and Metabolism,* Vol. 92, pp. 2038–2040.

Chanson P, Daujat F, Young J, Bellucci A, Kujas M, Doyon D, & Schaison G. (2001). Normal pituitary hypertrophy as a frequent cause of pituitary incidentaloma: a follow-up study. *Journal of Clinical Endocrinology & Metabolism,* Vol. 86, pp. 3009-3015.

Cheung C, Ezzat S, Smyth A, Asa SL. (2001). The spectrum and significance of primary hypophysitis. *Journal of Clinical Endocrinology and Metabolism,* Vol. 86, No. 3, pp. 1048-1053.

Choi SH, Kwon BJ, Na DG, Kim JH, Han MH, & Chang KH. (2007). Pituitary adenoma, craniopharyngioma, and Rathke cleft cyst involving both intrasellar and suprasellar regions: differentiation using MRI. *Clinical Radiology,* Vol. 62, pp. 453–462.

Civit T, Marchal JC, Pinelli C, Auque J, & Hepner H. (1999). Intrasellar epidermoid cysts. *Neurochirurgie,* Vol. 45, pp. 150–154.

Clayton R, Burden AC, Schrieber V, & Rosenthal FD. (1977). Secondary pituitary hyperplasia in Addison's disease. *Lancet,* Vol. 2, pp. 954-956.

Cohen-Gadol AA, Pichelmann MA, Link MJ, Scheithauer BW, Krecke KN, Young WF Jr, Hardy J, & Giannini C. (2003). Granular cell tumor of the sellar and suprasellar region: clinicopathologic study of 11 cases and literature review. *Mayo Clinic Proceedings,* Vol. 78, pp. 567–573.

Colao A. (2009). The prolactinoma. *Best Practice and Research in Clinical Endocrinology and Metabolism,* Vol. 23, pp. 575–596.

Cottier J-P, Destrieux C, Brunereau L, Bertrand P, Moreau L, Jan M, & Herbreteau D. (2000). Cavernous sinus invasion by pituitary adenoma: MR imaging. *Radiology,* Vol. 215, pp. 463-469.

Cozzi R, Baldelli R, Colao AM, Lasio G, Zini M, Attanasio R, Chanson P, Giustina A, Ghigo E, & Strasburger C. (2009a). AME Position Statement on clinical management of acromegaly. *Journal of Endocrinological Investigations,* Vol. 32, suppl 6, pp. 2-25.

Cozzi R, Lasio G, Cardia A, Felisati G, Montini M, & Attanasio R. (2009b). Perioperative cortisol can predict hypothalamus-pituitary-adrenal status in clinically non-functioning pituitary adenomas. *Journal of Endocrinological Investigation,* Vol. 32, pp. 460-464.

Curran JG, & O'Connor E. (2005). Imaging of craniopharyngioma. *Childs Nervous System,* Vol. 21, No. 8-9, pp. 635-639.

Daly AF, Rixhon M, Adam C, Dempegioti A, Tichomirowa MA, & Beckers A. (2006). High prevalence of pituitary adenomas: a cross-sectional study in the province of Liege, Belgium. *Journal of Clinical Endocrinology and Metabolism*, Vol. 91, No. 12, pp. 4769–4775.

Daly AF, Tichomirowa MA, Beckers A. (2009). The epidemiology and genetics of pituitary adenomas. *Best Practice & Research Clinical Endocrinology & Metabolism,* Vol. 23, pp 543–554.

Dan NG, Feiner RI, Houang MT, Turner JJ. (2002). Pituitary apoplexy in association with lymphocytic hypophysitis. *Journal of Clinical Neuroscience*, Vol. 9, No. 5, pp. 577–580.

Dash RJ, Gupta J, & Suri S. (1993). Sheehan's Syndrome: clinical profile, pituitary hormone responses, and computed sellar tomography. *Australia and New Zealand Journal of Medicine*, Vol. 23, pp. 26-31.

Davis FG, Kupelian V, Freels S, McCarthy B, & Surawicz T. (2001). Prevalence estimates for primary brain tumors in the United States by behavior and major histology groups. *Neuro-oncology*, Vol. 3, No. 3, pp. 152–158.

de Bruin WI, van't Verlaat JW, Graamans K, & De Bruin TW. (1991). Sellar granulomatous mass in a pregnant woman with active Crohn's disease. *Netherlands Journal of Medicine*, Vol. 39, No. 3-4, pp. 136–141.

De Marinis L, Bonadonna S, Bianchi A, Maira G, Giustina A. (2005). Primary empty sella. *Journal of Clinical Endocrinology and Metabolism*, Vol. 90, pp. 5471-5477.

Debeneix C, Bourgeois M, Trivin C, Sainte-Rose C, & Brauner R. (2001). Hypothalamic hamartoma: comparison of clinical presentation and magnetic resonance images. *Hormone Research*, Vol. 56, pp. 12-18.

Dekkers OM, Biermasz NR, Smit JW, Groot LE, Roelfsema F, Romijn JA, & Pereira AM. (2006) Quality of life in treated adult craniopharyngioma patients. *European Journal of Endocrinology*, Vol. 154, pp 483–489.

Dekkers OM, Hammer S, de Keizer RJW, Roelfsema F, Schutte PJ, Smit JW, Romijn JA, & Pereira AM. (2007). The natural course of non-functioning pituitary macroadenomas. *European Journal of Endocrinology*, Vol. 156, pp. 217–224.

Dekkers OM, Pereira AM, & Romijn JA. (2008). Treatment and follow-up of clinically non functioning pituitary macroadenomas. *Journal of Clinical Endocrinology and Metabolism*, Vol. 93, pp. 3717–3726.

Del Monte P, Foppiani L, Cafferata C, Marugo A, & Bernasconi D. (2006). Primary "empty sella" in adults: endocrine findings. *Endocrine Journal*, Vol. 53, pp. 803-809.

Domingues FS, de Souza JM, Chagas H, Chimelli L, & Vaisman M. (2002). Pituitary tuberculoma: an unusual lesion of sellar region. *Pituitary*, Vol. 5, No. 3, pp. 149-153.

Dubuisson AS, Beckers A, & Stevenaert A. (2007). Classical pituitary tumor apoplexy: clinical features, management, and outcome in a series of 24 patients. *Clinical Neurology and Neurosurgery*, Vol. 109, pp. 64-70.

Elster AD, Sanders TG, Vines FS, & Chen MY. (1991). Size and shape of the pituitary gland during pregnancy and postpartum: measurement with MR imaging. *Radiology*, Vol. 181, pp. 531–535.

Elster AD. (1993). Modern imaging of the pituitary. *Radiology*, Vol. 187, pp. 1-14.

Erdag N, Bhorade RM, Alberico RA, Yousuf N, & Patel MR. (2001). Primary lymphoma of the central nervous system: typical and atypical CT and MRI appearances. *AJR American Journal of Roentgenology*, Vol. 176, No. 5, pp. 1319-1326.

Erdem E, Angtuaco EC, Van Hemert R, Park JS, & Al-Mefty O. (2003). Comprehensive review of intracranial chordoma. *Radiographics*, Vol. 23, pp. 995-1009.

Ezzat S, Asa SL, Couldwell WT, Barr CE, Dodge WE, Vance ML, & McCutcheon IE. (2004). The prevalence of pituitary adenomas: a systematic review. *Cancer*, Vol. 101, No. 3, pp. 613–619.

Fahlbusch R, Honegger J, Paulus W, Huk W, & Buchfelder M. (1999). Surgical treatment of craniopharyngiomas: experience with 168 patients. *Journal of Neurosurgery*, Vol. 90, pp. 237–250.

Famini P, Maya MM, & Melmed S. (2011). Pituitary Magnetic Resonance Imaging for Sellar and Parasellar Masses: Ten-Year Experience in 2598 Patients. *Journal of Clinical Endocrinology & Metabolism*, Vol. 96, pp. 1633–1641.

Fernandez-Balsells MMM, Barwise A, Gallegos-Orozco J, Paul A, Lane M, Carpio I, Perestelo-Perez LI, Ponce de Leon Lovaton P, Erwin, P, Carey J, & Montori VM. (2011). The natural history of pituitary incidentalomas: a systematic review and meta-analysis. *Journal of Clinical Endocrinology and Metabolism*, Vol. 96, pp. 905-912.

Flanagan DE, Ibrahim AE, Ellison DW, Armitage M, Gawne-Cain M, & Lees PD. (2002). Inflammatory hypophysitis: the spectrum of disease. *Acta Neurochirurgica (Wien)*, Vol. 144, pp. 47-56.

Freda PU, & Post KD. (1999). Differential diagnosis of sellar masses. *Endocrinology and Metabolism Clinics of North America*, Vol. 28: pp. 81-117.

Freda PU, Beckers AM, Katznelson L, Molitch ME, Montori, VM, Post KD, & Vance ML. (2011). Pituitary Incidentaloma: An Endocrine Society Clinical Practice Guideline. *Journal of Clinical Endocrinology & Metabolism*, Vol. 96, pp. 894–904.

Freeman JL, Coleman LT, Wellard RM, Kean MJ, Rosenfeld JV, Jackson GD, Berkovic SF, & Harvey AS. (2004). MR imaging and spectroscopic study of epileptogenic hypothalamic hamartomas: analysis of 72 cases. *American Journal of Neuroradiology*, Vol. 25, pp. 450–462.

Frighetto L, De Salles AA, Behnke E, Smith ZA, & Chute D. (2003). Image-guided frameless stereotactic biopsy sampling of parasellar lesions. Technical note. *Journal of Neurosurgery*, Vol. 98, pp. 920–925.

Furlanetto TW, Faria Pitta Pinheiro C, Oppitz PP, de Alencastro LC, & Asa SL. (2009). Solitary Fibrous Tumor of the Sella Mimicking Pituitary Adenoma: An Uncommon Tumor in a Rare Location—A Case Report. *Endocrine Pathology* Vol. 20, pp. 56-61.

Fuyi L, Guilin L, Yong Y, Yi Y, Wenbin M, Yongning L, Gao C, & Renzhi W. (2010). Diagnosis and management of pituitary abscess: experiences from 33 cases. *Clinical Endocrinology*, Vol. 74, pp. 79–88.

Geddes JF, Jansen GH, Robinson SF, Gömöri E, Holton JL, Monson JP, Besser GM, & Révész T. (2000). "Gangliocytomas" of the pituitary: a heterogeneous group of lesions with differing histogenesis. *American Journal of Surgical Pathology*, Vol. 24, No. 4, pp. 607-613.

Gehanne C, Delpierre I, Damry N, Devroede B, Brihaye P, & Christophe C. (2005). Skull base chordoma: CT and MRI features. *JBR-BTR Belgian Journal of Radiology*, Vol. 88, pp. 325-327.

Gelabert-Gonzalez M. (1998). Intracranial epidermoid and dermoid cysts. *Reviews in Neurology*, Vol. 27, pp. 777-782.

Giustina A, Gola M, Doga M, & Agabiti Rosei E. (2001). Primary Lymphoma of the Pituitary: An Emerging Clinical Entity. *Journal of Clinical Endocrinology & Metabolism*, Vol. 86, pp. 4567–4575.

Giustina A, Aimaretti G, Bondanelli M, Buzi F, Cannavò S, Cirillo S, Colao A, De Marinis L, Ferone D, Gasperi M, Grottoli S, Porcelli T, Ghigo E, & degli Uberti E. (2010). Primary empty sella: Why and when to investigate hypothalamic-pituitary function. *Journal of Endocrinological Investigations*, Vol. 33, pp. 343-346.

Glezer A, Belchior Paraiba D, Bronstein MD. (2008). Rare Sellar Lesions. *Endocrinology and Metabolism Clinics of North America*, Vol. 37: pp. 195-211.

Goyal M, Kucharczyk W, & Keystone E. (2000). Granulomatosis hypophysitis due to Wegener's granulomatosis. *AJNR American Journal of Neuroradiology*, Vol. 21, pp. 1466–9.

Grois N, Prayer D, Prosch H, Minkov M, Pötschger U, & Gadner H. (2004). Course and clinical impact of magnetic resonance imaging findings in diabetes insipidus associated with Langerhans cell histiocytosis. *Pediatric Blood Cancer*, Vol. 43, pp. 59–65.

Guermazi A, Lafitte F, Miaux Y, Adem C, Bonneville JF, & Chiras J. (2005). The dural tail sign-beyond meningioma. *Clinical Radiology*, Vol. 60, pp. 171–88.

Guillamo JS, Doz F, & Delattre JY. (2001). Brain stem gliomas. *Current Opinion in Neurology*, Vol. 14, pp. 711–715.

Gutenberg A, Hans V, Puchner MJA, Kreutzer J, Brück W, Caturegli P, & Buchfelder M. (2006). Primary hypophysitis: clinical-pathological correlations. *European Journal of Endocrinology*, Vol. 155, pp. 101–107.

Gutenberg A, Larsen J, Lupi I, Rohde V, & Caturegli P. (2009). A radiologic score to distinguish autoimmune hypophysitis from nonsecreting pituitary adenoma preoperatively. *American Journal of Neuroradiology*, Vol. 30, pp. 1766 –1772.

Hald JK, Eldevik OP, Brunberg JA, & Chandler WF. (1994). Craniopharyngiomas - the utility of contrast medium enhancement for MR imaging at 1.5 T. *Acta Radiologica*, Vol. 35, pp. 520–525.

Hall WA, Luciano MG, Doppman JL, Patronas NJ, & Oldfield EH. (1994). Pituitary magnetic resonance imaging in normal human volunteers: occult adenomas in the general population. *Annals of Internal Medicine*, Vol. 120, pp. 817–20.

Haque TL, MikiY, Kashii S,Yamamoto A, Kanagaki M, Takahashi T, Fushimi Y, Asato R, Murase N, Shibasaki H, & Konishi J. (2004). Dynamic MR imaging in Tolosa-Hunt syndrome. *European Journal of Radiology*, Vol. 51, pp. 209–17.

Harrison MJ, Morgello S, & Post KD. (1994). Epithelial cystic lesions of the sellar and parasellar region: A continuum of ectodermal derivatives? *Journal of Neurosurgery*, Vol. 80, pp. 1018-1025.

Hartmann C, Bostrom J, & Simon M. (2006). Diagnostic and molecular pathology of meningiomas. *Expert Reviews of Neurotherapeutics*, Vol. 6, pp. 1671–1683.

Heinze HJ, & Bercu BB. (1997). Acquired hypophysitis in adolescence. *Journal of Pediatric Endocrinology and Metabolism*, Vol. 10, pp. 315-321.

Hofmann BM, Kreutzer J, Saeger W, Buchfelder M, Blumckel, Fahlbusch R, & Buslei R. (2006). Nuclear beta-catenin accumulation as reliable marker for the differentiation between cystic craniopharyngiomas and Rathke cleft cysts: a clinico-pathologic approach. *American Journal of Surgical Pathology*, Vol. 30, pp. 1595-1603.

Honegger J, Fahlbusch R, Bornemann A, Hensen J, Buchfelder M, Muller M, & Nomikos P. (1997). Lymphocytic and granulomatous hypophysitis: experience with nine cases. *Neurosurgery*, Vol. 40, pp. 713-723.

Honegger J, Barocka A, Sadri B, & Fahlbusch R. (1998). Neuropsychological results of craniopharyngioma surgery in adults: a prospective study. *Surgical Neurology*, Vol. 50, pp. 19-29.

Honegger J, Buchfelder M, & Fahlbusch R. (1999). Surgical treatment of craniopharyngiomas: endocrinological results. *Journal of Neurosurgery*, Vol. 90, pp. 251-257.

Honegger J, Zimmermann S, Psaras T, Petrick M, Mittelbronn M, Ernemann U, Reincke M, & Dietz K. (2008). Growth modeling of non-functioning pituitary adenomas in patients referred for surgery. *European Journal of Endocrinology*, Vol. 158, pp. 287-294.

Horn E, Coons SW, Spetzler RF, & Rekate HL. (2006). Isolated Langerhans cell histiocytosis of the infundibulum presenting with fulminant diabetes insipidus. *Child's Nervous System*, Vol. 22, pp. 542-544.

Huang BY, & Castillo M. (2005). Nonadenomatous tumors of the pituitary and sella turcica. *Top Magnetic Resonance Imaging*, Vol. 16, pp. 289-299.

Hutchins WW, Crues JV III, Miya P, & Pojunas KW. (1990). MR demonstration of pituitary hyperplasia and regression after therapy for hypothyroidism. *AJNR American Journal of Neuroradiology*, Vol. 11, pp. 410.

Iglesias A, Arias M, Brasa J, Paramo C, Conde C, & Fernandez R. (2000). MR imaging findings in granular cell tumor of the neurohypophysis: A difficult preoperative diagnosis. *European Radiology*, Vol. 10, pp. 1871-1873.

Isono M, Kamida T, Kobayashi H, Shimomura T, & Matsuyama J. (2001). Clinical features of symptomatic Rathke's cleft cyst. *Clinical Neurology and Neurosurgery*, Vol. 103: pp. 96-100.

Jaffrain-Rea ML, Di Stefano D, Minniti G, Esposito V, Bultrini A, Ferretti E, Santoro A, Faticanti SL, Gulino A, & Cantore G. (2002). A critical reappraisal of MIB-1 labelling index significance in a large series of pituitary tumours: secreting versus non-secreting adenomas. *Endocrine Related Cancer*, Vol. 9, pp. 103-113.

Jalalah S, Kovacs K, Horvath E, Couldwell W, Weiss MH, & Ezrin C. (1987). Rhabdomyosarcoma in the region of the sella turcica. *Acta Neurochirurgica*, Vol. 88, pp. 142-146.

Jalali R, Srinivas C, Nadkarni TD, & Rajasekharan P. (2008). Suprasellar haemangiopericytoma - challenges in diagnosis and treatment. *Acta Neurochirurgica*, Vol. 150, pp. 67-71.

Janmohamed S, Grossman AB, Metcalfe K, Lowe DG, Wood DF, Chew SL, Monson JP, Besser GM, & Plowman PN. (2002). Suprasellar germ cell tumours: specific problems and the evolution of optimal management with a combined chemoradiotherapy regimen. *Clinical Endocrinology*, Vol. 57, pp. 487–500.

Johnson BA, Fram EK, Johnson PC, & Jacobowitz R. (1997). The variable MR appearance of primary lymphoma of the central nervous system: comparison with histopathologic features. *AJNR American Journal of Neuroradiology*, Vol. 18, No. 3, pp. 563-572.

Judge DM, Kulin HE, Page R, Santen R, & Trapukdi S. (1977). Hypothalamic hamartoma: a source of luteinizing hormone-releasing factor in precocious puberty. New England Journal of Medicine, Vol. 296, pp. 7–10.

Kaltsas GA, Powles TB, Evanson J, Plowman PN, Drinkwater JE, Jenkins PJ, Monson JP, Besser GM, & Grossman AB. (2000). Hypothalamo-pituitary abnormalities in adult patients with Langerhans cell histiocytosis: clinical, endocrinological, and radiological features and response to treatment. *Journal of Clinical Endocrinology and Metabolism*, Vol. 85, pp. 1370–1376.

Kaltsas GA, Nomikos P, Kontogeorgos G, Buchfelder M, & Grossman AB. (2005). Diagnosis and management of pituitary carcinomas. *Journal of Clinical Endocrinology & Metabolism*, Vol. 90, pp. 3089–3099.

Kaltsas GA, Evanson J, Chrisoulidou A, & Grossman AB. (2008). The diagnosis and management of parasellar tumours of the pituitary. *Endocrine-Related Cancer*, Vol. 15, pp. 885–903.

Kanatani M, Nakamura R, Kurokawa K, Taoda M, Nemoto Y, Kamakura K, Kugai N, Nagata N, Takatani O, & Tsuchiya K. (1991). Hypopituitarism associated with Cogan's syndrome; high-dose glucocorticoid therapy reverses pituitary swelling. *Japanese Journal of Medicine*, Vol. 30, No. 2, pp. 164–169.

Karavitaki N, Brufani C, Warner JT, Adams CB, Richards P, Ansorge O, Shine B, Turner HE, & Wass JA. (2005). Craniopharyngiomas in children and adults: systematic analysis of 121 cases with long-term follow-up. *Clinical Endocrinology (Oxf)*, Vol. 62, No. 4, pp. 397-409.

Karavitaki N, Cudlip S, Adams CB, & Wass JA. (2006). Craniopharyngiomas. *Endocrine Reviews*, Vol. 27, pp. 371–397.

Karavitaki N, Collison K, Halliday J, Byrne JV, Price P, Cudlip S, & Wass JA. (2007). What is the natural history of nonoperated, nonfunctioning pituitary adenomas? *Clinical Endocrinology*, Vol. 67, pp. 938–943.

Karavitaki N, Wass JAH. (2009). Non-adenomatous pituitary tumours. *Best Practice & Research Clinical Endocrinology & Metabolism*, Vol. 23, pp 651–665.

Katsuta T, Inoue T, Nakagaki H, Takeshita M, Morimoto K, & Iwaki T. (2003). Distinctions between pituicytoma and ordinary pilocytic astrocytoma. Case report. *Journal of Neurosurgery*, Vol. 98, No. 2, pp. 404-406.

Kido G, Miyagi A, Shibuya T, Miyagami M, Tsubokawa T, & Sawada T. (1994). Turner's syndrome with pituitary hyperplasia: a case report. *No Shinkei Geka Neurological surgery*, Vol. 22, pp. 333-338.

Kim JE, Kim JH, Kim OL, Paek SH, Kim DG, Chi JG, & Jung HW. (2004). Surgical treatment of symptomatic Rathke cleft cysts: clinical features and results with special attention to recurrence. *Journal of Neurosurgery*, Vol. 100, pp. 33–40.

Kim K, Yamada S, Usui M, & Sano T. (2004). Preoperative identification of clearly separated double pituitary adenomas. *Clinical Endocrinology*, Vol. 61, pp. 26–30.

King Jr JT, Justice AC, & Aron DC. (1997). Management of incidental pituitary microadenomas: a cost-effectiveness analysis. *Journal of Clinical Endocrinology and Metabolism*, Vol. 82, pp. 3625-3632.

Kitange GJ, Templeton KL, & Jenkins RB. (2003). Recent advances in the molecular genetics of primary gliomas. *Current Opinion in Oncology*, Vol. 15, pp. 197–203.

Knosp E, Steiner E, Kitz K, & Matula C. (1993). Pituitary adenomas with invasion of the cavernous sinus space: a magnetic resonance imaging classification compared with surgical findings. *Neurosurgery*, Vol. 33, pp. 610-618.

Ko KW, Nam DH, Kong DS, Lee JI, Park K, & Kim JH. (2007). Relationship between malignant subtypes of meningioma and clinical outcome. *Journal of Clinical Neuroscience*, Vol. 14, pp. 747–753.

Komninos J, Vlassopoulou V, Protopapa D, Korfias S, Kontogeorgos G, Sakas DE, & Thalassinos NC. (2004). Tumors metastatic to the pituitary gland: case report and literature review. *Journal of Clinical Endocrinology & Metabolism*, Vol. 89, pp. 574–580.

Kontogeorgos G, Kovacs K, Horvath E, & Scheithauer BW. (1991). Multiple adenomas of the human pituitary. A retrospective autopsy study with clinical implications. *Journal of Neurosurgery*, Vol. 74, pp. 243–247.

Kontogeorgos G, Scheithauer BW, Horvath E, Kovacs K, Lloyd RV, Smyth HS, Rologis D. (1992). Double adenomas of the pituitary: a clinicopathological study of 11 tumors. *Neurosurgery*, Vol. 31, pp. 840–849.

Kornreich L, Blaser S, Schwarz M, Shuper A, Vishne TH, Cohen IJ, Faingold R, Michovitz S, Koplewitz B, & Horev G. (2001). Optic pathway glioma: Correlation of imaging findings with the presence of neurofibromatosis. *AJNR American Journal of Neuroradiology*, Vol. 22, pp. 1963-1969.

Korten AG, Berg HJ, Spincemaille GH, van der Laan RT, & Van de Wel AM. (1998). Intracranial chondrosarcoma: review of the literature and report of 15 cases. *Journal of Neurology, Neurosurgery, and Psychiatry*, Vol. 65, pp. 88–92.

Koutourousiou M, Kontogeorgos G, Wesseling P, Grotenhuis AJ, & Seretis A. (2010). Collision sellar lesions: experience with eight cases and review of the literature. *Pituitary*, Vol. 13, pp. 8-17.

Kovacs K, Horvath E, & Vidal S. (2001). Classification of pituitary adenomas. *Journal of Neuro-Oncology*, Vol. 54, pp 121–127.

Kovacs K, Bilbao JM, Fornasier VL, & Horvath E. (2004). Pituitary pathology in Erdheim-Chester disease. *Endocrine Pathology*, Vol. 15, No. 2, pp. 159–166.

Kowalski RJ, Pravson RA, & Mayberg MR. (2004). Pituicytoma. *Annals of Diagnostic Pathology*, Vol. 8, No. 5, pp. 290–4.

Kristjansdottir HL, Bodvarsdottir SP, & Sigurjonsdottir HA. (2011). Sheehan's syndrome in modern times: a nationwide retrospective study in Iceland. *European Journal of Endocrinology*, Vol. 164, pp. 349–354.

Kristopaitis T, Thomas C, Petruzzelli GJ, & Lee JM. (2000). Malignant craniopharyngioma. *Archives of Pathology & Laboratory Medicine*, Vol. 124, pp. 1356–1360.

Kurt G, Dogulu F, Kaymaz M, Emmez H, Onk A, & Baykaner MK. (2002). Hypothalamic lipoma adjacent to mamillary bodies. *Child's Nervous System*, Vol. 18, pp. 732-734.

Kyongsong K, Shozo Y, Masaaki U, & Toshiaki S. (2004). Preoperative identification of clearly separated double pituitary adenomas. *Clinical Endocrinology* ,Vol. 61, pp. 26–30.

Laigle-Donadey F, Taillibert S, Martin-Duverneuil N, Hildebrand J, & Delattre JY. (2005). Skull-base metastases. *Journal of Neuro-Oncology*, Vol. 75, pp. 63–69.

Laws ER. (2008). Endoscopic surgery for cystic lesions of the pituitary region. *Nature Clinical Practice in Endocrinology and Metabolism*, Vol. 4, pp. 662–663.

Levy A. (2003). Hazards of dynamic testing of pituitary function. *Clinical Endocrinology (Oxf)*, Vol. 58, pp. 543-544.

Levy MJ, Jäger HR, Powell M, Matharu MS, Meeran K, & Goadsby PJ. (2004). Pituitary volume and headache: size is not everything. *Archives of Neurology*, Vol. 61, pp. 721–725.

Liu F, Li G, Yao Y, Yang Y, Ma W, Li Y, Chen G, & Wang R. (2011). Diagnosis and management of pituitary abscess: experiences from 33 cases. *Clinical Endocrinology* ,Vol. 74, pp 79–88.

Liu JK, Sayama C, Chin SS, & Couldwell WT. (2007). Extranodal NK/T-cell lymphoma presenting as a pituitary mass. Case report and review of the literature. *Journal of Neurosurgery*, Vol. 107, pp. 660–665.

Lloyd RJ, Kovacs K, Young WF Jr, Farrell WE, Asa SL, Trouillas J, Kontogeorgos G, Sano T, Scheithauer BW, Horvath E, Watson RE, Jr, Lindell EP, Barkan AL, Saeger W, Nosé V, Osamura RY, Ezzat S, Yamada S, Roncaroli F, Lopes MBS, & Vidal Ruibal S. (2004a). Tumours of the pituitary gland. In: *Pathology and Genetics. Endocrine Tumours,* Eds. DeLellis RA, Lloyd RV, & Heitz PU, pp 9–48. International Agency for Research and Cancer (IARC), Lyon.

Lloyd RV, Kovacs K, Young Jr WF, Farrel WE, Asa SL, Truillas J, Kontogeorgos G, Sano T, Scheithauer BW, Horvath E, DeLellis RA, & Heitz PU. (2004b). Pituitary tumors. In: *Introduction. WHO classification of tumors of the endocrine organs: pathology and genetics of endocrine organs,* Eds. DeLellis R, Lloyd RV, Heitz PV, Eng C, pp. 10–13, International Agency for Research and Cancer (IARC), Lyon.

Lopes MB, Lanzino G, Cloft HJ, Winston DC, Vance ML, & Laws Jr ER. (1998). Primary fibrosarcoma of the sella unrelated to previous radiation therapy. *Modern Pathology*, Vol. 11, pp. 579–84.

Louis DN, Ohgaki H, Wiestler OD, Cavenee WK, Burger PC, Jouvet A, Scheithauer BW, & Kleihues P. (2007) The 2007 WHO classification of tumours of the central nervous system. *Acta Neuropathologica*, Vol. 114, pp. 97–109.

Lury KM, Smith JK, Matheus MG, & Castillo M. (2004). Neurosarcoidosis - review of imaging findings. *Seminars in Roentgenology*, Vol. 39, No. 4, pp. 495-504.

Lury KM. (2005). Inflammatory and infectious processes involving the pituitary gland. *Top Magnetic Resonance Imaging*, Vol. 16, pp. 301-306.

Makras P, Alexandraki KI, Chrousos GP, Grossman AB, & Kaltsas GA. (2007). Endocrine manifestations in Langerhans cell histiocytosis. *Trends in Endocrinology and Metabolism*, Vol. 18, pp. 252–257.

Matsutani M, Sano K, Takakura K, Fujimaki T, Nakamura O, Funata N, & Seto T. (1997). Primary intracranial germ cell tumors: a clinical analysis of 153 histologically verified cases. *Journal of Neurosurgery*, Vol. 86, pp. 446–455.

Matta MP, Kany M, Delisle MB, Lagarrigue J, & Caron PH. (2002). A relapsing remitting lymphocytic hypophysitis. *Pituitary*, Vol. 5, pp. 37-44.

Meij BP, Lopes MB, Ellegala DB, Alden TD, & Laws Jr ER. (2002). The long-term significance of microscopic dural invasion in 354 patients with pituitary adenomas treated with transsphenoidal surgery. *Journal of Neurosurgery*, Vol. 96, pp. 195-208.

Melmed S. (2006). Medical progress: Acromegaly. *New England Journal of Medicine*, Vol. 355, pp. 2558-2573.

Melmed S, Casanueva FF, Hoffman AR, Kleinberg DL, Montori VM, Schlechte JA, & Wass JAH. (2011). Diagnosis and treatment of hyperprolactinemia: An Endocrine Society clinical practice guideline. *Journal of Clinical Endocrinology and Metabolism*, Vol. 96, No. 2, pp. 273-288.

Meyers SP, Hirsch WL Jr, Curtin HD, Barnes L, Sekhar LN &, Sen C. (1992). Chondrosarcomas of the skull base: MR imaging features. *Radiologica*, Vol. 184, pp. 103-108.

Molitch ME. (2009). Pituitary incidentalomas. *Best Practice & Research Clinical Endocrinology & Metabolism*, Vol. 23, pp 667-675.

Möller-Goede DL, Brändle M, Landau K, Bernays Rl, & Schmid C. (2011). Pituitary apoplexy: re-evaluation of risk factors for bleeding into pituitary adenomas and impact on outcome. *European Journal of Endocrinology*, Vol. 164, pp. 37-43.

Moshkin O, Muller P, Scheithauer BW, Juco J, Horvath E, Patterson BJ, Kamel-Reid S, & Kovacs K. (2009). Primary pituitary lymphoma: a histological, immunohistochemical, and ultrastructural study with literature review. *Endocrine Pathology*, Vol. 20: pp. 46-49.

Mukherjee JJ, Islam N, Kaltsas G, Lowe DG, Charlsworth M, Afshar F, Trainer PJ, Monson JP, Besser GM, & Grossman AB. (1997). Clinical, radiological and pathological features of patients with Rathke's cleft cysts: tumors that may recur. *Journal of Clinical Endocrinology and Metabolism*, Vol. 82, pp. 2357-2362.

Mukhida K, Asa A, Gentili F, & Shannon P. Ependymoma of the pituitary fossa. (2006). Case report and review of the literature. *Journal of Neurosurgery*, Vol. 105, pp. 616-620.

Müller HL. (2011). Consequences of craniopharyngioma surgery in children. *Journal of Clinical Endocrinology and Metabolism*, Vol. 96, pp. 1981-1991.

Naggara O, Varlet P, Page P, Oppenheim C, & Meder JF. (2005). Suprasellar paraganglioma: a case report and review of the literature. *Neuroradiology*, Vol. 47, pp. 753-7.

Naing S, & Frohman LA. (2007). The empty sella. *Pediatric Endocrinology Reviews*, Vol. 4, pp. 335-42.

Nakasu Y, Nakasu S, Ito R, Mitsuya K, Fujimoto O, & Saito A. (2001). Tentorial enhancement on MR images is a sign of cavernous sinus involvement in patients with sellar tumors. *AJNR American Journal of Neuroradiology*, Vol. 22, pp. 1528-1533.

Nammour GM, Ybarra J, Naheedy MH, Romeo JH, & Aron DC. (1997). Incidental pituitary macroadenoma: a population-based study. *American Journal of Medical Sciences*, Vol. 314, pp. 287-291.

Nawar RN, AbdelMannan D, Selman WR, & Arafah BM. (2008). Pituitary Tumor Apoplexy: A Review. *Journal of Intensive Care Medicine*, Vol. 23, pp. 75-90.

Nelson GA, Bastian FO, Schlitt M, & White RL. (1988). Malignant transformation in craniopharyngioma. *Neurosurgery*, Vol. 22, pp. 427-429.

Newell-Price J. (2011). Whither Pituitary Incidentaloma? *Journal of Clinical Endocrinology & Metabolism*, Vol. 96, pp. 939–941.

Nielsen EH, Lindholm J, Bjerre P, Christiansen JS, Hagen C, Juul S, Jorgensen J, Kruse A & Laurberg P. (2006). Frequent occurrence of pituitary apoplexy in patients with nonfunctioning pituitary adenoma. *Clinical Endocrinology (Oxf)*, Vol. 64, pp. 319-322.

Nishioka H, Haraoka J, Izawa H, & Ikeda Y. (2006). Magnetic resonance imaging, clinical manifestations, and management of Rathke's cleft cyst. *Clinical Endocrinology (Oxf)*, Vol. 64, pp. 184–188.

Nomura M, Tachibana O, Hasegawa M, Kohda Y, Nakada M, Yamashima T, Yamashita J, & Suzuki M. (1996). Contrast-enhanced MRI of intrasellar arachnoid cysts: relationship between the pituitary gland and cyst. *Neuroradiology*, Vol. 38, pp. 566–568.

Ohba S, Yoshida K, Hirose Y, Ikeda E, & Kawase T. (2008). A supratentorial primitive neuroectodermal tumor in an adult: a case report and review of the literature. *Journal of Neuro-Oncology*, Vol. 86, pp. 217–224.

Onesti ST, Wisniewski T, & Post KD. (1990). Clinical versus subclinical pituitary apoplexy: presentation, surgical management, and outcome in 21 patients. *Neurosurgery*, Vol. 26, pp. 980-986.

Orakdogeny M, Karadereler S, Berkman Z, Ersahin M, Ozdogan C, & Aker F. (2004). Intra-suprasellar meningioma mimicking pituitary apoplexy. *Acta Neurochirurgica (Wien)*, Vol. 146, No. 5, pp. 511-515.

Packer RJ, Cohen BH, & Cooney K. (2000). Intracranial germ cell tumors. *The Oncologist*, Vol. 5, No. 4. pp. 312-320.

Pels H, Deckert-Schluter M, Glasmacher A, Kleinschmidt R, Oehring R, Fischer HP, Bode U, & Schlegel U. (2000). Primary central nervous system lymphoma: a clinicopathological study of 28 cases. *Hematological Oncology*, Vol. 18, pp. 21–32.

Perez-Nunez P, Miranda I, Arrese P, González P, Ramos A, & Lobato RD. (2005). Lymphocytic hypophysitis with cystic MRI appearance. Acta Neurochirurgica (Wien), Vol. 147, pp. 1297-1300.

Pinzer T, Reiss M, Bourquain H, Krishnan KG, & Schackert G. (2006). Primary aspergillosis of the sphenoid sinus with pituitary invasion - a rare differential diagnosis of sellar lesions. *Acta Neurochirurgica*, Vol. 148, No. 10, pp. 1085–1090.

Piotin M, Tampieri D, Rufenacht DA, Mohr G, Garant M, Del Carpio R, Robert F, Delavelle J, & Melanson D. (1999). The various MRI patterns of pituitary apoplexy. *European Radiology*, Vol. 9, pp. 918–923.

Pravdenkova S, Al-Mefty O, Sawyer J, & Husain M. (2006). Progesterone and estrogen receptors: opposing prognostic indicators in meningiomas. *Journal of Neurosurgery*, Vol. 105, pp. 163-173.

Prosch H, Grois N, Bokkerink J, Prayer D, Leuschner I, Minkov M, & Gadner H. (2006). Central diabetes insipidus: is it Langerhans cell histiocytosis of the pituitary stalk? A diagnostic pitfall. *Pediatric Blood Cancer*, Vol. 46, No. 3, pp. 363–366.

Rajasekaran S, Vanderpump M, Baldeweg S, Drake W, Reddy N, Lanyon M, Markey A, Plant G, Powell M, Sinha S, & Wass J. (2011). UK guidelines for the management of pituitary apoplexy Pituitary Apoplexy Guidelines Development Group: May 2010. *Clinical Endocrinology*, Vol. 74, pp. 9–20.

Randall BR, Kraus KL, Simard MF, & Couldwell WT. (2010). Cost of evaluation of patients with pituitary incidentaloma. *Pituitary*, Vol. 13, pp. 383–384.

Randeva HS, Schoebel J, Byrne J, Esiri M, Adams CB, & Wass JA. (1999). Classical pituitary apoplexy: clinical features, management and outcome. *Clinical Endocrinology (Oxf)*, Vol. 51, pp. 181-188.

Rennert J, & Doerfler A. (2007). Imaging of sellar and parasellar lesions. *Clinical Neurology and Neurosurgery*, Vol. 109, pp. 111–124.

Rivera JA. (2006). Lymphocytic hypophysitis: Disease spectrum and approach to diagnosis and therapy. *Pituitary*, Vol. 9, pp. 35–45

Roncaroli F, Bacci A, Frank G, & Calbucci F. (2004). Granulomatous hypophysitis caused by a ruptured intrasellar Rathke's cleft cyst: report of a case and review of the literature. *British Journal of Neurosurgery*, Vol. 18, No. 5, pp. 489-494.

Rousseau A, Bernier M, Kujas M, & Varlet P. (2005). Primary intracranial melanocytic tumor simulating pituitary macroadenoma: case report and review of the literature. *Neurosurgery*, Vol. 57, pp. E369.

Rumboldt Z, Gnjidic Z, Talan-Hranilovic J, & Vrkljan M. (2003). Intrasellar hemangioblastoma: characteristic prominent vessels on MR imaging. *AJR American Journal of Roentgenology*, Vol. 180, pp. 1480-1481.

Rumboldt Z. (2005). Pituitary adenomas. *Top Magnetic Resonance Imaging*, Vol. 16, pp. 277-288.

Ruscalleda J. (2005). Imaging of parasellar lesions. *European Radiology*, Vol. 15, pp. 549–559.

Saeger W, Lüdecke DM, Buchfelder M, Fahlbusch R, Quabbe HJ, & Petersen S. (2007). Pathohistological classification of pituitary tumors: 10 years of experience with the German Pituitary Tumor Registry. *European Journal of Endocrinology*, Vol. 156, pp. 203-216.

Sajko T, Rumboldt Z, Talan-Hranilovic J, Radic I, & Gnjidic Z. (2005). Primary sellar esthesioneuroblastoma. *Acta Neurochirurgica (Wien)*, Vol. 147, pp. 447-448.

Samandouras G, Kerr RS, & Milford CA. (2005). Minimally invasive biopsy of parasellar lesions: safety and clinical applications of the endoscopic, transnasal approach. *British Journal of Neurosurgery*, Vol. 19, pp. 338–344.

Sano T, Asa SL, & Kovacs K. (1988). Growth hormone-releasing hormone producing tumors: clinical, biochemical, and morphological manifestations. *Endocrine Reviews*, Vol. 9, pp. 357–373.

Sarma S, Sekhar LN, & Schessel DA. (2002). Nonvestibular schwannomas of the brain: A 7-year experience. *Neurosurgery*, Vol. 50, pp. 437-448.

Sartoretti-Schefer S, Wichmann W, Aguzzi A, & Valavanis A. (1997). MR differentiation of adamantinous and squamous-papillary craniopharyngiomas. *AJNR American Journal of Neuroradiology*, Vol. 18, pp. 77–87.

Sato N, Sze G, & Endo K. (1998). Hypophysitis: endocrinologic and dynamic MR findings. *AJNR American Journal of Neuroradiology*, Vol. 19, pp. 439–444.

Scanarini M, Rotilio A, Rigobello L, Pomes A, Parenti A, & Alessio L. (1991). Primary intrasellar coccidioidomycosis simulating a pituitary adenoma. *Neurosurgery*, Vol. 28, No. 5, pp. 748–51.

Scheithauer BW, Kovacs K, Horvath E, Kim DS, Osamura RY, Ketterling RP, Lloyd RV, & Kim OL. (2008). Pituitary blastoma. *Acta Neuropathologica*, Vol. 116, No. 6, pp. 657-666.

Semple PL, Jane Jr JA, & Laws Jr ER. (2007). Clinical relevance of precipitating factors in pituitary apoplexy. *Neurosurgery*, Vol. 61, pp. 956–961.

Shin JL, Asa SL, Woodhouse LJ, Smyth HS, & Ezzat S. (1999). Cystic lesions of the pituitary: clinicopathological features distinguishing craniopharyngioma, Rathke's cleft cyst, and arachnoid cyst. *Journal of Clinical Endocrinology and Metabolism*, Vol. 84, pp. 3972–3982.

Sibal L, Ball SG, Connolly V, James RA, Kane P, Kelly WF, Kendall-Taylor P, Mathias D, Perros P, Quinton R & Vaidya B. (2004). Pituitary apoplexy: a review of clinical presentation, management and outcome in 45 cases. *Pituitary*, Vol. 7, pp. 157-163.

Sinnott BP, Hatipoglu B, & Sarne DH. (2006). Intrasellar plasmacytoma presenting as a non-functional invasive pituitary macro-adenoma: Case Report & Literature Review. *Pituitary*, Vol. 9, pp. 65–72.

Smith JK. (2005). Parasellar Tumors: Suprasellar and Cavernous Sinuses. *Top Magnetic Resonance Imaging*, Vol. 16, pp. 307-315.

Spampinato MV, & Castillo M. (2005). Congenital pathology of the pituitary gland and parasellar region. *Top Magnetic Resonance Imaging*, Vol. 16, pp. 269-276.

Striano S, Striano P, Sarappa C, & Boccella P. (2005). The clinical spectrum and natural history of gelastic epilepsy-hypothalamic hamartoma syndrome. *Seizure*, Vol. 14, pp. 232-239.

Suh JH, & Gupta N. (2006). Role of radiation therapy and radiosurgery in the management of craniopharyngiomas. *Neurosurgery Clinics of North America*, Vol. 17, pp. 143–148.

Sumida M, Uozumi T, Kiya K, Mukada K, Arita K, Kurisu K, Sugiyama K, Onda J, Satoh H, Ikawa F, & Migita K. (1995). MRI of intracranial germ cell tumours. *Neuroradiology*, Vol. 37, No. 1, pp. 32-37.

Takao H, Doi I, & Watanabe T. (2006). Diffusion-weighted magnetic resonance imaging in pituitary abscess. *Journal of Computer Assisted Tomography*, Vol. 30, pp. 514–516.

Tatagiba M, Iaconetta G, & Samii M. (2000). Epidermoid cyst of the cavernous sinus: clinical features, pathogenesis and treatment. *British Journal of Neurosurgery*, Vol. 14, pp. 571–575.

Terada T, Kovacs K, Stefaneanu L, Horvath E. (1995). Incidence, pathology, and recurrence of pituitary adenomas: study of 647 unselected surgical cases. *Endocrine Pathology*, Vol. 6, pp. 301–310.

Teramoto A, Hirakawa K, Sanno N, & Osamura Y. (1994). Incidental pituitary lesions in 1,000 unselected autopsy specimens. *Radiology*, Vol. 193, pp. 161-164.

Thodou E, Kontogeorgos G, Scheithauer BW, Lekka I, Tzanis S, Mariatos P, & Laws ER Jr. (2000). Intrasellar chordomas mimicking pituitary adenoma. *Journal of Neurosurgery*, Vol. 92, pp. 976–982.

Tominaga JY, Higano S, & Takahashi S. (2003). Characteristics of Rathke's cleft cyst in MR imaging. *Magnetic Resonance Medical Science*, Vol. 2, pp. 1–8.

Toth M, Szabo P, Racz K, Szende B, Balogh I, Czirják S, Slowik F, & Gláz E. (1996). Granulomatous hypophysitis associated with Takayasu's disease. *Clinical Endocrinology*, Vol. 45, No. 4, pp. 499–503.

Tsunoda A, Okuda O, & Sato K. (1997). MR height of the pituitary gland as a function of age and sex: especially physiological hypertrophy in adolescence and in climacterium. *AJNR American Journal of Neuroradiology*, Vol. 18, pp. 551-554.

Turner HE, & Wass JA. (1999). Are markers of proliferation valuable in the histological assessment of pituitary tumours? *Pituitary*, Vol. 1: pp. 147-151.

Valassi E, Biller BMK, Klibanski A, & Swearingen B. (2010). Clinical features of nonpituitary sellar lesions in a large surgical series. *Clinical Endocrinology*, Vol. 73, pp. 798-807.

Van Effenterre R, & Boch AL. (2002). Craniopharyngioma in adults and children: a study of 122 surgical cases. *Journal of Neurosurgery*, Vol. 97, pp. 3-11.

Vates GE, Berger MS, & Wilson CB. (2001). Diagnosis and management of pituitary abscess: a review of twenty-four cases. *Journal of Neurosurgery*, Vol. 95, pp. 233-241.

Vernooij MW, Ikram A, Tanghe HL, Vincent AJPE, Hofman A, Krestin GP, Niessen WJ, Breteler MMB, & van der Lugt A. (2007). Incidental findings on brain MRI in the general population. *New England Journal of Medicine*, Vol. 357, pp. 1821-1828.

Whittle IR, Smith C, Navoo P, & Collie D. (2004). Meningiomas. *Lancet*, Vol. 363, pp. 1535-1543.

Yamada T, Nojiri K, Sasazawa H, Tsukui T, Miyahara Y, Nakayama K, Komatsu M, Aizawa T, & Komiya I. (2005). Correlation between the pituitary size and function in patients with asthenia. *Endocrine Journal*, Vol. 53, pp. 441-444.

Yamasaki F, Kurisu K, Satoh K, Arita K, Sugiyama K, Ohtaki M, Takaba J, Tominaga A, Hanaya R, Yoshioka H, Hama S, Ito Y, Kajiwara Y, Yahara K, Saito T, & Thohar MA. (2005). Apparent diffusion coefficient of human brain tumors at MRI. *Radiology*, Vol. 235, No. 3, pp. 985-991.

Yong TY, Li JY, Amato L, Mahadevan K, Phillips PJ, Coates PS, & Coates PT. (2008). Pituitary involvement in Wegener's granulomatosis. *Pituitary*, Vol. 11, No. 1, pp. 77-84.

Yoshino A, Katayama Y, Watanabe T, Ogino A, Ohta T, Komine C, Yokoyama T, Fukushima T, & Hirota H. (2007). Apoplexy accompanying pituitary adenoma as a complication of preoperative anterior pituitary function tests. *Acta Neurochirurgica (Wien)*, Vol. 149, pp. 557-565.

Young SC, Grossman RI, Goldberg HI, Spagnoli MV, Hackney DB, Zimmerman RA, & Bilaniuk LT. (1988). MR of vascular encasement in parasellar masses: comparison with angiography and CT. *American Journal of Neuroradiology*, Vol. 9, pp. 35-38.

Yue NC, Longsteth Jr. WT, Elster AD, Jungreis CA, O'Leary DH, & Poirier VC. (1997). Clinically serious abnormalities found incidentally at MR imaging of the brain: data from the Cardiovascular Health Study. *Radiology*, Vol. 202, pp. 41-46.

Yuen KCJ, Cook DM, Sahasranam P, Patel P, Ghods DE, Shahinian HK, Friedman TC. (2008). Prevalence of GH and other anterior pituitary hormone deficiencies in adults with nonsecreting pituitary microadenomas and normal serum IGF-1 levels. *Clinical Endocrinology*, Vol. 69, pp. 292-298.

Zada G, Lin N, Ojerholm E, Ramkissoon S, & Laws ER. (2010). Craniopharyngioma and other cystic epithelial lesions of the sellar region: a review of clinical, imaging, and histopathological relationships. *Neurosurgical Focus*, Vol. 28, pp. E4 1-12.

Zayour DH, Selman WR, & Arafah BM. (2004). Extreme elevation of intrasellar pressure in patients with pituitary tumor apoplexy: relation to pituitary function. *Journal of Clinical Endocrinology and Metabolism*, Vol. 89, pp. 5649–5654.

Zhang YQ, Wang CC, & Ma ZY. (2002). Pediatric craniopharyngiomas: clinicomorphological study of 189 cases. *Pediatric Neurosurgery*, Vol. 36, pp. 80–84.

8

# Pineal Region Tumors

Paolo Cipriano Cecchi[1], Giuliano Giliberto[2],
Angelo Musumeci[3] and Andreas Schwarz[1]
[1]*Unitá Operativa di Neurochirurgia, Ospedale San Maurizio, Bolzano,*
[2]*Dipartimento di Neurochirurgia, Ospedale Maggiore C.A. Pizzardi, Bologna,*
[3]*Unitá Operativa di Neurochirurgia, Ospedale Sant'Agostino Estense, Modena,*
*Italy*

## 1. Introduction

The pineal region can be affected by different types of lesions, ranging from benign masses (e.g. pineal cysts) to highly malignant tumors. These neoplasms are typical of the pediatric age, while they are rarer in adults. Due to the extreme heterogeneity of the cell types of the pineal gland and its surrounding structures, these tumors include several entities, namely germ cell tumors (GCTs), which are the most common (about 70% of the pineal region tumors, PRTs), primary parenchymal tumors (PPTs) arising from the pineal parenchyma (from pineocytoma to highly malignant pineoblastoma) and other tumors, including gliomas, metastases, and tumoral invasion of the gland by adjacent tumors (gliomas, meningiomas and others). GCTs, ependymomas and pineal cell tumors typically give "drop metastasis" through the cerebrospinal fluid (CSF). PRTs have no pathognomonic radiological features; CSF and serum markers can be helpful in this challenging differential diagnosis, which leads to different therapeutical approaches.

## 2. Epidemiology

Pineal masses, including benign pineal cysts, are common (up to 10% as incidental magnetic resonance imaging, MRI, finding) (Gaillard & Jones, 2010), while autoptic studies showed a prevalence of 20-40% (Hasegawa et al., 1987); the benign pineal cyst, which is beyond the goal of this chapter, is largely the most frequent pineal mass. Conversely, PRTs are relatively rare, accounting for 3-8% of intracranial pediatric tumors and <1% in adults (Regis et al., 1996). GCTs are the most common tumors of this region (70%), including germinomas (50%) and teratomas (15%) (Tab. 1); they account for 0.3-3.4% of brain tumors in western population, while in Asian population they are up to eight times more common; they are also more common in patients with Down syndrome; PPTs account for another 15% (Gaillard et al., 2010; Smirniotopopoulos et al., 1992).

## 3. Physiopathology and clinical features

The pineocyte is the main cell of the pineal gland; it produces melatonin, a hormone involved in wake/sleep and seasonal functions. The release of melatonin is triggered by sympathetic fibers originating from the retina, that reach the gland through the hypothalamus. Pineal gland is also involved in luteinizing (LH) and follicular stimulating hormone (FSH) production control. The blood-brain barrier is absent in the pineal region. Clinical symptoms associated with PRTs are non-specific (headache and seizures), endocrine disturbances and mass-related manifestations. The most common endocrine disturbance is precocious puberty; hypogonadism and diabetes insipidus are rarer. The origin of the precocious puberty is not clear, but it is probably due to the suppression of the antigonadotrophic effect of the gland itself or of the median eminence, or to the ectopic production of LH and FSH (Gaillard & Jones, 2010; Smirniotopopoulos et al., 1992). The mass-related disturbances are hydrocephalus, dorsal midbrain syndrome and direct compression of the surrounding structures. Obstructive hydrocephalus is the result of silvian aqueduct compression or distortion, with increased intracranial pressure signs, such as headache, vomiting and nausea. The dorsal midbrain syndrome, also known as Parinaud Syndrome, is due to the direct compression of the nuclei of the quadrigeminal plate; this syndrome consists of vertical upward gaze, convergence and accomodation palsy (Pearce, 2005; Jacobs & Galetta, 2007). Direct midbrain compression can give cerebellar, motor and sensory disturbances (Klein & Rubinstein, 1989).

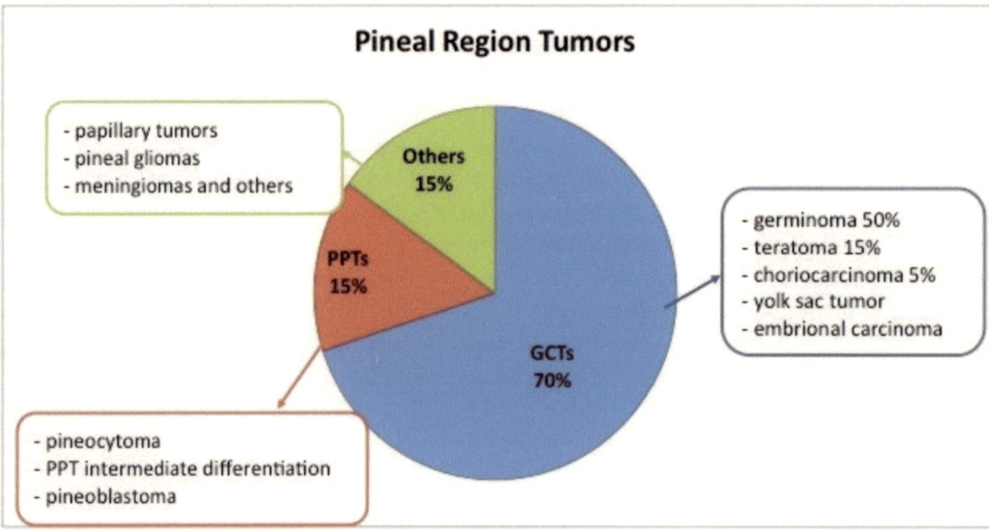


Table 1. Prevalence of various subtypes of PRTs

## 4. Pathology

Tumors of the pineal region can be divided into GCTs, including germinoma and non-germinomatous germ cell tumors (NGGCTs), PPTs, and others, such as papillary tumor of the pineal region, pineal gliomas, metastasis, and tumors from invasion of the gland by adjacent tumors.

### 4.1 Germ cell tumors

GCTs can be located both in the pineal region and in the suprasellar region; 13% of GCTs are bifocal and are called "synchronous GCTs" (Sugiyama et al., 1992). Pineal GCTs are more common in males, while the suprasellar ones appear more frequently in females. All of the

GCTs, excluding mature teratomas, are highly malignant and potentially metastatic. Germinoma (accounting for 50% of all pineal tumors) is an extra-gonadal seminoma, having a peak of incidence in the second decade of life (Villano et al., 2008). Alpha-fetoprotein (AFP) and beta-human chorionic gonadotrophin (β-hCG) are not typically increased, even if an elevation of β-hCG can occur (Horowitz & Hall, 1991). Germinomas have a better prognosis than NGGCTs, being generally radiation therapy-responding (Villano et al., 2008; Shibamoto et al., 2001) with a high rate of long term cure. NGGCTs include teratoma (15% of pineal tumors), choriocarcinoma (5% of pineal tumors), yolk sac tumor and embrional carcinoma (both rarer). They arise from a totipotential germ cell. Teratomas of the pineal region are more common in males and in childhood/early adulthood, and are classified as extra-axial teratomas. They can have different grades of differentiation, from well differentiated (mature) to indifferentiated and aggressive (immature) teratomas. AFP is only occasionally elevated in patients affected by these tumors. Choriocarcinomas are classically associated with the elevation of CSF and plasmatic β-hCG concentration; they are frequently metastatic and prone to hemorrhage. Yolk sac tumor, also known as endodermal sinus tumor, is usually malignant and is often (up to 50%) associated with other GCTs in the context of a mixed GCT (Smirniotopopoulos et al., 1992). CSF β-hCG and AFP are typically increased. Embryonal carcinoma is an aggressive and metastasis-prone tumor with an infrequent elevation of β-hCG and AFP. It is often the most aggressive component of a mixed GCT (Smirniotopopoulos et al., 1992).

### 4.2 Pineal parenchymal tumors

As stated above, PPTs account for 15% of the PRTs. They all derive from pineocytes and, accordingly with the World Health Organization (WHO) (Louis et al., 2007), can be divided into three groups: pineocytoma, pineal tumor of intermediate differentiation and pineoblastoma. Pineocytoma is a WHO grade I tumor, which affects young adults without significant gender difference. It is usually a solid mass, even if it can show hemorrhagic or cystic appearance; it is a highly differentiated, well circumscribed tumor, with a low growth rate and rarely gives metastases. The pineal tumor of intermediate differentiation, as its name suggests, has a biological behavior and a grade of differentiation which is intermediate between pineocytoma and pineoblastoma (WHO grade II/III). Pineoblastoma is a highly malignant tumor (WHO grade IV) which affects young patients without significant gender difference. It is biologically close to medulloblastoma and primitive neuroectodermal tumors and can be associated with retinoblastoma. It is prone to metastasize and to give obstructive hydrocephalus.

### 4.3 Other tumors

Papillary tumor of the pineal region is a rare and relatively new entity, having been introduced in the latest (2007) WHO Classification of Tumors of the Nervous System (Louis et al., 2007). It arises from ependimocytes of the subcommissural organ located in the lining of the posterior commissure (Chang et al., 2008; Jùnior et al., 2011), and is hardly distinguishable from other tumors. Pineal gliomas (fibrillar, pilocytic, anaplastic astrocytoma, glioblastoma, oligodendroglioma) and ependymomas of the pineal gland have been reported; they are more likely originating from adjacent structures rather than from the pineal gland. Epidermoid and dermoid cysts account for 3-4% of the intracranial tumors; 1% of them occur in the pineal region (Konovalov et al., 1999); dermoid cysts are much more common than epidermoid cysts. They are congenital inclusion cysts more than properly tumors, even if their neoplastic transformation has been rarely observed. The absence of the blood-brain barrier in this region makes metastases relatively common in this area. Up to 5% of patient with spread metastatic disease show metastases to the pineal gland; the most common arise from lung, breast, kidney, cervical, oesophageal, gastric and colonic primary tumors (Lassman et al., 2006). Any kind of tumors, such as meningiomas, choroid plexus papillomas, tectal gliomas, lymphomas and lipomas, originating from nearby structures, can involve the pineal region (Gaillard & Jones, 2010).

## 5. Neuroradiology

The variability of the shape of the pineal gland (Sener, 1995), the possible presence of calcification in a normal pineal gland context (about 10% of children between 11 and 14 years) (Kilgore et al., 1986) and the high prevalence of pineal cysts make it hard to diagnose a pineal gland tumor; in many cases it is not possible to achieve a correct diagnosis only by means of neuroradiological features. Pineal cysts is a non neoplastic mass which has to be distinguished from pineal tumors; it appears as a well circumscribed, CSF density/intensity lesions; their rim can show some calcifications and have some contrast enhancement. In atypical cases, a nodular enhancement can occur, making the differential diagnosis between a pineal cyst and a pineal tumor impossible (Gaillard & Jones, 2010). Germinomas are isodense or slightly hyperdense masses on computed tomography (CT); they are isointense to the brain in T1- and T2-weighted images on MRI. They can engulf calcifications and they are brightly enhancing after contrast in both CT and MRI. Up to half of them can have cystic components. The simultaneous involvement of the pineal and pituitary gland ("synchronous GCT") is a pathognomonic radiological feature of germinomas. NGGCTs have highly variable radiological findings, but some data can help narrowing the differential diagnosis: in general the presence of a cystic component is more common than in germinomas; fat and calcifications are more common in teratomas; hemorrhagic findings are more frequent in choriocarcinomas, appearing as blooming signal in T2-weighted images on MRI. PPTs differential diagnosis is problematic. Pineocytoma is a more defined and more homogeneous lesion than pineoblastoma, the latter being usually bigger, often showing local adjacent structures invasion and CSF metastases at presentation. They enhance on postcontrast images; calcifications, if present, are peripheral rather than engulfed, like it happens in germinomas. Papillary tumors of the pineal region do not have specific features: they have a high T1 signal on MRI, like other tumors; they show a moderate contrast enhancement and tend to content cystic areas. Pineal gliomas do not have specific radiological appearances, while metastases show frequently a coexistent leptomeningeal enhancement.

## 6. Treatment and prognosis

### 6.1 General principles

More than 50% of patients with a PRT have some degree of hydrocephalus due to compression of the cerebral aqueduct and, if symptomatic, control of CSF flow is a necessary initial step (Konovalov & Pitskhelauri, 2003; Yamini et al, 2004). The optimal surgical strategy for treating ventricular enlargement in these patients is endoscopic third ventriculostomy (ETV) even because, in selected cases and in experienced hands, this technique may be coupled with a biopsy of the tumor (Bruce & Ogden, 2004). Nevertheless, placement of an external ventricular drain (EVD), with a careful post-operative weaning, is still a reasonable procedure in those patients in whom a gross-total resection of the pineal neoplasm with restoration of CSF flow is highly probable, especially if mildly symptomatic. Due to a relatively high rate of infection, metastasis, malfunctioning and symptomatic overshunting, ventriculo-peritoneal shunt (VP-shunt) should be considered after an ETV failure or when the tumor involves the floor of the third ventricle to such a degree as to make ETV unsafe or unlikely to remain functional (Moise et al, 2011). Despite modern neuroradiological techniques, tumor histology cannot be reliably predicted based on radiographic features alone. Only high CSF and/or serum levels of malignant germ cell markers (AFP and/or β-hCG) make surgery and biopsy unnecessary (these patients should be treated with radio and chemotherapy) (Moise et al, 2011). Thus, for the vast majority of the cases, the first objective of surgical management of an unknown PRT is an accurate histological diagnosis. Given the wide spectrum of tumor histology in this anatomical region, a correct diagnosis is essential for determining the post-operative adjuvant therapy and the need for metastatic workup, for defining a reliable prognosis and for planning a long-term follow-up (Bruce & Ogden, 2004; Konovalov & Pitskhealuri, 2003). There are three surgical strategies to obtain tissue from a PRT: stereotactic biopsy, endoscopic biopsy and open microsurgical procedure. Stereotactic biopsy is associated with a minor degree of invasiveness and a low risk of complication and it should be strongly considered especially in those patients with a known primary systemic tumor, in case of multiple lesions or in patients with medical contraindications to lengthy surgery and general anesthesia (Bruce & Ogden, 2004). Furthermore, if the MRI appearance of the tumor is strongly compatible with a germinoma, a biopsy (stereotactic or endoscopic if feasible) should be the first choice in order to avoid an unnecessary craniotomy (De Tribolet, 2009). The main disadvantage of a simple bioptic procedure is the limited amount of tissue that can be obtained, thus increasing the possibility of an incorrect diagnosis even for experienced neuropathologists (Moise et al, 2011). In one study, where stereotactic biopsy was followed by open surgery for resection (also if not only for PRTs), bioptic diagnosis was incorrect with clinical implications in about 7% of the cases and incorrect without clinical implications in 30% of the cases (Chandrasama et al, 1989). Stereotactic biopsy, mainly with the use of frame-based image-guided systems, can be performed with mild sedation and local anesthesia. The most common trajectories are the anterolateral-superior approach, originating anterior to the coronal suture and lateral to the mid-pupillary line, and the posterolateral-superior approach through a parieto-occipital junction entry point, for tumors with a significant lateral extension. The hemorrhagic potential of a stereotactic biopsy in the pineal region is relatively high compared to other anatomical sites given the adjacent venous system, the presence of choroidal arteries, the multiple pial surfaces traversed with needle and the lack of tissue turgor provided by adjacent cisternal and ventricular spaces which limit the possibility to tamponade even minor bleeding (Bruce & Ogden, 2004; Moise et al, 2011). Nevertheless, there is no significant difference in clinical-evident complication rate between pineal region biopsies and biopsies of other regions of the brain. Peri-operative mortality is less than 2%, permanent major morbidity 0-1.2% and transient minor morbidity 7-8.4%. Diagnostic useful sample is 87-97% but diagnostic accuracy is around 90% (Moise et al, 2011). A bioptic specimen may be obtained also through an endoscopic approach in association with an ETV in case of hydrocephalus. If a rigid endoscope is used, two different trajectories are needed, but in selected cases a simultaneous procedure is possible with a flexible endoscope. There are only few reported series with a significant number of patients and the main limitations are the same of stereotactic procedures (hemorrhage and limited tissue sampling). Diagnostic yield is between 63 and 100%, and peri-operative mortality and morbidity seem acceptable (Bruce & Ogden, 2004; Moise et al, 2011). Open microsurgery, even if more invasive than stereotactic biopsy or endoscopy, permits to obtain an adequate amount of neoplastic tissue for a correct histological diagnosis in virtually all cases and offers a potential chance of cure for benign and low-grade lesions (pineocytoma, mature teratoma, meningioma, epidermoids) if a gross-total resection is achieved (Bruce & Ogden, 2004). For malignant tumors the oncological benefit of a maximal resection has not been definitely proved, but several studies found a correlation between the extent of tumor exeresis and an improved response to adjuvant therapy and increased survival, at least for certain histological subtypes. Furthermore, standard microsurgical techniques allow the restoration of CSF flow, obviating the need for CSF diversion procedures; moreover, a "second-look" surgery is also a potential useful strategy to remove residual tumor following radio and/or chemotherapy for malignant neoplasms (Moise et al, 2011). Two main surgical approaches are used to remove a PRT: the supracerebellar-infratentorial approach and the occipital-transtentorial approach. The choice between them is based on the anatomical features of the tumor but also on the experience and the preference of the surgeon (Bruce & Ogden, 2004; De Tribolet, 2009; Konovalov & Pitskhealuri, 2003). With the modern microsurgical skills and the neurocritical care, in the major series reported in the last 15 years mortality is less than 5%, major morbidity less than 6% but permanent minor morbidity is still reported in up to 28% of the cases (Moise et al, 2011). Hemorrhage is the most serious complication of any surgical approach to the pineal region, especially for malignant tumors with abnormal neovasculature incompletely resected. Bleeding in the surgical field may occur immediately after surgery as well as with a delay of several days. Specific neurological sequelae, generally transient and reversible over a period ranging from days to up to 1 year, are ataxia, papillary abnormalities and extraocular movement dysfunction because of cerebellar and/or brainstem manipulation, but also visual field disturbances after the occipital-transtentorial approach may occur. Prior radiation therapy, invasive/malignant tumors and pre-operative neurological symptoms, increase the risk and severity of post-operative complications (Bruce & Ogden, 2004; De Tribolet, 2009; Moise et al, 2011).

### 6.2 Germ cell tumors

Localized germinomas should be managed with radiation therapy alone, including ventricular or whole brain irradiation followed by a tumor boost for a total dose of 45-50 Gy (Haas-Kogan et al, 2003). Craniospinal irradiation is indicated if there are signs of CSF dissemination (Kyritis, 2010). Patients with germinoma had a 5-year survival rate of 96% and a 10-year survival rate of 91-93% (Brastianos et al, 2010; Kkyritis, 2010). For mature teratomas complete resection is the treatment of choice (Kyritis, 2010). In case of immature forms, maximal safe resection may be followed by radio and/or chemotherapy on an individual basis and evidence of residual disease (Kyritis, 2010). Malignant teratomas as well as choriocarcinomas, embryonal carcinomas, endodermal sinus tumors and mixed tumors with a malignant component should be maximally resected and then treated with radiotherapy and chemotherapy (Echevarria et al, 2008; Matsutani, 2004). As for germinomas, craniospinal irradiation is necessary only if the tumor is disseminated. In mixed germ cell tumors, response of the malignant component induced by radio and/or chemotherapy may spare the benign tumor part (Kyritis, 2010). This residual tumor is likely to be mature teratoma and operative resection is useful and safe, also if a stereotactic radiotherapy is a possible alternative for small intracranial residual disease (Friedman et al, 2001; Kohyama et al, 2001). The 10-year survival rate is estimated to be 78-93% for mature teratomas and 45-86% for immature teratomas, (Brastianos et al, 2010; Kkyritis, 2010). NGGCTs are associated with a 20-75% of 5-year survival rate following radiotherapy with or without chemotherapy (da Silva et al, 2010). The survival of patients with mixed tumors is dependent on the malignant component of the neoplasm, with a 3-year survival rate ranging from 94% of mixed germinoma and teratoma to only 10% of mixed tumors of predominantly pure malignant elements (Brastianos et al, 2010; Kkyritis, 2010). Application of very aggressive protocol including surgery (also for residual disease), radio and chemotherapy in selected cases may sporadically result in complete response and long survival also in cases of disseminated intracranial germ cell tumors (Kageji et al, 2007; Kochi et al, 2003).

### 6.3 Pineal parenchymal tumors

Gross-total resection is the standard of care for pineocytomas (Blakeley & Grossman, 2006) and is associated with a 5-year overall survival rate of 86-91% (Dahiya & Perry, 2010). Radiation therapy may be reserved for those patients with an incomplete resection or recurrent disease (Brastianos et al, 2010). Recently, a retrospective analysis of a small cohort of patients treated with up-front stereotactic radiosurgery documented a 1-, 3- and 5-year survival rate of 100, 92.3 and 92.3%, but this results should be interpreted with caution as susceptible to various biases (Kano et al, 2009). Pineal parenchymal tumors of intermediate differentiation are very rare so that a therapeutic treatment is not yet standardized. For high-grade lesions an aggressive management with a combination of surgery, radio and chemotherapy is reasonable, whereas for low-grade tumors the benefit of a postoperative radiotherapy remains unclear, at least after a gross-total exeresis (Anan et al, 2006; Senft et al, 2008). Pineoblastomas are very aggressive tumors with a high propensity to CSF dissemination and local recurrence. A correct management should include maximal safe surgical resection followed by chemo and radiotherapy (Brastianos et al, 2010; Dahiya & Perry, 2010). Lutterbach and collegues (Lutterbach et al, 2002) reported the largest series (retrospective and multicentric) to date regarding malignant PPTs (pineoblastoma and pineal parenchymal tumors of intermediate differentiation) in adult. Median overall survival of pineoblastomas was 77 months with a 5- and 10-year rate of 51% and 23% respectively. Median overall survival of pineal parenchymal tumors of intermediate differentiation was 165 months with a 5- and 10-year rate of 80% and 72%. Taken together, residual disease after initial treatment (no or minimal residual disease vs major residual disease), histology (pineoblastoma vs pineal parenchymal tumor of intermediate differentiation) and extent of disease (localized vs disseminated) were independent prognostic factors for overall survival. As for pineocytomas, also for pineoblastomas stereotactic radiosurgery has been investigated as a primary treatment modality with conflicting results. In one retrospective study seven patients with pineoblastomas or mixed pineal parenchymal tumors were submitted to stereotactic radiosurgery with a 1-, 3- and 5-year survival rate of 87.5, 57.1 and 28.6% respectively (Kano et al, 2009). In an older retrospective study stereotactic radiosurgery was used as the sole treatment or as an adjuvant therapy in four patients with pineoblastomas who died in a range of 7-56 months after diagnosis (Hasegawa et al, 2002). Finally, a possible alternative approach is interstitial brachytherapy but the number of patients treated with this strategy is too small to draw final conclusions (Julow et al, 2006).

### 6.4 Papillary tumor of the pineal region

Papillary tumor of the pineal region is a rare and recently described neoplasm with a tendency to local recurrence (51% in a recent series) (Fèvre-Montange et al, 2006). There is still no defined treatment protocol but aggressive local therapy with maximal surgical resection and adjuvant radiotherapy has been suggested (Dahiya & Perry, 2010). Nevertheless, the role of postoperative radiation therapy is debated. Despite clear-cut histological criteria have yet to be defined, most papillary tumors of the pineal region correspond to low-grade malignancy (WHO grade II) and 5-year estimated overall survival and progression-free survival are approximately 73% and 27% respectively. Mitotic index higher than 5 per 10 HPFs and residual disease after surgery are correlated with recurrence and decreased survival (Fèvre-Montange, 2006).

### 6.5 Other tumors

Pineal region meningiomas, originating at the level of the velum interpositum, should be surgically removed with a goal of gross-total resection as in all other sites (Brastianos et al, 2010). In a cohort of ten patients operated for a meningioma of the pineal region in all but one case there was no local recurrence at 3-year follow-up (Konovalov et al, 1996). There is still no general consensus for the treatment of gliomas of the pineal region. Given the fact that most of these tumors are small, localized in the tectal region, without contrast enhancement and with a very indolent course, the preferred approach seems to be a close radiological follow-up with surgical management of an eventual hydrocephalus (Daglioglu et al, 2003; Yeh et al, 2002). When a clinical and/or radiological progression is observed a stereotactic biopsy should be considered in order to properly define histology and radiotherapy and/or chemotherapy are recommended (Brastianos et al, 2010).

## 7. Surgical approaches

### 7.1 Anatomical background

Surgery of the pineal region tumours is a challenge for most neurosurgeons because of the variety of pathologies but mainly for the very deep anatomical location. Pineal region corresponds to the posterior tentorial incisural space (Rhoton, 2000). It lies in front of the cerebellum and behind the midbrain into the cerebello-mesencephalic fissure and is related with the quadrigeminal cistern (Rhoton & Ono, 1996; Yasargil, 1984). It extends upward to the lower surface of the splenium and backward to the level of the tentorial apex. Laterally its boundaries are the pulvinar of thalamus and the posterior parahippocampal gyrus but it continues in the middle or lateral incisural space.

### 7.2 Anesthesia considerations

Surgical procedures are done under standard general anesthesia. If sitting position is used, a central venous catheter should be placed and trans-oesophagel Doppler monitoring should

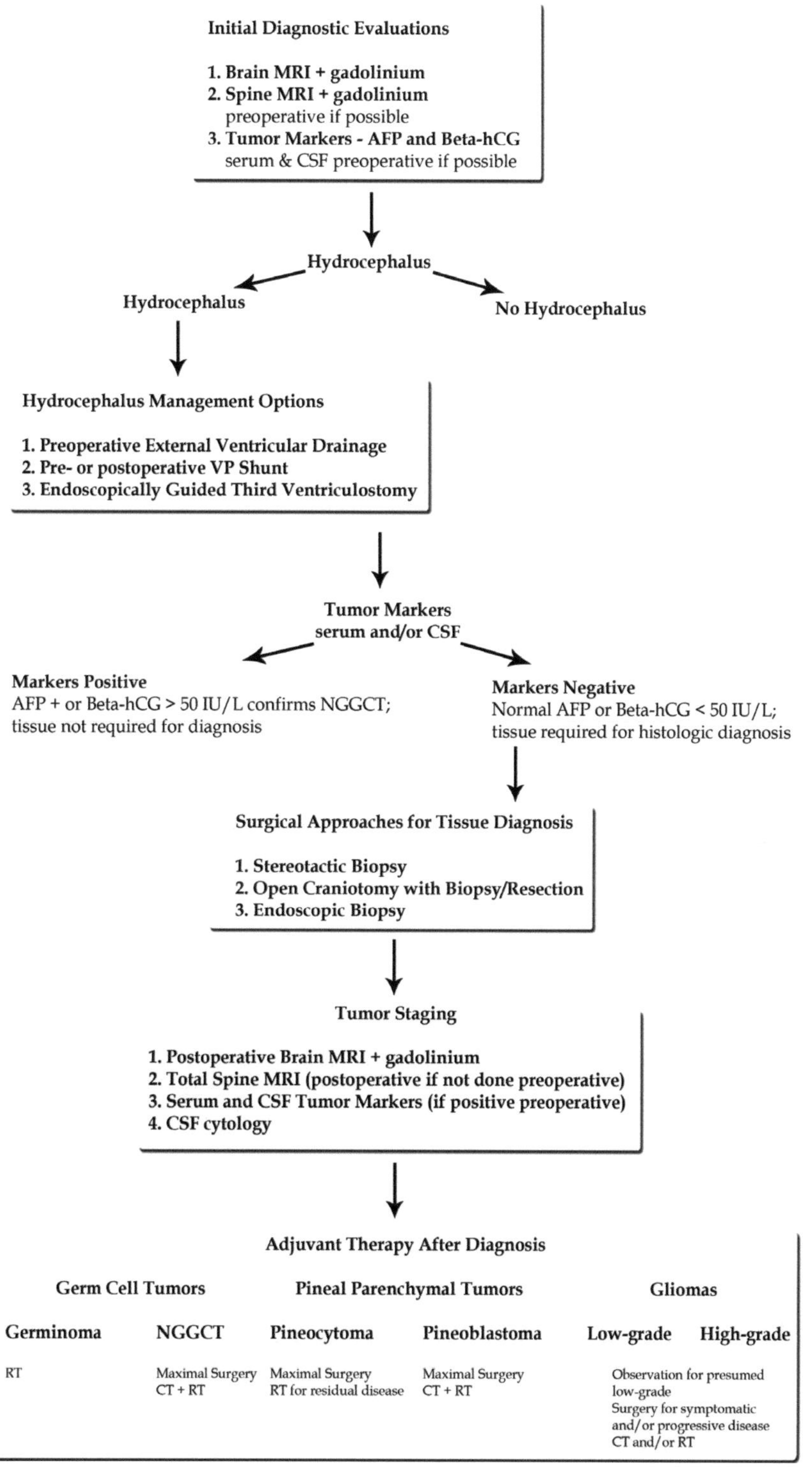


Table 2. Algorithm for diagnosis and treatment of PRTs (for more details see text)

be done for the risk of air embolism. When hydrocephalus is present, particular care should be reserved to increased intracranial pressure and a pre-operative external ventricular drainage, in sitting position, is preferable to prevent hypertensive pneumocephalus.

### 7.3 Operative approaches

Several approaches were so far developed to improve the exposure of the pineal region but basically they are categorized as either supratentorial or infratentorial approaches. The supratentorial approaches include the posterior interhemispheric trancallosal (Dandy, 1921), the occipital transtentorial (Foerster, 1928; Jamieson, 1971; Poppen, 1966; Lapras, 1987) and the very rarely used transtemporal-transventricular (Van Wagenen, 1931) approach. The exposure merely through the posterior fossa is achieved by the infratentorial-supracerebellar approach. Supra/infratentorial-transinus approach (Sekhar & Goel 1992; Ziyal et al, 1998), combining both supratentorial and infratentorial perspective, provide wider exposure of the pineal region but they are longer procedures with more risk of morbidity. Choosing amongst different surgical routes is mainly related to the size and location of the lesion to treat as well as to the surgeon's experience and preference with a specific approach. Generally supratentorial approaches are suitable for pineal lesions displacing downward the Galen's Vein complex; lesions developing below the level of the Galen's vein complex and displacing it upward are better managed through the infratentorial avenues. This allows dealing with pineal region tumors with less risks of damage of so crucial venous structures.

### 7.4 Patient positioning

Depending which approach is selected different position can be used, although the same position is suitable for more approaches.

#### 7.4.1 Sitting position

It is most commonly used for infratentorial-supracerebellar approach (Bruce, 1993). The head is fixed neutrally and moderately flexed, until tentorium is nearly parallel to the floor (Fig. 1). Caution should be taken to maintain two-finger breadth between chin and sternum to avoid compression of superior airways and jugular veins and consequent intracranial high venous pressure. After dural opening cerebellum spontaneously falls down offering a natural corridor below the inferior aspect of tentorium. At the depth of exposure anatomical landmarks are better recognizable, moreover fluids, CSF or blood, are continuously drained resulting in an always clean surgical field. On the other hand sitting position is often very tiring for the surgeon and complications are represented by air embolism, pneumocephalus and subdural haematoma (Bruce & Stein, 1993).

#### 7.4.2 Lateral position

Patient is positioned in lateral decubitus with the non-dominant hemisphere in dependent position (McComb & Apuzzo, 1988). The head is rotated 30 degrees toward the floor. A variation of lateral position is the three-quarter prone position, where the head is at an oblique 45 degrees angle with the non dominant hemisphere dependent (McComb & Apuzzo, 1987; Ausman et al, 1988). Both positions are used for occipital-transtentorial approach because the dependent hemisphere is easily retracted from the falco-tentorial junction with the aid of gravity. It is more comfortable for the surgeon but positioning could be time-consuming and demanding for O.R. personnel.

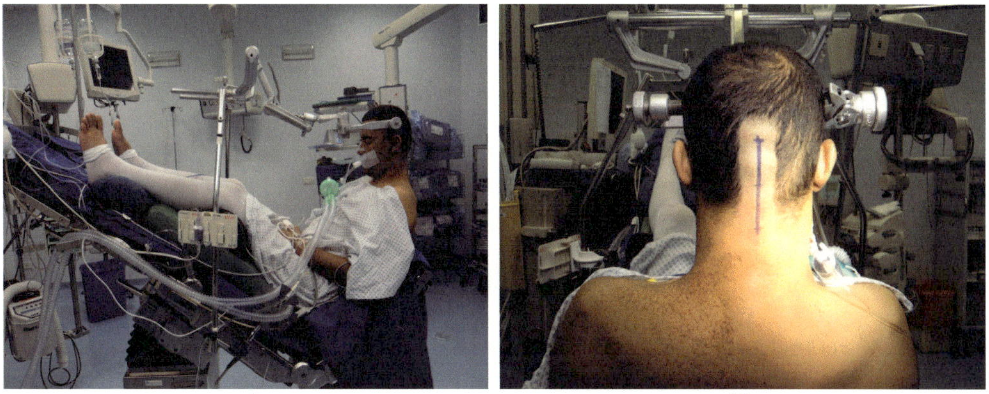

A B

Fig. 1. The sitting position for the infratentorial-supracerebellar approach. (A) The head is moderately flexed bringing the tentorium almost parallel to the floor. The inferior limbs are positioned higher than the level of heart to support venous pressure and prevent air embolism (B) The head is fixed with Mayfield head rest in neutral position. Median longitudinal skin incision is made from 2 cm above the inion down to C3 level.

### 7.4.3 Prone position

Is the simplest and fastest position to set up. Generally used for pediatric patients and for supratentorial approaches (Bruce et al., 1996). The head is neutrally fixed and slight flexed but the anatomical landmarks are inverted. Fluids stay in the field and need to be continuously aspirated getting the procedure slow. Venous drainage is not facilitated and brain or cerebellum swelling could occur. A variation is represented by Concorde position with the head rotated 15 degrees away from the side of craniotomy (Kobayashi et al, 1983).

## 7.5 Infratentorial procedures

### 7.5.1 Infratentorial-supracerebellar approach

The classic median infratentorial-supracerebellar approach was first described by Horsley, in 1910 and Krause in 1926; then it was refined and popularized by Stein in 1971. More recently extensions of the original approach were developed: the paramedian approach (Yasargil, 1984) and the extreme-lateral approach (Vishteh et al, 2000) to the lateral tentorial incisural region, the supracerebellar-transtentorial approach (Yonekawa et al., 2001) to the posterior parahyppocampal gyrus. For the median approach the sitting position is generally preferred. After a midline incision extending from 2 cm above the inion down to the level of C3 or C4 spinous process, a median suboccipital craniotomy is performed; the Torcular and adjacent transverse sinuses are skeletonized. Posterior edge of foramen magnum is not routinely opened but this maneuver facilitates opening the cisterna magna to release CFS. Every effort should be done to avoid air embolism waxing patent veins of the bone. The dura is opened in a gentle curvilinear fashion along the inferior margin of both transverse sinuses, and retracted upward via tacking suture. Almost complete exposure of transverse sinuses is necessary to avoid compression of the sinuses against the edge of craniotomy; moreover it permits a more angled vision through the microscope, in a cranio-caudal direction. If the posterior fossa is tight, opening arachnoid of cisterna magna allows releasing CFS. Cerebellum falls down spontaneously for gravity, opening the anatomical corridor below the tentorium. Under microscope magnification, severing the bridging veins between cerebellum and tentorium is a crucial point to gain the corridor carrying out the approach through. As some authors reported (Ueyama et al., 1998; Bruce & Stein, 1993; Fain et al., 1994; Page 1977), bridging veins in the midline can be sacrificed but this could lead to cerebellar venous infarction and consequent swelling. The arachnoidal adhesions should be released on the surface of cerebellum and all along the tentorial incisura as well, where they are particularly thickened. This allows pushing down the cerebellum and provides a large exposure of the region up to the apex of tentorium where the venous complex of Galen drains into the straight sinus, inferior to the splenium. Just below, the pineal gland and the posterior wall of third ventricle are visualized. Laterally the medial part of the pulvinar of thalamus borders the surgical field (Ammirati et al., 2002). Easy access to superior collicles is provided but the culmen vermis may limit the exposure of the inferior half of the quadrigeminal plate. Without splitting the vermis, a more angled vision through the microscope in a cranio-caudal direction together with an extensive and meticulous opening of the cerebello-mesencephalic fissure give the full exposure of the quadrigeminal plate down to the inferior collicles (Bricolo, 2000). Thus, the inferior limit of exposure would be considered the frenulum of inferior medullary velum with the origin of the trochlear nerve bilaterally (Fig. 2). The operative fields in very deep and extralong instruments are necessary together with a free-standing armrest to avoid surgeon's fatigue. When the tumor is encountered, posterior aspect of the capsule is sharply opened and internal debulking is done. Soft tumour could be easily decompressed by suction, after having taken some specimens for histological analysis. For decompression of solid tumors ultrasound aspirator is strongly recommended. Maintaining tumour capsule facilitate the dissection from surrounding structures. Whenever is possible total removal of the tumor should be achieved. When the lesion infiltrates the surrounding structures a sub-total or partial resection is justified, although residual tumor increases the risk of postoperative bleeding. A very careful hemostasis should be done and a watertight closure of the dura is mandatory. Craniotomy and skin closure are accomplished in the usual manner.

### 7.6 Supratentorial procedures

#### 7.6.1 Posterior interhemispheric transcallosal approach

The posterior interhemisferic transcallosal approach was proposed by Dandy in 1921 and popularized later by Yasargil for splenial and parasplenial lesions. It is suitable for lesions growing in pineal region below the level of the Galen's Vein complex (McComb et al., 1998). All positions could be used although sitting and prone positions have the advantage to allow a straight midline trajectory. Parieto-occipital craniotomy is performed, across the posterior third of superior sagittal sinus. Dura is opened in C-shaped fashion and reflected toward the midline. The approach in centered over the parietal lobe and every effort should be made to avoid tearing the bridging vein. It is preferable do not sacrifice more than one. Gently retracting the hemisphere laterally and releasing arachnoidal adherence with the falx, the interemispheric fissure is open. It is the surgical corridor leading to the splenium of corpus callosum identified by the white appearance. Retracting the parietal lobe instead of the occipital lobe allows avoiding visual field impairment. 2 cm callosotomy is made at the splenium and the lesion is identified in the velum interpositum, below the internal cerebral veins. Tumor occupied most of the exposure and it is interposed between the surgeon and caudal structure of the pineal region. Quadrigeminal plate and posterior choroidal artery are hidden until the tumor has been debulked and mostly removed at the end of the procedure. For this reason the posterior interhemisferic transcallosal approach is replaced in most case by the occipital-transtentorial approach or the infratentorial-supracerebellar approach and is used mainly for lesions expanding into the third ventricle as well as those extending upward in the corpus callosum (Hoffman, 1984; Rhoton et al., 1981).

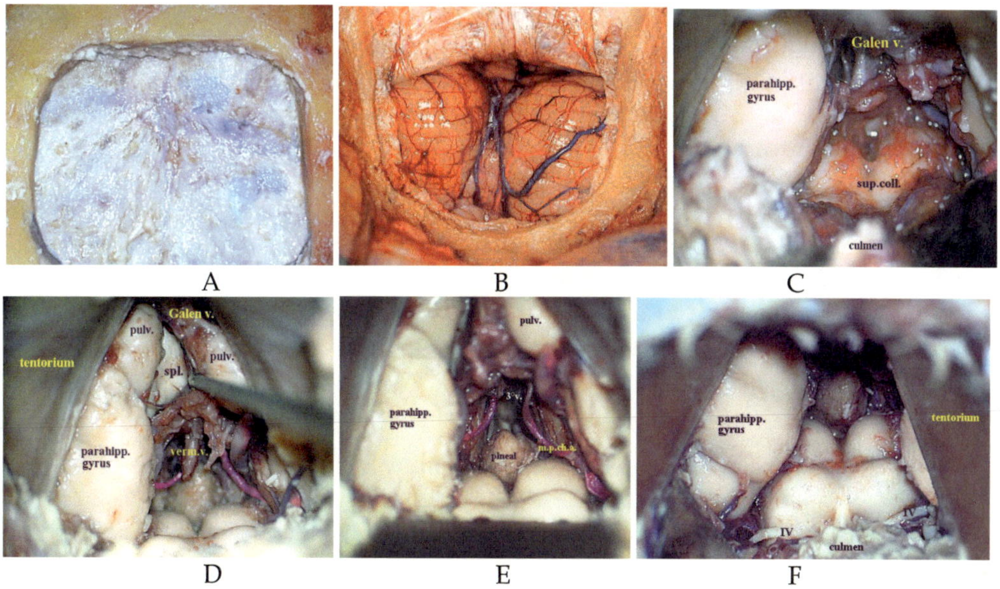


Fig. 2. Stepwise median infratentorial-supracerebellar approach in cadaveric specimen. (A) The median suboccipital craniotomy. The Torcular Herophili and the proximal part of both transverse sinuses are completely exposed. (B) After dural opening, bridging vein between the tentorial surface of cerebellum and the tentorium are severed allowing downward retraction, by self-retaining retractor, of the cerebellum. This gives access to the infratentorial-supracerebellar corridor. (C) Retraction of the culmen vermis exposes the Galen vein's complex (Galen v.) at tentorial apex and, below it, the superior collicles (sup.coll.) still covered by the deep arachnoidal layer of quadrigeminal cistern. Through the posterior tentorial incisura variable amount of the posterior parahippocampal gyrus (parahipp. gyrus) protrudes in the posterior incisural space. (D) Retraction of the vein of Galen (Galen v.) exposes the splenium of corpus callosum (spl.). Laterally both pulvinar thalami (pulv.) are evident. Severing the superior vermian veins (verm. v.) allows exposing the pineal gland and quadrigeminal plate. (E) Pineal gland (pineal) lies immediately above the quadrigeminal plate. Superiorly, dissecting the velum interpositum, the posterior third ventricle (3°v.) is entered. Laterally to the pineal gland the posterior medial choroidal arteries (p.m.ch.a) course toward the roof of the third ventricle. (F) Moving the microscope angle in a more cranio-caudal direction, through a careful and meticulous dissection of the cerebello-mesencephalic fissure, a complete exposure of quadrigeminal plate is achieved, down to the frenulum of superior medullary velum and the origin of both trochlear nerves (IV).

### 7.6.2 Occipital-transtentorial approach

The occipital-transtentorial approach was proposed by Foerster in 1928, described in detail by Poppen (1966) and popularized by Jamieson (1971). It is performed generally in lateral three-quarter prone position (Moshel et al., 2009) with non-dominant hemisphere dependent. Occipital craniotomy is carried out across superior sagittal sinus and Torcular. Dura is open in C-shaped fashion, reflected toward midline and retracted away from the Torcular via tack-up sutures. Lateral decubitus provides spontaneous falling down of occipital pole, minimizing retraction. The corridor along falco-tentorial junction is gained and the posterior tentorial incisura is reached. The Galen's vein complex comes into nice view but the exposure is widely enhanced by cutting the tentorium 1,5 cm lateral and parallel to the straight sinus, from the point anterior to the transverse sinus to the free edge (Moshel et al., 2009). Cutting the falx and the tentorium bilaterally, the exposure is enormously enlarged from the splenium cranially to the bottom of the cerebello-mesencephalic fissure caudally (Kawashima et al., 2002). All structures of the pineal region are well controlled as far as the quadrigeminal plate, although deep venous structures are somehow interposed between the surgeon and the tumor. The exposure is often excellent but the quite oblique perspective can disorient the surgeon. Moreover retraction of the occipital pole, although protected, gives the risk of visual field deficit. For the wide exposure of the pineal region that it can afford, the occipital-transtentorial approach represents an alternative to the infratentorial-supracerebellar approach.

## 8. Case report

A 60-year-old woman was admitted with two months history of headache and blurring vision. She complained of weakness of legs and balance disturbances. Neurological examination revealed only a slight ataxia. MRI of the brain showed a huge rounded well-enhanced lesion in the pineal region, suspected of meningioma, extending above and below the tentorium through the posterior tentorial incisura. Caudally dorsal midbrain was compressed and the Silvian aqueduct partially obstructed with consequent triventricular hydrocephalus. Cranially the lesion reached the splenium of corpus callosum, displacing the venous structures of Galen's vein complex (Fig. 3). According to Yasargil classification (Yasargil, 1996) the tumor looked a type 3 tentorial meningioma, arising from the posterior incisura. Digital angiography, after selective injection of the left internal carotid artery, showed a slight tumour blush, supplied by Bernasconi and Cassinari artery; in the venous phase a partial obstruction of the straight sinus was evident (Fig. 4). Considering the posterior attachment to the tentorium and the cranial displacement of the Galen's vein complex, the infratentorial-supracerebellar approach was believed the most appropriated to deal with the tumor. The patient was operated in sitting position and a median suboccipital craniectomy was carried out and extended to the torcular. The dura was opened flush to the torcular and proximal trasverse sinuses' inferior border that was lifted via tack up sutures. The huge meningioma was exposed through the infratentorial-supracerebellar corridor and gradually debulked with ultrasound aspirator. It was detached from the posterior tentorial edge, gently separated from the surrounding neuro-vascular structures and totally removed in a piecemeal fashion. Postoperative course was uneventful and the patient was discharged seven days after surgery. At discharge neurological ataxia was moderately worsened but recovered completely at six months follow-up. Histological examination documented a meningothelial meningioma (WHO Grade I). Postoperative and three year follow-up MRIs confirmed total removal and no recurrence of the lesion (Fig. 5).

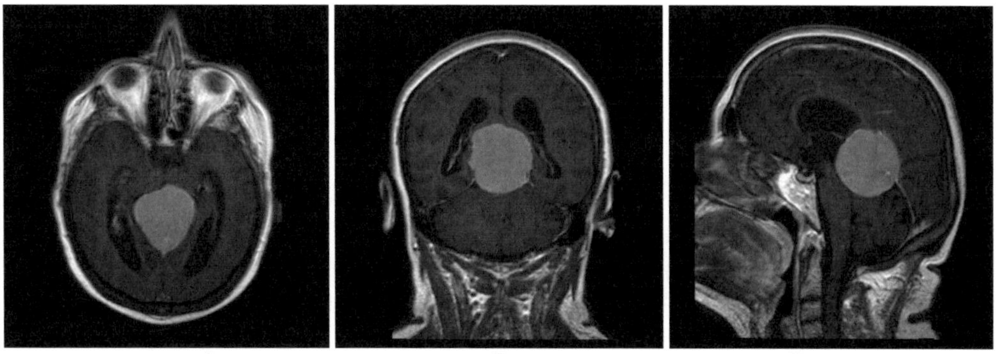

A B C

Fig. 3. Axial (A), coronal (B) and sagittal (C) preoperative MRI.

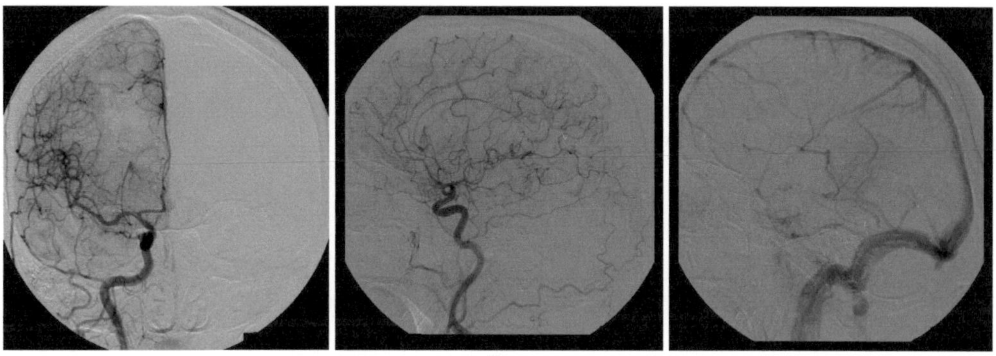

A B C

Fig. 4. Preoperative angiography. Slight tumor blush is visible supplied by Bernasconi and Cassinari artery (A-B). In venous phase straight sinus is minimally filled.

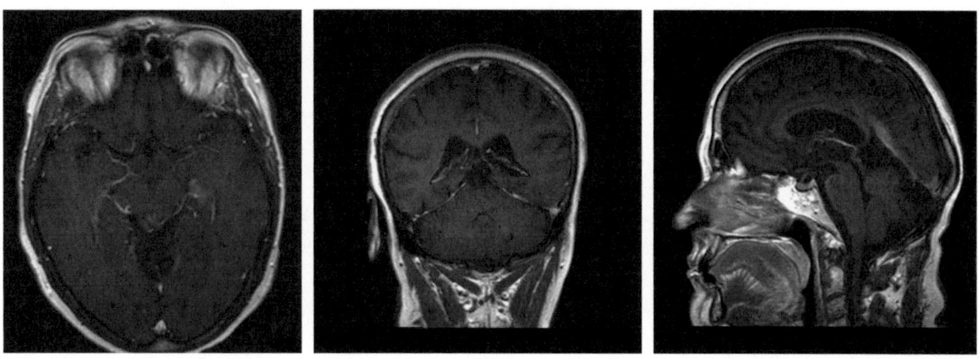

A B C

Fig. 5. Axial (A), coronal (B) and sagittal (C) three year follow-up MRI. The tumor was totally removed. No recurrence is evident.

## 9. References

Ammirati M, Bernardo A, Musumeci A & Bricolo A. (2002). Comparison of different infratentorial-supracerebellar approaches to the posterior and middle incisural space: a cadaveric study. *J. Neurosurg,* Vol. 97, No 4,(Oct. 2002), pp. 922-928

Anan M, Ishii K, Nakamura T, Yamashita M, Katayama S, Sainoo M, Nagatomi H & Kobayashi H. (2006). Postoperative adjuvant treatment for pineal parenchymal tumor of intermediate differentiation. *J Clin Neurosci,* Vol. 12, pp. 965-968

Ausman JI, Malik GM, Dujovniy M & Mann R. (1988). Three-quarter prone approach to the pineal-tentorial region. Surg. Neurol, Vol. 29, No 4, (Apr 1988), pp. 298-306

Blakeley JO & Grossman SA. (2006). Management of pineal region tumors. *Curr Treat Options Oncol,* Vol. 7, pp. 505-516

Pediatr Blood Cancer, Vol. 54, pp. 377-383

Brastianos HC, Brastianos PK & Blakeley JC. (2011). Pineal region tumors, In: *Primary central nervous system tumors. Pathogenesis and therapy.* Norden AD, deardon DA & Wen PYC (Ed), pp. 435-455, Humana Press, ISBN 978-1-60761-165-3, New York, USA

Bricolo A. (2000). Surgical management of intrinsic brain stem gliomas. *Op Tech Neurosurg,* Vol. 3, No 2, pp. 137-154

Bruce JN. (1993). Management of pineal region tumors. *Neurosurg Quart,* Vol. 3, pp. 103-119

Bruce JN & Stein BM. (1993). Supracerebellar approach in the pineal region, In: *Brain Surgery: Complication Avoidance and Management.* Apuzzo MLJ, pp. 511-536, Churchill-Livingstone, New York

Bruce JN, Fetell MR & Stein BM. (1996). Surgical approach to pineal tumors, In: *Neurosurgery.* Wilkins RH, Rengachary SS, pp. 1023-1033, McGraw-Hill, New York

Bruce JN & Ogden AT. (2004). Surgical strategy for treating patients with pineal region tumors. *J Neurooncol,* Vol. 69, pp. 221-236

Chandrasama PT, Smith MM & Apuzzo ML. (1989). Stereotactic biopsy in the diagnosis of brain masses: comparison of results of biopsy and resected surgical specimen. *Neurosurgery,* Vol. 24, No. 2, (Feb 1989), pp. 160-165

Chang AH, Fuller GN, Debnam JM, Karis JP, Coons SW, Ross JS, Dean BL. (2007). MR imaging of papillary tumor of the pineal region. *AJNR Am J Neuroradiol.,* Vol. 29, pp. 187-189

Dahiya S & Perry A. (2010). Pineal tumors. *Adv Anat Pathol,* Vol. 17, No. 6 (Nov 2010), pp. 419-427

Daglioglu E, Cataltepe O & Akalan N. (2003). Tectal gliomas in children: the implications for natural history and management strategy. *Pediatr Neurosurg,* Vol. 38, pp. 223-231

Dandy WE. (1921). An operation for removal of pineal tumors. *Surg Gynec Obstet,* Vol. 33, pp. 113-119

da Silva NS, Cappellano AM, Diez B, Cavalheiro S, Gardner S, Wisoff J, Kellie S, Parker R, Gawin J & Finlay J. (2010). Primary chemotherapy for intracranial germ cell tumors: results of the third international CNS germ cell tumor study. *Pediatr Blood Cancer.,* Vol. 54, No. 3, pp. 377-383

De Tribolet N. (2009). Management of pineal region tumors, In: *Practical handbook of neurosurgery. From Leading neurosurgeons.* Sindou M (Ed.), pp.287-300, Springer, Wien-New York

Echevarria ME, Fangusaro J & Goldman S. (2008). Pediatric central nervous system germ cell tumors: a review. *Oncologist,* Vol. 13, pp. 690-699

Fain JS, Tomlinson FH, Scheithauer BW, Parisi JE, Fletcher GP, Kelly PJ & Miller GM. (1994) Symptomatic glial cysts of the pineal gland. *J Neurosurg*, Vol. 80, pp. 454-460

Fèvre-Montange M, Hasselblatt M, Figarell-Branger D, Chauveinc L, Champier J, Saint-Pierre G, Taillander L, Coulon A, Paulus W, Fauchon F & Jouvet A. (2006). Prognosis and histopathologic features in papillary tumors of the pineal region: a retrospective multicenter study of 31 cases. *J Neuropathol Exp Neurol*, Vol. 65, pp. 1004-1011

Friedman JA, Lynch JJ, Buckner JC, Scheithauer BW & Raffel C (2001). Management of malignant pineal germ cell tumor with residual teratoma. *Neurosurgery*, Vol. 48, pp. 518-522

Gaillard F, Jones J. (2010). Masses of the pineal region: clinical presentation and radiographic features. *Postgrad Med J*. Vol. 86, pp. 597-607

Haas-Kogan DA, Misset BT, Wara WM, Donaldson SS, Lamborn KR, Prados MD, Fisher PG, Huhn SL, Fisch BM, Berger MS & Le QT. (2003). Radiation theraoy fro intracranial germ cell tumors. *Int J Radiat Oncol Biol Phys*, Vol. 56, pp. 511-518

Hasegawa A, Ohtsubo K, Mori W. (1987). Pineal gland in old age; quantitative and qualitative morphological study of 168 human autopsy cases. *Brain Res.*, Vol. 21, pp. 343-349

Hasegawa T, Kondziolka D, Hadjipanayis CC, Flickinger JC & Lunsford LD. (2002). The role of radiosurgery for the treatment of pineal parenchymal tumors. *Neurosurgery*, Vol. 51, pp. 880-889

Hoffman HJ. (1984). Transcallosal approach to pineal tumor and the Hospital for Sick Children series of pineal region tumors, In: *Diagnosis and treatment of pineal region tumors*. Neuwelt EA, pp. 223-235, Williams & Wilkins, Baltimore

Horowitz MB, Hall WA. (1991). Central nervous system germinomas: a review. *Arch Neurol*, Vol. 48, pp. 652-657

Lutterbach J, Fauchon F, Schield SE, Chang SM, Pagenstecher A, Volk B, Ostertag C, Momm F & Jovet A. (2002). Malignant pineal parenchymal tumors in adult patients: patterns of care and prognostic factors. *Neurosurgery*, Vol. 51, pp. 44-56

Jacobs DA, Galetta SL. (2007). Neuro-ophthalmology for neuroradiologists. *AJNR Am J Neuroradiol*. Vol. 28, pp. 3-8.

Jamieson KG. (1971). Excision of pineal tumors. *J Neurosurg*, Vol. 35, pp. 550-553

Julow J, Viola A & Major T. (2006). Review of radiosurgery of pineal parenchymal tumors. Long survival following 125-iodine brachytherapy of pineoblastomas in 2 cases. *Minim Inv Neurosurg*, Vol. 49, pp. 276-281

Júnior GV, Dellaretti M, de Carvalho GT, Brandão RA, Mafra A, de Sousa AA. (2011). Papillary tumor of the pineal region. *Brain Tumor Pathol*. [Epub ahead of print]

Kageji T, Nagahiro S, Matsuzaki K, Kanematsu Y, Nakatani M, Okamoto Y & Watanabe T. (2007). Successful neoadjuvant synchronous chemo- and radiotherapy for disseminated primary intracranial choriocarcinoma: case report. *J Neurooncol*, Vol. 83, pp. 199-204

Kano H, Niranjan A, Kondziolka D, Flickinger JC & Lunsford D. (2009). Role of stereotactic radiosurgery in the management of pineal parenchymal tumors. *Prog Neurol Surg*, Vol. 23, pp. 44-58

Kawashima M, Rhoton AL & Matsushima T. (2002). Comparison of posterior approaches to the posterior incisural space: microsurgical anatomy and proposal of a new method, the occipital bitranstentorial/falcine approach. *Neurosurgery,* Vol. 51, No 5, (Nov. 2002), pp. 1208-1221

Kilgore DP, Strother CM, Starshak RJ, Haughton VM. (1986). Pineal germinoma: MR imaging. *Radiology.,* Vol. 158, pp. 435-438

Klein P, Rubinstein LJ. (1989). Benign symptomatic glial cysts of the pineal gland: a report of seven cases and review of the literature. *J Neurol Neurosurg Psychiatry.,* Vol. 52, pp. 991-995

Kobayashi S, Sugita K, Tanaka Y & Kyoshima K. (1983). Infratentorial approach to the pineal region in the prone position: Concorde position. *J Neurosurg,* Vol. 58, pp. 141-143

Kochi M, Itoyama Y, Shiraishi S, Kitamura I, Mambayashi T & Ushio Y. (2003). Successful treatment of intracranial nongerminomatous malignant germ cell tumors by administering neoadjuvant chemotherapy and radiotherapy bifore excision of residual tumors. *J Neurosurg,* Vol. 99, pp. 106-114

Konovalov AN, Spallone A & Pitskhelauri DI. (1996). Meningioma of the pineal region: a surgical series of 10 cases. *J Neurosurg,* Vol. 85, pp. 586-590

Konovalov AN, Spallone A, Pitzkhelauri DI. (1999). Pineal epidermoid cysts: diagnosis and management. *J Neurosurg.,* Vol. 91, pp. 370-374

Konovalov AN & Pitskhelauri, DI. (2003). Principles and treatment of the pineall region tumors. *Surg Neurol,* Vol. 59, pp. 250-268

Kohyama S, Uematsu M. Ishihara S, Shima K, Tamai S & Kusano S. (2001). An experience of stereotactic radiation therapy for primary intracranial choriocarcinoma. *Tumori,* Vol. 87, pp. 162-165

Krause F. (1926). Operative freilegung der vierhugel, nebst beobachrungen uber hirndruch und dekompression. *Zentralbl Chir,* Vol. 53, pp. 2812-2819

Kyritis AP. (2010). Management of primary intracranial germ cell tumors. *J Neurooncol,* Vol. 96, pp. 143-149

Lapras C. (1984). Surgical therapy of pineal region tumors, In: *Diagnosis and treatment of pineal region tumors.* Neuwelt EA, pp. 289-299, Williams & Wilkins, Baltimore

Lapras C & Patet JD (1987). Controversies, techniques, and strategies for pineal tumor surgery, In: *Surgery of the third ventricle.* Apuzzo MLJ, pp. 649-662, Williams & Wilkins, Baltimore

Lapras C, Patet JD, Mottolese C & Lapras C Jr. (1987). Direct surgery for pineal tumours: occipital-trantentorial approach. *Progr Exp Tumour Res,* Vol. 30, pp. 268-280

Lassman AB, Bruce JN, Fetell MR. (2006). Metastases to the pineal gland. *Neurology.,* Vol. 67, pp. 1303-1304

Louis DN, Ohgaki H, Wiestler OD, Cavenee WK, Burger PC, Jouvet A, Scheithauer BW, Kleihues J. (2007). The 2007 WHO classification of tumours of the central nervous system. *Acta Neuropathol.,* Vol. 114:97-109. Review. Erratum in: *Acta Neuropathol.* 2007, Vol. 114, pp. 547

Matsutani M. (2004). Clinical management of primary central nervous system germ cell tumors. *Semin Oncol,* Vol. 31, pp. 676-683

McComb JG & Apuzzo MLJ. (1987). Posterior intrahemispheric retrocallosal and transcallosal approaches, In: *Surgery of the third ventricle.* Apuzzo MLJ, pp. 611-641, Williams & Wilkins, Baltimore

McComb J & Apuzzo M. (1988). The lateral decubitusposition for the surgical approach to pineal location tumors. *Concepts Pediat Neurosurg,* Vol. 8, pp. 186-199

McComb J, Levy M & Apuzzo M. (1998). Posterior intrahemispheric retrocallosal and transcallosal approaches, In: *Surgery of the third ventricle,* 2nd ed, Apuzzo MLJ, pp. 486-511, Williams & Wilkins, Baltimore

Moise G, Ogden AT & Bruce JN. (2011). Pineal gland tumors, In: *Principles and practice of Neuro-Oncology.* Metha MP (Ed.), pp. 485-495, demosMEDICAL, New York

Moshel AM, Parker EC & Kelly PJ. (2009). Occipital transtentorial approach to the precentral cerebellar fissure and posterior incisural space. *Neurosurgery,* Vol. 65, No 3, (Sept. 2009), pp. 554-564

Page LK. (1977). The infratentorial-supracerebellar exposure of tumors in pineal area. *Neurosurgery,* Vol. 1, pp. 36-40

Pearce JM. (2005). Parinaud's syndrome. *J Neurol Neurosurg Psychiatry.,* Vol. 76, pp. 99

Poppen JL. (1966). The right occipital approach to a pinealoma. *J Neurosurg,* Vol. 25, pp. 706-710

Regis J, Bouillot P, Rouby-Volot F, Figarella-Branger D, Dufour H,Peragut JC. (1996). Pineal region tumors and the role of stereotactic biopsy: review of the mortality, morbidity, and diagnostic rates in 370 cases. *Neurosurgery.,* Vol. 39, pp. 907-912

Rhoton AL Jr. (2000). Tentorial Incisura. *Neurosurgery,* Vol. 47, suppl, (Sept 2000), pp. S131-S153

Rhoton AL Jr, Yamamoto I & Peace DA. (1981). Microsurgery of the third ventricle, 2: operative approaches. *Neurosurgery,* Vol. 8, pp. 357-373

Rhoton AL Jr & Ono M. (1996). Microsurgical anatomy of the region of the tentorial incisura, In: *Neurosurgery.* Wilkins RH, Rengachary SS, pp. 897-915, McGraw-Hill, New York

Sekhar LN & Goel A. (1992). Combined supratentorial and infratentorial approach to large pineal-region meningioma. *Surg Neurol,* Vol. 37, pp. 197-201

Sener RN. (1995). The pineal gland: A comparative MR imaging study in children and adults with respect to normal anatomical variations and pineal cysts. *Pediatr Radiol.,* Vol. 25, pp. 245-248

Senft C, Raabe A, Hattingen E, Sommerlad D, Seifert V & Franz K. (2008). Pineal parenchymal tumor of intermediate differentiation: diagnostic pitfalls and discussion of treatment options of a rare tumor entity. *Neurosurg Rev,* Vol. 31, No. 2, (Apr 2008), pp. 231-236

Shibamoto Y, Sasai K, Oya N, Hiraoka M. (2001). Intracranial germinoma: radiation therapy with tumor volume-based dose selection. *Radiology.,* Vol. 218, pp. 452-456

Smirniotopoulos JG, Rushing EJ, Mena H. (1992). Pineal region masses: differential diagnosis. *Radiographics.,* Vol. 12, pp. 577-596

Stein BM. (1971). The infratentorial supracerebellar approach to the pineal lesions. *J Neurosurg,* Vol. 35, pp. 197-202

Sugiyama K, Uozumi T, Kiya K, Mukada K, Arita K, Kurisu K, Hotta T, Ogasawara H, Sumida M. (1992). Intracranial germ-cell tumor with synchronous lesions in the pineal and suprasellar regions: report of six cases and review of the literature. *Surg Neurol.,* Vol. 38, pp. 114-120

Ueyama T, Al-Mefty O & Tamaki N. (1998). Bridging veins on the tentorial surface of the cerebellum: A microsurgical anatomic study and operative considerations. *Neurosurgery,* Vol. 43, pp. 1137-1145

Van Wagenen WP. (1931). A surgical approach for the removal of certain pineal tumors: report of a case. *Surg Gynecol Obstet,* Vol. 53, pp. 216-220

Villano JL, Propp JM, Porter KR, Stewart AK, Valyi-Nagy T, Li X, Engelhard HH, McCarthy BJ. (2008) Malignant pineal germ-cell tumors: an analysis of cases from three tumor registries. *Neuro Oncol.*, Vol. 10, pp. 121-130

Vishteh AG, David CA, Marciano FF, Coscarella E & Spetzler RF. (2000). Extreme lateral supracerebellar infratentorial approach to the posterolateral mesencephalon: technique and clinical experience. *Neurosurgery*, Vol. 46, pp. 384-389

Yamini B, Refai D, Rubin CM, & Frim DM. (2004). Initial endoscopic management of pineal region tumors and associated hydrocephalus: clinical series and literature review. *J Neurosurg*, Vol. 100, pp. 437-441

Yasargil MG. (1984). Paramedian supracerebellar approach, In: *Microneurosurgery*, Yasargil MG, Vol. I, p. 242, Georg Thieme Verlag, New York

Yasargil MG. (1994). Mesencephalic lesion and parasplenial lesion, In: *Microneurosurgery*, Yasargil MG, Vol. IVA, pp. 308-309, Georg Thieme Verlag, New York

Yasargil MG. (1996). Meningiomas, In: *Microneurosurgery*, Yasargil MG, Vol. IVB, pp. 137, Georg Thieme Verlag, New York

Yonekawa Y, Imhof HG, Taub E, Curcic M, Kaku Y, Roth P, Wieser HG & Groscurth P. (2001). Supracerebellar transtentorial approach to posterior temporomedial structures. *J Neurosurg*, Vol. 94, pp. 339-345

Yeh DD, Warnick RE & Ernst RJ. (2002). Management strategy for adult patients with dorsal midbrain gliomas. *Neurosurgery*, Vol. 50, pp. 735-738

Ziyal IM, Sekhar LN, Salas E, Olan WJ. (1998). Combined supra/infratentorial-transinus approach to large pineal region tumors. *J Neurosurg*, Vol. 88, pp. 1050-1057

# Section 3

## Management of Neurovascular Diseases

# 9

# Cerebral Aneurysms

Mohammad Jamous, Mohammad Barbarawi and Hytham El Oqaili
*Department of Neurosurgery, Faculty of Medicine,*
*Jordan University of Science and Technology, Irbid,*
*Jordan*

## 1. Introduction

Intracranial aneurysms (IAs) occur in 0.2%-9% of adults (18, 35, 54). This wide range probably reflects methodological differences between studies: prospective or retrospective designs, diagnostic tools (angiography or autopsy) and study populations. IAs are present with subarachnoid haemorrhage (SAH) in the majority of cases. Aneurismal subarachnoid haemorrhage is a sudden and often catastrophic event with high mortality and morbidity rates: 15% die before hospitalisation and 36% die within 48 hours of its onset, 43% in the first week and 57% within six months (3). Furthermore, half of the survivors manifest physical or psychosocial deficits one year after SAH (22).

In the USA, it is estimated that SAH accounts for over 25% of all stroke-related years of potential life lost before the age of 65 (37). In Japan, SAH inflicts as many people as automobile accidents (AMA), about 13,000 per year (60). Recent improvements in the management of patients with aneurismal SAH have slightly reduced fatality rates over the last three decades (28). However, the severity of the initial bleeding and the clinical condition of the patients following SAH remain the main predictors for their outcome. Therefore, we believe that the treatment of unruptured aneurysms and the prevention of their formation and progression represent the best practical measures to avoid the grim outcomes of SAH. This requires a good understanding of the pathogenesis of IAs and the role of the various risk factors in their formation and progression.

## 2. Definition of cerebral aneurysm

The word aneurysm comes from the Latin word *aneurysma,* which means dilatation. Aneurysm is a persistent localised dilatation of the vessel wall, usually an artery. Saccular aneurysms account for the vast majority (98%) of all intracranial aneurysms, and the word aneurysm in this work refers to this form. Other types of aneurysms are fusiform, dissecting, infectious (mycotic) and traumatic aneurysms.

Saccular aneurysms consist of three main regions: the neck, the sac and the dome. The neck is that part of an aneurysm where it joins the parent artery, while the sac represents the cavity of the aneurysm and the dome relates to the convex wall facing the neck of the aneurysm. The size of an aneurysm is usually described as the maximum distance between the neck and the dome, and more detailed description of an aneurysm's size requires the measurement of its two dimensions: the maximum distance between the neck and the dome and the maximum distance between the sides of the aneurysm (figure 1). Saccular aneurysms are specific to the intracranial arteries because their walls lack an external elastic lamina and contain very thin adventitia factors that may predispose to the formation of aneurysms. An additional feature is that they lie unsupported in the subarachnoid space.

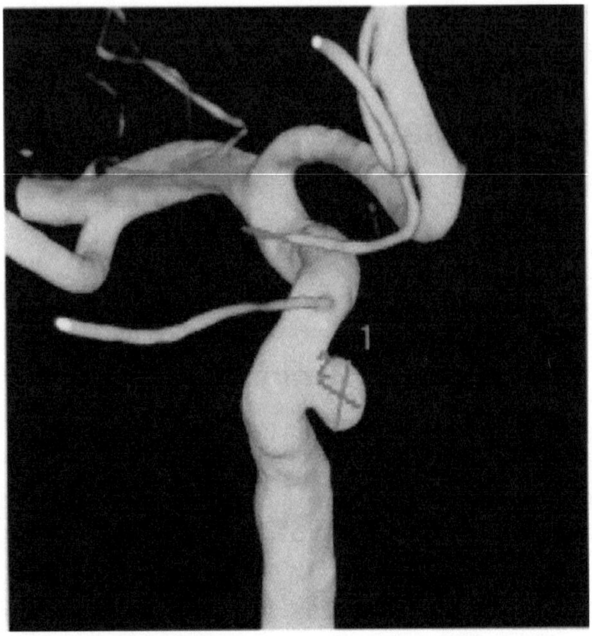


Fig. 1. 3D DSA image of a left ICA showing a left ICA saccular aneurysm, measuring 22.7 mm (1) X 13.5 mm (2) and projecting medially

## 3. Historical background

The first description of saccular cerebral aneurysm in the medical literature was made in the eighteenth century (1761) by Morgagni (58) and Biumi (2), who first described the dilatation of the cerebral arteries and showed that their rupture might lead to SAH. Morgagni and Biumi's observations were not further evaluated until 1859, when Sir William Gull (21) offered recognition of the pathological nature of the lesion by his often quoted statement: "whenever young persons die with apoplexy, and after death a large effusion of blood is found, especially if the effusion be over the surface of the brain, in the meshes of the pia matter, the presence of aneurysm is probable."

In 1927, Egas Moniz (57) introduced cerebral angiography to the medical community and the clinician finally developed a method to diagnose CA. In 1933, Dott (10) presented a series of 8 patients who had undergone angiography with a diagnosis of subarachnoid haemorrhage, describing the location of their aneurysms and reporting his operative results. This was followed by many reports describing different methods for the management of CA, among which was that of Dandy (9) who described a series of 108 patients, 30 of them having had an intracranial procedure while others had carotid ligation. The technique of angiography is considered to be the key for all research in the field of cerebral aneurysm.

## 4. Epidemiology of cerebral aneurysms

Intracranial aneurysms are reported to be present in about 5% (range: 0.2%-9.0%) of the general population (18, 35, 54). The prevalence figures are clearly related with the method employed and the region and population studied. The true prevalence of intracranial aneurysms remains unknown, since most aneurysms remain undiagnosed until they rupture or produce neurological deficits. In one series of 72 consecutive patients undergoing coronary angiography, incidental intracranial aneurysms were found in 5 cases (6.9%) (36); another series reported a 2.8% prevalence of asymptomatic incidental aneurysms in 4518 patients undergoing magnetic resonance angiography (31). Reviewing 3684 cerebral arteriograms, Winn et al. reported a 0.65% prevalence of asymptomatic IAs (100).

A high incidence of IA has been reported in Japan and Finland (14, 36); on the other hand, a low incidence was reported in India, Iran, the Middle East and many parts of Africa (39, 61, 62), and it is difficult to determine whether this regional variation is genuine or related to the difference in diagnostic workup among these countries.

Aneurysms are typically diagnosed in people aged 40-60 years, reaching a peak in people aged 55-60 years (23, 60). Intracranial aneurysms are uncommon in children, accounting for fewer than 2% of all cases. When aneurysms occur in the paediatric age group, they are more often post-traumatic or mycotic rather than degenerative, and they have a slight male predilection. Aneurysms in children are also larger than those found in adults (55, 67).

Cerebral aneurysms affect women more frequently than men. In an autopsy study from Japan, the prevalence of aneurysms for women was 2.4 times higher than that for men (35). Among men, the prevalence of aneurysms remained unchanged across the range of age groups. In contrast, there were 2 peaks in the prevalence of aneurysms for women falling in the 40-49 and 60-69-year age groups (35). A cerebral angiogram based on a retrospective study showed that 67% of the patients harbouring asymptomatic aneurysms were women (100).

## 5. Location and nomenclature

Aneurysms commonly arise at the branching site of major arteries. It also occurs at a turn or curve of the artery, and points in the direction that the blood would have gone if the curve at the aneurysm site were not present (71). Aneurysm is usually referred to by the name of the parent artery from which they originate. Cerebral aneurysms occur more frequently in arteries of the anterior circulation. In large forensic clinical and autopsy series, the locations of intracranial aneurysms are the internal carotid artery (ICA) (24%-41%), the anterior cerebral artery (ACA) (30%-39%), the middle cerebral artery (MCA) (20%-33%) and the vertebrobasilar arteries (VBA) (4%-12%) (95) (Figure 2).

## 6. Presentation of unruptured cerebral aneurysms

Due to the recent spread of non-invasive diagnostic modalities (CTA and MRA), the majority of unruptured IAs are diagnosed incidentally. Here are some specific syndromes associated with particular aneurismal locations.

- *Anterior communicating artery:* Usually, ACoA aneurysms are silent until they rupture. Suprachiasmatic pressure may cause altitudinal visual field deficits, aboulia or akinetic mutism, amnestic syndromes and hypothalamic dysfunction.

- *Anterior cerebral artery:* Most are asymptomatic until they rupture, although frontal lobe syndromes, anosmia and motor deficits may be noted.
- *Middle cerebral artery:* This typically affects the first or second division in the sylvan fissure. Aphasia, hemiparesis, hemisensory loss, anosognosia and visual field defects may be noted.
- *Posterior communicating artery:* These are directed laterally, posteriorly and inferiorly. Pupillary dilatation, ophthalmoplegia, ptosis, mydriasis and hemiparesis may result.
- *Internal carotid artery:* Supraclinoid aneurysms may cause ophthalmoplegia due to the compression of the cranial nerve (CN) III or variable visual defects and optic atrophy due to the compression of the optic nerve. Chiasmal compression may produce bilateral temporal hemianopsia. Hypopituitarism or anosmia may be seen with giant aneurysms. Cavernous-carotid aneurysms exert mass effects within the cavernous sinus, producing ophthalmoplegia and facial sensory loss.
- *Basilar artery:* The clinical findings are usually those associated with SAH, although bitemporal hemianopsia or an oculomotor palsy may occur. Dolichoectatic aneurysms may cause bulbar dysfunction, respiratory difficulties and neurogenic pulmonary oedema.
- *Vertebral artery or posterior inferior cerebellar artery:* Aneurysms at these arterial segments typically result in ataxia, bulbar dysfunction or spinal involvement.

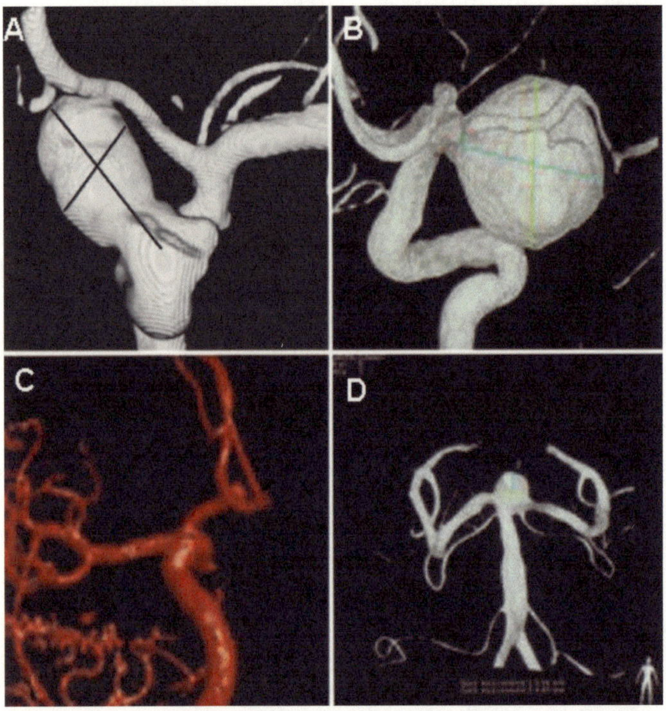


Fig. 2. 3D DSA images demonstrating common sites of IAs. A: Right ICA, demonstrating right giant ICA saccular aneurysm, measuring 22 mm X 11.8 mm (A). B: Right MCA trifurcation aneurysm (26X19 mm). C: Anterior communicating artery small aneurysm. D: 3D DSA image of the vertebrobasilar arteries showing basilar top aneurysm measuring 24X16

## 7. The natural course of incidental aneurysms

The increased sensitivity of neuroimaging techniques has enabled the more frequent diagnosis of unruptured aneurysms. Because the most devastating complication of an unruptured aneurysm is subarachnoid haemorrhage, it has been considered desirable to treat these aneurysms before they rupture. However, the optimal treatment strategy for patients with unruptured aneurysms remains controversial. The management decision requires knowledge of the natural history of the patient and an accurate assessment of the risks related to various treatment options.

No consensus exists regarding the natural course of unruptured aneurysms. Unruptured aneurysms may remain asymptomatic and static; they may grow and or rupture. On the other hand, there are some reports describing the spontaneous regression of aneurysms (82, 97).

A systematic review of the literature on the risk of the rupture of aneurysms identified nine studies with a total of 3907 patient years of follow-up (72). During follow-up, 75 of 495 (15.2%) patients suffered an SAH, giving an annual rupture rate of 1.9%. Aneurysms were significantly more likely to rupture in women than in men (RR 2.1, 95% CI 1.1-3.9) and the risk of rupture increased with age, e.g., in the group of patients aged 60-79 years, the RR of rupture was 1.7 (95% CI 0.7-4.0) compared with those aged 40-59 years. The review also showed higher RR in symptomatic aneurysms when compared to asymptomatic aneurysms (6.5% versus 0.8% respectively) (72).

The initial size of the intact aneurysm and the subsequent rupture rate is a complex issue. In Juvela's study (38), there was no disparity in the size of the aneurysm on digital subtraction angiography (DSA) at the start of follow-up between patients who later had a SAH and those who did not (median 4 mm, range 2-25 mm in those with later SAH versus median 4 mm, range 2-26 mm in those without). Of the aneurysms which later ruptured, 67% were <6 mm in diameter.

In a study by Yasui et al., (103) 234 patients with and without SAH were evaluated during a period of 6.25 years. Thirty-four patients (14.5%) bled, with an average annual rupture rate of 2.3%. In a separate study, these authors evaluated aneurysm size in 25 patients with the rupture of a previously unruptured aneurysm (102).Twenty-two of the newly ruptured aneurysms were <9 mm in diameter at initial diagnosis, and 16 were <5 mm in diameter. The authors concluded that even the smallest UIAs require "radical treatment or careful follow-up."

The largest ever study to follow-up unruptured aneurysms is the ISUIA, with 2621 patients (33, 34). This studied two groups of patients retrospectively: (i) patients with asymptomatic aneurysms with no prior SAH, and (ii) those with multiple aneurysms who had previously sustained an aneurismal SAH. The investigators also studied prospectively the risks of the treatment of asymptomatic unruptured aneurysms (34). The results of the ISUIA indicate a tiny rupture risk of 0.05% per annum for small aneurysms (<I 0 mm diameter) in patients who have not had an SAH previously, and 0.5% per annum for large aneurysms and for all aneurysms in patients who had previously sustained SAH from another aneurysm. Of the 1449 included patients with 1937 unruptured saccular aneurysms <12 mm diameter, 32 patients had confirmed aneurysm rupture during follow-up; the mean duration of follow-up was 8.3 years (12023 patient years in total). In the cohort that had previously not had an SAH, only one of 12 aneurismal ruptures occurred in an aneurysm <10 mm in diameter, compared with 17 of 20 patients in the cohort who had previously had an SAH. This study also found that the only significant predictors of rupture were the size and location of the aneurysm: aneurysms >10 mm diameter had an RR of rupture of 11.6; for posterior circulation aneurysms, the RR was 13.8 and 13.6 for basilar tip and vertebrobasilar locations, respectively, and 8.0 for posterior communicating artery aneurysms.

The discrepancy in aneurismal rupture rates between the systematic reviews (38, 72, 102, 103) and the ISUIA (33, 34) requires explanation. The majority of ISUIA patients were identified retrospectively from hospital records (1981 onwards, with the identification process commencing in 1992) and only survivors with persistently asymptomatic aneurysms - in whom a complete set of angiograms could be traced - were eligible for inclusion. These patients might not be entirely representative of the natural history of all aneurysms: e.g., subjects who had suffered a fatal episode of SAH, or where an asymptomatic aneurysm had been treated since 1981, or else who had incomplete angiograms, could not be included in the ISUIA. The prospective analysis and follow-up of patients with asymptomatic aneurysms provides less biased data.

Although many authors tried to define a critical size for saccular aneurysm rupture, we believe that a critical size below which SAH does not occur does not appear to exist. Other risk factors for IA rupture include age, sex, hypertension, and multiple aneurysms and previous SAH. Identifying the mechanism of aneurysm formation, growth and rupture will explain the role of the various risk factors - including aneurismal size - in the rupture of IAs.

## 8. Treatment of unruptured IAs

Aneurysms may be treated by surgical clipping (or wrapping) or by interventional neuroradiology. Surgical treatment, having been in use routinely for >40 years, has fairly clearly defined the risks and morbidity.

A systematic review of surgical treatment for unruptured aneurysms was performed by Raaymakers and colleagues, who identified 61 studies including 2460 patients and at least 2568 aneurysms published between 1966 and June 1996 (69).

Only studies in which at least 90% of patients were treated by clipping (as opposed to wrapping or other surgical techniques) were included. Unfortunately, only eight of the studies were prospective, the rest being retrospective and - in virtually all studies - the neurosurgeon performing the operation was also the observer of the outcome. The median follow-up was only 24 weeks (range 2-234 weeks) in the 21 studies which reported the time of outcome assessment. The overall permanent morbidity occurred in 10.9% (95% CI 9.6%-12.2%) of patients and mortality was 2.6% (95% CI 2.0%-3.3%). The lowest morbidity and mortality was found with small anterior circulation aneurysms (mortality 0.8%, morbidity 1.9%), and the worst with large posterior fossa aneurysms (mortality 9.6%, morbidity 37.9%).

The prospective arm of the ISUIA also addressed the issue of the risks of surgical intervention in unruptured aneurysms (34). This enrolled 1172 patients (211 of whom had a history of previous SAH) and 996 underwent surgery. The surgery-related mortality at 1 year was 3.8% (95% CI) in patients with no prior SAH and 2% in patients who had previously suffered an SAH from a different aneurysm which had already been treated. The morbidity was 12.0% and 12.1%, respectively. The mortality figures at 1 month in the ISUIA study were similar to those in the systematic review, at a median of 24 weeks, 2.3% versus 2.6%, respectively. Age was the only independent predictor of outcome in the ISUIA study: the RR of surgery-related morbidity and mortality at 1 year was X5 in the group >64 years of age compared with patients <45 years of age.

The effectiveness and risks of aneurysm coiling are less certain because the technique is newer and still developing. The USA Multicenter Study Group identified a 1% mortality and a 4% morbidity for unruptured aneurysm treatment, with 78% of aneurysms being completely occluded. The rupture rate of partially coiled aneurysms was 0.5% per annum from the limited follow-up data available (91). There is some evidence that even partial treatment by GDC confers benefits in the early post-rupture period; post-GDC treatment haemorrhage occurred in only nine of 403 patients, although the length of follow-up was very limited in many patients (91).

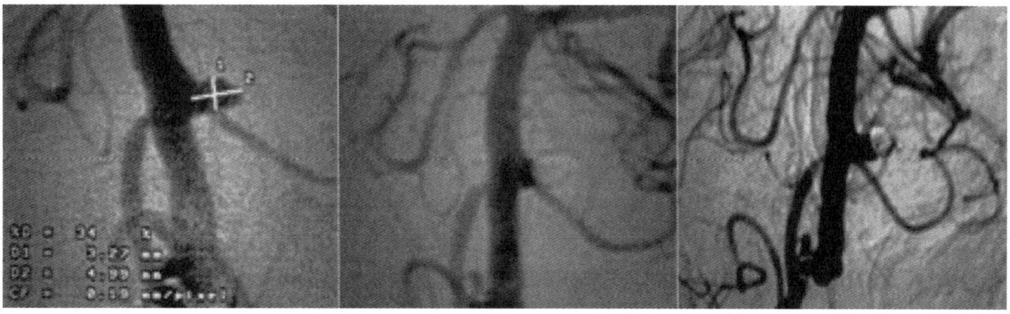

Fig. 3. Demonstrating the enlargement of BA AICA aneurysm following coiling with GDC. A: Initial Left VADSA; B: DSA following coiling; C: DSA six months after coiling showing coil impaction and enlargement of the aneurismal cavity.

In the case of an unruptured aneurysm, should one decide treatment was necessary then the long-term results of coiling are particularly relevant because coiling could provide a less invasive alternative to surgery. It is worth noting that the published rupture rate of partially coiled aneurysms is the same as that reported from the ISUIA study for untreated unruptured aneurysms >10 mm diameter or for any unruptured aneurysm in a patient with a previous SAH. The regrowth rate of partially coiled aneurysms is still being defined, and so there are considerable uncertainties about the long- and short-term effectiveness of coiling.

Apart from direct treatment of the aneurysm, it is likely that there are other ways of reducing the risk of rupture for incidentally discovered aneurisms, which could - collectively - have a useful effect. The cessation of smoking, careful control of blood pressure and the avoidance of risk factors for atherosclerosis (careful diet, regular exercise, etc.), while unproven, may help reduce both the risk of formation of aneurysms and the risk of rupture, as well as improving general health.

### 8.1 Management considerations and recommendations

Aneurismal SAH is a devastating condition for which prevention has been advocated as the most effective strategy aimed at lowering mortality rates. However, all current treatments carry risks, and recommendations for treatment versus observation are often difficult and controversial. Treatment complications generally occur at around the time of the procedure, but they could potentially improve during the patient's remaining lifetime. In contrast, the risk of rupture of an untreated aneurysm is cumulative but may provide a period of unimpaired life. Non-lethal complications in both settings can potentially improve over time.

Deliberations must take into account important characteristics of the aneurysm and the patient in whom it exists. Of the former, particular consideration must be given to aneurysm size, form and location and its symptomatic versus incidental status. As a general rule, exclusively extradural, intracavernous (internal carotid artery) aneurysms, even if symptomatic with pain or ophthalmoparesis, do not carry a major risk for intracranial haemorrhage, and thus management decisions are primarily aimed at symptom relief rather than haemorrhage prevention.

Among patient factors, the patient's age, general medical condition, previous history of SAH and family history of aneurismal SAH are prime considerations in the treatment analysis. Symptoms due to UIAs should be discriminated relative to those developing rapidly and related to smaller aneurysms, presumably due to acute aneurismal expansion. Generally, symptomatic aneurysms are larger, occasionally giant in size and sometimes partially thrombosed, producing subacute symptoms due to adjacent cranial nerve or brain compression. Such lesions carry a major risk for both progressive neurological deficit and aneurysm rupture.

The existing body of knowledge supports the following recommendations (options) regarding the treatment of UIAs:

1. The treatment of small incidental intracavernous ICA aneurysms is not generally indicated. For large symptomatic intracavernous aneurysms, treatment decisions should be individualised on the basis of the patient's age, the severity and progression of symptoms and treatment alternatives. The higher risk of treatment and shorter life expectancy in older individuals must be considered in all patients, and it favours observation in older patients with asymptomatic aneurysms.
2. Symptomatic intradural aneurysms of all sizes should be considered for treatment, with relative urgency for the treatment of acutely symptomatic aneurysms. Symptomatic large or giant aneurysms carry higher surgical risks that require a careful analysis of individualised patient and aneurismal risks and surgeon and centre expertise.
3. Coexisting or remaining aneurysms of all sizes in patients with SAH due to another treated aneurysm carry a higher risk for future haemorrhage than do similar sized aneurysms without a prior SAH history, and they warrant consideration for treatment.
4. If a decision is made for observation, re-evaluation on a periodic basis with CT/MRA or selective contrast angiography should be considered so as to check for changes in aneurismal size and shape.
5. In consideration of the apparent low risk of haemorrhage from incidental small (<10 mm) aneurysms in patients without previous SAH, treatment rather than observation cannot generally be advocated. However, special consideration for treatment should be given to young patients in this group. Likewise, small aneurysms approaching the 10 mm diameter size, those with daughter sac formation and other unique hemodynamic

features, and patients with a positive family history for aneurysms or aneurismal SAH deserve special consideration for treatment.

6. Asymptomatic aneurysms of ->10 mm (ISUIA) or >7mm (ISUIA-II) in diameter warrant strong consideration for treatment, taking into account the patient's age, existing medical and neurological conditions and the relative risks of treatment.

These recommendations are based on our limited knowledge concerning the natural history of unruptured aneurysm. In our clinical practice, we recommend - whenever possible - the active management of these lesions

## 9. Subarachnoid haemorrhage (SAH)

Primary SAH is defined as a bleeding which takes place primarily in the intracranial subarachnoid space and is not secondary to some other intracranial haemorrhage (66). In a recent systematic review of the literature, the worldwide overall incidence of SAH was 10.5 per 100,000 person years (85). However, the incidence in Japan was 21.0 per 100,000 person years and in Finland it was 22.0 per 100,000 person years (63). The overall incidence of aneurismal SAH has remained constant during recent decades (50), but increases almost linearly with increasing age (16).

### 9.1 The aetiology of SAH

In more than 80% of cases, the cause of primary SAH is the rupture of an intracranial aneurysm (77, 85). SAHs of unknown origin represent 9%-15% of cases (75). The source of the bleeding of unknown origin can be the rupture of a small perforating artery or a micro-arteriovenous malformation (AVM) which is not identifiable in diagnostic imaging (75). Intracranial artery dissections, cerebral AVMs, dural AVMs, trauma, bleeding disorders, substance abuse, a spinal origin of the haemorrhage and other rare conditions account for primary SAH in less than 5% of cases (85).

### 9.2 Clinical presentation

This is characterised by the acute onset of severe headache, which patients often describe as "the worst headache of my life." The sudden elevation of intracranial pressure associated with aneurismal rupture may lead to a precipitous decline in cerebral perfusion pressure, causing syncope (50% of cases), confusion or mild impairment in alertness. Other symptoms include:

- Seizures: Focal or generalised seizures are present in 25% of aneurismal SAH cases, with most events occurring within 24 hours of onset.
- Manifestations of meningeal irritation: Neck pain or stiffness, photophobia, sonophobia or other hyperesthesia may be noted with SAH.
- Autonomic disturbances: The subarachnoid accumulation of the products of blood degradation may elicit fever, nausea or vomiting, sweating, chills and cardiac arrhythmias.
- Focal neurological complaints: Haemorrhage or ischemia may manifest with focal deficits, including weakness, hemisensory loss, language disturbances, neglect, memory loss or olfactory disturbances. Focal symptoms are more common with giant aneurysms.

- Respiratory dysfunction or cardiovascular instability: These are ominous signs of brainstem compression.
- SAH can be associated with myocardial stunning (transient), sometimes with the features of tako-tsubo syndrome (transient left ventricular apical ballooning syndrome), and with lethal ventricular arrhythmia, all probably caused by SAH-induced catecholamine surge.

The physical examination of patients with aneurismal SAH may reveal nuchal rigidity, a decreased level of consciousness, subhyaloid haemorrhages, pupillary abnormalities (i.e., typically dilated), ophthalmoplegia, cranial neuropathies and other focal deficits. Giant aneurysms may cause mass effects or distal thromboembolism with prominent focal deficits, optic atrophy or other cranial neuropathies as well as brainstem compression.

### 9.3 The diagnosis of SAH

CT and MRI

If SAH is suspected, CT scanning is the first line in investigation because of the characteristically hyperdense appearance of extravasated blood in the basal cisterns. The pattern of haemorrhage often suggests the location of any underlying aneurysm (86) (Figure 4). CT studies performed within 12 h after the haemorrhage were found to be negative in 2% of patients with SAH (84).

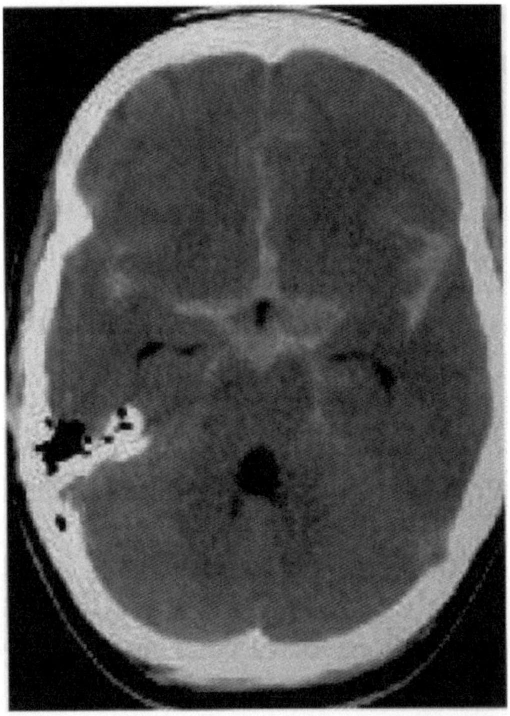

Fig. 4. CT scan of a 47-year-old woman presented with headache and vomiting; her CT scan in the emergency department revealed subarachnoid haemorrhage involving the sylvan and interhemispheric fissure, the interpeduncular and the ambient cistern.

MRI with FLAIR (fluid attenuated inversion recovery) techniques demonstrates SAH in the acute phase as reliably as CT (59), but MRI is impracticable because the facilities are less readily available than CT scanners, and restless patients cannot be studied unless anaesthesia is given. In the subacute cases, however, MRI is increasingly superior to CT in detecting SAH (59).

Lumbar puncture

Lumbar puncture is still an indispensable step in the exclusion of SAH in patients with a convincing history and negative brain imaging. Lumbar puncture should not be carried out rashly or without some background knowledge. The first rule is that at least 6 h and preferably 12 h should have elapsed between the onset of headache and the spinal tap. The delay is essential because if there are red cells in the CSF, sufficient lysis will have taken place during that time for bilirubin and oxyhaemoglobin to have formed (90). The pigments give the CSF a yellow tinge after centrifugation (xanthochromia) - a critical feature in the distinction of SAH from a traumatic tap - and are invariably detectable until at least 2 weeks later. The 'three tube test' (a decrease in red cells in consecutive tubes) is notoriously unreliable, and a false-positive diagnosis of SAH can be almost as invalidating as a missed one. Spinning down the blood-stained CSF should be done immediately, otherwise oxyhaemoglobin will form *in vitro*. If the supernatant appears crystal-clear, the specimen should be stored in darkness until the absence of blood pigments is confirmed by spectrophotometry.

### 9.4 Diagnosis of intracranial aneurysm

The gold standard for detecting aneurysms is conventional angiography, but this is not an innocuous procedure. A systematic review of three prospective studies in which patients with SAH were distinguished from other indications for catheter angiography found a complication rate (transient or permanent) of 1.8% (6).

Other imaging modalities are MR angiography (MRA) and CT angiography (CTA), which are non-invasive. A recent review of studies comparing MRA and intra-arterial angiography in patients with recent SAH, under blinded-reader conditions, showed a sensitivity in the range of 69%-100% for detecting at least one aneurysm per patient and 70%-97% for the detection of all aneurysms, with specificity in the range 75%-100% (93). The sensitivity of CTA (compared with catheter angiography) is 85-98%, which is in the same range as that of MRA (1). Hashimoto et al, reported the ability of CTA to detect aneurysms that were missed by conventional angiography (25).

### 9.5 The grading of SAH

The Fisher (15) grading method (Table 1) is dependent on findings by CT-scan and has been found to be useful in predicting vasospasm after SAH; patients with a thick layer of blood in the subarachnoid space were found to have a higher incidence of cerebral vasospasm (46).

The most common system for grading the clinical condition after SAH is the Hunt and Hess (H&H) (32) scale (Table 2). In the original classification according to Hunt&Hess, the patient grade was increased by one level in the presence of serious underlying medical disorders. On this scale, a higher grade at presentation correlates with increasingly poor clinical outcomes.

| *Fisher Grade* | *Blood on CT* | *No of Pts* | *Angiographic vasospasm* | *Clinical vasospasm* |
|---|---|---|---|---|
| 1 | none | 11 | 4 | 0 |
| 2 | Diffuse or vertical layer >1 mm thick | 7 | 3 | 0 |
| 3 | Localised clot or vertical layer >1 mm thick | 24 | 24 | 23 |
| 4 | Intracerebral or intraventricular blood | 5 | 2 | 0 |

Table 1. The Fisher CT grade

| *H&H Grade* | *Description* |
|---|---|
| 1 | Asymptomatic or mild H/A and slight nuchal rigidity |
| 2 | Moderate to severe H/A, nuchal rigidity, no deficit except Cr. N. palsy (e.g., III, VI) |
| 3 | Mild focal deficit, lethargy or confusion |
| 4 | Stupor, moderate to severe hemiparesis, early decerebrate rigidity |
| 5 | Deep coma, decerebrate rigidity, moribund appearance |
| Add one grade for serious systemic disease (D.M, HTN, Atherosclerosis, COPD) | |

Table 2. Hunt and Hess classification of SAH

In 1987, the World Federation of Neurological Surgeons (WFNS) (70) proposed a new grading system (Table 3) in which two factors have been assigned to differentiate grades: the level of consciousness - classified with the Glasgow coma scale (GCS) - and focal neurological deficits. The timing of the grading is important because the patient's worst clinical grade is the best predictor of the outcome.

| *WFNS grade* | *Glasgow Coma Scale Score* | *Major focal deficit** |
|---|---|---|
| 0 (intact aneurysm) | - | - |
| 1 | 15 | absent |
| 2 | 13-14 | absent |
| 3 | 13-14 | present |
| 4 | 7-12 | present or absent |
| 5 | 3-6 | present or absent |

*Aphasia and/or hemiparesis or hemiplegia

Table 3. World Federation of Neurologic Surgeons (WFNS) SAH grade

### 9.6 The outcome of ruptured intracranial aneurysms

Case fatality ranged between 32% and 67% in a review of population-based studies from 1960 onward. The weighted average was 51%. Of patients who survive the haemorrhage, approximately one-third remain dependent (28). Recovery to an independent state does not necessarily mean that the outcome is good. In a study of quality of life in patients after SAH, only 9 of 48 (19%; 95% CI 9%-33%) patients who were independent 4 months after the haemorrhage had no significant reduction in quality of life (29). All in all, only a small minority of all patients with SAH have a truly good outcome. The relatively young age at which SAH occurs and its poor outcome together explain why the loss of years of potential life before the age of 65 from SAH is comparable to that of ischaemic stroke (37).

**Factors that influence prognosis**

The predictors for mortality include the patient's decreased level of consciousness, their increased age, the thickness of the subarachnoid haemorrhage clot on computerised tomography, elevated blood pressure, pre-existing medical illnesses and basilar aneurysms (42, 79). A decreased level of consciousness, with the initial haemorrhage or after early rebleeding, may be caused by intracerebral haematoma, subdural haematoma or hydrocephalus. Only by exclusion should it be assumed that the cause is global brain damage as a result of high pressure and subsequent ischaemia.

Rebleeding

In the first few hours after admission for the initial haemorrhage, up to 15% of patients have a sudden episode of clinical deterioration that suggests rebleeding (17). As such, sudden episodes often occur before the first CT scan, or even before admission to hospital - a firm diagnosis is difficult and the true frequency of rebleeding on the first day is invariably underestimated.

In the prospective Cooperative Aneurysm Study (44), the risk of rebleeding with conservative therapy was highest (4%) on the first day after SAH and then remained constant at a rate of 1%-2% per day during the subsequent two weeks. In his earlier series, Pakarinen (66) reported a cumulative frequency of rebleeding of 7%, 16%, 23% and 33% at week 1, week 2, week 3 and week 4 respectively. The mortality at first recurrence was 63.6%, and at second recurrence it had risen to 86%.

Intracerebral haematoma

Intraparenchymal haematomas occur in up to 30% of patients with ruptured aneurysms (87). Not surprisingly, the average outcome is worse than in patients with purely subarachnoid blood (26). When a large haematoma is the most likely cause of the poor condition on admission, the immediate evacuation of the haematoma should be seriously considered (with simultaneous clipping of the aneurysm if it can be identified), often with the aneurysm having been demonstrated only by MR angiography or CT angiography.

Acute subdural haematoma

An acute subdural haematoma, which is usually associated with recurrent aneurismal rupture, but can also occur with the initial haemorrhage, may be life threatening; in these cases, immediate evacuation is also called for (65).

Acute hydrocephalus

Gradual obtundation within 24 h of haemorrhage, sometimes accompanied by slow pupillary responses to light and downward deviation of the eyes, is fairly characteristic of acute hydrocephalus (73). If the diagnosis is confirmed by CT, this can be a reason for early ventricular drainage, although some patients improve spontaneously in the first 24 h.

Global cerebral ischaemia

The most likely explanation is the elevation of the pressure in the cerebrospinal fluid spaces to the level of that in the arteries at the time of haemorrhage, resulting in a prolonged period of global cerebral ischemia. Such an immediate and potentially lethal arrest of the circulation to the brain is indeed suggested by autopsy evidence and by the recording of intracranial pressure or transcranial Doppler sonography at the time of recurrent aneurismal haemorrhage (19, 78). This is quite distinct from delayed ischaemia, which is either focal or multifocal (see below).

Cerebral vasospasm

The most feared complication of SAH is a form of delayed-onset cerebral arterial narrowing, known as VSP (13). Angiographic VSP is detected in 50%-70% of patients in the first two weeks after SAH (94). In about one-half of cases, angiographic VSP manifests itself by the occurrence of a delayed ischemic neurological deficit, which may resolve or progress to permanent cerebral infarction (53). The development of delayed ischemic deficit (DID) is still considered to be the major cause of morbidity and mortality in those patients who survive long enough to reach the neurosurgical unit. In a recent large multicentre study, DID killed 7% of patients with aneurismal SAH and left another 7% with severe permanent neurological deficits (42).

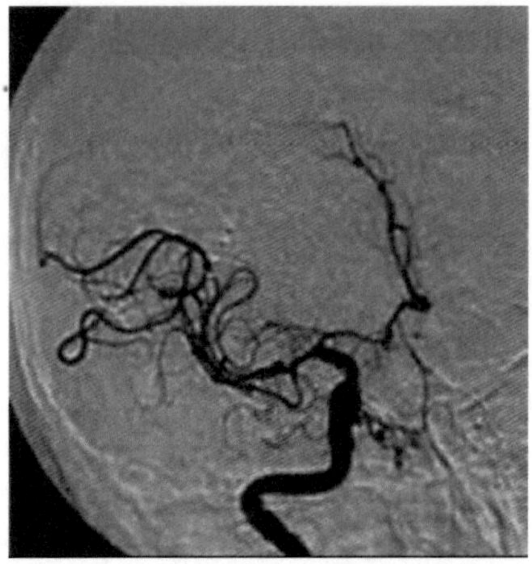

Fig. 5. Left carotid DSA performed postoperatively and demonstrating cerebral vasospasm affecting both ACA and MCA.

## 9.7 Treatment guidelines for ruptured IA

### 9.7.1 The prevention of rebleeding

#### 9.7.1.1 Antifibrinolytic drugs

Medical treatment for preventing rebleeding has not yet been successful; treatment with antifibrinolytic agents does reduce the rebleed rate, but fails to improve overall outcome.

A systematic review of antifibrinolytic agents included eight trials published before 2000 that met predefined inclusion criteria and totalled 937 patients (76). By far the largest study was a Dutch-Scottish trial (89). In this meta-analysis, antifibrinolytic treatment did not provide any evidence of benefit on outcome. The risk of rebleeding was significantly reduced by antifibrinolytic therapy, but this was offset by a similar increase of the risk of secondary cerebral ischaemia.

### 9.7.1.2 Operative clipping of the aneurysm

The results of operative treatment were poor until advances in microsurgical techniques and neuroanaesthesia in the late 1960s allowed neurosurgeons to successfully treat the majority of intracranial aneurysms. The goal for surgical treatment of intracranial aneurysms is to eliminate the aneurysm from the circulation while preserving blood flow through the parent artery and branch vessels. This treatment is best accomplished by direct clip placement across the aneurysm neck.

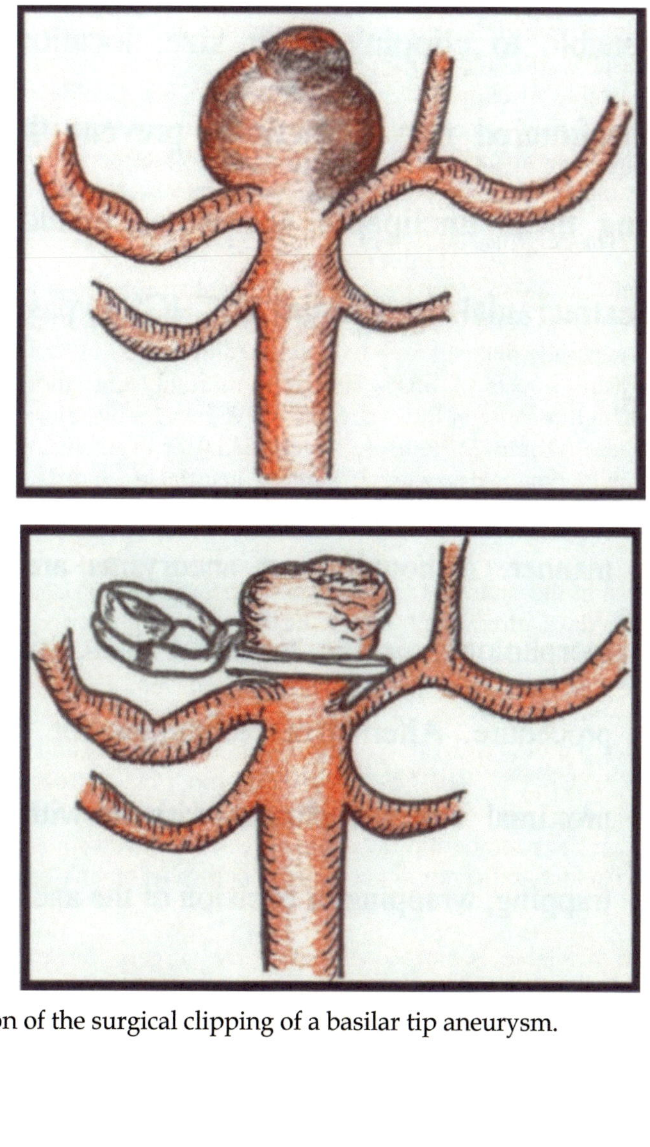

Fig. 6. Illustration of the surgical clipping of a basilar tip aneurysm.

*9.7.1.2.1 Technical aspects of the surgical repair of ruptured aneurysms*

An operative approach must take into account the location of the aneurysm, and it should allow minimal brain retraction. According to Yasargil (101), the most useful approaches are: 1) pterional craniotomy for aneurysms of the anterior circulation and upper basilar artery; 2) paramedian frontal craniotomy for pericallosal artery aneurysms; 3) lateral suboccipital craniotomy for aneurysms of the vertebral circulation below the origin of the superior cerebellar arteries. The clips for the temporary occlusion of the parent artery have a low closing force so as not to cause permanent damage to the vessel wall. To achieve permanent clipping, there are multiple choices of clips of different sizes, shapes and closing forces. The modern clips are MRI compatible.

Using gentle brain retraction, the arachnoid cisterns are entered with sharp dissection and finally the aneurysm and the adjacent vessels are exposed with a meticulous dissection. Prior to the application of the clip, the aneurysm neck must be free of adhesions to the surrounding arteries and neural structures. In narrow-necked aneurysms, the clip can be placed across the aneurysm neck. However, in complex aneurysms several clips may be needed to appropriately occlude the aneurysm in a stepwise manner. Although most aneurysms are amenable to clipping, their size, location, morphology and the technical difficulties encountered may sometimes prevent the procedure. Alternative techniques for treating these unclippable aneurysms include proximal vessel occlusion with or without extracranial intracranial (EC IC) bypass, trapping, wrapping and excision of the aneurysm.

*9.7.1.2.2 The timing of the surgical treatment of ruptured aneurysms*

The optimal timing for the surgical treatment of acutely ruptured aneurysms has been under constant investigation and is the subject of major controversy. In the 1960s, operative treatment was still generally delayed for 3 to 4 weeks following SAH so that the brain could recover from the acute effects of SAH. However, mortality and morbidity during the waiting period was high because of the occurrence of VSP and rebleeding (43). An operation during an early phase (within 72 hours following SAH) or even during the acute phase (within 24 hours following SAH) was considered justifiable in order to prevent early rebleeding and allow for the aggressive treatment of VSP, and thus improve the outcome for the patients.

In a randomised trial of the timing of the operation performed, 216 patients were allocated to operation within 3 days, after 7 days or else in the intervening period (64). The outcome tended to be better with the early operations rather than after intermediate or late operations, but the difference was not statistically significant. The same result - i.e., no difference in outcome after early or late operations - has emerged from various observational studies: a multi-centre study from North America (43) and a single institution review in Cambridge, UK (96). The US study found the worst outcome among patients operated on between day 7 and day 10 after the initial haemorrhage. This disadvantageous period for performing the operation in the second week after SAH coincides with the peak time of cerebral ischaemia and cerebral vasospasm, both phenomena being most common between days 4-12.

Although the data available is not consistent, early surgery for patients in a good preoperative clinical grade (Hunt&Hess Gr I-III) has gradually been accepted as a treatment policy by many institutions. Delayed surgery for patients in a poor preoperative clinical grade, however, may be advisable unless immediate surgical intervention is required because of large haematoma or severe hydrocephalus.

### 9.7.1.3 Endovascular treatment of ruptured intracranial aneurysms

Until a few years ago, endovascular treatment was restricted to patients in whom the aneurysm was unsuitable for clipping because of the size or location of the aneurysm, or in whom surgical clipping was contraindicated because of the general medical condition of the patient. Since the introduction of controlled detachable coils for the endosaccular packing of aneurysms (20), endovascular embolisation is increasingly used. In some institutes, endovascular embolisation is even proposed as the initial method of treatment (7).

**The Guglielmi Detachable Coil system**

In 1991, Guglielmi et al. (20) introduced an electrically detachable coil system (GDC) that permitted the readjustment of the coil position before its final detachment. The GDC system consists of a platinum coil attached to a stainless steel delivery wire (pusher). The pusher is coated for electrical isolation with the exception of the most distal part: the detachment zone. A guiding catheter is used in advancing to the ICA or the vertebral artery. A microcatheter with 2-tip-markers and a guidewire are used for hyperselective catheterisation of the aneurismal sac. The distal end of the microcatheter is shaped with steam to tailor the vascular geometry before catheterisation. Digital road mapping may be used so as not to touch the aneurismal wall with the guidewire or catheter. A continuous pressurised flush of heparinised saline is maintained in both the guiding catheter and the microcatheter. The aneurysm sac is then filled with coils of selected shapes and sizes. The system allows for the removal of the coil as well as the repositioning of the mesh to an optimal position. When the coil is seen to be in a suitable position inside the aneurysm, a positive direct electric current is applied to the proximal end of the stainless steel guidewire. The current provokes thrombus formation in the aneurismal cavity and dissolves the uninsulated stainless steel coil closest to the platinum coil, resulting in the detachment of the coil.

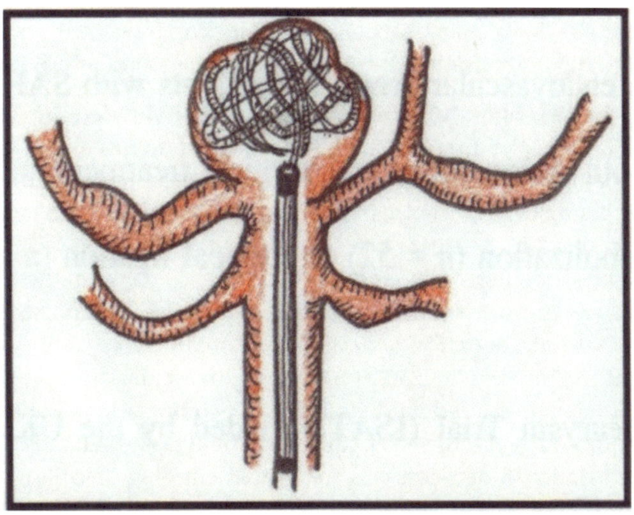

Fig. 7. Of c: Illustration of the oiling procedure with coils filling the aneurismal cavity.

Numerous observational studies have published complication rates, occlusion rates and short-term follow-up results. These have been summarised - up to March 1997 - in a systematic review of 48 eligible studies of 1383 patients (4). Permanent complications in the procedure occurred in 3.7% of 1256 patients in whom this was recorded (95% CI 2.7%-4.9%). A >90% occlusion of the aneurysm was achieved in almost 90% of patients. The most frequent complication was procedure-related ischaemia, even if patients were treated with heparin. The second most frequent complication was aneurysm perforation, which occurred in 2% of patients. Most of the aneurysms treated with controlled detachable coils were located at the basilar artery, followed by the carotid and anterior communicating arteries. Pericallosal arteries are difficult to reach and another problematic site is the trifurcation of the middle cerebral artery because one or more of the branches often originate from the aneurysm.

### 9.7.1.4 Clipping versus coiling

Indirect comparisons between endovascular and surgical treatment are inappropriate, if only because there are so many differences in study design and among the patients and aneurysms. Moreover, the rerupture of aneurysms may occur even months after apparently successful coiling (52), and the long-term rates of rebleeding after endovascular coiling still need to be established. A first report from a single centre in which >300 patients were followed-up after aneurysm embolisation for a median period of almost 2 years showed rebleeding rates of 0.8% in the first year, 0.6% in the second year and 2.4% in the third year, with no rebleeding in subsequent years (5).

Similarly surgical treatment is not always definitive: in a retrospective review of postoperative angiograms in a series of 66 patients with ruptured aneurysms and 12 additional aneurysms, all treated by surgical clipping, 8% of patients showed aneurysms with a residual lumen or aneurysms that were previously undetected (51). Controlled trials are urgently needed in patients with aneurysms for which it is uncertain whether surgical clipping or endovascular coiling should be the preferred treatment. The first such study, although a small one (109 patients), found no difference in outcome at 3 months between the surgical group and the endovascular group for patients with SAH. All of the patients were suitable candidates for both endovascular and surgical treatment and were randomly assigned to undergo coil embolisation ($n$ = 52) or surgical ligation ($n$ = 57) (88).

The International Subarachnoid Aneurysm Trial (ISAT), funded by the UK's Medical Research Council (56), is the first large multi-centre randomised study in the world to compare the two methods. The ISAT trial enrolled 2143 patients with ruptured intracranial aneurysms in 43 neurosurgical centres in Europe, North America and Australia, and randomly assigned them to neurosurgical clipping ($n$ = 1070) or GDC coils ($n$ = 1073). Because interim analysis demonstrated a striking difference between these groups in favour of coiling, the trial was stopped short of its planned goal of 2500 patients. At 1 year follow-up, the risk of death or significant disability (Rankin score 3-6) was 30.6% in the neurosurgical group compared to 23.7% in the endovascular group. There was a 6.9% absolute and 22.6% relative risk reduction in favour of coiling. Many patients were screened but excluded from the study. Of the 9559 patients initially assessed, only 20% were actually enrolled. In the remainder, a decision was made that clipping or coiling was clearly more favourable, and thus the patient could not be subjected to a random treatment choice. Considerable bias could have been introduced into the study during this screening process.

The ISAT patients are not completely representative of the SAH population at large. 88% were of good clinical status (Hunt and Hess grade I or II), 93% of aneurysms were 10 mm or smaller in diameter and 97% were in the anterior circulation. The generalisability of the ISAT data is therefore limited. There was a significant occurrence of post-treatment rebleeding. This was found in 2.4% (26/1048) of endovascular cases compared with 1.0% (10/994) of clipped patients. While these results clearly favour neurosurgery, such an incidence of incompletely treated aneurysms is unusual for either therapy in experienced hands. In conclusion, the ISAT tells us that in patients with a ruptured intracranial aneurysm - for which endovascular coiling and neurosurgical clipping are therapeutic options - the outcome in terms of survival free from disability at 1 year is significantly better with endovascular coiling. Long-term follow-up is very important since rebleeding rates were found to be significantly higher in patients undergoing endovascular coiling.

### 9.7.2 The prevention of vasospasm

Angiographic VSP is detected in 50%-70% of patients within the first two weeks after SAH (94). In about one-half of cases, angiographic VSP manifests itself by the occurrence of a delayed ischemic neurological deficit (53). Delayed cerebral ischaemia (DID) is still considered to be the major cause of morbidity and mortality in those patients who survive long enough to reach the neurosurgical unit. Despite many years of intensive research, the pathogenesis of secondary cerebral ischaemia following SAH has not been elucidated. It is a generally held belief that after haemorrhage a thus far unidentified factor is released in the subarachnoid space, which induces vasoconstriction and thereby secondary ischaemia. Also, an often quoted study from Boston (of 41 patients in total) postulates a close relationship between the location of subarachnoid blood and the 'thickness' of the clot on the one hand, and the occurrence of vasospasm and delayed cerebral ischaemia on the other (46). Several observations argue against this popular notion. Firstly, the presence of subarachnoid blood, though a powerful predictor of delayed cerebral ischaemia, is not in itself a sufficient factor for the development of secondary ischaemia - secondary ischaemia does not occur in patients with a perimesencephalic (non-aneurismal) SAH (74) and it is rare in patients with SAH secondary to intracerebral haematoma or a ruptured arteriovenous malformation. Secondly, in a larger series of patients than in the Boston study, the site of delayed cerebral ischaemia did not correspond with the distribution or even with the side of subarachnoid blood (30). Thirdly, many patients with vasospasm never develop secondary ischaemia. These observations collectively suggest not only the presence of subarachnoid blood *per se*, but also that its combination with other factors determines whether and where secondary ischaemia will develop.

Classically, the clinical symptoms of VSP have consisted of the impairment of consciousness, confusion, disorientation and worsening neurological deficits such as dysphasia and hemiplegia. The clinical diagnosis of VSP is traditionally based on the time of the onset of the deficits, the rate of the development of the deficits (hours), the nature of the deficits and the exclusion of other factors that may cause the gradual deterioration of the patient or focal neurological signs. The diagnosis is therefore not always definitive. It is especially difficult to differentiate symptoms of VSP from other causes that worsen the clinical state in patients with impaired consciousness.

Despite this lack of pathophysiological insight, some progress has been made in the prevention of secondary ischaemia after aneurismal SAH through changes in general medical care (notably, increased fluid intake and the avoidance of antihypertensive drugs) as well as through specific drug treatment. Transcranial Doppler sonography may suggest impending cerebral ischaemia by means of the increased blood flow velocity from arterial narrowing in the middle cerebral artery or in the posterior circulation; however, narrowing in distal branches often escapes detection. Only velocities >120 cm/s or >200 cm/s are reasonably accurate in excluding or predicting delayed ischaemia, but almost 60% of patients are in the intermediate range (92).

Early surgery

Early surgery was introduced after it was considered that the early clipping of the aneurysm not only prevented rebleeding but also allowed for the surgical removal of spasmogenic clot from the basal cisterns (80). The aim of intrathecal fibrinolytic treatment after SAH is to promote the rapid dissolution of blood clot prior to haemolysis and the release of spasmogenic intermediates.

The management of blood pressure

The management of hypertension is a difficult issue in patients with SAH, especially if their blood pressure rises above 200/110 mmHg. Following intracranial haemorrhage, the range between the upper and lower limits of the autoregulation of cerebral blood flow becomes narrower, which makes the perfusion of the brain more dependent on arterial blood pressure. Consequently, the aggressive treatment of surges of blood pressure entails a definite risk of ischaemia in areas with a loss of autoregulation. The rational approach would, therefore, be to advise against treating hypertension following aneurismal rupture. An observational study from the 1980s showed that the rate of rebleeding was lower but that the rate of cerebral infarction was higher than in untreated patients (99). A further observational study suggested that the combined strategy of avoiding antihypertensive medication and increasing fluid intake may decrease the risk of cerebral infarction (24).

Fluid balance and electrolytes

Fluid management in SAH is important for preventing a reduction in plasma volume, which may contribute to the development of cerebral ischaemia. In approximately one-third of patients, plasma volume drops by >10% within the preoperative period, which is significantly associated with a negative sodium balance. Moreover, fluid restriction in patients with hyponatraemia is associated with an increased risk of cerebral ischaemia. Fluid restriction was applied in the past because hyponatraemia was erroneously attributed to water retention via the inappropriate secretion of antidiuretic hormones.

Despite the incomplete evidence, it seems reasonable to prevent hypovolaemia. We favour giving 2.5-3.5L/day of normal saline, unless contraindicated by signs of impending cardiac failure

Calcium antagonists

Initially, the rationale for the use of calcium antagonists in the prevention or treatment of secondary ischaemia was based on the assumption that these drugs reduce the frequency of vasospasm by counteracting the influx of calcium in the vascular smooth muscle cell.

Clinical trials have been undertaken with three types of calcium antagonists: nimodipine, nicardipine and AT877 (of which nimodipine is the most extensively studied and used). A recent systematic review of all randomised controlled trials on calcium antagonists in patients with SAH showed a significant reduction in the frequency of poor outcomes, which resulted from a reduction in the frequency of secondary ischaemia (12). When analysed separately, the nimodipine trials showed a significant reduction in the frequency of poor outcomes, but the nicardipine and AT877 trials did not. While, nicardipine and AT877 significantly reduce the frequency of vasospasm, the nimodipine trials showed only a trend towards the reduction of vasospasm, despite the fact that a larger number of patients were included. In brief, the administration of nimodipine improves outcomes in patients with SAH, but it is uncertain whether nimodipine acts through neuroprotection or through reducing the frequency of vasospasm, or both. Nicardipine and AT877 definitely reduce the frequency of vasospasm, but the effect on the overall outcome remains unproven, which again underlines the weak relation between vasospasm and outcomes.

Since the systemic administration of vasoactive drugs has been associated with significant side effects and insufficient efficacy, the intrathecal administration of nicardipine prolonged-release implants (NPRI) has been developed. At the time of the surgical clipping of the ruptured aneurysm, NPRIs are positioned next to the large cerebral arteries. Several clinical protocols revealed that NPRIs dramatically reduce the incidence and severity of angiographic vasospasm, which was matched by a reduction in cerebral infarction and delayed ischaemic neurologic deficit. On average, the incidence of angiographic vasospasm decreased from approximately 70% to less than 10%. Its efficacy seemed to be dose-dependent and reduced for peripheral vasospasm, and large controlled trials are needed to further confirm these results.

### 9.7.3 The treatment of delayed cerebral ischaemia

Treatment with hypervolaemia, haemodilution and induced hypertension - the so-called 'triple H therapy' - has become widely used, although evidence from clinical trials is still lacking. In a series of patients with progressive neurological deterioration and angiographically confirmed vasospasm, the deficits could be permanently reversed in 43 of 58 cases (41). In 16 patients who had responded to this treatment, the neurological deficits recurred when the blood pressure transiently dropped but again resolved when the pressure increased. The most plausible explanation for these phenomena is a defect of cerebral autoregulation that makes the perfusion of the brain passively dependent on systemic blood pressure. The risks of deliberately increasing the arterial pressure and plasma volume include the rebleeding of an unclipped aneurysm, increased cerebral oedema or haemorrhagic transformation in areas of infarction, myocardial infarction and congestive heart failure.

Recent developments in endovascular treatments have enabled the direct dilatation of constricted cerebral arteries by transluminal angioplasty (48). Since angioplasty is not effective in dilating the distal arteries, superselective intra-arterial papaverine administration was proposed as an alternative or adjunctive method of treatment (40). Subsequently, the use of intra-arterial papaverine has been found to not provide additional benefits when compared with the medical treatment of vasospasm alone (68). Studies comparing the effects of transluminal angioplasty with intra-arterial papaverine have found angioplasty to be superior in reversing DID and in improving CBF (11, 14).

### 9.8 Other complications of subarachnoid haemorrhage

Hydrocephalus

Acute hydrocephalus is frequently associated with SAH. In the International Cooperative Study on the Timing of Aneurysm Surgery (43), early hydrocephalus was initially noted in 15% of the overall population (3521 patients). During the course of treatment, 18% of the patients received ventricular CSF drainage, 8% had lumbar CSF drainage and 8% received a permanent shunt device. In the surgical series of 835 consecutive patients with aneurismal SAH, Tapaninaho et al. (81) reported a frequency of 35% of early hydrocephalus. 10% of patients finally developed a shunt-dependent hydrocephalus. Severe bleeding into the CSF cisterns or intraventricularly was the basic prognostic factor in the development of chronic hydrocephalus. Shunt-dependent hydrocephalus had a clear adverse effect on outcomes.

Seizures

There was frequency of 4.5% in the occurrence of seizures during the primary hospital course in the International Cooperative Study on the Timing of Aneurysm Surgery (43). In the series of Hernesniemi et al. (27), epilepsy was seen in approximately 14% of patients with acute aneurismal SAH who were treated surgically and who were still alive two months after treatment. Keranen et al. (45) reported an overall frequency of 14% of late epilepsy in surgically treated patients with supratentorial aneurysms; 2.5% in patients with preoperative Hunt&Hess grade I and 33% in patients with Hunt&Hess grade III-V. Ukkola et al. (83) reported a lower frequency of 8% of secondary epilepsy in their series of 183 consecutive patients operated on for ruptured aneurysms. They noted that the development of secondary epilepsy was associated with MCA aneurysms, temporary clipping during surgery, the wrapping technique used to treat the aneurysm and postoperative angiographic VSP.

## 10. Screening for occult IA

Screening for occult IA is a complex issue, it being of arguable effectiveness and very expensive. Unless a screening test is very highly sensitive and specific, inexpensive, easy to administer and can be delivered in practice to the appropriate population successfully, it is unlikely to produce worthwhile results and is more likely to increase health care costs and stress among the population and healthcare staff alike. Furthermore, unless one can differentiate between diseases that are likely to remain sub-clinical and those that are likely to cause significant symptoms, the treatment of disease following a screening program may have less of an impact than expected on cumulative mortality rates. In the case of intracranial aneurysms, because we cannot yet tell when aneurysms are going to rupture or form *de novo*, it would be difficult to know which to treat, which to leave alone and how often to screen, etc. The stress of being screened is difficult to quantify and probably depends in part upon the seriousness (in the minds of the screened population) of the disease being sought.

As with any screening exercise, multiple factors need to be considered, such as raising anxieties in the patient or the patient's family, confidentiality issues, 'the right not to know', the problems raised by false-positive and false-negative diagnoses, what age to start investigating patients and how often to repeat the investigations, etc. For intracranial aneurysms, many of these factors remain uncertain. There may be financial costs for the individuals who are screened. If conservative management is advised, knowledge of the presence of an aneurysm may be worrying to the individual concerned (and to his/her family and employer). Bearing all of these factors in mind, ignorance (of the presence or absence of an aneurysm) may actually be the best course of action for an individual at present.

Several groups have recommended screening for intracranial aneurysms in high-risk groups, namely ADPKD patients and those with a strong family history of aneurismal SAH (47, 49, 98). The efficacy of screening for aneurysms depends crucially on certain parameters relating to the natural history of aneurysms, particularly the prevalence and the annual risk of rupture. The analysis of rupture risk is complicated further by the pattern of aneurysm rupture - some aneurysms appear to develop and rupture rapidly whilst others stabilise (38). Screening will tend to detect the low-risk stable type rather than the high-risk aneurysms. The other critical consideration is the safety and effectiveness of treating a silent aneurysm in a healthy patient. A recent study found that the screening of individuals with a family history of L2 first-degree relatives with intracranial aneurysm with magnetic resonance angiography (MRA), followed by digital subtraction angiography (DSA) and surgery, is not an effective way of reducing morbidity and mortality from ruptured intracranial aneurysm (8).

## 11. References

[1] Alberico RA, Patel M, Casey S, Jacobs B, Maguire W, Decker R: Evaluation of the circle of Willis with three-dimensional CT angiography in patients with suspected intracranial aneurysms. AJNR Am J Neuroradiol 16: 1571-8, 1995

[2] Biumi F: Observationes Anatomicae. Observatio V; in Sandifort: Thesaurus Dissertationum. Lugd. Bat. S. and J. Lichtmans 3: 373, 1778

[3] Bonita R, Thomson S: Subarachnoid hemorrhage: epidemiology, diagnosis, management, and outcome. Stroke 16: 591-4, 1985

[4] Brilstra EH, Rinkel GJ, van der Graaf Y, van Rooij WJ, Algra A: Treatment of intracranial aneurysms by embolization with coils: a systematic review. Stroke 30:470-6,1999

[5] Byrne JV, Sohn MJ, Molyneux AJ: Five-year experience in using coil embolization for ruptured intracranial aneurysms: outcomes and incidence of late rebleeding. J Neurosurg 90: 656-63, 1999

[6] Cloft HJ, Joseph GJ, Dion JE: Risk of cerebral angiography in patients with subarachnoid hemorrhage, cerebral aneurysm, and arteriovenous malformation: a meta-analysis. Stroke 30: 317-20, 1999

[7] Cognard C, Pierot L, Boulin A, Weill A, Tovi M, Castaings L, Rey A, Moret J: Intracranial aneurysms: endovascular treatment with mechanical detachable spirals in 60 aneurysms. Radiology 202: 783-92, 1997

[8] Crawley F, Clifton A, Brown MM: Should We Screen for Familial Intracranial Aneurysm? Stroke 30: 312-316, 1999

[9] Dandy WE: Intracranial arterial Aneurysms. Comstock Ithacal N.Y. 1944

[10] Dott NM: Intracranial aneurysms: cerebral arteriography and surgical treatment. Trans. Med.-chir. Soc. Edinb. 112: 219-240, 1933

[11] Elliott JP, Newell DW, Lam DJ, Eskridge JM, Douville CM, Le Roux PD, Lewis DH, Mayberg MR, Grady MS, Winn HR: Comparison of balloon angioplasty and

papaverine infusion for the treatment of vasospasm following aneurysmal subarachnoid hemorrhage. J Neurosurg 88: 277-284, 1998
[12] Feigin VL, Rinkel GJE, Algra A, Vermeulen M, van Gijn J. Calcium antagonists for aneurysmal subarachnoid haemorrhage [Cochrane Review]. Cochrane Database of Systematic Reviews 2000; issue 2. Oxford: Update Software
[13] Findlay JM: Current management of aneurysmal subarachnoid hemorrhage guidelines from the Canadian Neurosurgical Society. Can J Neurol Sci 24: 161-170, 1997
[14] Firlik AD, Kaufmann AM, Jungreis CA, Yonas H: Effect of transluminal angioplasty on cerebral blood flow in the management of symptomatic vasospasm following aneurysmal subarachnoid hemorrhage. J Neurosurg 86: 830-839, 1997
[15] Fisher CM, Kistler JP, Davis JM: Relation of cerebral vasospasm to subarachnoid hemorrhage visualized by computerized tomographic scanning. Neurosurgery 6: 1-9, 1980
[16] Fogelholm R: Subarachnoid hemorrhage in middle Finland: incidence, early prognosis and indications for neurosurgical treatment. Stroke 12: 296-301, 1981
[17] Fujii Y, Takeuchi S, Sasaki 0, Minakawa T, Koike T, Tanaka R: Ultra-early rebleeding in spontaneous subarachnoid hemorrhage. J Neurosurg 84: 35-42, 1996
[18] Griffiths PD, Worthy S, Gholkar A: Incidental intracranial vascular pathology in patients investigated for carotid stenosis. Neuroradiology 38: 25-30, 1996
[19] Grote E, Hassler W: The critical first minutes after subarachnoid hemorrhage. Neurosurgery 22: 654-61, 1988
[20] Guglielmi G, Vinuela F, Duckwiler G, Dion J, Lylyk P, Berenstein A, Strother C, Graves V, Halbach V, Nichols D: Endovascular treatment of posterior circulation aneurysms by electrothrombosis using electrically detachable coils. J Neurosurg 77: 515-24, 1992
[21] Gull W:Cases of aneurysm of the cerebral vessels. Guy's Hosp. Rep. 5:281-304, 1859
[22] Hackett ML, Anderson CS: Health outcomes 1 year after subarachnoid hemorrhage: An international population-based study. The Australian Cooperative Research on Subarachnoid Hemorrhage Study Group. Neurology 55: 658-62, 2000
[23] Hamada J, Morioka M, Yano S, Kai Y, Ushio Y: Incidence and early prognosis of aneurysmal subarachnoid hemorrhage in Kumamoto Prefecture, Japan. Neurosurgery 54: 31-7, 2004
[24] Hasan D, Vermeulen M, Wijdicks EF, Hijdra A, van Gijn J: Effect of fluid intake and antihypertensive treatment on cerebral ischemia after subarachnoid hemorrhage. Stroke 20: 1511-5, 1989
[25] Hashimoto H, Iida J, Hironaka Y, Okada M, Sakaki T: Use of spiral computerized tomography angiography in patients with subarachnoid hemorrhage in whom subtraction angiography did not reveal cerebral aneurysms. J Neurosurg 92: 278-83, 2000
[26] Hauerberg J, Eskesen V, Rosenorn J: The prognostic significance of intracerebral haematoma as shown on CT scanning after aneurysmal subarachnoid haemorrhage. Br J Neurosurg 8: 333-9, 1994
[27] Hernesniemi J, Vapalahti M, Niskanen M, Tapaninaho A, Kari A, Luukkonen M, Puranen M, Saari T, Rajpar M: One year outcome in early aneurysm surgery: a 14 years experience. Acta Neurochir (Wien) 122: 1-10, 1993
[28] Hop JW, Rinkel GJ, Algra A, van Gijn J: Case-fatality rates and functional outcome after subarachnoid hemorrhage: a systematic review. Stroke 28: 660-4, 1997

[29] Hop JW, Rinkel GJ, Algra A, van Gijn J: Quality of life in patients and partners after aneurysmal subarachnoid hemorrhage. Stroke 29: 798-804, 1998a
[30] Hop JW, Rinkel GJ: Secondary ischemia after subarachnoid hemorrhage. Cerebrovasc Dis 6: 264-5, 1996
[31] Horikoshi T, Akiyama I, Yamagata Z, Nukui H: Retrospective analysis of the prevalence of asymptomatic cerebral aneurysm in 4518 patients undergoing magnetic resonance angiography when does cerebral aneurysm develop? Neurol Med Chir (Tokyo) 42: 105-12, 2002
[32] Hunt WE, Hess RM: Surgical risk as related to time of intervention in the repair of intracranial aneurysms. J Neurosurg 28: 14-20, 1968
[33] International Study of Unruptured Intracranial Aneurysms (ISUIA) Investigators. Factors related to the development and detection of single versus multiple unruptured intracranial aneurysms. Stroke 1996; 27: 178.
[34] International Study of Unruptured Intracranial Aneurysms Investigators. Unruptured intracranial aneurysms-risk of rupture and risks of surgical intervention. N Engl J Med 339: 1725-33, 1998
[35] Iwamoto H, Kiyohara Y, Fujishima M, Kato I, Nakayama K, Sueishi K, Tsuneyoshi M: Prevalence of intracranial saccular aneurysms in a Japanese community based on a consecutive autopsy series during a 30-year observation period. The Hisayama study. Stroke 30: 1390-5, 1999
[36] Iwata K, Misu N, Terada K, Kawai S, Momose M, Nakagawa H: Screening for unruptured asymptomatic intracranial aneurysms in patients undergoing coronary angiography. J Neurosurg 75: 52-5, 1991
[37] Johnston SC, Selvin S, Gress DR: The burden, trends, and demographics of mortality from subarachnoid hemorrhage. Neurology 50: 1413-1418, 1998.
[38] Juvela S, Porras M, Heiskanen O: Natural history of unruptured intracranial aneurysms: a long4erm follow-up study. J Neurosurg 79: 174-82, 1993
[39] Kapoor K, Kak VK: Incidence of intracranial aneurysms in north-west Indian population. Neurol India 51: 22-6, 2003
[40] Kassell NF, Helm G, Simmons N, Phillips CD, Cail WS: Treatment of cerebral vasospasm with intra-arterial papaverine. J Neurosurg 77: 848-852, 1992
[41] Kassell NF, Peerless SJ, Durward QJ, Beck DW, Drake CG, Adams HP: Treatment of ischemic deficits from vasospasm with intravascular volume expansion and induced arterial hypertension. Neurosurgery 11: 337-43, 1982
[42] Kassell NF, Torner JC, Haley EC, Jr., Jane JA, Adams HP, Kongable GL: The International Cooperative Study on the Timing of Aneurysm Surgery. Part 1: Overall management results. J Neurosurg 73: 18-36, 1990
[43] Kassell NF, Torner JC, Jane JA, Haley EC, Jr., Adams HP: The International Cooperative Study on the Timing of Aneurysm Surgery. Part 2: Surgical results. J Neurosurg 73: 37-47, 1990
[44] Kassell NF, Torner JC: Aneurysmal rebleeding: a preliminary report from the Cooperative Aneurysm Study. Neurosurgery 13: 479-481, 1983
[45] Keranen T, Tapaninaho A, Hernesniemi J, Vapalahti M: Late epilepsy after aneurysm operations. Neurosurgery 17: 897-900, 1985
[46] Kistler JP, Crowell RM, Davis KR, Heros R, Ojemann RC~ Zervas T, Fisher CM: The relation of cerebral vasospasm to the extent and location of subarachnoid blood visualized by CT scan: a prospective study. Neurology 33: 424-36, 1983

[47] Kojima M, Nagasawa S, Lee YE, Takeichi Y, Tsuda E, Mabuchi N. Asymptomatic familial cerebral aneurysms. Neurosurgery 43: 776-81, 1998.

[48] Le Roux PD, Newell DW, Eskridge J, Mayberg MR, Winn HR: Severe symptomatic vasospasm: the role of immediate postoperative angioplasty. J Neurosurg 80: 224-229, 1994

[49] Levey AS. Screening for occult intracranial aneurysms in polycystic kidney disease: interim guidelines [editorial]. J Am Soc Nephrol 1: 9-12, 1990

[50] Linn FH, Rinkel GJ, Algra A, van Gijn J: Incidence of subarachnoid hemorrhage: role of region, year, and rate of computed tomography: a meta-analysis. Stroke 27: 625-629, 1996

[51] Macdonald RL, Wallace MC, Kestle JR: Role of angiography following aneurysm surgery. J Neurosurg 79: 826-32, 1993

[52] Manabe H, Fujita S, Hatayama T, Suzuki S, Yagihashi S: Rerupture of coil-embolized aneurysm during long-term observation. Case report. J Neurosurg 88: 1096-8, 1998

[53] Mayberg MR: Intracranial Arterial Spasm, in Wilkins RH, Rengachary SS (eds): Neurosurgery. St. Louis, McGraw-Hill, 1996, 2245-2254

[54] McCormick WF, Nafzinger JD: Saccular intracranial aneurysms: an autopsy study. J Neurosurg 22:155-159, 1965

[55] Meyer FB, Sundt TM Jr, Fode NC, Morgan MK, Forbes GS, Mellinger JF: Cerebral aneurysms in childhood and adolescence. J Neurosurg 70: 420-5, 1989

[56] Molyneux A, Kerr R, Stratton I, Sandercock P, Clarke M, Shrimpton J, Holman R: International Subarachnoid Aneurysm Trial (ISAT) of neurosurgical clipping versus endovascular coiling in 2143 patients with ruptured intracranial aneurysms: a randomised trial. Lancet 360: 1267-74, 2002

[57] Moniz E: L'encephalographie arterielle, son importance dans la localization des tumeurs cerebrales. Rev Neurol 2: 72-90, 1927

[58] Morgagni JB: De sedibus et causis morborum per anatomen indagatis. Venetiis ex typog. Remondiniana 1761

[59] Noguchi K, Ogawa T, Seto H, Inugami A, Hadeishi H, Fujita H, Hatazawa J, Shimosegawa E, Okudera T, Uemura K: Subacute and chronic subarachnoid hemorrhage: diagnosis with fluid-attenuated inversion-recovery MR imaging. Radiology 203: 257-62, 1997

[60] Noguchi M: Subarachnoid hemorrhage in 'Vital Statistics of Japan', 1993-1995: variability with age and sex. No Shinkei Geka 26: 225-32, 1998

[61] Nogueira GJ: Spontaneous subarachnoid haemorrhage and ruptured aneurysms in the Middle East. A myth revisited. Acta Neurochir (Wien) 114: 20-5, 1992

[62] Ohaegbulam SC: Racial bias in intracranial arterial aneurysms? Trop Geogr Med 30: 305-11, 1978

[63] Ohkuma H, Fujita S, Suzuki S: Incidence of aneurysmal subarachnoid hemorrhage in Shimokita, Japan, from 1989 to 1998, Stroke 33: 195-9, 2002

[64] Ohman J, Heiskanen 0: Timing of operation for ruptured supratentorial aneurysms: a prospective randomized study. J Neurosurg 70: 55-60, 1989

[65] O'Sullivan MG, Whyman M, Steers JW, Whittle IR, Miller JD: Acute subdural haematoma secondary to ruptured intracranial aneurysm: diagnosis and management. Br J Neurosurg 8: 439-45, 1994

[66] Pakarinen S: Incidence, aetiology, and prognosis of primary subarachnoid haemorrhage. A study based on 589 cases diagnosed in a defined urban population during a defined period. Acta Neurol Scand 29: 1-28, 1967

[67] Pasqualin A, Mazza C, Cavazzani P, Scienza R, DaPian R: Intracranial aneurysms and subarachnoid hemorrhage in children and adolescents. Childs Nerv Syst 2: 185-90, 1986
[68] Polin RS, Hansen CA, German P, Chadduck JB, Kassell NF: Intra-arterially administered papaverine for the treatment of symptomatic cerebral vasospasm. Neurosurgery 42: 1256-1267, 1998
[69] Raaymakers TW, Rinkel GJ, Limburg M, Algra A: Mortality and morbidity of surgery for unruptured intracranial aneurysms: a meta-analysis. Stroke 29: 1531-8, 1998
[70] Report of World Federation of Neurological Surgeons Committee on a Universal Subarachnoid Hemorrhage Grading Scale. J Neurosurg 68: 985-986, 1988
[71] Rhoton AL Jr, Saeki N, Perlmutter D, Zeal A: Microsurgical anatomy of common aneurysm sites. Clin Neurosurg 26: 248-306, 1979
[72] Rinkel GJ, Djibuti M, van Gijn J: Prevalence and risk of rupture of intracranial aneurysms: a systematic review. Stroke 29: 251-6, 1998
[73] Rinkel GJ, Wijdicks EF, Ramos LM, van Gijn J: Progression of acute hydrocephalus in subarachnoid haemorrhage: a case report documented by serial CT scanning. J Neurol Neurosurg Psychiatry 53: 354-5, 1990
[74] Rinkel GJ, Wijdicks EFM, Vermeulen M, Hasan D, Brouwers PJ, van Gijn J: The clinical course of perimesencephalic nonaneurysmal subarachnoid hemorrhage. Ann Neurol 29: 463-8, 1991
[75] Ronkainen A, Hernesniemi J: Subarachnoid haemorrhage of unknown aetiology. Acta Neurochir (Wien) 119: 29-34, 1992
[76] Roos Y: Antifibrinolytic treatment in subarachnoid hemorrhage: a randomized placebo-controlled trial. STAR Study Group. Neurology 54: 77-82, 2000
[77] Schievink WI: Intracranial aneurysms. N Engl J Med 336: 28-40, 1997
[78] Smith B: Cerebral pathology in subarachnoid haemorrhage. J Neurol Neurosurg Psychiatry 26: 535-9, 1963
[79] Soucy JP, McNamara D, Mohr G, Lamoureux F, Lamoureux J, Danais S: Evaluation of vasospasm secondary to subarachnoid hemorrhage with technetium 99m-hexamethyl-propyleneamine oxime (HM PAO) tomoscintigraphy. J Nucl Med 31: 972-977, 1990
[80] Taneda M: Effect of early operation for ruptured aneurysms on prevention of delayed ischemic symptoms. J Neurosurg 57: 622-628, 1982
[81] Tapaninaho A, Hernesniemi J, Vapalahti M, Niskanen M, Kari A, Luukkonen M, Puranen M: Shunt-dependent hydrocephalus after subarachnoid haemorrhage and aneurysm surgery: timing of surgery is not a risk factor. Acta Neurochir (Wien) 123: 118-124, 1993
[82] Ueta T, Ichi S, Ochi T, Suzuki I: Spontaneous regression of an aneurysm at a nonbranching site of the supraclinoid internal carotid artery. Case report. J Neurosurg 101: 1070 2, 2004
[83] Ukkola V, Heikkinen ER: Epilepsy after operative treatment of ruptured cerebral aneurysms. Acta Neurochir Wien 106: 115-118, 1990
[84] van der Wee N, Rinkel GJ, Hasan D, van Gijn J: Detection of subarachnoid haemorrhage on early CT: is lumbar puncture still needed after a negative scan? J Neurol Neurosurg Psychiatry 58: 357-9, 1995
[85] van Gijn J, Rinkel GJ: Subarachnoid haemorrhage: diagnosis, causes and management. Brain 124: 249-278, 2001

[86] van Gijn J, van Dongen KJ: Computed tomography in the diagnosis of subarachnoid haemorrhage and ruptured aneurysm. Clin Neurol Neurosurg 82: 11-24,1980

[87] van Gijn J, van Dongen KJ: The time course of aneurysmal haemorrhage on computed tomograms. Neuroradiology 23: 153-6, 1982

[88] Vanninen R, Koivisto T, Saari T, Hernesniemi J, Vapalahti M: Ruptured intracranial aneurysms: acute endovascular treatment with electrolytically detachable coils - a prospective randomized study. Radiology 211: 325-36, 1999

[89] Vermeulen M, Lindsay KW, Murray GD, Cheah F, Hijdra A, Muizelaar JP, Schannong M, Teasdale GM, van Crevel H, van Gijn J: Antifibrinolytic treatment in subarachnoid hemorrhage. N Engl J Med 311: 432-7, 1984

[90] Vermeulen M, van Gijn J: The diagnosis of subarachnoid haemorrhage. J Neurol Neurosurg Psychiatry 53: 365-72, 1990

[91] Vinuela F, Duckwiler Q Mawad M: Guglielmi detachable coil embolization of acute intracranial aneurysm: perioperative anatomical and clinical outcome in 403 patients. J Neurosurg 86: 475-82, 1997

[92] Vora YY, Suarez Almazor M, Steinke DE, Martin ML, Findlay JM: Role of transcranial Doppler monitoring in the diagnosis of cerebral vasospasm after subarachnoid hemorrhage. Neurosurgery 44: 1237-47, 1999

[93] Wardlaw JM, White PM: The detection and management of unruptured intracranial aneurysms. Brain 123: 205-21, 2000

[94] Weir B, Grace M, Hansen J, Rothberg C: Time course of vasospasm in man. J Neurosurg 48: 173-178, 1978

[95] Weir B, Macdonald L: Intracranial aneurysms and subarachnoid hemorrhage: an overview, in Wilkins RH, Rengachary SS (eds): Neurosurgery. St. Louis, McGraw-Hill, 1996, 2191-2213.

[96] Whitfield PC, Moss H, O'Hare D, Smielewski P, Pickard JD, Kirkpatrick PJ: An audit of aneurysmal subarachnoid haemorrhage: earlier resuscitation and surgery reduces inpatient stay and deaths from rebleeding. J Neurol Neurosurg Psychiatry 60: 301-6,1996

[97] Whittle IR, Williams DB, Halmagyi GM, Besser M: Spontaneous thrombosis of a giant intracranial aneurysm and ipsilateral internal carotid artery. Case report. J Neurosurg 56: 287-9, 1982

[98] Wiebers DO, Torres VE. Screening for unruptured intracranial aneurysms in autosomal dominant polycystic kidney disease [editorial]. N Engl J Med 327: 953-5, 1992

[99] Wijdicks EF, Vermeulen M, Murray GD, Hijdra A, van Gijn J: The effects of treating hypertension following aneurysmal subarachnoid hemorrhage. Clin Neurol Neurosurg 92: 111-7, 1990

[100] Winn HR, Jane JA Sr, Taylor J, Kaiser D, Britz GW: Prevalence of asymptomatic incidental aneurysms: review of 4568 arteriograms. J Neurosurg 96: 43-9, 2002

[101] Yasargil MG: Microsurgical anatomy of the basal cisterns and vessels of the brain, diagnostic studies, general operative techniques and pathological considerations of the intracranial aneurysms. New York, Georg Thieme Verlag Stuttgart -New York, 1984, vol 1.

[102] Yasui N, Magarisawa S, Suzuki A, Nishimura H, Okudera T, Abe T: Subarachnoid hemorrhage caused by previously diagnosed, previously unruptured intracranial aneurysms: a retrospective analysis of 25 cases. Neurosurgery 39: 1096-100, 1996

[103] Yasui N, Suzuki A, Nishimura H, Suzuki K, Abe T: Long-term follow-up study of unruptured intracranial aneurysms. Neurosurgery 40: 1155-9, 1997

# 10

# Ruptured Cerebral Aneurysms: An Update

Ming Zhong, Bing Zhao, Zequn Li and Xianxi Tan
*Department of Neurosurgery, The First Affiliated Hospital of Wenzhou Medical College*
*China*

## 1. Introduction

A Cerebral aneurysm is an abnormal bulging outward of one of cerebral arteries and is common lesion in the adult population. Cerebral aneurysm occurs in 1~5% of people which translates to 10 million to 12 million persons in the United States [1, 2]Approximately 0.2 to 3 percent of people with an aneurysm suffer from rupture per year. Ruptured aneurysm is the leading cause of subarachnoid hemorrhage (SAH) in 85% of cases. SAH is a common devastating condition and the age-adjusted annual incidence of SAH 2.0 cases per 100 000 population in China[3]. SAH accounts for 5% of stroke, but the case fatality is as high as 45% and some patients have significant morbidity among survivors [1, 4] Rebleeding is the most imminent danger. The first treatment purpose is therefore complete occlusion of aneurysms and prevention of rebleeding.

Treatment for a ruptured aneurysm includes microsurgical clipping and endovascular coiling. Although microsurgery is the traditional and standard treatment for aneurysms with a high complete obliteration, endovascular treatment has been widely used to treat aneurysm and has displaced surgical clipping in many centers[1, 2, 5-7]. With the development of microsurgical technique and intraoperative monitoring technique, microsurgical clipping still remains a definitive treatment for ruptured cerebral aneurysms[8, 9].Now we will review the pathology of ruptured cerebral aneurysm, clinical manifestations for SAH, preoperative evaluation and improvement of surgical techniques.

## 2. Pathology of ruptured aneurysm

Cerebral aneurysms are very common in the population and considered to be sporadically acquired lesions. Acquired factors include atherosclerosis, hypertension and hemodynamic stress. Certain genetic syndromes such as polycystic kidney disease, connective tissue disorders fibromuscular dysplasia, and Marfan's syndrome have also been associated with an increased risk of SAH and support the concept of inherited susceptibility to aneurysm formation[10-12] Aneurysms may also result from congenital defects, weakness of cerebral artery, a decrease in the tunica media, the middle muscular layer of the artery, are thought to have a major role[2].

Most studies on risk of rupture and pathology have been reported, and the mechanism of aneurysmal rupture also is unknown at present[1, 4]. A recent meta-analysis yields an annual rupture risk of 0.6% to 1.3% of intracranial aneurysms. The Size of aneurysms is the most important risk factor for rupture, with smaller risks for smaller aneurysms. Other risk factors are the site, age, female gender. Posterior circulation aneurysms have higher risk of bleeding than anterior circulation[13]. A Statement for healthcare professionals from the Stroke Council, American Heart Association recommends cessation of smoking is reasonable to reduce the risk of SAH, although evidence for this association is not direct[4]. A new study found chronic inflammatory reaction is going on in the aneurysmal wall, and susceptibility of the aneurysm to bleeding is associated with the degeneration of the aneurysmal wall [14]

## 3. Clinical classification of SAH

Aneurysmal SAH is a neurosurgical emergency and devastating event. These symptoms include severe headache, nausea, vomiting, vision impairment, and loss of consciousness. But symptoms are different from every patient with an onset of aneurysm rupture, followed in about one third of the patients by severe confusion or coma. A retrospective study found of 109 patients with SAH, headache was in 74%, nausea or vomiting in 77%, loss of consciousness in 53%, and nuchal rigidity in 35%. As many as 12% die before receiving medical attention[1].Many patients present with an acute onset of severe headache, often described by patients as the "worst headache of my life" .

Numerous grade systems have been reported for grading the clinical condition of patients with SAH from a ruptured cerebral aneurysm. These include the Hunt and Hess Scale[15] (Table 1), Glasgow Coma Scale, and World Federation of Neurological Surgeons Scale[16] (Table 2), but the current literature remains deficient regarding the grading of patients with SAH. Recently Hunt and Hess scale and World Federation of Neurological Surgeons grading scale are commonly used to describe the neurologic condition on admission and severity of SAH. These grading scales are considered good predictors of ultimate outcome. Computed tomography (CT) of the head can diagnose SAH and be used to describe the amount of blood in the brain. The Fisher grading scale has been shown to correlate with symptomatic vasospasm. Delayed cerebral ischemia (DCI) from vasospasm is an important cause of complications and death after SAH. A new and easy-to-use SAH rating scale accounts for the independent predictive value of subarachnoid and ventricular blood for delayed cerebral ischemia, superior to the Fisher Scale for differentiation between different levels of risk for DCI[17] (Table 3).

| Grade | Symptoms |
|---|---|
| Grade I | Asymptomatic or minimal headache and slight nuchal rigidity; |
| Grade II | Moderate to severe headache; nuchal rigidity; no neurologic deficit except cranial nerve palsy. |
| Grade III | Drowsiness, confusion, or mild focal deficit. |
| Grade IV | Stupor, moderate to severe hemiparesis, and early decelerate rigidity and vegetative disturbances. |
| Grade V | Deep coma, decelerate rigidity; moribund. |

Table 1. Hunt and Hess grading scale for SAH

| Grade | Glasgow coma score | Motor deficit* |
|---|---|---|
| Grade I | 15 | Absent |
| Grade II | 13 or 14 | Absent |
| Grade III | 13 or 14 | Present |
| Grade IV | 7 to 12 | – |
| GradeV | 3 to 6 | – |

*Excludes cranial neuropathies but includes dysphasia.

Table 2. World Federation of Neurological Surgeons grading system for SAH

| Grade | Demonstration | Correlations with DCI |
|---|---|---|
| Grade 1 | minimal or diffuse thin SAH without bilateral IVH | low risk |
| Grade 2 | minimal or thin SAH with bilateral IVH | indicating intermediate risk |
| Grade 3 | cisternal clot without bilateral IVH | indicating intermediate risk |
| Grade 4 | cisternal clot with bilateral IVH | high risk |

Table 3. CT scan scales for SAH and its correlations with DCI

## 4. Alternative procedures

### 4.1 Microsurgical clipping and endovascular coiling

Surgical clipping or endovascular coiling techniques can be used in the treatment of ruptured aneurysms. Most studies on the clipping and coiling of cerebral aneurysms were either small-scale studies or were retrospective studies until the multi-center prospective randomized clinical trial has been reported[6]. The International Subarachnoid Aneurysm Trial (ISAT) study which selected 2143 of 9559 SAH patients for randomization into endovascular or surgical aneurysm treatment found that endovascular coiling treatment produced substantially better patient outcomes than surgical clipping in patients with ruptured aneurysms equally suited for both treatment options[6]. The relative risk of death or severe disability at one year for patients treated by coiling (15.6%) was lower than in patients treated by open surgery (22.6%).

The results suggest that endovascular coiling is associated with better outcomes at one year than surgical clipping[6, 7]. Unfortunately, most patients in ISAT presented with a favorable clinical grade (>90 percent) and had aneurysms in the anterior circulation (97.3 percent) that were smaller than 10 mm (nearly 95 percent). In general, the incidence of recanalization is higher with coiling and complete aneurysm occlusion is more likely to be achieved with clipping. Long-term follow-up on risks of death, disability, and rebleeding in patients randomly assigned to clipping or endovascular coiling after rupture of an intracranial aneurysm in ISAT, found 24 rebleeding had occurred more than 1 year after treatment and the risk of death at 5 years was significantly lower in the coiling group (11% , 112 of 1046) than in the clipping group (14%, 144 of 1041)[9].

Complex intracranial aneurysms are frequently treated with surgical and endovascular methods. These aneurysms are fusiform or complex wide-necked structure, giant size, or involvement with critical perforating or branch vessels and are not treated with direct surgical clipping or endovascular treatment. Strategies include surgery followed by endovascular therapy or endovascular therapy followed by surgery[18, 19] . In fact, Medical conditions and severity from an initial SAH influence the selection of treatment. A poor grade aneurysmal SAH may increase the risk of surgical retraction but has less influence on the difficulty of endovascular therapy[20].A large life-threatening hematoma related to ruptured aneurysms may favor a decision to perform open surgery to reduce intracranial pressure by evacuation of the hematoma. Combined treatment involving acute aneurysm coiling and surgical decompression of brain swelling or hemorrhage can also be used successfully. For example, the initial treatment of large clot of blood without mass effect from an aneurysm includes aneurysm clipping with hematoma evacuation, endovascular coiling with hematoma evacuation. In summary, optimal treatment requires availability of both experienced cerebrovascular surgeons and endovascular surgeons working in a collaborative effort to evaluate each case of SAH[1]. In summary, microsurgical treatment with endovascular approach can achieve the best outcomes for patients with ruptured cerebral aneurysms.

## 5. Preoperative planning

Pretreatment planning needs identification of a ruptured aneurysm and delineation of the size and morphologic features of aneurysms. A ruptured cerebral aneurysm commonly leads to SAH or brain hematoma, which is found on a head CT scan. If a CT scan is negative, a ruptured aneurysm is still suspected, a lumbar puncture is performed to detect blood in the cerebrospinal fluid (CSF). Cerebral angiography, computed topographic angiography (CTA) or magnetic resonance angiography (MRA) are commonly used to determine the exact location, size and shape of a ruptured aneurysm before treatment.

MRA in SAH has evolved as the initial test for aneurysm identification and localization over the past decade. The sensitivity of MRA for cerebral aneurysms is only between 55% and 99.2%, because with aneurysms 5 mm , the sensitivity is 85% to 100% and the sensitivity of MRA for detecting aneurysms <5 mm drops to 56%[21, 22] . MRA has practical limitations in the characteristics of the aneurysm neck and its relationship to the parent vessels[1, 23]. MRA takes considerably longer to perform than does CTA and does not replace CT tomography and cerebral angiography to identify the ruptured cerebral aneurysms before treatment[23, 24].

CTA images show cerebral vessels in three-dimensional directions and the vasculature to be visualized relative to the brain and the skull base, facilitating surgical planning. CTA can provide three dimensional images for aneurysm detection, aneurysm location and size[25]. Some studies evaluating CTA in the management of intracranial aneurysms have reported sensitivities ranging from 77% and 100% and specificities ranging from 79% and 100%[2, 23]. Among aneurysms detected on CTA and then undergoing surgery, 100% correlation was observed between CTA and catheter angiography[26]. CTA, as a less invasive alternative to cerebral angiography, is a widely accepted method for detection and characterization of cerebral aneurysms when planning surgical intervention[27].

The sensitivity and specificity of CTA for aneurysm detection depend on radiologist experience, image acquisition, and the presentation of the images. Disadvantages of CTA include the need for iodinated contrast dye administration, the possibility of bony artifact that interferes with image quality, and the inability to study small distal vessels. We should have not overestimated the diagnostic accuracy of CT angiography[28] because of the features, the possibility of bony artifact and the inability to study small distal vessels. 74% patients did not reveal any additional information, when catheter angiography was performed after CTA. Therefore, s small number of neurosurgeons have used these images to perform routine surgery on CTA alone[29].

Digital subtraction angiography (DSA) is currently the standard to document the presence and anatomic features of aneurysms. The three-dimensional cerebral angiography was developed to demonstrate the aneurysm and its relation to other vessels to be assessed in three dimensions, overcoming prior to two dimensional angiography limitations [30]. Actually, CTA is better able to define aneurysmal wall calcification, intraluminal aneurysm thrombosis, orientation of aneurysm with respect to intraparenchymal hemorrhage, and the relationship of the aneurysm with bony landmarks. CTA can also be used to supplement information obtained by catheter angiography[1].

## 6. Surgical technique

Surgical treatment includes aneurysm clipping, aneurysmorrhaphy, trapping, coating, and arterial reconstruction. Carotid ligation was commonly used to treat recently ruptured intracranial aneurysms before 1970. Carotid ligation did not lead to a significant improvement in mortality or rebleeding in the acute period compared with regulated bedrest in the intent-to-treat analysis[31]. Compared with conservative therapy, carotid ligation may produce a decrease in rebleeding; however, the rate of treatment failures of rebleeding plus complications likely exceeds that of direct surgical treatment of the aneurysm[1].

Clipping approach and techniques were introduced by Prof. Yaşargil and have been widely used since 1970s. The current principle of clipping requires microsurgical dissection and clipping of the ruptured aneurysm neck whenever possible. Most patients with anterior or posterior circulation aneurysms, patients in the grades Hunt and Hess IV or V can be treated by clipping in our department[32]. At present it is not necessary to use the large conventional pterional fronto-temporal craniotomies in regular cerebral aneurysm surgery. With developments in visualization of operative microscope, surgical techniques, and the introduction of neuroendoscopy have led to less invasive methods in cerebral base surgery. The keyhole approach has been used for the treatment of a ruptured cerebral aneurysm[33-37].

As we know, the size and location of the cerebral aneurysm is not always proportionate to the extent of brain exposure. Cerebral aneurysms surgery is apt to be treated by the keyhole approach. Keyhole approaches include supraorbital keyhole, the eyebrow keyhole and other keyhole associated with the location of aneurysms. Most supratentorial or basilar tip aneurysms are treated with the supraorbital keyhole approach[34] The concept and technique of the keyhole approach are presented in detail by Prof. Perneczky A [38] The supraorbital keyhole approach offers equal surgical possibilities with less intraoperative accidental rupture and less approach-related morbidity as conventional approaches in the treatment of supratentorial aneurysms. A study comparing the results of minimally invasive keyhole craniotomy and standard larger craniotomies found both surgical approaches had reached almost similar morbidity and mortality rates, and overall surgical results[36].

With the development of the endoscope to the microsurgical management, endoscopic-assisted microsurgery is an exceptional aid to the surgeon and become part of the operating theatre equipment with no complications[39]. The use of the endoscope to assist the microsurgical clipping of cerebral aneurysm has been reported[40, 41].The rigid endoscope has been increasingly used during aneurysm surgery to plan surgical strategies and verify the regional anatomic features, neck anatomic features and perforators and verification of the optimal clip position. However, it is necessary for the surgeon to be familiar with the endoscope instrumentation and fully prepared for the risks and inconveniences of procedures. Five ways of observing the endoscopic and microscopic images at the same time were introduced[38].Endoscope-assisted microsurgery during keyhole approaches may provide maximum efficiency to clip the cerebral aneurysm, maximum safety for the patient, and minimum invasiveness.

Fusiform and dolichoectatic aneurysms are often not treated with direct clipping and require alternative surgical strategies such as the wrapping technique, arterial reconstruction. These aneurysms are commonly located on the middle cerebral artery, carotid ophthalmic. Clip-wrap techniques for the treatment of fusiform aneurysms seem to be safe to prevent rebleeding and represent an improvement with a low rate of acute or delayed postoperative complications[42]. In some lesions of giant or large internal carotid artery-ophthalmic artery aneurysm which cannot be trapped, proximal and distal occlusion (trapping) is the most effective strategy, however, occlusion of parent arteries has a high incidence of transient complications and may lead to ischemia [1]. Many patients with proximal parent artery occlusion with surgical clips or endovascular techniques will be consider necessary to perform brain cerebral blood flow alteration or an extracranial-intracranial arterial bypass. Bypass technique is an important and increasing aspect of these alternative treatments.

Temporary vascular occlusion has been frequently used during aneurysm surgery prevent intraoperative rupture of large or difficult-to-approach aneurysms. The length of time of temporary clips is dependent on the capability of a low brain perfusion. In selected patients with giant aneurysms, particularly of the basilar artery, deep hypothermia with circulatory arrest under cardiopulmonary extracorporeal circulation has been shown to be an acceptable technique[43]. However, there is no reliable method of predicting the possibility of ischemia due to extended regional circulatory interruption by the temporary clipping technique during surgery.

## 7. Intraoperative monitoring method

The routine monitoring methods includes continuous EKG monitoring, and frequent determinations of blood pressure, electrolytes, fluid balance, in many centers. These monitoring and intervention may belong to neuroanesthetic management. In addition to microsurgical dissection and clipping aneurysm, correct intraoperative assessment of aneurysm occlusion, perforating artery patency, and parent artery reconstruction are possible in all patients with ruptured aneurysms. At present there are no reliable and standard method to assess regional anatomic features, verification of the optimal clipping and other ischemia events after surgery. The assisted neuroendoscope technique, the intraoperative microvascular doppler probe (IMD)[44, 45] [42] and fluorescence angiography [46]have been used intraoperative microsurgical treatment of cerebral aneurysms.

Microvascular doppler sonography with a 20-MHz probe (1-mm diameter) was used in 1990s[44]before and after clip application, to confirm the obliteration of aneurysms. Now many studies showed IMD is a safe, instantaneous, effective, reliable method instead of moreover intraoperative angiography for the surgical treatment of aneurysms. IMD is also used for assessment of a blood flow reduction for adjusting the clip placement[45].Intraoperative angiography (IOA) has proven to be a safe and effective adjunct to cerebral aneurysms surgery[47]. Although an argument for routine use of IOA exists during cerebral aneurysm surgery and substantial practice variation exists regarding use of this modality in different centers, including use of IOA routinely, selectively, or rarely. IOA should be standard in cerebral aneurysm surgery[42].Fluorescence angiography method is a microscope integrated intraoperative near-infrared indocyanine green angiography (ICG) technique and microscope-integrated light source containing infrared excitation light illuminates the operating field. ICG provides real-time information of the cerebral vasculature about aneurysms[46, 48] Summarily the intraoperative monitoring and vascular imaging methods compared were complementary rather than competitive in nature method.

The occurrence of brain ischemia during surgery due to temporary arterial occlusion or incorrect placement of the clip is a major complication of aneurysm surgery. At present, no method exists to predict the possibility of ischemia cased by aneurysm surgery. A study reported brain tissue oxygen concentration (PtiO(2)) was monitored during surgery of middle cerebral artery (MCA) aneurysm with SAH and found intraoperative monitoring of PtiO(2) may be a useful method of detection of changes in brain tissue oxygenation during MCA aneurysm surgery for detection of changes in brain oxygenation due to reduced blood flow, as a predictor of ischemic events[49] .

## 8. Complications

### 8.1 Rebleeding

Rebleeding remains a serious consequence of aneurysmal SAH, with a case fatality rate of 70%, and is currently the most treatable cause of poor outcomes[1]. Previous studies delineated the re-bleedings in the first days were thought to be related to the unstable nature of the aneurysmal thrombus. The incidence of rebleeding in unoperated patients is greatest in the first 2 weeks. In the prospective Cooperative Aneurysm Study [50], the rate of rebleeding was 4% on the first day after SAH and then constant at a rate of 1% per day to 2% per day over the following 4 weeks. Recent studies found that all preoperative rebleeding occurred within 12 hours of initial SAH and 70% of ultraearly rebleeds occurred within 2 hours of initial SAH[51, 52].A large retrospective study reported a rebleeding rate of 6.9% after admission but no relationship to blood pressure[53].

Although older studies demonstrated an overall negative effect of antifibrinolytics, recent evidence suggests that early treatment with a short course of antifibrinolytic agents combined with a program of early aneurysm treatment followed by discontinuation of the antifibrinolytic and prophylaxis against hypovolemia and vasospasm may be reasonable (Class IIb, Level of Evidence B). Antifibrinolytics, and other medical measures alone are not enough to prevent rebleeding after SAH except early treatment of ruptured cerebral aneurysms[1].

Procedural efficacy for treatment of a cerebral aneurysm is determined by the rebleeding and the residuals and recurrences of the treated aneurysm. One study reported all rebleeding occurred in the first 12 months after treatment and overall rebleeding with endovascular treatment was somewhat more common than with surgical treatment[54]. Case reports have demonstrated that even when aneurysms appear to be completely occluded after surgery, rebleeding may occur later[55]. However, the majority of hemorrhages after treatment reported in patients with postoperative angiography have occurred in incompletely occluded aneurysms.

### 8.2 Cerebral vasospasm

Cerebral vasospasm is the most common cause of death and disability after aneurysmal SAH. In one half of patients, vasospasm is manifested by the occurrence of a delayed neurological ischemic deficit. 15% to 20% of such patients suffer stroke or die of vasospasm despite maximal therapy[1]. Vasospasm leads to additional artery lumen narrowing, impaired vascular reactivity, a fall in cerebral blood flow which causes ischemia and following infarction. The development of a new focal deficit or the obvious symptoms in comatose unexplained by hydrocephalus or rebleeding, is the first objective sign of symptomatic vasospasm.

Monitoring for vasospasm typically include the clinical neurologic exams, serial measurement of blood flow and catheter angiography. Detection of signs of vasospasm is particularly difficult in poor grade patients. Many centers, including our department, rely on cerebral angiography for the diagnosis of vasospasm. However, the American Academy of Neurology Expert Committee believes the use of TCD on the basis of the fact that although sensitivity and specificity are quite variable and depend on the vessel of interest, severe spasm can be identified with fairly high reliability[56].Recently perfusion computed tomography, diffusion weighted magnetic resonance imaging, and single photon emission computed tomography (SPECT) in detecting vasospasm is under investigation[57]. However, the effect of microsurgical treatment on incidence of vasospasm is not exactly known.

The management of vasospasm involves medical drugs, aggressive volume expanse interventions and hemodilution. Calcium channel blockers, particularly Nimodipine (oral) 60 mg every four hours reduces the risk of poor outcome and secondary ischemia related to aneurysmal SAH (Class I, Level of Evidence A)[5].The use of triple-H therapy (hypervolemia, hypertension and hemodilution) induces hypertension and improves cerebral blood flow, and then improves patients' clinical symptoms. Therefore, Volume expansion therapy becomes a mainstay in the management of cerebral vasospasm[5]. However, recent studies found there was no any difference between the prophylactic volume expansion and hyperdynamic therapy group and the normovolemic therapy group[58, 59].Moreover, the initiation of prophylactic volume expansion is associated with significant risks, including the possibility of cardiac failure, electrolyte abnormality, cerebral edema. The prophylactic hemodynamic therapy needs further study before it can be commonly used[60].

Endovascular techniques frequently play a role in the aggressive treatment of vasospasm, including transluminal angioplasty, balloon angioplasty, and intra-arterial infusion of vasodilators [61], Spastic cerebral vessels are dilated mechanically via microcatheters. The theoretical goal of balloon angioplasty is to increase the CBF distal to the area of stenosis. However, interventional procedures have their unique associated risks and the optimal timing of angioplasty in relation to medical therapy is uncertain[62].

With microcatheter technology improving and superselective techniques having advanced over the last decade, it has become possible to selectively catheterize third- and fourth-order cerebral vessels and to administer high doses of vasodilators such as papaverine into vessels that cannot be treated with balloon angioplasty[63]. The doses of papaverine reported in the literature are infused at a concentration of 3 mg/mL at 6 to 9 L/min for a total dose of up to 300 mg per vascular territory[64]. Alternatively, cerebral angioplasty and/or selective intraarterial vasodilator therapy may be reasonable after, together with, or in the place of triple-H therapy, depending on the clinical scenario (Class IIb, Level of Evidence B)[1]. Despite recent advances in the treatment of the vasospasm of aneurysmal SAH, few effective treatments exist, and further research is needed.

### 8.3 Postoperative image evaluation

Surgery claims to exclude aneurysms completely from the circulation and rates of aneurysms rupture is significantly decreased relative to the natural history of the lesions. However, Aneurysm residuals and recurrences are not uncommon after microsurgery. A risk of rupture is still present even after surgical clipping. Rates of aneurysm residuals are not negligible, ranging from 3.8% to 8 %.[65]. In a small number of patients treated by surgery, the aneurysm is incompletely clipped and has a risk of rupture and regrowth. Case reports and series have found that even when aneurysms appear to be completely occluded after surgery, recurrence and rupture may occur later. The incidence of recurrent aneurysms after complete clipping was approximately 0.02% per year; aneurysms recurred after 13.3 years on average with 25 years the longest duration from initial clipping to recurrence[66] . Repeat craniotomy may be performed to prevent the rebleeding.

Follow-up imaging provides an opportunity to identify incompletely treated aneurysms by the conventional DSA. Computed tomography angiography (CTA) is a time and cost saving investigation for postoperative evaluation of clipped cerebral aneurysm patient[67]. In one study up to 85% of postoperative CTA images were of excellent quality with absent or minimal artefacts in 81% and seem adequate to detect small aneurysm remnants[68]. Three-dimensional DSA also allows us to detect more residual aneurysms after surgical clip placement than what is indicated in the existing literature, the conventional DSA[69].Three-dimensional DSA may provide baseline data for the long-term follow-up of postsurgical aneurysms[70].

## 9. Outcome

In a population-based study by Broderick et al, the 30-day mortality rate among all patients who suffered from SAH was 45%, with the majority of deaths occurring in the first days after SAH[71]. The prospective, randomized trial to date comparing surgery and endovascular techniques is ISAT, which selected 2143 of 9559 SAH patients for randomization into endovascular or surgical aneurysm treatment Evaluation at one year demonstrated mortality rate was 10.1%; greater disability rate was 21.6% in surgical patients [6, 7]. The prognosis for a patient with a ruptured cerebral aneurysm treated by microsurgery depends on brain injury severity from initial bleeding, the extent and location of the aneurysm. The most significant factors in determining outcome are GCS and increasing age. Generally patients with Hunt and Hess grade I and II on admission can anticipate a good outcome, and Hunt and Hess grade IV and V have a poor outcome, death, or permanent severe disability.

## 10. Expert suggestions

In general, all patients with aneurysmal SAH frequently get CTA and selective three-dimensional DSA to plan the individual therapeutic strategy in our hospital: microsurgical, endovascular. CTA has advantages of rapid image acquisition and its widespread availability, which can make it suitable for critically ill patients. Patients with life-threatening hematoma and with suspected the ruptured aneurysms only receive CTA, which are used for emergency surgery for clipping. Postoperative angiography is usually recommended and performed, including CTA and three-dimensional cerebral angiography. Three-dimensional angiography is the best method for evaluation of aneurysm residuals or recanalisation, providing detailed information from all different angles.

## 11. Explicative cases

**Case 1.** A 46-year-old woman with SAH was diagnosed with a ruptured anterior communicating artery aneurysm using CTA and DSA, and then treated with microsurgical clipping. C and D: The aneurysm neck was completely clipped by the pterional approach.

**Case 2.** A 52-year-old woman was diagnosed with a brain hematoma due to a ruptured middle artery aneurysm on admission and received emergency open surgery after CTA.

**Case 3.** Postoperative 3D-CTA was performed 10 days after surgical clipping and showed the complete occlusion of a posterior communicating artery aneurysm.

**Case 4** Postoperative 3D-DSA showed two aneurysms on the posterior communicating and A1 segment of anterior cerebral artery were clipped completely.

## 12. Conclusion

Aneurysmal SAH is a common and devastating condition, with a high mortality and morbidity rate. Despite recent advances in microsurgical treatment, endovascular coiling and preoperative management, the outcome of ruptured aneurysm remains poor. Although microsurgical treatment and intraoperative motoring procedures are developed rapidly, outcome of patients treated by microsurgery involves many factors: ruptured severity, Hunt and Hess grade, aneurysm location, size and characteristics. Decisions about microsurgery, the surgical approach, and specific technical adjuncts must be based on the individual clinical setting.

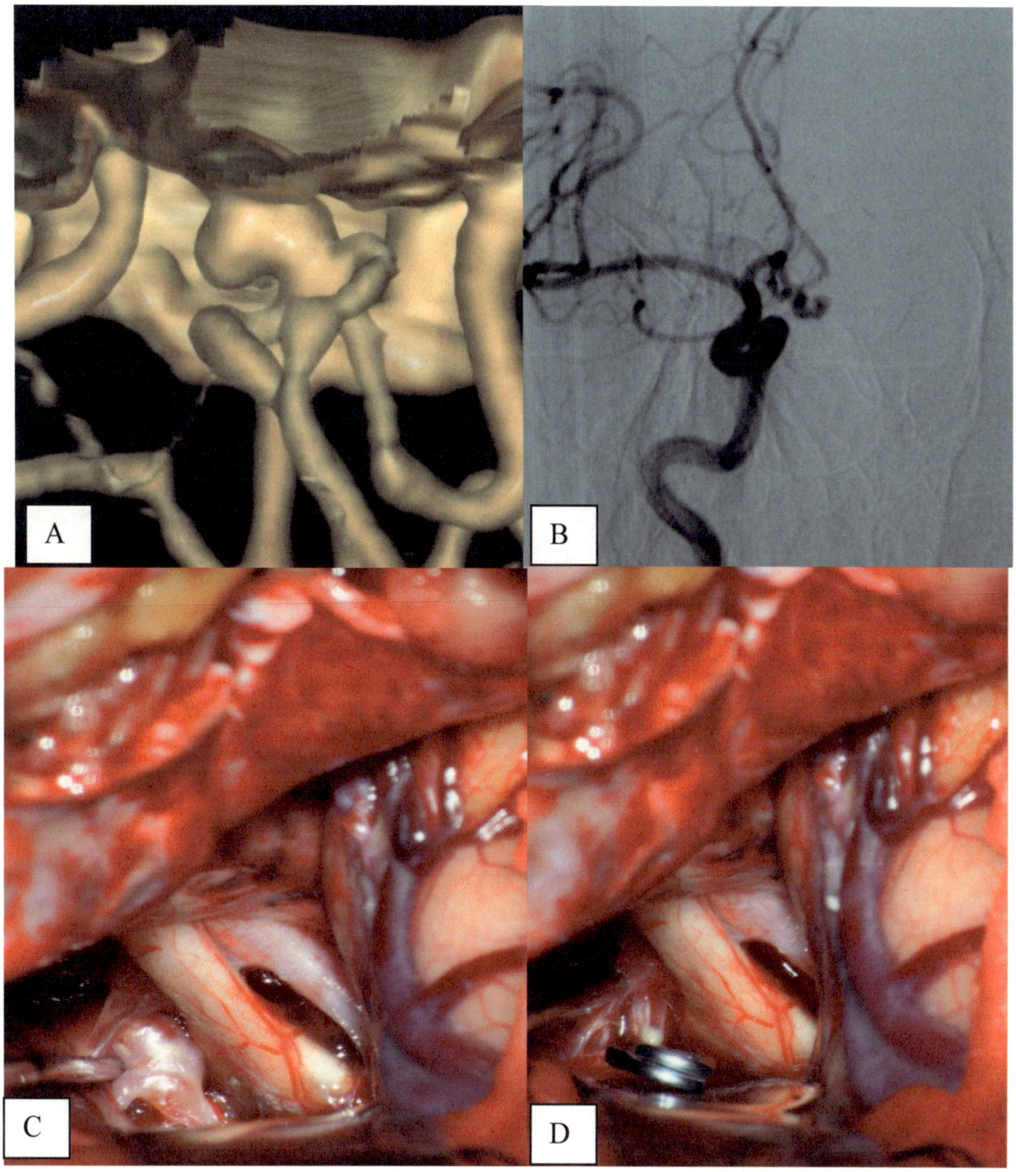


Fig. 1. Case 1: A and B: Preoperative CTA and DSA showed a saccular aneurysm (arrow) on ACoA. C and D: The aneurysm neck was completely clipped by the pterional approach.

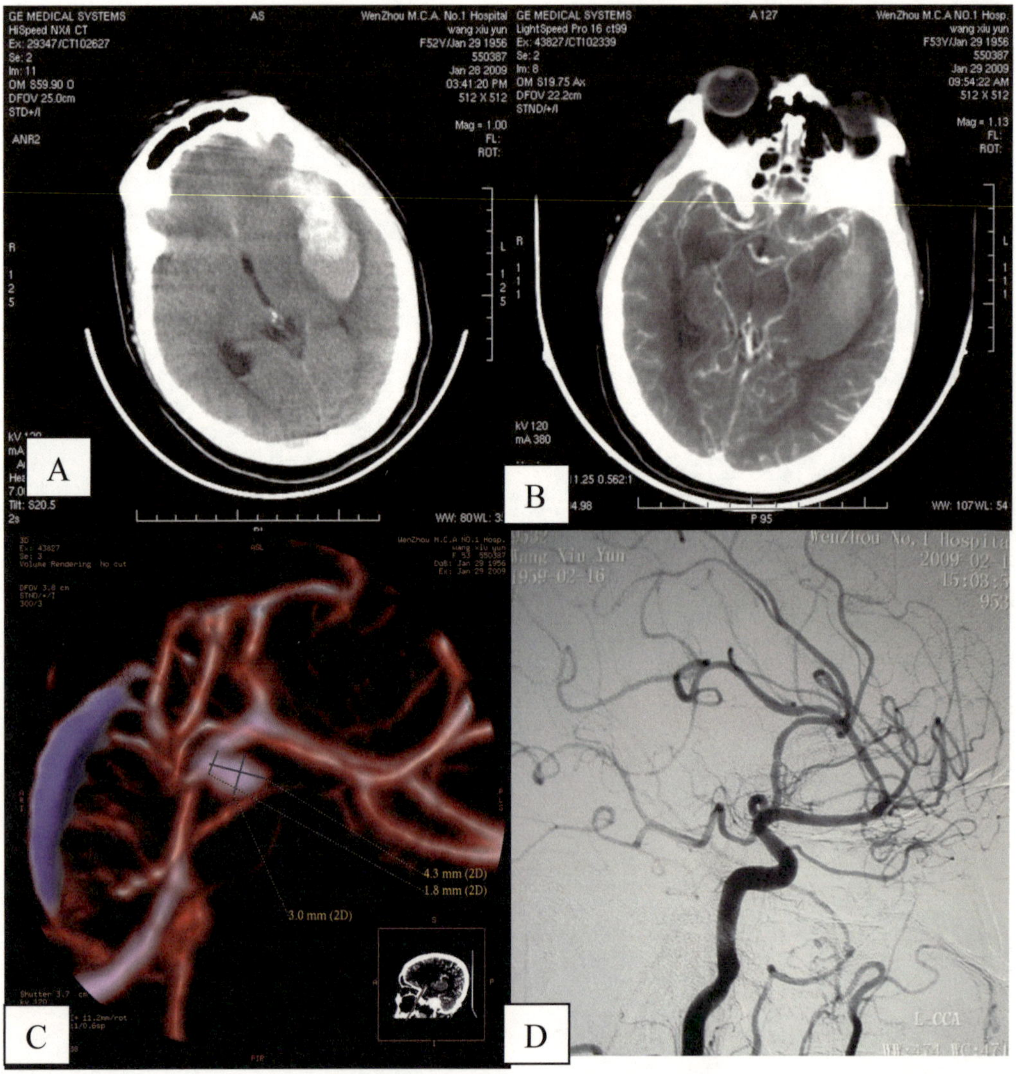

Fig. 2. Case 2: A. CT scan demonstrated a massive intracranial hematoma in the left temporal lobe B and C: CTA MIP and VR images demonstrated a saccular middle artery aneurysm surrounding the hematoma. D: DSA showed the complete occlusion of the aneurysm.

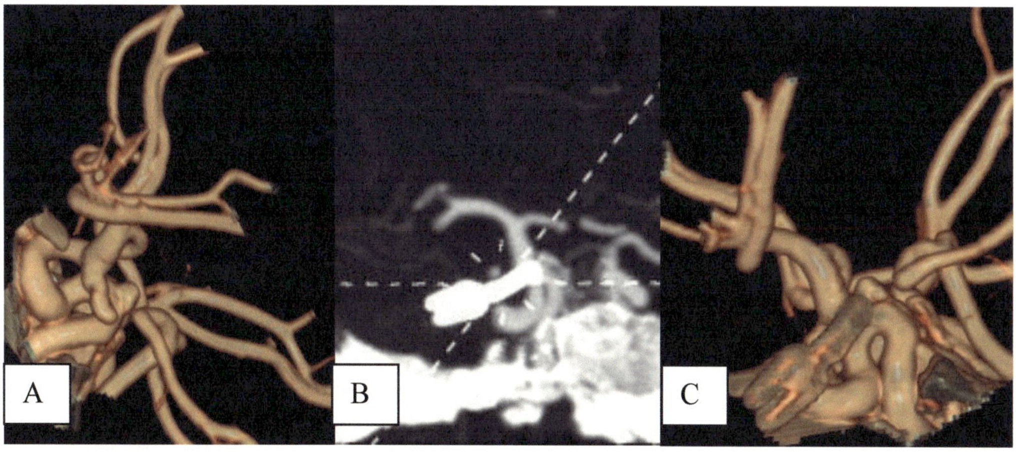


Fig. 3. Case 3: A: Preoperative CTA showed a saccular aneurysm on posterior communicating artery B and C: CTA MIP and VR images demonstrated the complete occlusion of the aneurysm .

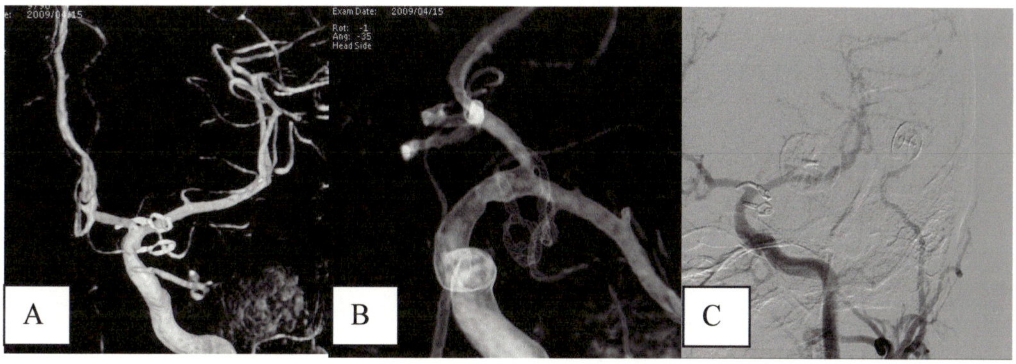


Fig. 4. Case 4: A and B: 3D-DSA was performed 7 days after surgical clipping completely C: The remnant of aneurysms were not visible on the 2D-DSA.

## 13. Acknowledgments

Funding for this chapter was from: Ministry of Health, China (20102-016); Department of Health, Zhejiang Province science funding (2008A142); Bureau of Science and Technology, Wenzhou (Y20090005).

## 14. References

[1] Bederson JB, Connolly ES, Jr., Batjer HH, Dacey RG, Dion JE, Diringer MN, Duldner JE, Jr., Harbaugh RE, Patel AB, Rosenwasser RH: Guidelines for the management of aneurysmal subarachnoid hemorrhage: a statement for healthcare professionals from a special writing group of the Stroke Council, American Heart Association. *Stroke; a journal of cerebral circulation* 2009, 40(3):994-1025.

[2] Brisman JL, Song JK, Newell DW: Cerebral aneurysms. *The New England journal of medicine* 2006, 355(9):928-939.

[3] Ingall T, Asplund K, Mahonen M, Bonita R: A multinational comparison of subarachnoid hemorrhage epidemiology in the WHO MONICA stroke study. *Stroke; a journal of cerebral circulation* 2000, 31(5):1054-1061.

[4] van Gijn J, Rinkel GJ: Subarachnoid haemorrhage: diagnosis, causes and management. *Brain* 2001, 124(Pt 2):249-278.

[5] Al-Shahi R, White PM, Davenport RJ, Lindsay KW: Subarachnoid haemorrhage. *BMJ (Clinical research ed* 2006, 333(7561):235-240.

[6] Molyneux A, Kerr R, Stratton I, Sandercock P, Clarke M, Shrimpton J, Holman R: International Subarachnoid Aneurysm Trial (ISAT) of neurosurgical clipping versus endovascular coiling in 2143 patients with ruptured intracranial aneurysms: a randomised trial. *Lancet* 2002, 360(9342):1267-1274.

[7] Molyneux AJ, Kerr RS, Yu LM, Clarke M, Sneade M, Yarnold JA, Sandercock P: International subarachnoid aneurysm trial (ISAT) of neurosurgical clipping versus endovascular coiling in 2143 patients with ruptured intracranial aneurysms: a randomised comparison of effects on survival, dependency, seizures, rebleeding, subgroups, and aneurysm occlusion. *Lancet* 2005, 366(9488):809-817.

[8] Colby GP, Coon AL, Tamargo RJ: Surgical management of aneurysmal subarachnoid hemorrhage. *Neurosurgery clinics of North America*, 21(2):247-261.

[9] Molyneux AJ, Kerr RS, Birks J, Ramzi N, Yarnold J, Sneade M, Rischmiller J: Risk of recurrent subarachnoid haemorrhage, death, or dependence and standardised mortality ratios after clipping or coiling of an intracranial aneurysm in the International Subarachnoid Aneurysm Trial (ISAT): long-term follow-up. *Lancet neurology* 2009, 8(5):427-433.

[10] Butler WE, Barker FG, 2nd, Crowell RM: Patients with polycystic kidney disease would benefit from routine magnetic resonance angiographic screening for intracerebral aneurysms: a decision analysis. *Neurosurgery* 1996, 38(3):506-515; discussion 515-506.

[11] Kojima M, Nagasawa S, Lee YE, Takeichi Y, Tsuda E, Mabuchi N: Asymptomatic familial cerebral aneurysms. *Neurosurgery* 1998, 43(4):776-781.

[12] Kissela BM, Sauerbeck L, Woo D, Khoury J, Carrozzella J, Pancioli A, Jauch E, Moomaw CJ, Shukla R, Gebel J *et al*: Subarachnoid hemorrhage: a preventable disease with a heritable component. *Stroke; a journal of cerebral circulation* 2002, 33(5):1321-1326.

[13] Wermer MJ, van der Schaaf IC, Algra A, Rinkel GJ: Risk of rupture of unruptured intracranial aneurysms in relation to patient and aneurysm characteristics: an updated meta-analysis. *Stroke; a journal of cerebral circulation* 2007, 38(4):1404-1410.

[14] Tulamo R, Frosen J, Laaksamo E, Niemela M, Laakso A, Hernesniemi J: [Why does the cerebral artery aneurysm rupture?]. *Duodecim; laaketieteellinen aikakauskirja*, 127(3):244-252.

[15] Hunt WE, Hess RM: Surgical risk as related to time of intervention in the repair of intracranial aneurysms. *Journal of neurosurgery* 1968, 28(1):14-20.

[16] Report of World Federation of Neurological Surgeons Committee on a Universal Subarachnoid Hemorrhage Grading Scale. *Journal of neurosurgery* 1988, 68(6):985-986.

[17] Claassen J, Bernardini GL, Kreiter K, Bates J, Du YE, Copeland D, Connolly ES, Mayer SA: Effect of cisternal and ventricular blood on risk of delayed cerebral ischemia

after subarachnoid hemorrhage: the Fisher scale revisited. *Stroke; a journal of cerebral circulation* 2001, 32(9):2012-2020.

[18] Hacein-Bey L, Connolly ES, Jr., Mayer SA, Young WL, Pile-Spellman J, Solomon RA: Complex intracranial aneurysms: combined operative and endovascular approaches. *Neurosurgery* 1998, 43(6):1304-1312; discussion 1312-1303.

[19] Hoh BL, Putman CM, Budzik RF, Carter BS, Ogilvy CS: Combined surgical and endovascular techniques of flow alteration to treat fusiform and complex wide-necked intracranial aneurysms that are unsuitable for clipping or coil embolization. *Journal of neurosurgery* 2001, 95(1):24-35.

[20] Kremer C, Groden C, Hansen HC, Grzyska U, Zeumer H: Outcome after endovascular treatment of Hunt and Hess grade IV or V aneurysms: comparison of anterior versus posterior circulation. *Stroke; a journal of cerebral circulation* 1999, 30(12):2617-2622.

[21] Li MH, Li YD, Tan HQ, Gu BX, Chen YC, Wang W, Chen SW, Hu DJ: Contrast-free MRA at 3.0 T for the detection of intracranial aneurysms. *Neurology*.

[22] Hacein-Bey L, Provenzale JM: Current imaging assessment and treatment of intracranial aneurysms. *Ajr*, 196(1):32-44.

[23] Roth C: [Value of CT and MR angiography for diagnostics of intracranial aneurysms]. *Der Radiologe*, 51(2):106-112.

[24] Okahara M, Kiyosue H, Yamashita M, Nagatomi H, Hata H, Saginoya T, Sagara Y, Mori H: Diagnostic accuracy of magnetic resonance angiography for cerebral aneurysms in correlation with 3D-digital subtraction angiographic images: a study of 133 aneurysms. *Stroke; a journal of cerebral circulation* 2002, 33(7):1803-1808.

[25] Tan XX, Zhong M, Zheng K, Zhao B: Computed tomography angiography based emergency microsurgery for massive intracranial hematoma arising from arteriovenous malformations. *Neurology India*, 59(2):199-203.

[26] Velthuis BK, Rinkel GJ, Ramos LM, Witkamp TD, Berkelbach van der Sprenkel JW, Vandertop WP, van Leeuwen MS: Subarachnoid hemorrhage: aneurysm detection and preoperative evaluation with CT angiography. *Radiology* 1998, 208(2):423-430.

[27] Chen CY, Hsieh SC, Choi WM, Chiang PY, Chien JC, Chan WP: Computed tomography angiography in detection and characterization of ruptured anterior cerebral artery aneurysms at uncommon location for emergent surgical clipping. *Clinical imaging* 2006, 30(2):87-93.

[28] Westerlaan HE, van Dijk MJ, Jansen-van der Weide MC, de Groot JC, Groen RJ, Mooij JJ, Oudkerk M: Intracranial aneurysms in patients with subarachnoid hemorrhage: CT angiography as a primary examination tool for diagnosis--systematic review and meta-analysis. *Radiology*, 258(1):134-145.

[29] Velthuis BK, Van Leeuwen MS, Witkamp TD, Ramos LM, Berkelbach van Der Sprenkel JW, Rinkel GJ: Computerized tomography angiography in patients with subarachnoid hemorrhage: from aneurysm detection to treatment without conventional angiography. *Journal of neurosurgery* 1999, 91(5):761-767.

[30] Anxionnat R, Bracard S, Ducrocq X, Trousset Y, Launay L, Kerrien E, Braun M, Vaillant R, Scomazzoni F, Lebedinsky A *et al*: Intracranial aneurysms: clinical value of 3D digital subtraction angiography in the therapeutic decision and endovascular treatment. *Radiology* 2001, 218(3):799-808.

[31] Dyste GN BD: De novo aneurysm formation following carotid ligation: case report and review of the literature. *Neurosurgery* 1989, 24(1):88-92.

[32] Zhao Bing ZM, TAN Xian-xi, ZHENG Kuang, LI Jiang,ZHAO Jian-ting, CHENG Wei Surgical management of high-grade aneurysmal subarachnoid hemorrhage. *Chinese Journal of Cenebrovascular Diseases* 2010, 7(8):406－410.

[33] van Lindert E, Perneczky A, Fries G, Pierangeli E: The supraorbital keyhole approach to supratentorial aneurysms: concept and technique. *Surgical neurology* 1998, 49(5):481-489; discussion 489-490.

[34] Ramos-Zuniga R, Velazquez H, Barajas MA, Lopez R, Sanchez E, Trejo S: Trans-supraorbital approach to supratentorial aneurysms. *Neurosurgery* 2002, 51(1):125-130; discussion 130-121.

[35] Reisch R, Perneczky A, Filippi R: Surgical technique of the supraorbital key-hole craniotomy. *Surgical neurology* 2003, 59(3):223-227.

[36] Paladino J, Mrak G, Miklic P, Jednacak H, Mihaljevic D: The keyhole concept in aneurysm surgery--a comparative study: keyhole versus standard craniotomy. *Minim Invasive Neurosurg* 2005, 48(5):251-258.

[37] Lan Q, Chen J, Qian ZY, Zhang QB, Huang Q: [Microsurgical treatment of complex intracranial aneurysms via keyhole approaches]. *Zhonghua yi xue za zhi* 2007, 87(13):872-876.

[38] Perneczky A, Fries G: Endoscope-assisted brain surgery: part 1--evolution, basic concept, and current technique. *Neurosurgery* 1998, 42(2):219-224; discussion 224-215.

[39] Profeta G, De Falco R, Ambrosio G, Profeta L: Endoscope-assisted microneurosurgery for anterior circulation aneurysms using the angle-type rigid endoscope over a 3-year period. *Childs Nerv Syst* 2004, 20(11-12):811-815.

[40] Taniguchi M, Takimoto H, Yoshimine T, Shimada N, Miyao Y, Hirata M, Maruno M, Kato A, Kohmura E, Hayakawa T: Application of a rigid endoscope to the microsurgical management of 54 cerebral aneurysms: results in 48 patients. *Journal of neurosurgery* 1999, 91(2):231-237.

[41] Kalavakonda C, Sekhar LN, Ramachandran P, Hechl P: Endoscope-assisted microsurgery for intracranial aneurysms. *Neurosurgery* 2002, 51(5):1119-1126; discussion 1126-1117.

[42] Figueiredo EG, Foroni L, Monaco BA, Gomes MQ, Sterman Neto H, Teixeira MJ: The clip-wrap technique in the treatment of intracranial unclippable aneurysms. *Arquivos de neuro-psiquiatria*, 68(1):115-118.

[43] Solomon RA, Smith CR, Raps EC, Young WL, Stone JG, Fink ME: Deep hypothermic circulatory arrest for the management of complex anterior and posterior circulation aneurysms. *Neurosurgery* 1991, 29(5):732-737; discussion 737-738.

[44] Bailes JE, Tantuwaya LS, Fukushima T, Schurman GW, Davis D: Intraoperative microvascular Doppler sonography in aneurysm surgery. *Neurosurgery* 1997, 40(5):965-970; discussion 970-962.

[45] Cui H, Wang Y, Yin Y, Wan J, Fei Z, Gao W, Jiang J: Role of intraoperative microvascular Doppler in the microsurgical management of intracranial aneurysms. *J Clin Ultrasound*, 39(1):27-31.

[46] Raabe A, Nakaji P, Beck J, Kim LJ, Hsu FP, Kamerman JD, Seifert V, Spetzler RF: Prospective evaluation of surgical microscope-integrated intraoperative near-

infrared indocyanine green videoangiography during aneurysm surgery. *Journal of neurosurgery* 2005, 103(6):982-989.

[47] Nanda A, Willis BK, Vannemreddy PS: Selective intraoperative angiography in intracranial aneurysm surgery: intraoperative factors associated with aneurysmal remnants and vessel occlusions. *Surgical neurology* 2002, 58(5):309-314; discussion 314-305.

[48] Gruber A, Dorfer C, Standhardt H, Bavinzski G, Knosp E: Prospective comparison of intraoperative vascular monitoring technologies during cerebral aneurysm surgery. *Neurosurgery*, 68(3):657-673; discussion 673.

[49] Cerejo A, Silva PA, Dias C, Vaz R: Monitoring of brain oxygenation in surgery of ruptured middle cerebral artery aneurysms. *Surgical neurology international*, 2:70.

[50] Kassell NF, Torner JC: Aneurysmal rebleeding: a preliminary report from the Cooperative Aneurysm Study. *Neurosurgery* 1983, 13(5):479-481.

[51] Ohkuma H, Tsurutani H, Suzuki S: Incidence and significance of early aneurysmal rebleeding before neurosurgical or neurological management. *Stroke; a journal of cerebral circulation* 2001, 32(5):1176-1180.

[52] Laidlaw JD, Siu KH: Poor-grade aneurysmal subarachnoid hemorrhage: outcome after treatment with urgent surgery. *Neurosurgery* 2003, 53(6):1275-1280; discussion 1280-1272.

[53] Naidech AM, Janjua N, Kreiter KT, Ostapkovich ND, Fitzsimmons BF, Parra A, Commichau C, Connolly ES, Mayer SA: Predictors and impact of aneurysm rebleeding after subarachnoid hemorrhage. *Archives of neurology* 2005, 62(3):410-416.

[54] Rates of delayed rebleeding from intracranial aneurysms are low after surgical and endovascular treatment. *Stroke; a journal of cerebral circulation* 2006, 37(6):1437-1442.

[55] David CA, Vishteh AG, Spetzler RF, Lemole M, Lawton MT, Partovi S: Late angiographic follow-up review of surgically treated aneurysms. *Journal of neurosurgery* 1999, 91(3):396-401.

[56] Sloan MA, Alexandrov AV, Tegeler CH, Spencer MP, Caplan LR, Feldmann E, Wechsler LR, Newell DW, Gomez CR, Babikian VL *et al*: Assessment: transcranial Doppler ultrasonography: report of the Therapeutics and Technology Assessment Subcommittee of the American Academy of Neurology. *Neurology* 2004, 62(9):1468-1481.

[57] Suarez JI, Qureshi AI, Yahia AB, Parekh PD, Tamargo RJ, Williams MA, Ulatowski JA, Hanley DF, Razumovsky AY: Symptomatic vasospasm diagnosis after subarachnoid hemorrhage: evaluation of transcranial Doppler ultrasound and cerebral angiography as related to compromised vascular distribution. *Critical care medicine* 2002, 30(6):1348-1355.

[58] Egge A, Waterloo K, Sjoholm H, Solberg T, Ingebrigtsen T, Romner B: Prophylactic hyperdynamic postoperative fluid therapy after aneurysmal subarachnoid hemorrhage: a clinical, prospective, randomized, controlled study. *Neurosurgery* 2001, 49(3):593-605; discussion 605-596.

[59] Lennihan L, Mayer SA, Fink ME, Beckford A, Paik MC, Zhang H, Wu YC, Klebanoff LM, Raps EC, Solomon RA: Effect of hypervolemic therapy on cerebral blood flow after subarachnoid hemorrhage : a randomized controlled trial. *Stroke; a journal of cerebral circulation* 2000, 31(2):383-391.

[60] Keyrouz SG, Diringer MN: Clinical review: Prevention and therapy of vasospasm in subarachnoid hemorrhage. *Critical care (London, England)* 2007, 11(4):220.

[61] Jestaedt L, Pham M, Bartsch AJ, Kunze E, Roosen K, Solymosi L, Bendszus M: The impact of balloon angioplasty on the evolution of vasospasm-related infarction after aneurysmal subarachnoid hemorrhage. *Neurosurgery* 2008, 62(3):610-617; discussion 610-617.

[62] Diringer MN: Management of aneurysmal subarachnoid hemorrhage. *Critical care medicine* 2009, 37(2):432-440.

[63] Cross DT, 3rd, Moran CJ, Angtuaco EE, Milburn JM, Diringer MN, Dacey RG, Jr.: Intracranial pressure monitoring during intraarterial papaverine infusion for cerebral vasospasm. *Ajnr* 1998, 19(7):1319-1323.

[64] Clouston JE, Numaguchi Y, Zoarski GH, Aldrich EF, Simard JM, Zitnay KM: Intraarterial papaverine infusion for cerebral vasospasm after subarachnoid hemorrhage. *Ajnr* 1995, 16(1):27-38.

[65] Macdonald RL, Wallace MC, Kestle JR: Role of angiography following aneurysm surgery. *Journal of neurosurgery* 1993, 79(6):826-832.

[66] el-Beltagy M, Muroi C, Roth P, Fandino J, Imhof HG, Yonekawa Y: Recurrent intracranial aneurysms after successful neck clipping. *World neurosurgery*, 74(4-5):472-477.

[67] ZHAOBing YH, LIU Jian,ZHONG Ming,TAN Xiang-xin,ZHANG Ming-sheng Value of three-dimensional CT angiography in postoperative evaluation of intracranial aneurysm clipping. *Chinese Jounal of Neuromedicine* 2009, 8(2):157-160.

[68] Zachenhofer I, Cejna M, Schuster A, Donat M, Roessler K: Image quality and artefact generation post-cerebral aneurysm clipping using a 64-row multislice computer tomography angiography (MSCTA) technology: A retrospective study and review of the literature. *Clinical neurology and neurosurgery*, 112(5):386-391.

[69] Kang HS, Han MH, Kwon BJ, Jung SI, Oh CW, Han DH, Chang KH: Postoperative 3D angiography in intracranial aneurysms. *Ajnr* 2004, 25(9):1463-1469.

[70] Ahn SS, Kim YD: Three-dimensional digital subtraction angiographic evaluation of aneurysm remnants after clip placement. *Journal of Korean Neurosurgical Society*, 47(3):185-190.

[71] Broderick JP, Brott TG, Duldner JE, Tomsick T, Leach A: Initial and recurrent bleeding are the major causes of death following subarachnoid hemorrhage. *Stroke; a journal of cerebral circulation* 1994, 25(7):1342-1347.

11

# Surgical Management of Posterior Circulation Aneurysms: Defining the Role of Microsurgery in Contemporary Endovascular Era

Leon Lai* and Michael Kerin Morgan
*The Australian School of Advanced Medicine, Macquarie University, Sydney, Australia*

## 1. Introduction

In the period between 1930 and 1960, surgical treatment of posterior circulation aneurysms were only possible by indirect trapping or parent vessel ligation. Olivecrona was said to have performed the first unplanned trapping of a posterior inferior cerebellar artery (PICA) aneurysm in 1932. In 1937, Tonnis inadvertently opened a cerebellopontine angle aneurysm having assumed that it was a tumour preoperatively[1]. Dandy performed the first vertebral artery ligation beneath the atlas to treat a vertebral aneurysm in 1944 [2]. In 1948, Schwartz[3] reported his experience with direct surgical approach to a large basilar artery aneurysm and successfully trapped it using silver clips. Logue[4] and Mount[5] formally described the techniques of vertebral artery and basilar artery ligation in 1958 and 1962, respectively.

By the 1960s, neurosurgeons were attempting direct surgical clipping of vertebrobasilar aneurysms. Early attempts, however, were not met with great success. Dr Charles Drake from Canada published his initial experience with direct surgical clipping of four ruptured basilar bifurcation aneurysms in 1961[6]. Although two of his patients died postoperatively, the two survivors made dramatic functional recoveries. He concluded that 'direct surgical attack was feasible and worthwhile under exceptional circumstances, when life was threatened by repeated haemorrhages'. Dr Ken Jamieson from Australia reported 19 surgical cases in 1964, 10 of whom had died and 5 were left with severe morbidity[7]. He commented 'it is clear that the basilar bifurcation is no place for the faint of heart. Only time and greater experience will indicate whether it is a place for neurosurgeons at all.'

The introduction of the surgical microscope to neurosurgery in the late 1960s and their propagation in the 1970s, 1980s and through to the 1990s greatly influenced the results of aneurysm surgery. Perhaps the greatest impact of the operating microscope was not just in enhancing the results of experienced aneurysm surgeons, but in accelerating the learning curve of young neurosurgeons that enabled them to master microsurgical skills and achieved competitive results within a shorter period of time. Worldwide reported surgical mortality rates for posterior circulation aneurysms have dropped from 34.4% in the 1960s to

---

* Correspondig Author

7.5% (1970s), 5.6% (1980s), 6.0% (1990s) and 5.0% in the new millennium. Surgical morbidity averaged between 9.8% and 12.8% throughout this time period.

The invention by Guglielmi[8] in the early 1990s to treat intracranial aneurysms by detachable platinum coils once again revolutionised the practice of cerebrovascular neurosurgery. This change was most dramatic and rapid for aneurysms located in the posterior circulation where surgical approaches continued to impose significant morbidities to the patients. By the end of 1990s, endovascular treatments of posterior circulation aneurysms were already well established in many centres across the United States[9,10,11,12] and Europe[13,14]. The International Subarachnoid Aneurysm Trial (ISAT)[15], which compared endovascular coiling to microsurgical clipping, included only 58 patients (2.7%) with posterior circulation aneurysms from their cohort of 2143 because most authors by that stage did not perceived clinical equipoise between the two treatment modalities for aneurysms in this location. Endovascular procedures were regarded as the new promises for treatment of posterior circulation aneurysms.

Two decades on, we learnt that the effectiveness of endovascular treatment, measured by its durability, is a major technical limitation. Complete obliteration is frequently not achieved. Overall, recurrent filling is seen in 15% of aneurysms on angiograms obtained at 6 months after treatment. Longer term follow up in most series suggest complete obliteration rate is possible in just over 50% of coiled posterior circulation aneurysms. This carries significant implications on retreatments, monitoring and risk of rebleeding for many patients.

Until endovascular techniques evolve to a point where recurrence and rebleeding rates are within acceptable limits, surgery remains a viable and competitive treatment option for aneurysms of the vertebrobasilar system. The challenge for contemporary vascular neurosurgeons is to understand the differing but complementary role each treatment modality currently has to offer, and to maintain the proficiency and technical skills to deal with an emergence of complex and recurrence of previously coiled aneurysms.

## 2. The role of endovascular coiling for posterior circulation aneurysms

Endovascular therapy has changed the way we practice cerebrovascular neurosurgery. In the past, endovascular techniques were used to occlude aneurysms when there is 'anticipated surgical difficulty', 'failed clipping', 'patient or physician preference', and 'poor medical condition'. Today, the reverse appears to be true. Endovascular therapy has largely replaced microsurgery as the firstline treatment modality for aneurysms located in the posterior circulation. In many neurosurgical centres in recent years, this trend is even more evident for unruptured posterior circulation aneurysms.

The essential characteristic and therapeutic goal of the endovascular procedure is to induce thrombosis within the aneurysm by the deployment of platinum microcoils. From a neurointerventional perspective, the key determinant for success is aneurysmal morphology, not so much location. Small aneurysms with small necks and those at a right angle to blood flow are considered appropriate for endovascular procedures. Because of the complexity or the infrequency (therefore negative impact upon confidence of competence) of surgical access to the posterior circulation, endovascular repair has gained dominant mode of treatment in this location. Other important factors to consider whether to treat or not and which mode of treatment to employ include the patient's clinical status and the available institutional expertise. Elderly patients, or those in poor clinical grade post subarachnoid haemorrhages, may be better treated using endovascular techniques irrespective of aneurysm morphology.

Although good data is available regarding endovascular repair by means of coiling, many aneurysms are now repaired with more complex techniques including additional stents, bioactive coils, balloon re-modelling, and the addition of ethylene-vinyl alcohol copolymer and flow diversion stents. Each of these techniques offers promise to deal with problems that the simple coiling procedure was found wanting. However, with complexity comes complications, and their risks and expectations of treatment await further experience and analysis.

Not all aneurysms are amenable to endovascular treatment. For large or wide-necked aneurysms, or where the dome-to-neck ratio is less than 2, coiling is less effective. In this situation, aneurysm neck and parent vessel may be best reconstructed by microsurgical techniques. Other factors that may limit successful endovascular aneurysm occlusion include inadequate endovascular access or the presence of unstable intraluminal thrombus. When an arterial branch is incorporated in the neck of an aneurysm, as in the case of many basilar bifurcation lesions, effective endovascular treatment can be difficult.

Observational studies suggest that endovascular occlusion of ruptured aneurysms is comparable to that of conventional microsurgery in the short term and can prevent early rebleeding. These studies suggest that endovascular techniques provide protection against rebleeding in the first few months, when rebleeding occurs most frequently. A review of the literature on endovascular treatment outcomes for both ruptured and unruptured posterior circulation aneurysms is demonstrated in Table 1.

In summary, around 70 to 91% of patients with posterior circulation aneurysms achieve independence (mean 85%) if treated by endovascular techniques. The overall morbidity is 4.4% (range 0 to 9.6%) and mortality is 9.1% (range 0 to 18.2). The risk of post coiling haemorrhage is 1.5% out of the 961 reported cases between 1990 to 2005 (Table 1).

The rate of complete occlusions is 52.1% (compared to >90% in most surgical series)[16 17]. The degree of initial occlusion has important ramifications on retreatments, monitoring, and risks of rehemorrhages. Long-term results of the ISAT suggested that rebleeding rate is 3 times more likely in patients who have recurrent aneurysms from incomplete coiling than patients with completely treated aneurysms. Of those patients that experienced rebleeds, mortality rate was up to 70%[18]. It is therefore prudent that younger patients with unruptured posterior circulation aneurysms be recommended for surgical management where long-term durability by this technique is an advantage.

## 3. The role of microsurgery for posterior circulation aneurysms

According to the International Study of Unruptured Intracranial Aneurysms (ISUIA), unruptured posterior circulation aneurysms, particularly at the basilar bifurcation, carry a more aggressive risk of rupture than that of similarly sized lesion located in the anterior circulation[19]. Over a five-year period, aneurysms over 6mm diameter bear a cumulative risk of rupture of at least 15%. This compares to 2.6% for those in the anterior circulation.

Therefore, Younger patients (age <50 years) with unruptured posterior circulation aneurysms should be treated, given the accumulated risk of rupture during a period of many years. Although endovascular treatment options must be considered in all cases, higher partial obliteration rates and recurrence rates make microsurgical obliteration more favourable in relatively young patients without extenuating medical circumstances.

| Author/Year | Study Period | No. of patients | % SAH | Mean follow up (months) | % Complete occlusion | Post GDC haemorrhage | Independent (%) | Morbidity (%) | Mortality (%) |
|---|---|---|---|---|---|---|---|---|---|
| Guglielmi 1992[20] | 1990-1991 | 43 | 56 | 2 | 40 | 1/43 | 83 | 4.8 | 7 |
| McDougall 1996[21] | 1991-1995 | 33 | 70 | 15 | 21 | 1/33 | NA | 3 | 12.1 |
| Pierot 1996[22] | 1993-1994 | 35 | 91 | 4.8 | 73 | 0/35 | 91 | 0 | 8.8 |
| Klein 1997[23] | 1993-1996 | 21 | 76 | 9.8 | 67 | 0/21 | 91 | 4.8 | 4.8 |
| Nichols 1997[24] | 1992-1995 | 28 | 100 | 6 | 61 | 0/28 | 80 | 0 | 15.4 |
| Raymond 1997[25] | 1992-1995 | 31 | 74 | 15.5 | 42 | 0/31 | 87 | 3.2 | 6.5 |
| Vinuela 1997[26] | 1990-1995 | 403 | 100 | NA | NA | NA | 84.3 | 9.6 | 6.1 |
| Eskridge 1998[27] | 1991-1995 | 150 | 49 | 12 | 75* | 4/150 | 78 | 6.7 | 18.2 |
| Bavinzski 1999[28] | 1992-1998 | 45 | 75 | 27.4 | 54 | 1/45 | 73 | 4.4 | 15.5 |
| Gruber 1999[29] | 1993-1996 | 21 | 52 | 26 | 14 | 0/21 | 90 | 9.5 | 0 |
| Steiger 1999[30] | 1990-1998 | 16 | 69 | 6 | 69 | 0/16 | 88 | 6.3 | 6.3 |
| Lempart 2000[31] | 1991-1998 | 112 | 100 | 13.1 | 54 | 1/112 | 83 | 2.8 | 15 |
| Tateshima 2000[32] | 1990-1999 | 75 | 58 | 31.3 | 45 | 1/75 | 86 | 4.1 | 8.4 |
| Birchall 2001[33] | 1992-1998 | 35 | 46 | 42.7 | 46 | 1/35 | 86 | 3.4 | 8.6 |
| Uda 2001[34] | 1990-1999 | 41 | 69 | 21 | 32 | 1/41 | 90 | 2.6 | 7.7 |
| Pandey 2007[35] | 1995-2005 | 275 | 61.5 | 31.8 | 87.8** | 3/275 | 87.4 | 5.1 | 4.9 |
| | *Summary* | *1364* | *71.7* | *17.6* | *52.1* | *1.5 (14/961)* | *85.2* | *4.4* | *9.1* |

*% complete occlusion defined as >90% by source author; **% complete occlusion defined as >95% by source author

Table 1. Endovascular treatment outcomes of posterior circulation aneurysms: analysis of published series.

Unlike endovascular treatment that depends on aneurysmal morphology, microsurgical success relies critically on

1. The specific aneurysmal location along the vertebrobasilar system.
2. Aneurysm size and patient's age

**Location**

Location determines surgical approaches, which largely affects the outcomes. In general, surgical approaches to posterior circulation aneurysms are difficult because:

1. Surgical exposure is deep. This translates into long surgical corridor with narrow confines, thus limiting manoeuvrability and the proficiency to which a clip can be optimally placed on the aneurysm. The ability to attain good proximal and distal control may be restricted, further increasing the operative risk in the presence of subarachnoid haemorrhage.
2. The margin of error is small. The close proximity of posterior circulation aneurysms to the brainstem with interposing cranial nerves and perforator arteries makes the anatomy around this region complex and unforgiving.
3. The infrequency of these lesions. Posterior circulation aneurysms account for approximately 10 to 15% of all intracranial aneurysms, thereby giving few surgeons the opportunity to gain the necessary experience to manage them well. The emergence of endovascular therapy in the last 20 years further reduces the number of posterior circulation aneurysms available for surgical repair.

**Size and patient's age**

Raaymakers et al[36], in a meta-analysis of case series published between 1966 and 1996 found that the morbidity and mortality of surgery for non-giant unruptured posterior circulation aneurysms was 12.9% and 3.0% respectively. They found that age; aneurysm size and location of the aneurysms (anterior versus posterior) were factors that predicted a greater chance of a favourable outcome. In ISUIA II, patients' age was an important factor in overall surgical outcome. Other predictors of poor outcome included large aneurysmal size, history of ischaemic cerebrovascular disease, and presence of aneurysmal symptoms other than rupture. In Ogilvy and Carter's logistic regression model[37], posterior circulation, size of aneurysm and age of the patient were associated with poor outcome. Eftekhar et al[38] reminded us of the overall low risk associated with surgical clipping at dedicated cerebrovascular centres, when treating patients with small unruptured posterior circulation aneurysms. In their surgical treatment of 136 unruptured vertebrobasilar aneurysms in 120 patients, the combined surgical mortality and morbidity for aneurysms <9mm in size was 3.2%. They emphasized that younger age patients and smaller sized aneurysms were favourable surgical predictive factors. This view is well supported by the works at other dedicated cerebrovascular centres[39].

In general, aneurysms that are most suitable to surgical clipping are:

1. Superior cerebellar artery (SCA) aneurysms
2. P1 Posterior cerebral artery (PCA) aneurysms
3. Distal anterior inferior cerebellar artery (AICA) aneurysms
4. PICA aneurysms

Aneurysms that are difficult to approach microsurgically are:

1. P2 Posterior cerebral artery aneurysms
2. Basilar trunk
3. Proximal AICA
4. Vertebral-basilar junctions

## 4. Preoperative consideration

A wide variety of operative approaches exist and the surgeon must select the most appropriate for the aneurysm location, size and projection. A number of critical factors must be considered prior to making the decision to operate.

1. *Imaging*: An angiogram combined with bone imaging reveals important anatomical features, of value not just in determining the optimal approach but also in indicating the operative risks. Note the
    a. Height of the aneurysm neck in relation to the posterior clinoids or clivus
    b. Size and direction of the aneurysm fundus.
    c. Any associated crucial perforator anatomy
    d. Any co-existent anterior circulation aneurysms that may alter the side of intended approach
2. *Neuro-anesthesia and cerebral protection*: Mild hypothermia and barbiturate-induced electroencephalographic burst suppression are necessary for complex basilar bifurcation and trunk aneurysms. Both techniques are essential when considering using temporary clipping as an adjunct to final aneurysm dissection and permanent clipping. It is important that these are thoroughly communicated with the anaesthetists and the rest of the neurosurgical team throughout the case.
3. *Side of approach:* In general, access to the parent artery immediately prior to the aneurysm dictates the side. For midline locations, a right-sided approach is preferable if either side provides equal access to the parent artery. Other factors may be taken into consideration but only if access to the parent artery is ensured. These factors include:
    a. Coexistent left-sided anterior circulation aneurysm.
    b. Hearing loss where a medial petrosectomy is required.
4. *Types of approach:* In considering the approach, it is important to keep in mind the principles underlying most cranial base surgical strategies including
    a. Shortest trajectory to the lesion
    b. Bone removal rather than brain retraction
    c. Maximization of extradural exposure
    d. Skeletonization/decompression of cranial nerves and vascular structures
    e. Reconstitution of all dural openings.

From an anatomical perspective, it is useful to subdivide the vertebrobasilar arterial system into 3 compartments (Table 2).

1. *Upper vertebrobasilar*: incorporating basilar bifurcation, posterior cerebral artery (PCA) and superior cerebellar artery (SCA).
2. *Middle vertebrobasilar*: incorporating low-lying basilar bifurcation, basilar trunk, proximal Anterior Inferior Cerebellar Artery (AICA), and vertebra-basilar junction (VBJ).

3. *Lower vertebrobasilar*: incorporating vertebral and PICA arteries aneurysms.

The selection of a particular approach depends on a number of important factors

1. Location of aneurysm along the vertebrobasilar system
2. Size and projection of fundus of aneurysm
3. Surgeon's familiarity with specific approaches

| Compartments | Aneurysms | Surgical corridor | Approach Options |
|---|---|---|---|
| Upper vertebrobasilar | Basilar bifurcation<br>Posterior cerebral artery<br>Superior cerebellar artery<br>Upper basilar trunk | Anterolateral | Pterional approach<br>Orbitozygomatic approach<br>Subtemporal approach |
| Middle vertebrobasilar | Midbasilar trunk<br>Anterior inferior cerebellar artery | Lateral | Transpetrosal approach<br>Combined supra- and infratentorial approach<br>Extended middle fossa approach<br>Transoral approach |
| Lower vertebrobasilar | Vertebrobasilar junction<br>Vertebral artery<br>Posterior inferior cerebellar artery | Posterolaterally | Far-lateral approach<br>Extended far-lateral approach<br>Midline suboccipital approach |

Table 2. Surgical approaches to posterior circulation aneurysms

## 5. Skull base approaches for aneurysm occlusion

In vascular neurosurgery, exposure is extremely important. Only with adequate exposure can neurosurgeons directly visualize vascular anatomy, obtain proximal and distal control, apply meticulous microsurgical technique, and manoeuvre a clip to occlude an aneurysm successfully with a good outcome.

In the last 3 decades, skull base neurosurgeons have disassembled and reassembled the skull in every possible way with the intention to maximise exposure and minimise neurological injury. These techniques have been designed to reduce the distance between the surgeon and the aneurysm, increase surgical manoeuvrability, and reduce retraction on neighbouring neurovascular structures to improve safe aneurysm clipping. In this section, we described only a selected few approaches that are practised by the senior author (MKM) in approaches to aneurysms of the posterior circulation.

**Orbitozygomatic approach**

The *orbitozygomatic* (OBZ) approach dramatically enhances the standard pterional craniotomy. It allows exposure of, and access to, the medial end of the sphenoid wing and middle fossa floor, providing a much greater scope for manoeuvre in the vertical dimension than through conventional anterolateral techniques.

The "orbito" aspect involves removing the superior and lateral orbit, which opens up the roof of the operative corridor when the patient's head is rotated away from the aneurysm and extended. In addition, extending the zygomatic removal by removing the zygomatic arch is utilised when there is an advantage in creating a flat trajectory with the middle cranial fossa floor (e.g. for medial petrosectomy). A widened operative corridor improves illumination, eliminates the need for brain retraction, and optimises manoeuvrability. A good OBZ approach gives the neurosurgeon a wide sweep of surgical trajectories ranging from supraorbital to transsylvian to pretemporal to subtemporal. Surgical trajectory can then be tailored to the pathology at hand.

There are a number of important limitations to this technique, although the risks are low:

1. Cosmetic concerns including
    a. Temporalis atrophy
    b. Subtle orbital asymmetries that bother some patients
    c. Frontalis nerve injury,
    d. Pulsatile enophthalmos,
2. Orbital problems such as
    a. Orbital entrapment,
    b. Diplopia from extraocular muscle or nerve injury,
    c. Blindness
3. Infection: communication with the frontal or ethmoidal sinus may increase the risk of infection or cerebrospinal fluid leakage.

**Key steps in an orbitozygomatic approach**

1. Patient's head is placed in a 3-point fixation head frame in slight extension such that the malar process is upper most. An imaginary line, starting from the lateral canthus of the ipsilateral eye to the external occipital protuberance, should be positioned perpendicular to the floor. This will ensure the Sylvian fissure remains vertical, such that after wide splitting of the fissure, the frontal and temporal lobe fall away from the operative field.
2. A curvilinear incision is planned from just anterior to the ipsilateral tragus up to the superior temporal line. The incision then gently curves to terminate at the hairline superior to the contralateral midpupillary line. A small strip of hair is shaved with clippers along the course of the planned incision.
3. The skin is incised and haemostasis is obtained with Raney clips. The inferior limb of the incision is complete after the scalp is dissected from the temporalis fascia with a periosteal elevator.
4. The scalp flap is mobilised anteriorly and the temporalis fascia is exposed. The fascia is sharply incised and elevated separately in a subfascial dissection to protect the frontalis branch of the facial nerve running along the superficial surface of this fascial plane.
5. Dissection continues anteriorly to expose the orbital rim, malar eminence, and the zygomatic arch.
6. The temporalis muscle is raised separately, exposing the zygomatic root and pterion. The muscle flap is left attached to the cranium at its vascular pedicle in the infratemporal fossa.

7. The scalp flaps and temporalis muscle are retracted anteriorly and inferiorly using surgical hooks.
8. The periorbital is a delicate lining and can be carefully stripped from the undersurface of the orbit with a Mitchell dissector. Periorbita can be preserved by beginning the dissection where it is thickest inferolaterally near the inferior orbital fissure, by using side-to-side sweeps with a round-tipped dissector, and by advancing circumferentially along the orbital roof and the lateral wall. This dissection gradually deepens towards the orbital apex.
9. Two burrholes are placed over the temporal bone near the root of the zygoma and a pterional craniotomy is performed.
10. The OBZ unit consists of the orbital rim, orbital roof, lateral orbital wall, and zygomatic arch. Removal of the zygoma is optional. The OBZ unit can be removed with the cranial flap as one integrated piece, which provides a better cosmetic result than a two-piece technique, although more difficult.
11. Additional bone is removed around the orbital apex, resecting what remains of the orbital roof, lateral orbital wall, and medial sphenoid wing, back to superior orbital fissure.
12. The dura is then opened in a semicircular incision, and reflected anteriorly and inferiorly over the periorbita and temporalis and tacked to the over lying scalp. This way, the profile of the periorbital contents is flattened to enhance the exposure.

**Arachnoid dissection**

The Sylvian fissure is the gateway to aneurysms along the circle of Willis. Separating the frontal and temporal lobes with the fissure split is one of the most important skills a vascular neurosurgeon needs to master. It is important, when performing the Sylvian fissure split, to keep the following principles in mind:

1. No retraction should be used.
2. Superficial Sylvian veins are the guardians of the Sylvian fissure. Knowing which way to dissect beyond the veins is an important skill. In general, superficial Sylvian veins course inferiorly and bridge to the sphenoparietal sinus under the sphenoid ridge. Dissection, therefore, should be along the frontal side to preserve these connections. However, it is important to maintain the venous connections of the larger veins in the region of the frontal operculum to minimise the risk of venous infarction in this region.
3. Cortical and deep arachnoid dissection must always be sharp, precise and controlled, using only the inverted tip of a No. 11 scalpel blade. Blunt dissection places stress on arachnoid-bound structures and increases the risk of complications from bleeding and neural injuries.
4. The Sylvian fissure is entered from distal to medial, and from deep to superficial along the direction of the middle cerebral artery branches.
5. All cisterns must be opened maximally to allow CSF egression and optimise brain relaxation. This manoeuvre eliminates the need for fix brain retraction. The Sylvian cistern is entered first, followed by the opticocarotid and the chiasmal cisterns. Fenestration of the lamina terminalis is encouraged to allow more CSF drainage from the third ventricle in cases where CSF outflow obstruction due to haemorrhage may be present. This further enhances brain relaxation.
6. The deep Sylvian cistern is opened and the carotico-oculomotor triangle is dissected.

7. Arachnoid adhesions to the oculomotor nerve lying along the edge of the tentorium are dissected as the temporal lobe is retracted gently. The course of the posterior communicating artery is then visible as it pierces the membrane of Liliequist. Incising the attachment of the tentorium at the posterior clinoid process is usually not of help in further facilitating exposure of the distal basilar complex. In the senior author's experience, this has not been a necessary manoeuvre.
8. Liliequist's membrane is opened sharply with a no. 11 blade. Through this space the course of the posterior communicating artery (PComA) can be observed to its junction with the ipsilateral PCA.
9. Further dissection along the PCA towards midline will expose the basilar bifurcation and the four-vessel complex, exposing the distal basilar compartment in the interpeduncular cistern.

**Skull base extension for low-lying distal basilar complex aneurysms**

For low-lying basilar apex aneurysms or SCA aneurysms, skull base extensions may be performed through the transcavernous route as originally described by Dolenc[40]. This extended basal approach widens the distal surgical corridor near the lesion, and allows exposure of the basilar artery and its proximal branches as far as the AICAs, with minimal retraction of the brain. The demands of this approach involve drilling of the anterior clinoid, freeing the ICA from the proximal and distal dural rings, opening of the cavernous sinus and drilling of the posterior clinoid process. This manoeuvre enhances the corridor between the ICA and the oculomotor nerve, and is useful for low-lying distal basilar complex lesions, and giant or recurrent BA aneurysms in which proximal control may be necessary during aneurysm dissection and clip placement.

**Far-lateral approach**

The *far-lateral approach* is also known as the lateral suboccipital approach, the extreme lateral approach, and the extreme lateral inferior transcondylar exposure (ELITE). These approaches are best suited for aneurysms along the lower third of the basilar artery.

**Key steps in a Far-lateral approach**

1. The patient is positioned semi-prone (or lateral), with the head held in 3-pin fixation and square to the shoulders and the chin tucked in to tighten the nuchal ligament.
2. A 'hockey-stick' incision is made beginning in the cervical midline over the C4 spinous process. It extends cranially to the inion, courses laterally along the superior nuchal line to finish immediately above the ear.
3. The paraspinous muscle is split in the avascular plane of the nuchal ligament.
4. Retraction of soft tissue is facilitated by exposure down to and around the C2 spinous process.
5. The vertebral artery (VA) is identified and protected as it courses from the transverse foramen of the lateral mass of C1, through the sulcus arteriosus of the C1 vertebral arch, to its dural entry point.
6. The lateral epidural venous plexus can cause troublesome bleeding and is best preserved by blunt dissection and packing with surgicel.
7. Bone removal consists of 3 parts
   a. Lateral occipital craniotomy,

   b. C1 laminotomy, and
   c. Partial condylectomy
8. A suboccipital craniotomy is extended unilaterally from the foramen magnum in the midline, up to the muscle cuff at the level of the transverse sinus, as far laterally as possible, and then back around the foramen magnum. In elderly patients with adherent dura, a suboccipital burrhole with subsequent cut-downs to the foramen magnum may help to preserve dura. The rim of the foramen magnum is rongeured to extend the opening across the midline and laterally toward the occipital condyle.
9. The craniectomy extends from the midline to the edge of the transverse/sigmoid sinus and includes a rim of foramen magnum.
10. The arch of C1 is removed with the drill, making a cut just medial to the sulcus arteriosus and another across the contralateral arch. These cuts are made in a rostral-to-caudal direction to keep any lurching of the drill away from the VA. Additional atlantal bone can be removed under the VA laterally to the transverse foramen.
11. The lateral aspect of the foramen magnum and the postero-medial two thirds of the occipital condyle are removed. The anterior extent of the condylar resection is defined either by the condylar emissary vein or by dura that begins to curve antero-medially, giving a tangential view along this dural plane.
12. Condylar resection enables the dural flap reflected against the condyle to be completely flat.
13. The dural incision curves from the cervical midline, across the circular sinus, to the lateral edge of the craniotomy. An inferior dural incision laterally under C1 mobilizes the flap further laterally against the margin of the craniotomy.
14. Multiple dural packing sutures hold the flap against the condyle under tension. Condylectomy is sufficient if there is no bony prominence obstructing the view of the lateral medulla.
15. The arachnoid of the cisterna magna is preserved until the microscope is brought into the field to keep blood out of the subarachnoid space.
16. After opening the arachnoid layer and taking care to minimize any retraction of the nerves, the vertebral artery is followed rostrally until the origin of the PICA. Alternatively PICA may be easily identified running around and under the cerebellar tonsils and this can be followed down to its origin and the aneurysm.

## 6. Revascularization

Direct surgical clipping remains the best treatment of aneurysms. It approximates normal arterial walls to promote endothelialisation that seals the aneurysm orifice. Parent vessels can be reconstructed and normal blood flow restored around the base of the aneurysm. However, not all aneurysms can be treated by direct clipping. Giant saccular aneurysm and complex fusiform or dolichoectactic aneurysms may lack a clippable neck. In these situations, it has been advocated that surgical bypass and trapping of the aneurysms would be a less invasive alternative treatment option.

In revascularization procedures to treat complex aneurysms in the posterior circulation, it is important to understand that the surgical approach is largely dependent on the exposure required to perform the arterial bypass. In most cases, this is often a less extensive exposure than that needed for direct clipping, making the overall surgery less traumatic for the patients. In addition, endovascular occlusion of parent vessel is a safe and feasible option in most centres, thus reducing the exposure required to only that needed for the bypass.

The surgical approaches for posterior circulation revascularisation are no different from the techniques discussed above. However, the strategy is important, and depends on:

1. Which aspect of the posterior circulation requires revascularization (i.e. upper, middle or lower vertebrobasilar territory)
2. How much blood flow is required – high or low flow strategies.

Possible posterior circulation bypasses to treat complex aneurysms are listed in Table 3.

| Compartments | EC-IC low flow | EC-IC high flow | IC-IC low flow | Approach |
|---|---|---|---|---|
| Upper Basilar | STA-SCA<br>STA-PCA | ECA-SCA<br>ECA-PCA | PCA-SCA | Orbitozygomatic |
| Mid Basilar | OA-AICA | ECA-AICA | AICA-PICA | Retrosigmoid<br>Retrolabyrinthine |
| Low Basilar | OA-PICA | VA-VA<br>VA-PICA | PICA-PICA | Far-Lateral |

Adapted from Youman's Neurological Surgery, 5th edition.

Table 3. Surgical bypass options for posterior circulation aneurysms

## 7. Postoperative care

1. Patients are managed in a dedicated neurosurgical intensive care unit for a minimum of 24-hours post-operatively.
2. Patients should be kept in a euvolemic state, with blood pressure allowed to rise to the patient's high normal pressure without the use of inotropes of vasopressors unless the patient shows clinical evidence of vasospasm.
3. Corticosteroids and anticonvulsants medications are not routinely used.
4. A CT/CT-angiogram is performed on day 1 post-operatively. If clipping is incomplete, surgical as well as endovascular options should be considered to obliterate the aneurysm remnant.
5. CSF leak can be treated with bed rest and lumbar CSF drainage; in cases where this fails to resolve, surgical re-exploration and repair of CSF fistula may be required.
6. A dedicated digital subtraction angiography (DSA) should be performed for cerebral revascularization cases to assess the adequacy of flow in the bypass.

## 8. Complications and their treatment

### 8.1 Cranial nerve damage

*Upper basilar territory*: The most common complication after surgical clipping of aneurysms in this region is an ipsilateral third nerve palsy, which may occur transiently in as many as 70 percent of patients. Damage may be peripheral which has an excellent chance of recovery. For central third nerve palsy, mostly from injury to the oculomotor nucleus in the brainstem, complete recovery is rare.

In the transsylvian approach, the third nerve needs to be dissected away from the tent to avoid retraction injury. The opposite should be employed in a subtemporal approach, where third nerve needs to be protected and tugged under the temporal lobe to avoid direct injury during retraction.

*Mid basilar* territory: The transtentorial approach to the basilar trunk risks damage to the $4^{th}$ and $5^{th}$ and $6^{th}$ nerves and the combined petrosal approach also risk damage to the $7^{th}$ and $8^{th}$ nerves.

*Lower basilar territory:* Approaches in this region risk damage to the lower cranial nerves, particularly when dissecting and clipping PICA aneurysms. Great care and delicacy is required when retracting these nerves to gain access. Damage can lead to potentially fatal aspiration pneumonia.

### 8.2 Perforator injuries

The most common cause of permanent morbidity for surgical management of posterior circulation aneurysms is perforator injury or occlusion. The importance of recognizing and preserving perforator damages at all case was well recognised by Dr Drake early on in his experience. Depending on the level of perforator involvement, patient may have significant cranial nerve deficits due to damage of cranial nuclei. Other complications may involve pseudobulbar palsy, ataxia, memory loss, a variable degree of hemiparesis and, in severe cases, disturbance of consciousness.

### 8.3 Venous infarction

Inadequate surgical exposure or inappropriate approach inevitably leads to the need for brain retraction. This significantly increases the risk of venous infarction, particularly for the subtemporal and petrosal route, where the vein of Labbe may be at risk. It is therefore important that when not necessary, retraction should be avoided at all cost. Furthermore, coagulating veins should be avoided during the approach as much as possible. If bleeding occurs, particular at the point where the vein of Labbe inserts into the sinus, do not coagulate; pack, irrigate, and dissect elsewhere until bleeding spontaneously stopped.

### 8.4 Vessel occlusion

An important lesson that neurosurgeons must learn from our endovascular colleagues is that it is always safer to compromise on the aneurysm sac than the parent artery. The pursuit of perfect clipping across an aneurysm neck at the compromise of constricting the parent artery and inflicting postoperative ischaemia is not acceptable. A microdoppler probe can provide a guide to patency, but intraoperative indocyanine green (ICG) fluorescence videoangiography if available should be used to ensure that the aneurysm is safely clipped. ICG fluorescence videoangiography can also reveal perforator occlusion.

### 8.5 Failure to use temporary clipping

Inadequate surgical exposure can compromise the ability to proximal and distal vessel control with temporary clipping. While the confines of the surgical corridor are limited, the role of temporary clipping for posterior circulation aneurysms is critical. Temporary clipping of the proximal vessel softens the aneurysmal wall, minimises the risk of clip closure, prevent proximal clip migration, and allows manipulation of the sac to identify critical perforators and adjacent vessels. Over the years, several authors have reported the use of circulatory arrest in the treatment of giant intracranial aneurysms[41]. These techniques enable longer period of temporary clipping up to 60 minutes, thus helping both the dissection and clipping of such complex aneurysms.

## 9. Outcome and prognosis (including results of author's series)

There is a popular trend in contemporary published surgical series to combine all treatment outcomes of posterior circulation aneurysms into one category. This method of classification conceals the unique features, management strategies, surgical approaches and outcomes that are distinctive to the individual aneurysm along the various parts of the vertebrobasilar system.

Like anterior circulation aneurysms, the outcome following direct clipping of aneurysms in the posterior circulation depends on a number of key factors:

1. Patient's preoperative grade
2. Aneurysm size and shape and related factors (e.g. degree of atheroma at the neck, extent of mural thrombosis, direction of the fundus)
3. Specific anatomical location along the vertebrobasilar system
4. Surgical expertise

In the senior author's aneurysm series (MKM) over a 20-year period from 1989 to 2010, 256 aneurysms in the posterior circulation were operated in 239 operations. 120 (46.9%) of the aneurysms were ruptured and 136 (53.1%) unruptured. Mean age was 51.2 +/- 13.1 years (range 9 to 77). There were 144 basilar bifurcation, 30 basilar trunk and 82 vertebral-PICA aneurysms. Aneurysms sizes were <7mm in 132 cases (53%), 7 to 12mm in 60 (24.1%), 13-24mm in 37 (14.9%) and >24mm in 20 (8%). The overall mortality was 9.2% and surgical morbidity was 12.9%.

Table 4 summarises the senior author's own surgical results and the results from the literature for surgical outcomes of posterior circulation aneurysms according to their location along the vertebrobasilar system.

| **Basilar Bifurcation Aneurysms** | | | | | |
|---|---|---|---|---|---|
| | No. of studies | No. of patients | % Independent | % Morbidity | % Mortality |
| 1960-69 | 6 | 37 | 48.6 (18/37) | 10.8 (4/37) | 37.8 (14/37) |
| 1970-79 | 10 | 408 | 77.2 (315/408) | 15.9 (65/408) | 6.9 (28/408) |
| 1980-89 | 12 | 1177 | 82.3 (969/1177) | 12.6 (148/1177) | 5.1 (60/1177) |
| 1990-99 | 13 | 2859 | 82.4 (2357/2859) | 10.8 (308/2859) | 6.2 (178/2859) |
| 2000-09 | 10 | 644 | 76.4 (492/644) | 14.4 (93/644) | 6.1 (39/644) |
| Author's series | 1 | 144 | 77.9 (109/140) | 12.5 (18/144) | 5.6 (8/144) |
| **Overall** | **52** | **5269** | **80.9 (4260/5265)** | **12.1 (636/5269)** | **6.2 (327/5269)** |

| **Basilar Trunk Aneurysms** | No. of studies | No. of patients | % Independent | % Morbidity | % Mortality |
|---|---|---|---|---|---|
| 1960-69 | 4 | 18 | 61.1 (11/18) | 16.7 (3/18) | 22.2 (4/18) |
| 1970-79 | 5 | 144 | 88.2 (127/144) | 6.9 (10/144) | 4.9 (7/144) |
| 1980-89 | 7 | 208 | 84.1 (175/208) | 7.2 (15/208) | 8.7 (18/208) |
| 1990-99 | 16 | 471 | 86.0 (405/471) | 8.7 (41/471) | 5.3 (25/471) |
| 2000-09 | 5 | 59 | 81.4 (48/59) | 13.6 (8/59) | 5.1 (3/59) |
| Author's series | 1 | 30 | 65.4 (17/26) | 20.7 (6/29) | 20.7 (6/29) |
| **Overall** | **38** | **930** | **84.6 (783/926)** | **8.9 (83/929)** | **6.8 (63/929)** |

| Vertebral-PICA Aneurysms | No. of studies | No. of patients | % Independent | % Morbidity | % Mortality |
|---|---|---|---|---|---|
| 1960-69 | 2 | 9 | 66.7 (6/9) | 0 (0/9) | 33.3 (3/9) |
| 1970-79 | 5 | 165 | 86.7 (143/165) | 1.8 (3/165) | 11.5 (19/165) |
| 1980-89 | 9 | 304 | 89.2 (248/278) | 5.4 (15/278) | 5.4 (15/278) |
| 1990-99 | 11 | 370 | 91.6 (329/359) | 3.6 (13/359) | 4.7 (17/359) |
| 2000-09 | 13 | 259 | 88.8 (222/250) | 8.4 (21/250) | 2.4 (6/250) |
| Author's series | 1 | 82 | 78.5 (62/79) | 9.1 (7/77) | 8.9 (7/79) |
| **Overall** | **41** | **1189** | **88.6 (1010/1140)** | **5.2 (59/1138)** | **5.9 (67/1140)** |

Table 4. Surgical Outcomes of Posterior Circulation Aneurysms 1960-2011

When the outcomes from major published series in both the surgical arm and the endovascular arm are combined (Table 5), a number of important points are noted:

| **Posterior Circulation Aneurysms: Coiling vs Clipping** | Study period | No. of studies | No. of patients | Independent (%) | Morbidity (%) | Mortality (%) |
|---|---|---|---|---|---|---|
| Endovascular | 1990-2005 | 16 | 1364 | 85.2 | 4.4 | 9.1 |
| Microsurgery | 1960-2009 | 56 | 7132 | 82.8 (5865/7086) | 10.5 (747/7086) | 9.1 (437/7086) |

Table 5. Comparison of outcomes for coiling versus clipping of posterior circulation aneurysms.

1. Contrary to contemporary belief, endovascular treatments and surgical treatments share similar rates of mortality and independence outcomes post procedures for posterior circulation aneurysms.
2. Morbidity is significantly lower in the endovascular group (absolute 6.1% difference), reflecting the better ease of access from an endovascular view point.

3. However, reduced morbidity in the endovascular arm is compromised by inefficient coiling rate with high recurrence and rebleeding rates, which has a negative impact in the long term for younger patients.

## 10. Expert suggestions

1. *Brain relaxation.* A relaxed brain is critical when operating on aneurysms in the posterior fossa. The key factors in ensuring a relaxed brain and avoid brain retraction include correct patient head positioning, maximal Sylvian fissure dissection, and optimal opening of the Sylvian and basal cisterns to promote CSF drainage.
2. *Distance of aneurysm from the clivus.* The transsylvian approaches to the basilar bifurcation involve a downward directed angle, therefore the closer the aneurysm neck is to the clivus the more hidden it becomes from the surgeon's view. Conversely, while it may be more desirable that the aneurysm is distanced from the clivus, the more posterior it is, the more likely it is adherent to the brain stem.
3. *Perforators.* A hypoplastic P1 carries as many and as vital perforators as a normal-sized P1 and therefore demands equal respect and preservation. If the ipsilateral P1 carries no perforators, then the contralateral P1 almost certainly carries perforators that supply both sides. Basilar bifurcation perforators emerge from the posterior aspect and not anteriorly. It is therefore vital to meticulously separate these perforating branches not only in the neck but also up to their adhesion to the fundus. It is possible that during clip occlusion of the neck, the resulting traction and aneurysm decompression can kink these branches distal to the clip site.
4. *Division of the posterior communicating artery.* Division of the PComA has been described in the literature and can be useful in maximising exposure to the posterior circulation. This manoeuvre, however, is often not necessary in the senior author's experience. We cautioned that division of the PComA should be done only judiciously. The anterior thalamoperforators generally leave the PComA from its medial-dorsal aspect and ascend rostroposteriorly. The decision to divide the PComA cannot be made without first confirming this and the exclusion of a fetal circulation.
5. *Aneurysm dissection.* Microdissection around the aneurysm should not be limited by a fear of intraoperative rupture. The morbidity caused by suboptimal exposure and insufficient circumferential dissection around the aneurysm can outweigh the morbidity related to a rupture. When appropriate preoperative and operative strategies are utilized, most intraoperative ruptures can be controlled.
6. *Placement of clips.* Careful selection of an appropriate aneurysm clip is important. Blade length should match the width of the aneurysm neck, which may widen as the blades close. Clips can be removed and reapplied as many times as necessary to optimally obliterate aneurysm, while preserving the parent vessels. Some aneurysms cannot be clipped directly. In such situations, it is important to recognize the challenges and consider alternative strategies.
7. *Utilize available technologies to ensure safe aneurysm surgery.* There are a number of major advances in vascular microsurgery in recent years, such as the use of ICG fluorescence videoangiography, endoscopic assisted aneurysm clipping and the utilization of intraoperative electrophysiological monitoring. These options should be exploited to reduce operative complications.

## 11. Explicative case

An 18 year-old girl presented with several months history of progressive left sided paraesthesia and difficulty walking. Subsequent investigations revealed a large middle basilar trunk aneurysm measuring 2cm in maximal diameter. The fundus of this aneurysm was projecting toward the right side (Figure. 1).

Fig. 1

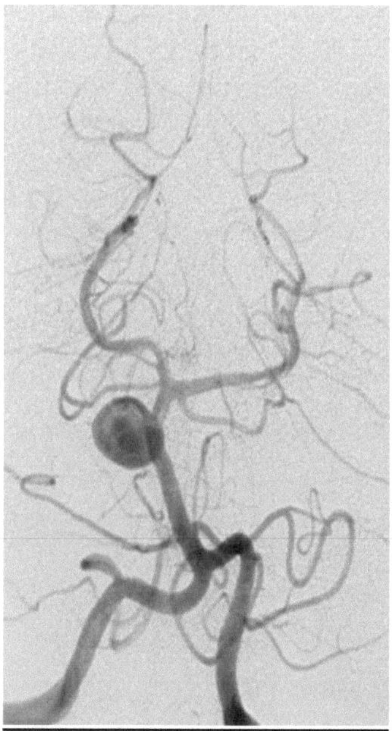

Fig. 2

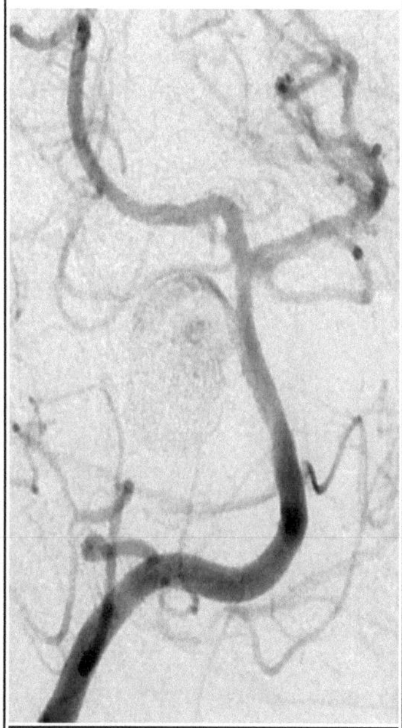

Fig. 3

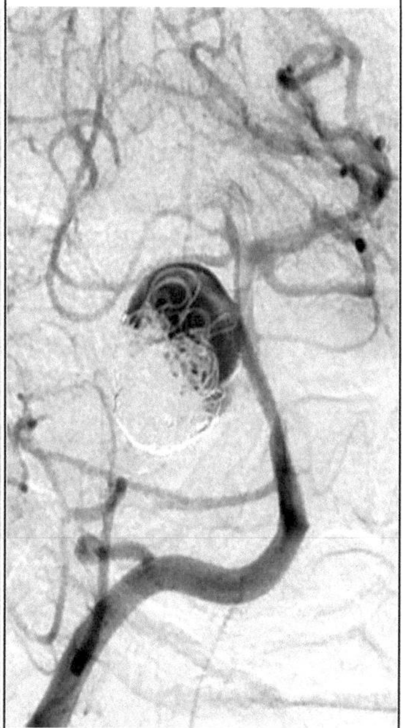

Due to its location, this aneurysm was initially treated by endovascular coiling with near complete occlusion (Figure. 2). At 3-month post-coiling follow-up, a repeat cerebral angiogram revealed coil compaction and recurrence of the aneurysm along (Figure. 3). A further attempt at recoiling with stent was carried out but this failed to robustly repair the aneurysm (Figure 4). At this point, surgical option was chosen for definitive treatment.

Surgery was carried out via a right sided orbitozygomatic approach with the zygomatic arch removed. A medial petrosectomy was made extradurally having first unroofed the ipsilateral internal carotid artery. The dura was then opened and reflected on to superior orbital fissure continuing the dural opening down to the superior petrosal sinus, communicating this with an opening of the dura in the posterior fossa, dividing the superior petrosal sinus and bringing the dural opening across the tentorium to the free edge of the tent behind the fourth cranial nerve.

The Sylvian fissure was then widely split, followed by isolation of the fourth nerve with intact dura drawing and placing tension on the cavernous sinus. This allowed full access to the aneurysm that was well exposed both proximally and distally. Direct clipping of the aneurysm neck was rendered problematic as the stent protruded through the basilar artery wall as the clip was closed. At this point, the aneurysm was trapped by necessity to control bleeding. Having assessed the posterior communicating arteries were of small calibre, it was deemed appropriate to supplement the patient's posterior circulation with a vein bypass.

The vein graft was harvested from the long Saphenous below the left knee and a right anterior sternomastoid approach was made to the common carotid artery. The vein was tunnelled into a subcutaneous location and then an end-to-side anastomosis was performed between the vein and the right P2 segment of the posterior cerebral artery. Following this an end-to-side anastomosis was performed onto the common carotid artery with the fish-mouth. A post-operative computed tomography angiogram is demonstrated in Figure 5. Patient remained well posteropatively and the large basilar trunk aneurysm was cured on followed up imaging.

Fig. 4

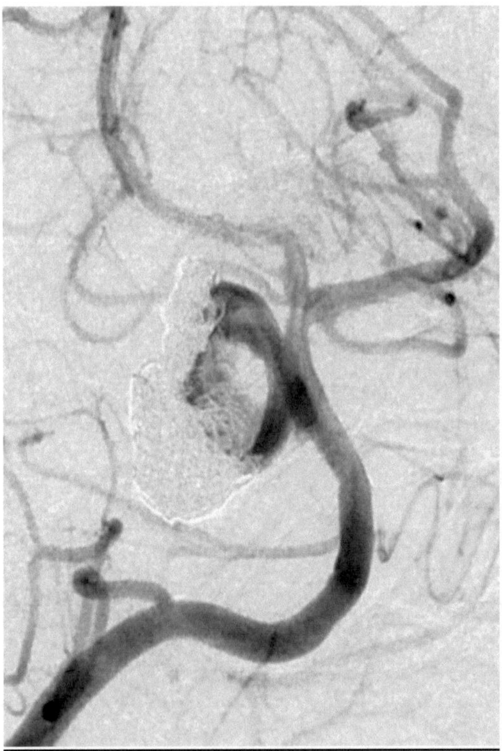

Fig. 5

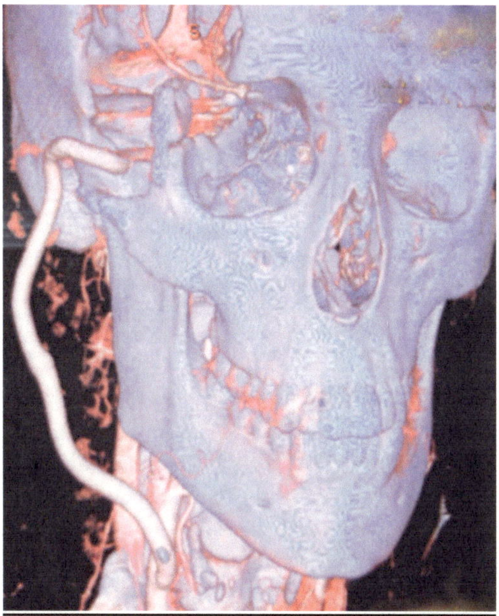

## 12. Conclusions

Over the last 5 decades, neurosurgeons have worked tirelessly to tackle with aneurysms in the posterior circulation. The skull have been deconstructed and reconstructed in every feasible way to minimise neurological injuries in a territory where surgical corridors are deep, manoeuvrability is limited, and mistakes are unforgivable. At this instance, there is little room for microsurgical innovation. The next phase of breakthroughs for posterior circulation aneurysm treatments will likely transpire from endovascular and endoscopic skull base advancements. At some point, endovascular techniques will reach their limits and will not replace the role of open surgical clipping, as had previously anticipated. The responsibility for future generations of vascular neurosurgeons, therefore, is to embrace and integrate these innovations while maintaining technical proficiency in all aspects of microsurgical skull base approaches. This will be to ensure that the increasing emergence of complex aneurysms can be safely treated with microsurgical methods.

## 13. References

[1] Tonnis W. Zur Behandlung intracranieller Aneurysme. Langenbecks Arch Klin Chir 1937; 189: 474.
[2] Dandy WE: Intracranial Arterial Aneurysms. New York. Hafner 1944 (reprinted 1969).
[3] Schwartz HG. Arterial aneurysms of the posterior fossa. J Neurosurg 1948; 5: 312-6.
[4] Logue V. Posterior fossa aneurysms. Clin Neurosurg 1964; 11: 183-219.

[5] Mount LA, JM Taveras. Ligature of the basilar artery in treatment of an aneurysm of the basilar-artery bifurcation. J Neurosurg 1962; 19: 167-170.

[6] Drake CG. Bleeding aneurysms of the basilar artery. Direct surgical management in four cases. J Neurosurg 1961; 18: 230-8.

[7] Jamieson KG. Aneurysms of the vertebrobasilar system. J Neurosurg 1964; 21: 781-797.

[8] Guglielmi G, Vinuela F, Dion J, Duckwiller G. Electrothrombosis of saccular aneurysms via endovascular approach. Part 2: Preliminary clinical experience. J Neurosurg 1991; 75:8-14.

[9] Eskridge JM, Song JK. Endovascular embolization of 150 basilar tip aneurysms with Guglielmi detachable coils: results of the Food and Drug Administration multicenter clinical trial. J Neurosurg 1998; 89: 81-86.

[10] Guglielmi G, Vinuela F, Duckwiler G, Dion J, Lylyk P, Berenstein A, Strother C, Graves V, Halback V, Nichols D, et al. Endovascular treatment of posterior circulation aneurysms by electrothrombosis using electrically detachable coils. J Neurosurg 1992; 77: 515-524.

[11] Vinuela F, Duckwiler G, Mawad M. Guglielmi detachable coil embolization of acute intracranial aneurysm: perioperative anatomical and clinical outcome in 403 patients. J Neurosurg 1997; 86: 475-482.

[12] Tateshima S, Murayama Y, Gobin YP, Duckwiler GR, Guglielmi G, Vinuela G. Endovascular treatment of basilar tip aneurysms using Guglielmi detachable coils: anatomic and clinical outcomes in 73 patients from a single institution. Neurosurgery 2000; 47: 1332-1339.

[13] Bavinzski G, Killer M, Gruber A, Reiinprecht A, Gross CE, Richling B. Treatment of basilar artery bifurcation aneurysms by using Guglielmi detachable coils: a 6-year experience. J Neurosurg 1999; 90: 843-52.

[14] Pierot L, Boulin A, Castaings L, Rey A, Moret J. Selective occlusion of basilar artery aneurysms using controlled detachable coils: report of 35 cases. Neurosurgery 1996; 38: 948-53.

[15] Molyneux A, Kerr R, Stratton I, Sandercock P, Clarke M, Shrimpton J, Holman R. International Subarachnoid Aneurysm Trial (ISAT) Collaborative Group: International Subarachnoid Aneurysm Trial (ISAT) of neurosurgical clipping versus endovascular coiling in 2143 patients with ruptured intracranial aneurysms: A randomized trial. Lancet 2002; 360: 1267-74.

[16] David CA, Vishteh G, Spetzler RF, et al: Late angiographic follow-up of surgically treated aneurysms. J Neurosurg 1999; 91: 396-401.

[17] Le Roux P, Elliott JP, Eskridge JM, et al: Risk and benefits of diagnostic angiography following aneurysm surgery: A retrospective analysis of 597 studies. Neurosurgery 1998; 42: 1248-1255.

[18] Molyneux AJ, kerr RSC, Birks J, Ramzi N, Yarnola J, Sneade M, Rischmiller Jl for the ISAT collaborators. Risk of recurrent subarachnoid hemorrhage, death, or dependence, and standardized mortality ratios after clipping or coiling of an intracranial aneurysm in the International Subarachnoid Aneurysm Trial (ISAT): long-term follow-up. Lancet Neurol. 2009; 9:427-33.

[19] Wiebers DO, Whisnant JP, Huston J III, Meissner I, Brown RD Jr, Piepgras DG, Forbes GS, Thielen K, Nichols D, O'Fallon WM, Peacock J, Jaeger L, Kassell NF, Kongable-Beckman GL, Torner JC: International Study of Unruptured Aneurysms Investigators: Unruptured Intracranial aneurysms - Natural history, clinical outcome, and risks of surgical and endovascular treatment. Lancet 2003; 362: 103-110.

[20] Guglielmi G, Vinuela F, Duckwiler G, Dion J, Lylyk P, et al: Endovascular treatment of posterior circulation aneurysms by electrothrombosis using electrically detachable coils. J Neurosurg 1992; 77: 515-524.

[21] McDougall CG, Halbach VV, Dowd CF, Higashida RT et al: Endovascular treatment of basilar tip aneurysms using electrolytically detachable coils. J Neurosurg 1996; 84: 393-399.

[22] Pierot L, Boulin A, Castaings L, Rey A, Moret J. Selective occlusion of basilar artery aneurysms using controlled detachable coils: report of 35 cases. Neurosurgery 1996; 38: 948-953.

[23] Klein GE, Szolar DH, Leber KA, Karaic R, Hausegger KA. Basilar tip aneurysm: endovascular treatment with Gugluelmi detachable coils - midterm results. Radiology 1997; 205: 191-196.

[24] Nichols DA, Brown RD Jr, Thielen KR, Meyer FB, Atkinson JL, Piepgras DG. Endovascular treatment of ruptured posterior circulation aneurysms using electrolytically detachable coils. J Neurosurg 1997; 87: 374-380.

[25] Raymond J, Roy D, Bojanowski M, Moumdjian R, L'Esperance G. Endovascular treatment of acutely ruptured and unruptured aneurysms of the basilar bifurcation. J Neurosurg 1997; 86: 211-219.

[26] Vinuela F, Duckwiler G, Mawad M. Guglielmi detachable coil embolization of acute intracranial aneurysm: perioperative anatomical and clinical outcome in 403 patients. J Neurosurg 1997; 86: 475-482.

[27] Eskridge JM, Song JK. Endovascular embolization of 150 basilar tip aneurysms with Guglielmi detachable coils: results of the Food and Drug Administration multicenter clinical trial. J Neurosurg 1998; 89: 81-86.

[28] Bavinzski G, Killer M, Gruber A, Reinprecht A, Gross CE, Richling B. Treatment of basilar artery bifurcation aneurysms by using Guglielmi detachable coils: a 6-year experience. J Neurosurg 1999; 90: 843-852.

[29] Gruber DP, Zimmerman GA, Tomsick TA, van Loveren HR, Link MJ, Tew JM Jr. A comparison between endovascular and surgical management of basilar artery apex aneurysms. J Neurosurg 1999; 90: 868-874.

[30] Steiger HJ, Medele R, Bruckmann H, Schroth G, Reulen HJ. Interdisciplinary management results in 100 patients with ruptured and unruptured posterior circulation aneurysms. Acta Neurochir (Wien) 1999; 141: 359-366.

[31] Lempert TE, Malek AM, Halbach VV, Phatouoros CC, Meyers PM, Dowd CF, Higashida RT. Endovascular treatment of ruptured posterior circulation cerebral aneurysms: clinical and angiographic outcomes. Stroke 2000; 31: 100-110.

[32] Tateshima S, Murayama Y, Gobin YP, Duckwiler GR, Guglielmi G, Vinuela F. Endovascular treatment of basilar tip aneurysms using Guglielmi detachable coils:

anatomic and clinical outcomes in 73 patients from a single institution. Neurosurgery 2000; 47: 1332-1339.
[33] Birchall D, Khangure M, McAuliffe W, Apsimon H, Knuckey N. Endovascular treatment of posterior circulation aneurysms. Br J Neurosurg 2001; 15: 39-43.
[34] Uda K, Murayama Y, Gobin YP, Duckwiler GR, Vinuela F. Endovascular treatment of basilar artery trunk aneurysms with Guglielmi detachable coils: clinical experience with 41 aneurysms in 39 patients. J Neurosurg 2011; 95: 624-632.
[35] Pandey AS, Koebbe C, Rosenwasser RH, Veznedaroglu E. Endovascular coil embolization of ruptured and unruptured posterior circulation aneurysms: Review of a 10-year experience. Neurosurgery 2007; 60: 626-636.
[36] Raaymakers TW, Rinkel GJ, Limburg M, et al. Mortality and morbidity of surgery for unruptured intracranial aneurysms: a meta-analysis. Stroke 1998; 29: 1531-8.
[37] Ogilvy CS, Carter BS. Stratification of outcome for surgically treated unruptured intracranial aneurysms. Neurosurgery 2003; 52: 82-8.
[38] Eftekhar B, Morgan MK. Preoperative factors affecting the outcome of unruptured posterior circulation aneurysm surgery. J Clin Neurosc 2011; 18:85-89.
[39] Hauck EF, White JA, Samson D. The small "surgical aneurysm" at the basilar apex. J Neurosurg 2010; 112; 1216-1221.
[40] Dolenc VV, Skrap M, Sustersic J, Skrbec M, Morina A: A transcavernous-transsellar approach to the basilar tip aneurysms. Br J Neurosurg 1987; 1: 251-259.
[41] Spetzler RF, Hadley MN, Rigamonti D, Carter LP, Raudzens PA, Shedd SA, Wilkinson E. Aneurysms of the basilar artery treated with circulatory arrest, hypothermia, and barbiturate cerebral protection. J Neurosurg 1988; 68: 868-879.

# 12

# Skull Base Approaches for Vertebro-Basilar Aneurysms

Renato J. Galzio[1,2], Danilo De Paulis[2] and Francesco Di Cola[1]
[1]*Department of Health Sciences (Neurosurgery), Medical School of the University of L'Aquila, L'Aquila*
[2]*Department of Neurosurgery, "San Salvatore" City Hospital, L'Aquila, Italy*

## 1. Introduction

Posterior circulation aneurysms are deeply embedded in very limited subarachnoidal spaces surrounded by heavy bony structures and in intimate relationship with both the brainstem and its vasculature. These lesions, if compared to anterior circulation aneurysms, more frequently present large dimensions, intraluminal thrombosis and sclerotic changes of the sac and of the parental artery. Both vertebro-basilar (VB) aneurysms' intrinsic characteristics and their location make every kind of treatment a challenge. Endovascular therapy has gained a special and effective role in the management of these lesions, but it is not always indicated or possible, hence surgery still represents the best therapeutic option, especially in case of complex and giant lesions. We have revised our casuistic from January 1990 to December 2010 to discuss the approaches that have been used in the surgically treated 150 vertebro-basilar aneurysms.

## 2. Clinical materials and methods

### 2.1 Patient population

From January 1990 to December 2010, 1056 patients harbouring 1193 aneurysms have been operated by the senior author (RJG) up to a total of 1114 surgical procedures. 118 of the patients harboured multiple aneurysms that have been treated in single or multiple surgical sessions, or with combined treatments (surgical for one or more lesions and endovascular for others). 144 patients were surgically treated for VB lesions; 4 of them presented 2 different aneurysms in the posterior circulation and 1 of them showed 3 lesions all located in the VB system. 10 patients harboured at least 1 VB aneurysm together with 1 or more aneurysms located in the anterior circulation. A total of 150 aneurysms of the posterior circulation have been operated; 48 lesions showed a diameter larger than 2.0 cm: 24 of them (16%) presented a diameter larger than 2.5 cm (giant aneurysms) and 24 of them (16%) presented a diameter between 2.0 cm and 2.5 cm (very large aneurysms). Clinical presentation of our patients (144) with posterior circulation aneurysms was hemorrhagic in 95 cases (63.3%) and not hemorrhagic in 49 subjects (32,6%). Because of the introduction of the endovascular treatment, this series is not homogeneous; endovascular therapy began to be routinely used in our department since the year 2000, thereafter, the number of surgically treated patients has progressively reduced, while the percentage of surgical procedures for complex aneurysms has relatively increased. From January 1990 to December 1999, 94 patients harbouring 98 VB aneurysms have been operated; 27 aneurysms (27.5%) presented a diameter larger than 2.0 cm. Only 50 patients harbouring 52 VB aneurysms were operated after January 2000, but 21 lesions (42%) were very large or giant aneurysms. In the present study we have only considered lesions treated by direct microsurgical approach, hence cases treated exclusively by endovascular approach or by extra- to intra-cranial bypass and trapping (2 giant aneurysms of the distal prejunctional vertebral artery) have been excluded. Table 1 summarizes location and characteristics of the lesions. Table 2 summarizes the number of treated aneurysms before and after the introduction of endovascular therapy in our institute. Table 3 summarizes the outcomes in the presented series.

| | *N° of Aneurysms* | *Giants (Ø ≥ 2.5 cm)* | *Very large (2cm< Ø <2.5cm)* |
|---|---|---|---|
| Basilar tip | 75 | 9 | 12 |
| PCA/SCA | 16 | 2 | 3 |
| Midbasilar (AICA) | 12 | 2 | 3 |
| Vertebro-basilar Junction | 13 | 3 | 2 |
| Vertebral (PICA) | 22 | 3 | 2 |
| Distal branches | 12 | 5 | 2 |
| **Total** | **150 (100%)** | **24 (16%)** | **24 (16%)** |
| | | **Total (Giant & Very large): 48 (32%)** | |

Table 1. Locations and characteristics of the 150 treated aneurysms.

| | *N° of Patients* | *N° of Aneurysms* | *N° of Giant & Very Large Aneurysms* |
|---|---|---|---|
| **Global (1999-2008)** | **144 (100%)** | **150 (100%)** | **48 (32%)** |
| **First period (1990-1999)** | **94 (65,2%)** | **98 (65,3%)** | **27 (27,5%)** |
| **Last period (2000-2008)** | **50 (34,8%)** | **52 (34,7%)** | **21 (42%)** |

Table 2. Number of treated aneurysms before and after the introduction of the endovascular therapy in our Institute.

| | *N° of Patients* | *No or Minimal deficit* | *Moderate deficit* | *Severe deficit or Vegetative* | *Death* |
|---|---|---|---|---|---|
| **Global** | **144** | **94 (65,3%)** | **28 (19,5%)** | **10 (6,9%)** | **12 (8,3%)*** |
| **Unruptured Aneurysms**** | **49** | **33 (67,4%)** | **7 (14,3%)** | **5 (10,2%)** | **4 (8,1%)** |
| **Giant Aneurysms** | **24** | **15 (62,6%)** | **3 (12,5%)** | **2 (8,3%)** | **4 (16,6%)*** |

Table 3. Outcome of the presented series (* 2 Giants aneurysms operated in grade IV Hunt-Hess scale for impending life hematoma; ** 10 Giant aneurysms comprised).

## 2.2 Surgical procedure

Successful direct surgical treatment of VB aneurysms, specially of complex ones, is mainly based on the choice of an adequate approach and on the application of specific surgical adjuncts.

Approaches have to provide a wide working room, short working distance, straight access and the possibility of handling the lesion from different points of view with minimal manipulation and retraction of critical perilesional neurovascular structures; exposure of the parental artery and efferent vessels (to achieve eventual temporary occlusion), complete exposure of the implant base (to get best clip positioning) and wide exposure of the aneurismal sac, at least of its proximal portion, (to manipulate the lesion from different directions) have to be achieved through an adequate access to the lesion. These goals are, in most instances, achieved by performing skull base approaches, which are essentially based on the principle of removing as much bone as possible to minimize retraction and manipulation of critical perilesional structures. We have used standardized approaches and the choice was essentially performed taking into consideration the location and the specific intrinsic features of the lesion (Figure 1).

Many intraoperative surgical techniques may result truly effective in the treatment of VB aneurysms; temporary clipping or trapping of the parental vessel allows, in many instances, an effective decompression of the aneurismal sac and the possibility to expose the implant base of the lesion which has to be dissected from perforators and efferent arteries before definitively clipping [Taylor, 1996; Baussart, 2005]; the "stacking-seating" technique, which consists in the use of differently shaped and sized clips which are progressively apposed and eventually removed until obtaining definitive exclusion of the sac, may prevent injuries to perforators and perilesional vasculature and may avoid constriction of flow through the parent vessel [Levy, 1995; Giannotta, 2002]; intraluminal decompression is often necessary to achieve a definitive exclusion of the aneurysm, and in case of thrombosed lesions it can be obtained using the ultrasonic aspirator [de Oliveira, 2009]; the use of multiple, variously shaped and sized clips apposed in embricated way ("tandem" clipping, "dome" clipping) results especially helpful when dealing with giant and very large VB aneurysms [Lawton, 1998; Kato, 2003; Sharma, 2008]; bipolar coagulation to reconstruct the parental vessels in wide based lesions; definitive trapping has been used in 2 cases of massively thrombosed aneurysms located in the distal branches, one in the superior cerebellar artery (SCA) and the other in the P2 tract of the posterior cerebral artery (PCA); aneurismorraphy has been used in one case of giant partially thrombosed aneurysm of the P1 tract of the left PCA [Hosobuchi, 1979; Samii, 1985].

The application of other intraoperative additional methodologies also turned out to be especially useful in the treatment of VB aneurysms; intraoperative doppler to test patency of afferent vessels after clipping has been used in nearly every case [Akdemir, 2006; Kapsalaki, 2008]; more recently, we have used intraoperative fluoroangiography [Raabe, 2005; Dashti, 2009] and endoscopic assistance to microneurosurgery, which has revealed particularly effective in the treatment of lesions located in the distal portion of basilar artery [Taniguchi, 1999; Kalavakonda, 2002; Galzio and Tschabitscher, 2010].

We have operated on 144 patients harbouring 150 VB aneurysms. Four of these subjects harboured 2 aneurysms in the VB system and one patient harboured 3 posterior circulation aneurysms: two patients harbouring 2 aneurysms respectively located in the top of the basilar artery and in the junction between basilar artery (BA) and SCA were operated on through a fronto-temporo-orbital (FTO) approach (one of these patients also harboured an internal carotid artery/posterior communicating artery aneurysm); one subject harbouring a basilar top and PCA (P2) aneurysm was operated at first through a pterional approach and successively through a subtemporal controlateral approach; one patient harbouring a BA/SCA aneurysm and a posterior inferior cerebellar artery (PICA) aneurysm underwent a pterional approach and successively a far lateral approach; the patient with 3 lesions was operated at first through a FTO approach (to clip a basilar top and a BA/SCA aneurysms) and successively through a far lateral controlateral approach to treat a PICA aneurysm; none of multiple aneurysms was a giant one.

Thereafter, we have performed 147 procedures to treat 150 posterior circulation aneurysms in 144 patients.

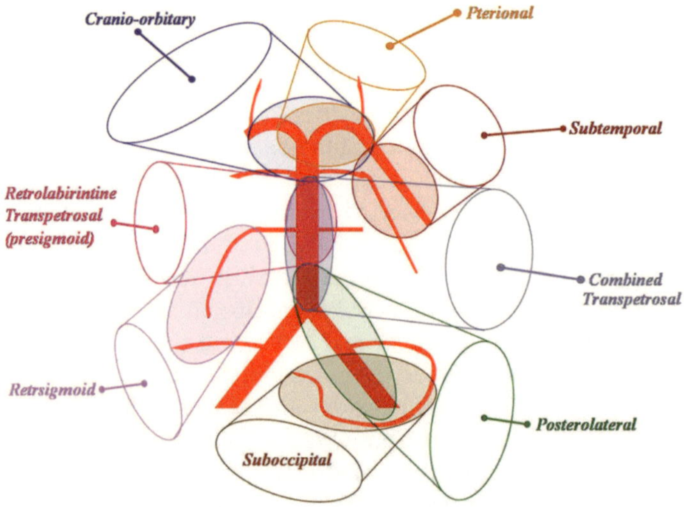


Fig. 1. Schematic drawing defining the surgical approaches used for 150 posterior circulation aneurysms, essentially based on their location.

### 2.2.1 Pterional approach

The pterional approach has been used in 75 patients harbouring lesions located in the distal portion of the basilar artery: 65 lesions were located in the basilar artery bifurcation/P1 tract (basilar top) and 10 lesions were located in the BA, at the level of the origin of the SCA to the origin to the PCA (PCA/SCA aneurysms). 4 of the basilar top aneurysms that we treated through the pterional approach, were giant ones. The pterional approach has been essentially used for medium sized, not very complex lesions (Figure 2).

We prepare the pterional approach in the submuscular fashion, as described by Spetzler [Coscarella, 2000; Oikawa, 1996]. In any case a drilling of the sphenoid wing was accomplished until opening the sphenoid fissure and drilling the orbital crests; an extradural anterior clinoidectomy and optic canal unroofing was also accomplished to have the possibility to achieve a wider mobilization of the optic nerve (ON) and of the internal carotid artery (ICA) during the operation [Sato, 2001; Noguchi, 2005]. After opening the dura, the sylvian fissure was widely dissected and basal cisterns exposed [Yasargil, 1976]. Two main surgical corridors allow access to the distal portion of the basilar artery; the first, between ON and ICA, is usually narrow and it has been rarely used; the second, between ICA and 3rd cranial nerve (CN), is normally wider and it has been used in most instances: this corridor may be further widened by incising the attachment of the tentorial notch (Figure 3).

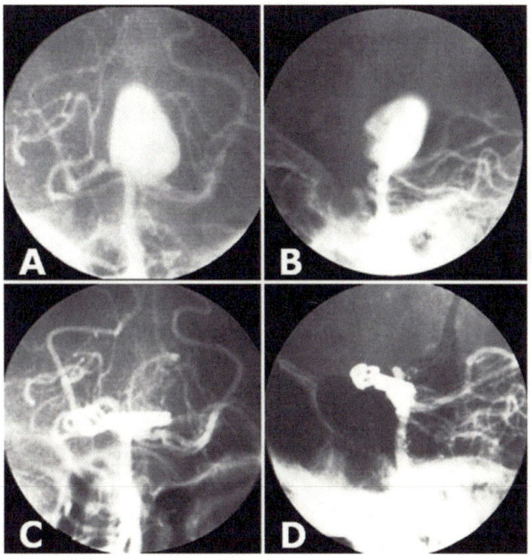


Fig. 2. Preoperative (A,B) and postoperative (C,D) angiography of a basilar tip aneurysm treated through a pterional approach.

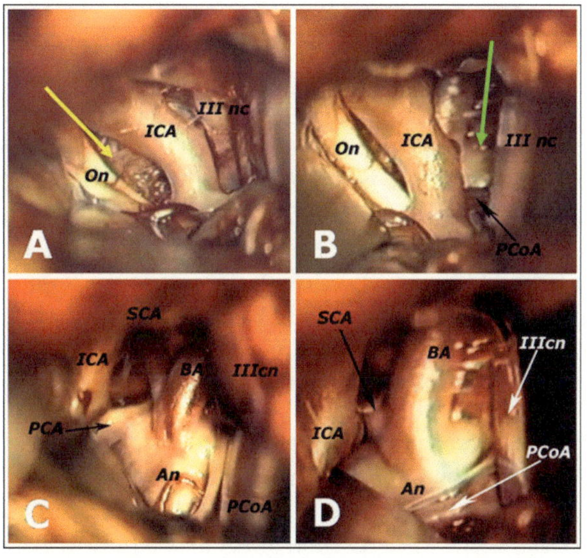


Fig. 3. Intraoperative images: after the preparation of a right pterional approach, the dura is opened and the sylvian fissure widely dissected, exposing the structures located in the

anterior basal cisterns: the surgical corridor (yellow arrow) between the optic nerve (ON) and the internal carotid artery (ICA) is normally narrower than the corridor (green arrow) located between the internal carotid artery and the third cranial nerve (III CN) (A,B); the corridor between ICA and III CN can be further widened by incising the attachment of the tentorial notch to better expose the basilar artery (BA) with its terminal branches, posterior cerebral artery (PCA) and superior cerebellar artery (SCA) and the implant base of the aneurysm (An); the posterior communicating artery (PCoA) remains in the right infero-lateral sector of the operative field (C,D).

Sometimes, a short posterior communicating artery (PcoA) inhibits the exposure of the distal portion of the BA and it has to be sectioned to allow a vision of the aneurysmal implant base [Yasargil, 1976; Inao, 1996]; when the aneurysm has a wide neck, it may be useful to prepare the parental vessel in a way to apply a temporary clip, if necessary in a safe location without endangering perforators or other adherent vessels (Figure 4).

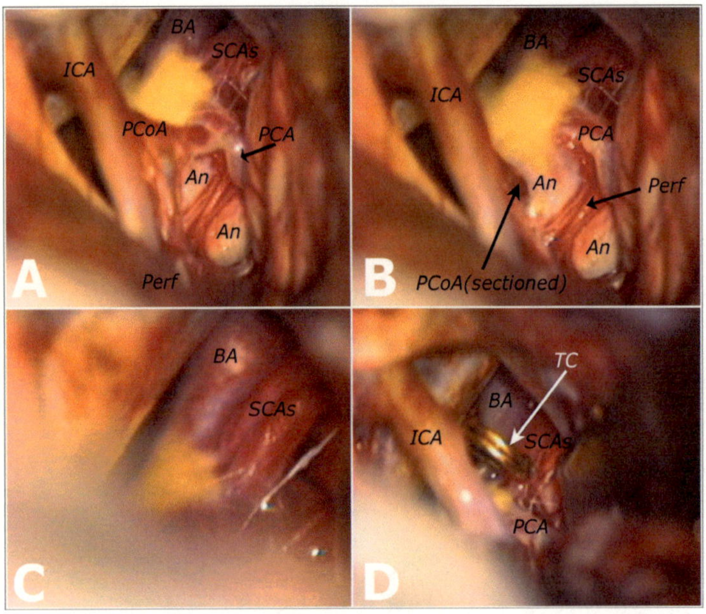


Fig. 4. Intraoperative images (same case of Fig.3): a short posterior communicating artery (PCoA) sometimes inhibits the exposure of the distal portion of the basilar artery (BA) (A); it may be sectioned, avoiding damage to perforators, to get a sight of the implant base of the aneurysm (An) (B); control of the parental basilar artery (BA) and of its distal branches, superior cerebellar artery (SCA) and posterior cerebral artery (PCA), has to be achieved (C); a temporary clip (TC) may be placed in a safe position (D).

The use of differently sized and shaped clips to perform transitory and definitively clipping is, in case of wide based lesions, the only way to preserve perforators (Figure 5); after definitive clipping, the sac has to be opened and evacuated to confirm a complete exclusion (Figure 6). For aneurysms of the distal portion of BA located below the posterior biclinoidal line (Figure 7), a posterior clinoidectomy has to be performed to visualize the parent vessels and the implant base [Fujitsu, 1985; Dolenc, 1987] (Figure 8).

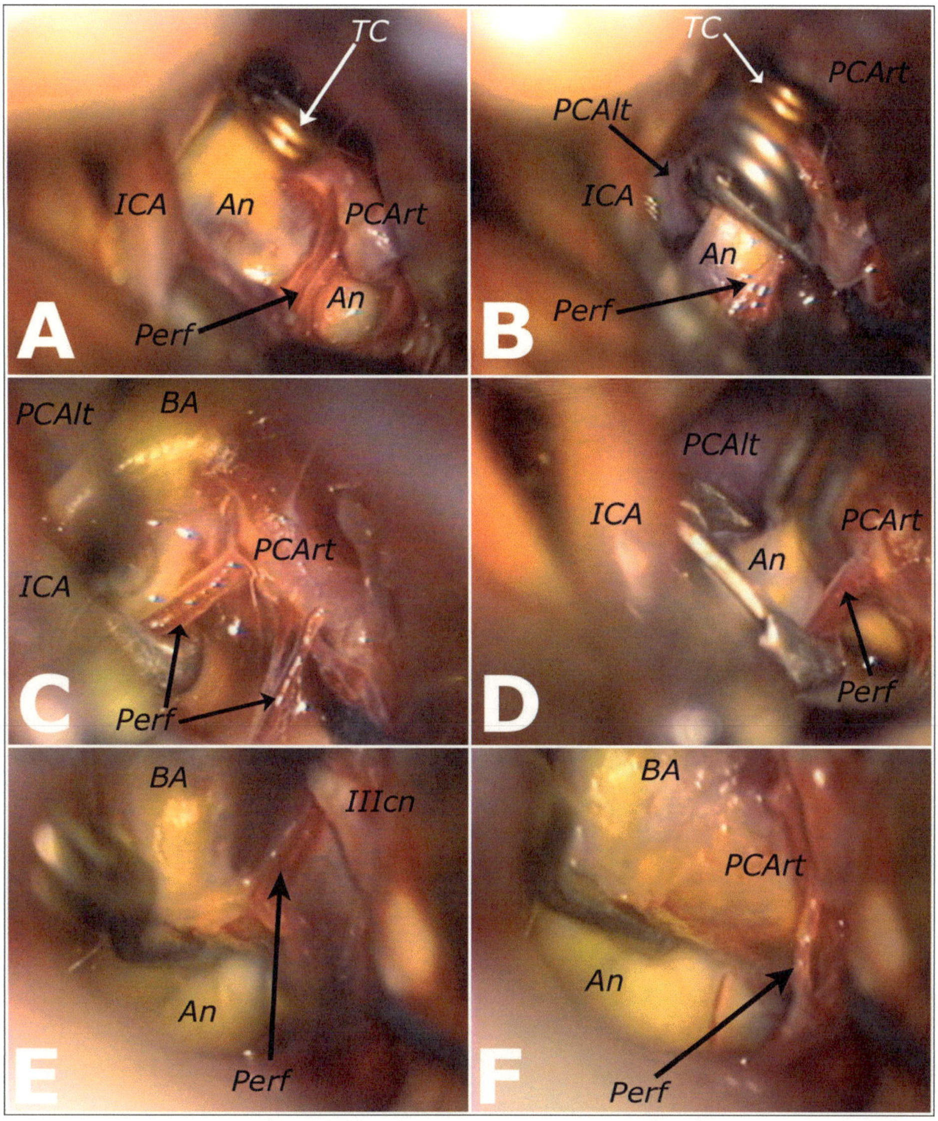


Fig. 5. Intraoperative images (same case of Figs.3 and 4): the temporary clip (TC) is applied on the basilar artery (BA) to reduce the intraluminal pressure into the aneurysmal sac and differently shaped and sized clips are progressively apposed and removed, both to avoid damage to perforators (Perf) and efferent arteries and to avoid constriction of flow through the parent vessel, until obtaining a definitive exclusion of the aneurysm ("stacking-seating technique") (A,B,C,D); the aneurysm has been definitively excluded with a bayonet shaped clip, preserving integrity of the left posterior cerebral artery (PCAlt), of the right one (PCArt) and of perforators, which have been progressively separated from the aneurysmal sac; the temporary clip initially placed on the basilar artery has been removed (E,F).

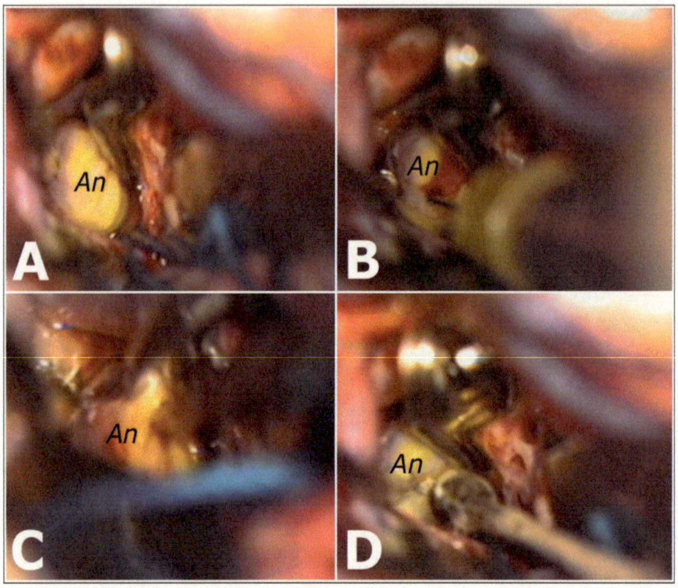


Fig. 6. Intraoperative images (same case of Figs.3, 4 and 5): the definitive clip has been reinforced with a second bayonet shaped clip applied parallel (A) and the aneurysmal sac is evacuated by puncture (B), shrunk with the bipolar coagulator (C) and opened with a microknife (D).

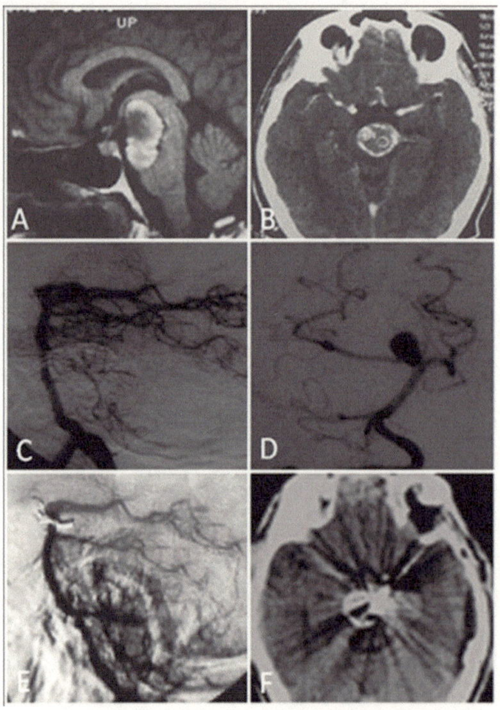


Fig. 7. Preoperative MRI (A), preoperative CT scan (B), preoperative angiography (C,D), postoperative angiography (E) and postoperative CT scan (F) of a very large massively

thrombosed aneurysm with the implant base located low with respect to the posterior biclinoidal line, in the distal portion of the basilar artery between the origin of the right superior cerebellar artery and the origin of the right posterior cerebral artery; this lesion was approached through a right pterional approach.

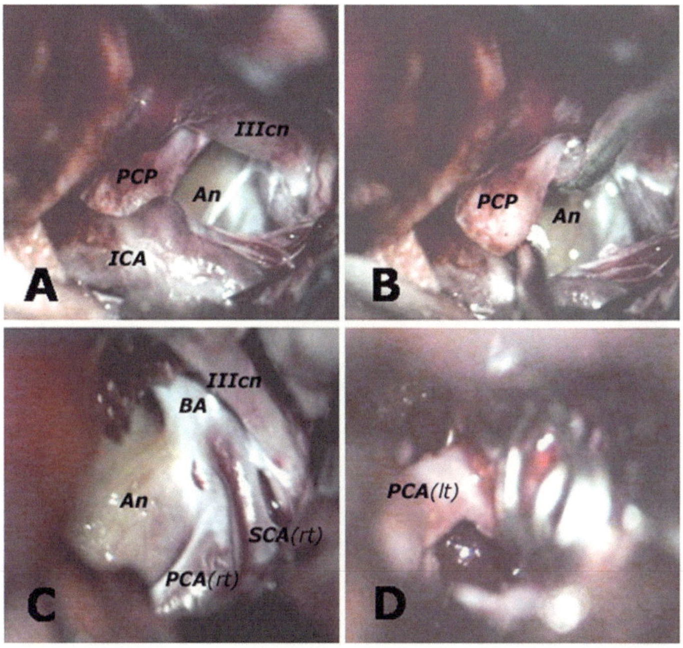


Fig. 8. Intraoperative images of the same case of Fig.7: the posterior clinoid process (PCP) limits the inspection of the implant base of the aneurysm (A,B);after resection of the PCP, the basilar artery (BA) with its right (rt) distal branches, superior cerebellar artery (SCA) and posterior cerebral artery (PCA), and the proximal portion of the aneurysm are completely displayed (C); after definite clipping of the aneurysm, also the left (lt) PCA is clearly patent (D).

### 2.2.2 Fronto-temporo-orbital approach

The fronto-orbito-temporal (FTO) approach has been used in 10 cases: 5 giant aneurysms located in the basilar top, 5 SCA/PCA aneurysms, among which 2 were giant lesions.

We usually prefer to perform the FTO approach as a two-piece, non osteoplastic craniotomy [Zabramski, 1998; Lemole, 2003; Galzio, 2010]. The FTO approach has been essentially used for more complex and very large and giant aneurysms; in effect this approach allows a very wide working room, with the possibility to use three different surgical corridors: not only the normally used two corridors, the first between ON and ICA and the second between ICA artery and the third cranial nerve, which are widely exposed, but it is also possible to open the anterior border of the tentorium to work laterally to the third cranial nerve. This third surgical corridor is especially useful to treat complex aneurysms of the distal BA directed laterally or mainly implanted in the P1 segment of the PCA (Figures 9 and 10).

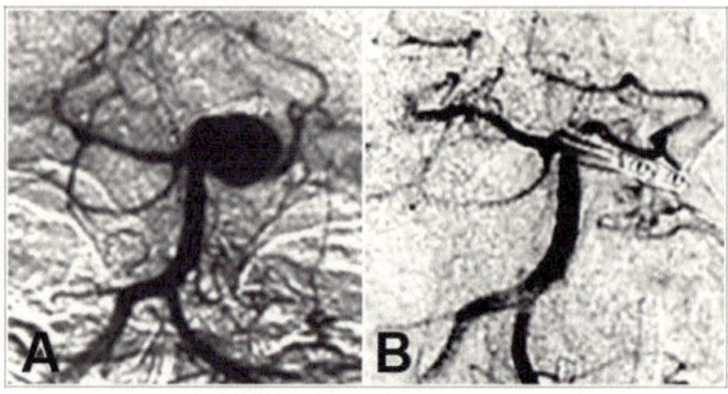


Fig. 9. Preoperative (A) and postoperative (B) angiography of a very large basilar tip aneurysm directed toward the left side, treated through a left fronto-temporo-orbital approach.

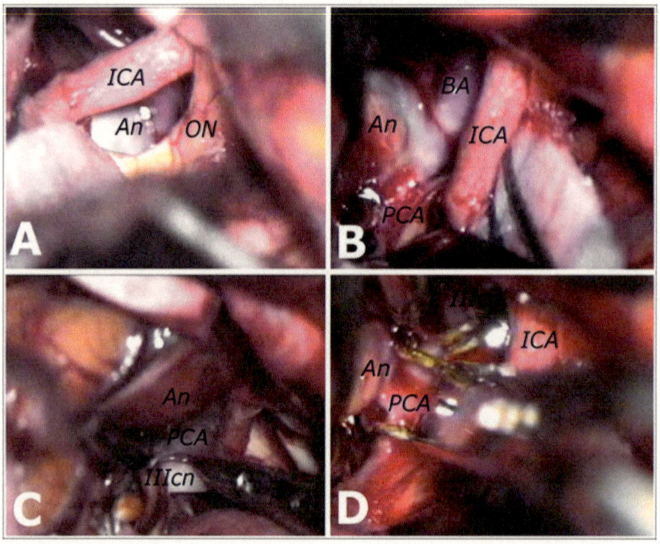


Fig. 10. Intraoperative images of the same case of Fig 9: the aneurysm (An) is visible in the surgical corridor between optic nerve (ON) and internal carotid artery (ICA) (A); changing the direction of view, the aneurysm, the parental basilar artery (BA) and the posterior cerebral artery (PCA) are visualized (B); after the incision of the tentorial edge, the implant base of the aneurysm at the angle between the basilar artery and the posterior cerebral artery is better evidentiated (C); the aneurysm is clipped working laterally to the third cranial nerve (D).

### 2.2.3 Fronto-temporo-orbito-zygomatic approach

The fronto-temporo-orbito-zygomatic (FTOZ) approach has been used in 5 cases of basilar top aneurysm, including a giant one, and in 1 case of BA/SCA aneurysm.

This approach is performed in a two-pieces fashion, exactly as FTO, by adding the resection of the zygomatic arch which is left attached to the masseter muscle [Galzio, 2010]. This approach has been used for lesions located very high with respect to posterior biclinoidal line [Jennett, 1975; Kasdon, 1979; Ikeda, 1991; Bowles, 1995; Sindou, 2001] because both zygomatic arch and orbital roof translocation together allow the complete observation of the implant base and the possibility of manipulating these aneurysms from different directions (Figures 11 and 12).

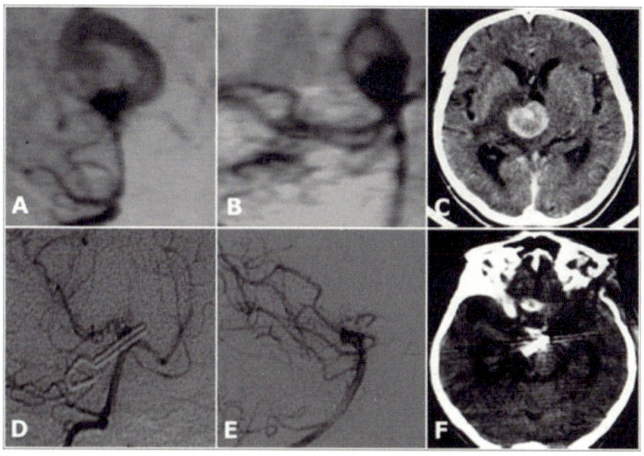


Fig. 11. Preoperative angiography (A,B), preoperative CT scan (C), postoperative angiography (D,E) and postoperative CT scan (F) of a giant basilar tip aneurysm, located high with respect to the posterior biclinoidal line, embedded into the third ventricular room, exposed through a fronto-temporo-orbito-zygomatic approach.

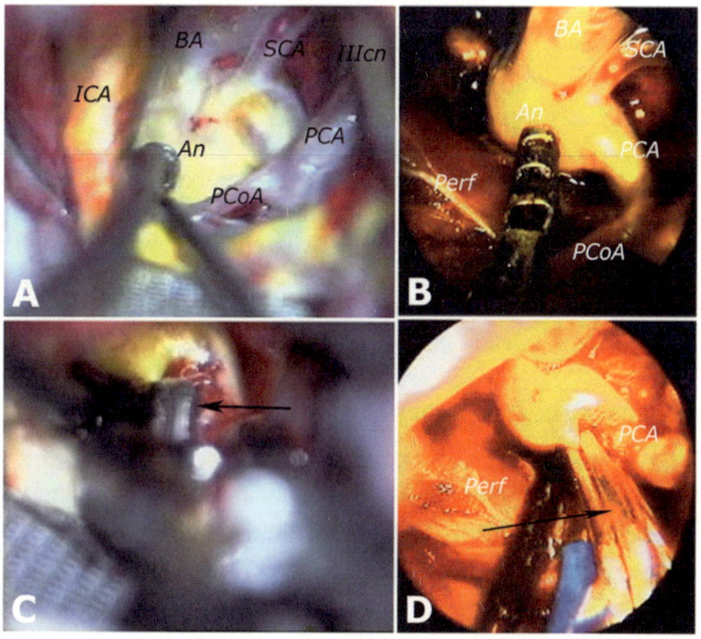


Fig. 12. Intraoperative images (same case of Fig.11): microsurgical images (A,C) and endoscopic images (B,D) performed during the endoscope-assisted microsurgical treatment of a basilar tip aneurysm through a right FTOZ approach; it is clear that the endoscope allows a better panoramic vision of the aneurysm (An) with minimal retraction of the internal carotid artery (ICA) and of the short posterior communicating artery (PCoA) from which a critical perforator (Perf), not visible in pure microscopic vision, enters the mesencephalon; the parental basilar artery (BA) with its distal branches, superior cerebellar artery (SCA) and posterior cerebral artery (PCA), are also better controlled by the endoscope; the scope also allows a better control of the distal portion of the clip (arrows).

### 2.2.4 Retrolabyrinthine presigmoid approach

The retrolabyrinthine transpetrosal presigmoid approach [Lawton, 1997; Motoyama, 2000] has been used in 6 cases of middle basilar artery aneurysm (lesions located at the junction of the basilar artery with anterior inferior cerebellar artery-AICA), none of which was a giant lesion.

The most important point in preparing this approach is the preservation of the labyrinth; in 2 cases we violated the labyrinthine bone with post-operative hearing troubles. This approach gives a tangential sight of the middle basilar trunk and allows an adequate clipping of small and medium sized aneurysms, but provides a very narrow surgical corridor which is not useful for more complex lesions (Figure 13).

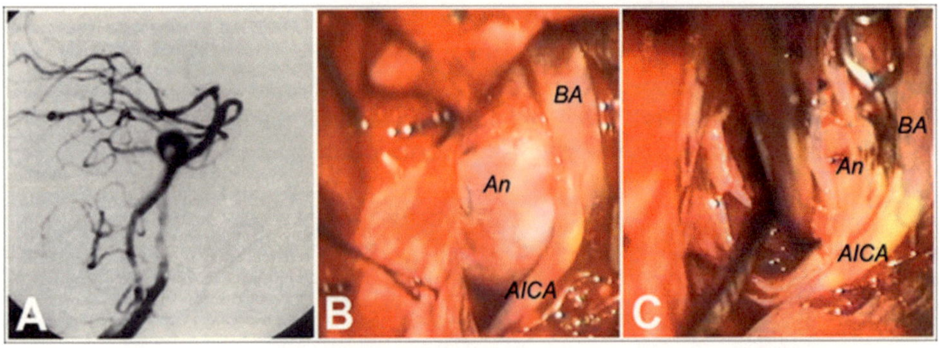


Fig. 13. Preoperative angiography of a large partially thrombosed middle basilar aneurysm (A); intraoperative view of the intact aneurysm (An), exposed through a right retrolabirinthine transpetrosal presigmoid approach, which allows a tangential vision of the lesion originating from the junction between the basilar artery (BA) and the anterior inferior cerebellar artery (AICA) (B); intraoperative image: the aneurysm has been clipped at the implant base and the sac completely opened (C).

### 2.2.5 Combined transpetrosal approach

The combined transpetrosal approach [Kawase, 1985; Seifert, 1996; Seifert, 2003] has been used in 10 cases: 5 complex middle basilar arteries aneurysms (2 of them were giant ones) and 5 aneurysms located in the vertebro-basilar junction (VBJ).

We prepared this approach as described by Fukushima and Sekhar [Harsh, 1992; Fukushima, 1996]. Nowadays we prefer using this approach to treat middle basilar/AICA aneurysms instead of the retrolabyrinthine approach, because it allows a wider working room, where multiple clips can be apposed to treat more complex lesions, and always allows the preservation of the labyrinthine bone (Figure 14). Moreover, we have used this approach in case of junctional aneurysms, specially when the VBJ was high located.

### 2.2.6 Far lateral approach

The far lateral approach has been used in 30 cases: 8 aneurysms in the VBJ, including 3 giant ones, and 22 aneurysms located in the intradural VA (VA/PICA aneurysms), including 3 giant lesions. Multiple variations of this approach have been described [Salas, 1999]: it allows the complete control of the VA along the full length of its intradural portion until the basilar junction.

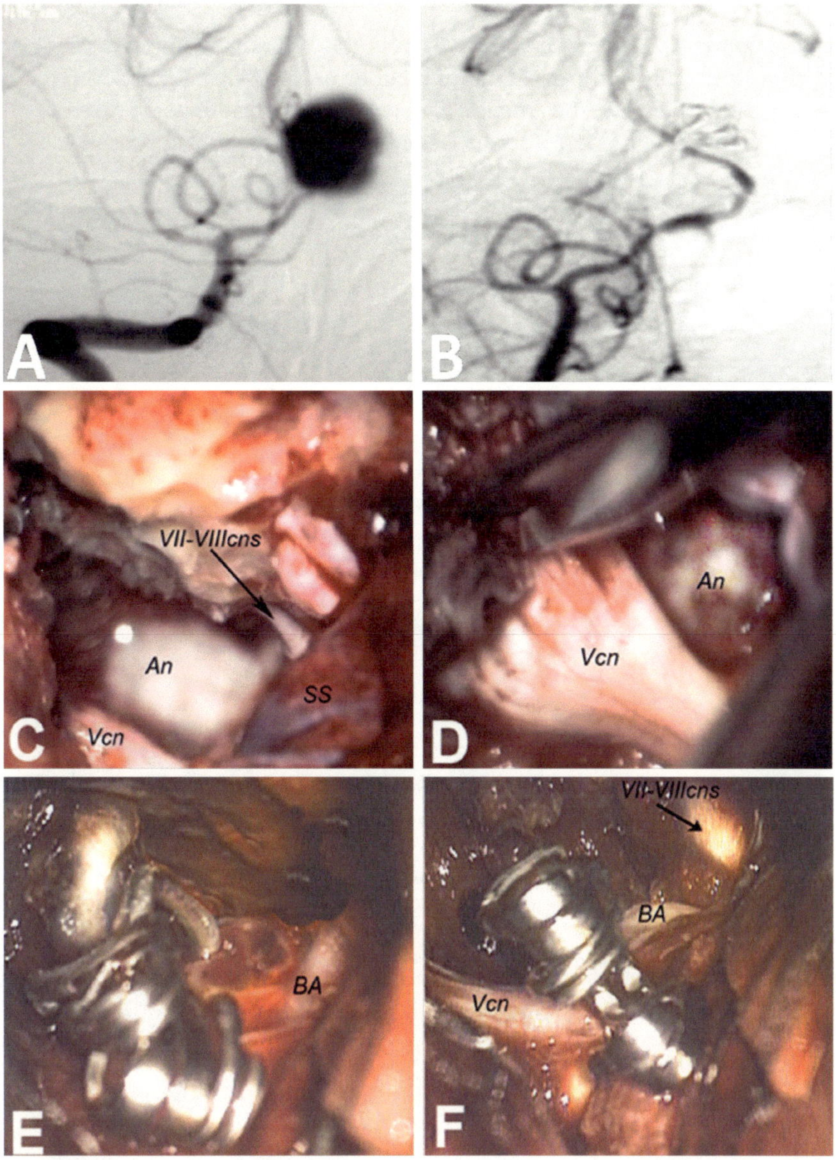


Fig. 14. Preoperative and postoperative angiography of a very large BA/AICA aneurysm, approached through a right combined transpetrosal presigmoid approach (A,B); intraoperative images: the aneurysm (An) is visible after opening the dura located anterior to the sigmoid sinus (SS) deeply embedded between the complex of seventh and eight cranial nerves (VII-VIIIcns) and the fifth cranial nerve (Vcn) which appears flattened by the underlying aneurysm (C,D); intraoperative images: after the definitive clipping with multiple differently shaped and sized clips, the sac was opened, thus highlighting its complete exclusion with preservation of the parental basilar artery (BA) (E,F).

We performed the approach as originally described by B. George, who defines it as the "postero-lateral" approach to the cranio-vertebral junction [George, 1980; Heros, 1986; George, 2000].

The far lateral approach is the ideal choice to treat the VBJ aneurysms because it provides a tangential view of the junction itself with minimal or no cerebellar retraction (Figures 15 and 16). This is specially true when the junction is not very high positioned: in case of high located VB junction or in case of evident platybasia a combined transpetrosal approach is preferable.

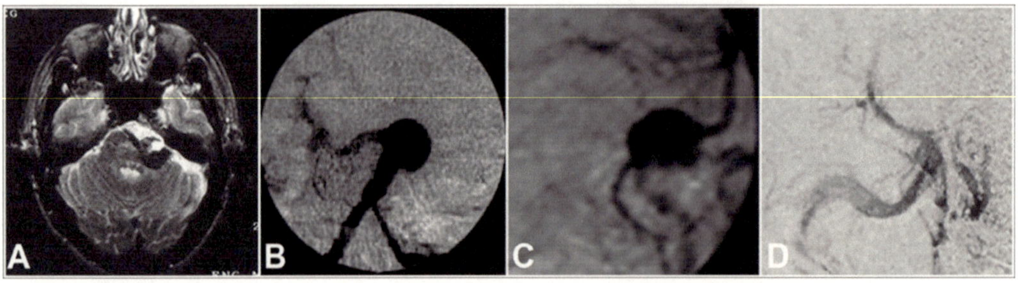


Fig. 15. Preoperative CT scan (A), preoperative angiography (B,C) and intraoperative angiography (D) of a very large aneurysm located at level of the vertebro-basilar junction and prevalently located in the lower portion of the left ponto-cerebellar angle because of the dolichotis deviation of the vertebrobasilar arteries.

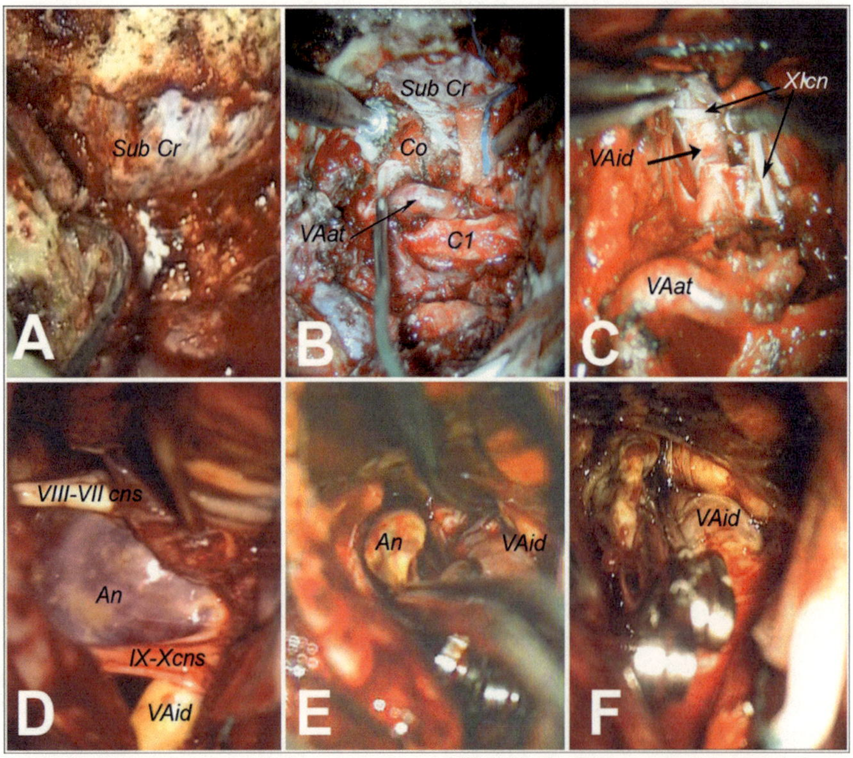


Fig. 16. Intraoperative images of the same case of Fig.15: the lesion was exposed through a right far lateral approach; after skeletonizing the squama occipitalis, the occipital condyle,

the lamina and lateral mass of the first cervical vertebra (C1), a suboccipital craniectomy (sub Cr) is perfomed (A) and the condyle (Co) is partially drilled to expose the atlantal portion of vertebral artery (VAat) (B); after opening the dura, the eleventh cranial nerve (XIcn) and the intradural portion of the left vertebral artery (VAid) are exposed (C); the dissection is superiorly directed and the cerebellar hemisphere is medialized thus displaying the aneurysm (An) embedded between the inferior cranial nerves (IX-X cns) and the facio-uditive complex (VIII-VIIcns) (D); the aneurysm has been clipped with two long straight clips apposed in "tandem" fashion and the sac was opened and shrinked with bipolar coagulation (E,F).

It is also the approach of choice for aneurysms located in the intradural vertebral artery (VA/PICA region), where it may be necessary to dissect the implant base of the aneurysmal wall from the inferior cranial nerves and from PICA; this method provides the complete control of the posterolateral aspect of this kind of aneurysms which is, on the other hand, the real necessity because the VA has not important perforators in its anterior wall in this portion (Figures 19 and 20). This approach allows complete exposure of the implant base of the aneurysm and of the parental artery also in case of lesions deeply located in the midline (Figures 19 and 20) or in case of very large lesions (Figures 17 and 18). Thereafter, it is not necessary, in our opinion, to use an extreme lateral approach as suggested by other authors [Day, 1997].

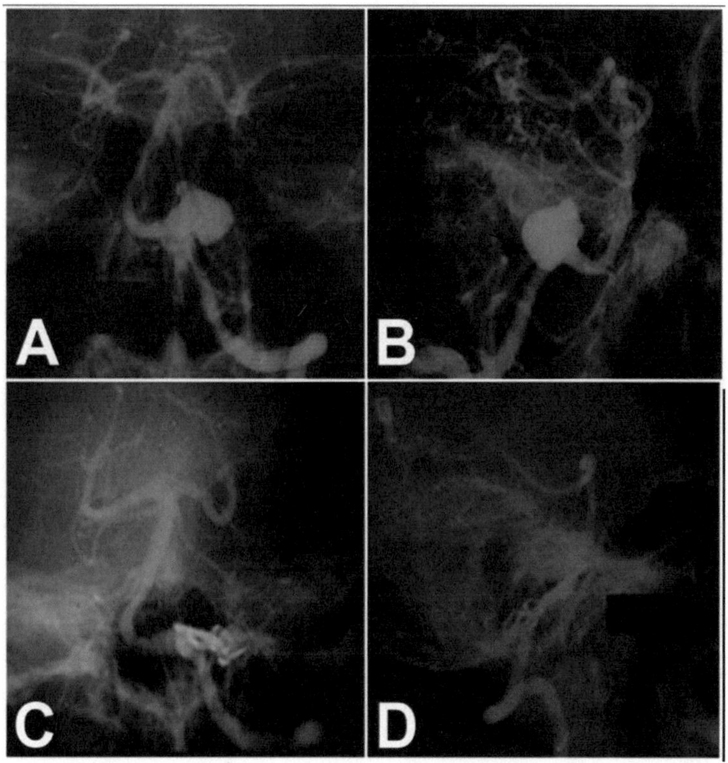


Fig. 17. Preoperative (A,B) and postoperative angiography (C,D) of a multilobulated very large left sided VA/PICA aneurysm.

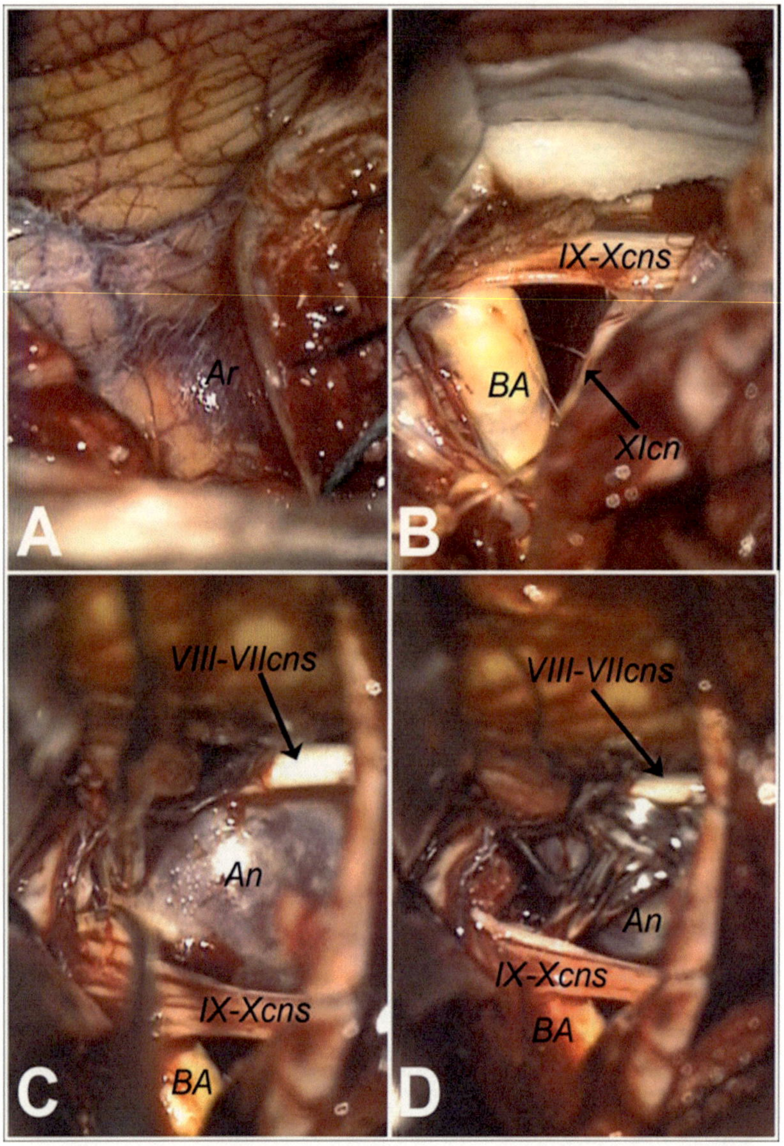


Fig. 18. Intraoperative images of the same case of Fig.17: the lesion was exposed through a left far lateral retrocondylar approach; after opening the dura mater of the posterior cranial fossa, the arachnoid (Ar) of the lateral inferior perimedullary cistern is opened and the spinal accessory nerve (XIcn) as well as the glossopharingeal and vagus nerves (IX-Xcns) and the intradural vertebral artery are exposed (A,B); the cerebellar hemisphere is medialized, evidentiating the aneurysm (An) between the inferior cranial nerves (IX-X cns) and the facio-uditive complex (VIII-VIIcns) (C); the aneurysm has been clipped with two clips parallel to the vertebral artery (D).

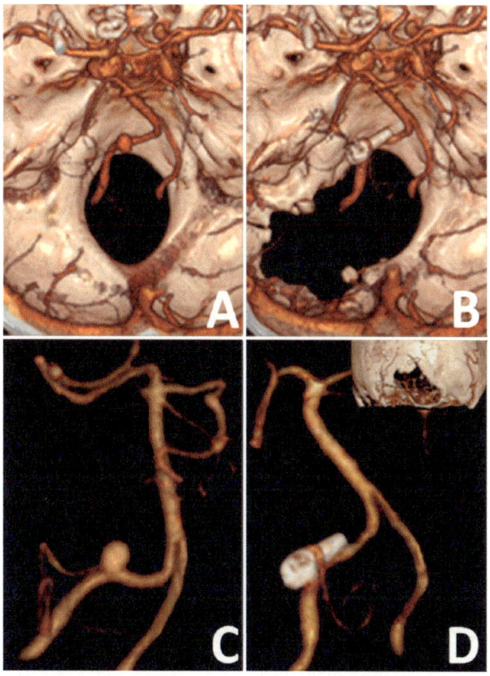


Fig. 19. Preoperative (A,B) and postoperative (C,D) 3D angio-CT reconstructions of a left VA/PICA aneurysm reached through a left far-lateral supracondylar approach. Because of the dolichotis course of the left vertebral artery, the aneurysm was deeply located at the level of the midline; it was exposed and treated with a limited bone removal of the occipital squama, without drilling of the occipital condyle.

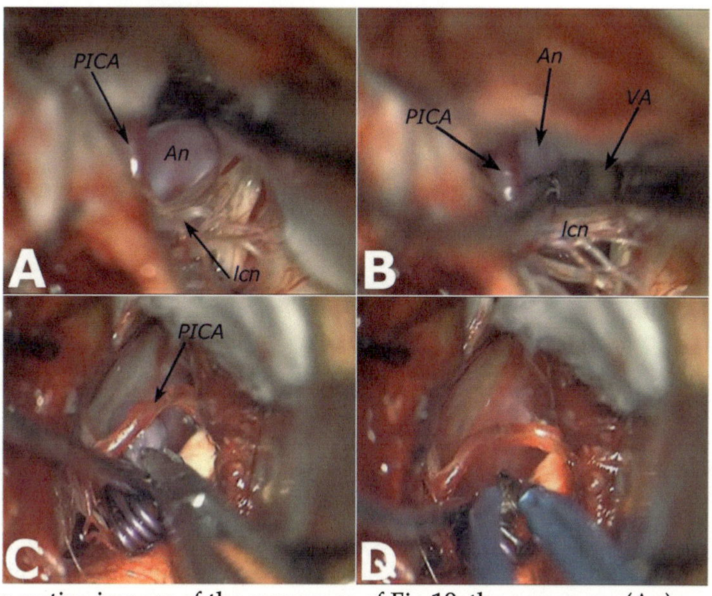


Fig. 20. Intraoperative images of the same case of Fig.19: the aneurysm (An) was exposed through a left far-lateral supracondylar approach, which gives a tangential view of the

aneurismal implant base and allows its dissection from the PICA and the lower cranial nerves (lcn) (A). The aneurysm is mobilized to visualize the prejunctional course of the VA (B). The clip was positioned parallel to the course of the VA, preserving the PICA: thereafter the sac is opened with microscissors and shrunk with bipolar coagulation (C,D).

### 2.2.7 Subtemporal approach

The sub-temporal approach has been used in the treatment of 5 aneurysms located in the P1/P2 and P2/P3 tracts of the PCA (4 of them were giant lesions) and of 3 aneurysms located in the distal portion of the SCA (none of them was a giant one).

To gain a wide subtemporal working room it may be necessary to dissect the vein of Labbè subpially to avoid stretching of the vein itself which can leave postoperative infarctions. To highlight the distal portion of PCA/SCA it is necessary to section the medial tentorial edge; this maneuver has to be performed posteriorly to the entrance of the 4th CN into the tentorium itself (Figure 21).

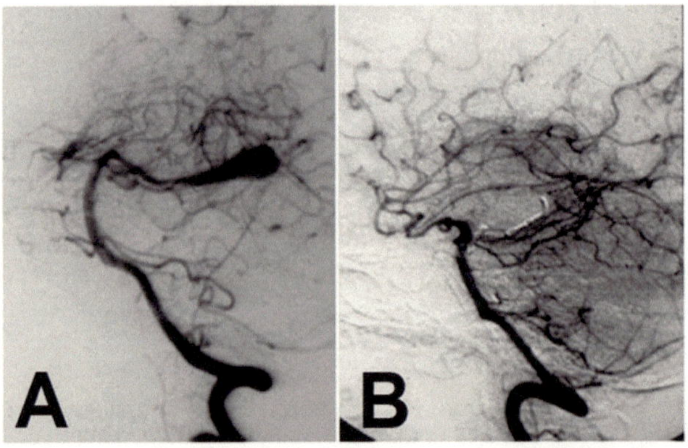


Fig. 21. Preoperative(A) and postoperative angiography (B) of a giant partially thrombosed aneurysm of the P2-P3 tract of the right posterior cerebral artery.

It has to be remarked that in three cases of giant massively thrombosed aneurysms of the distal portion of the PCA, the lesions were excluded by trapping with no additional postoperative deficit (Figures 21 and 22).

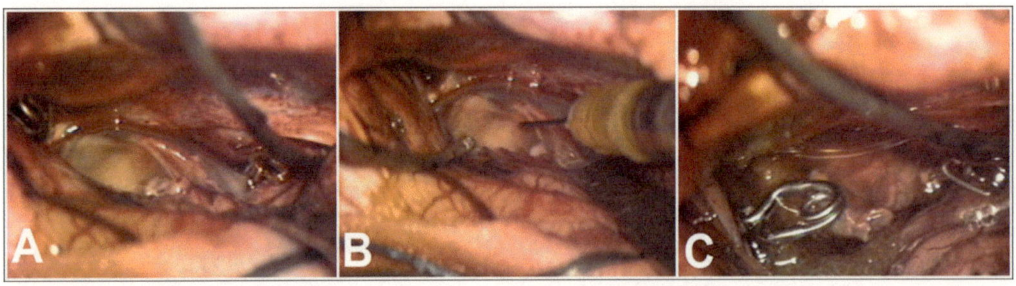


Fig. 22. Intraoperative images of the same case of Fig.21: the lesion was treated through a right subtemporal approach; the temporal lobe is retracted and the aneurysm exposed and trapped between two clips (A), evacuated (B) and completely opened (C).

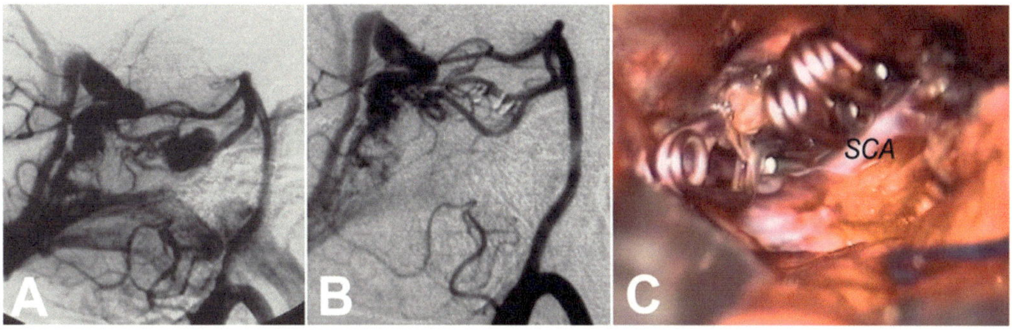


Fig. 23. Preoperative(A), postoperative angiography (B) and intraoperative image (C) of a large aneurysm of the distal portion of the superior cerebellar artery (SCA), excluded with multiple cerebral clips thus preserving flow in the parental artery. In the angiograms it is visible an artero-venous malformation partly irrorated by the SCA, where the aneurysm was located, which was successively treated by a suboccipital approach.

### 2.2.8 Retrosigmoid approach

The retrosigmoid approach has been used to treat a giant completely thrombosed aneurysm located in the premeatal portion of the AICA (Figure 24) and of an aneurysm of the labyrinthine artery, intrameatally located and thus requiring the drilling of the posterosuperior wall of the meatus to be exposed (Figure 25) [Zotta, 2011]. It has also been used in 1 case of BA/AICA aneurysm, but for this kind of lesion this approach seems inadequate because it only provides a narrow opening with an angle of attack parallel to the petrous bone with a limited exposure of the anterolateral wall of the basilar tract.

### 2.2.9 Suboccipital approach

The suboccipital approach has been used in the treatment of 2 aneurysms located in the distal portion of the PICA. The telovelar corridor has allowed to clip an aneurysm deeply embedded into the lateral recess of the fourth ventricle (Figures 26 and 27) [Kellogg, 1997; Mussi, 2000].

## 3. Discussion

The impressive advances of the endovascular technique have progressively shifted the management of intracranial aneurysms away from direct microsurgical clipping. Both the International Subarachnoid Aneurysm Trial (ISAT) [Molineux, 2001] and the International Study of Intracranial Aneurysms (ISUIA) [ISUIA, 1998] have reported better outcomes with endovascular coiling if compared with microsurgical clipping. In any case, the conclusions of these studies are significant only for aneurysms whose anatomy was suitable for both techniques and this is not the case for most of posterior circulation aneurysms. Only 58 patients from the cohort of 2143 patients enrolled in the ISAT harboured vertebro-basilar aneurysms and among the 7416 excluded patients, those with posterior circulation aneurysms had an anatomical configuration not equally suitable for both clipping and coiling or had factors excluding therapeutic equipoise. Also data regarding vertebro-basilar aneurysms reported in the ISUIA showed an apparent therapeutic advantage of coiling only in the treatment of large and very large (13-24 mm in diameter) aneurysms. Thereafter, neither ISAT nor ISUIA have definitively reported a clear evidence that endovascular therapy is superior to microsurgical clipping for posterior circulation aneurysms. A revision of follow-up data from ISAT has highlighted decreased rebleeding and potentially more favourable results for younger patients (less than 40 year old) treated by microsurgery [Mitchell, 2008].

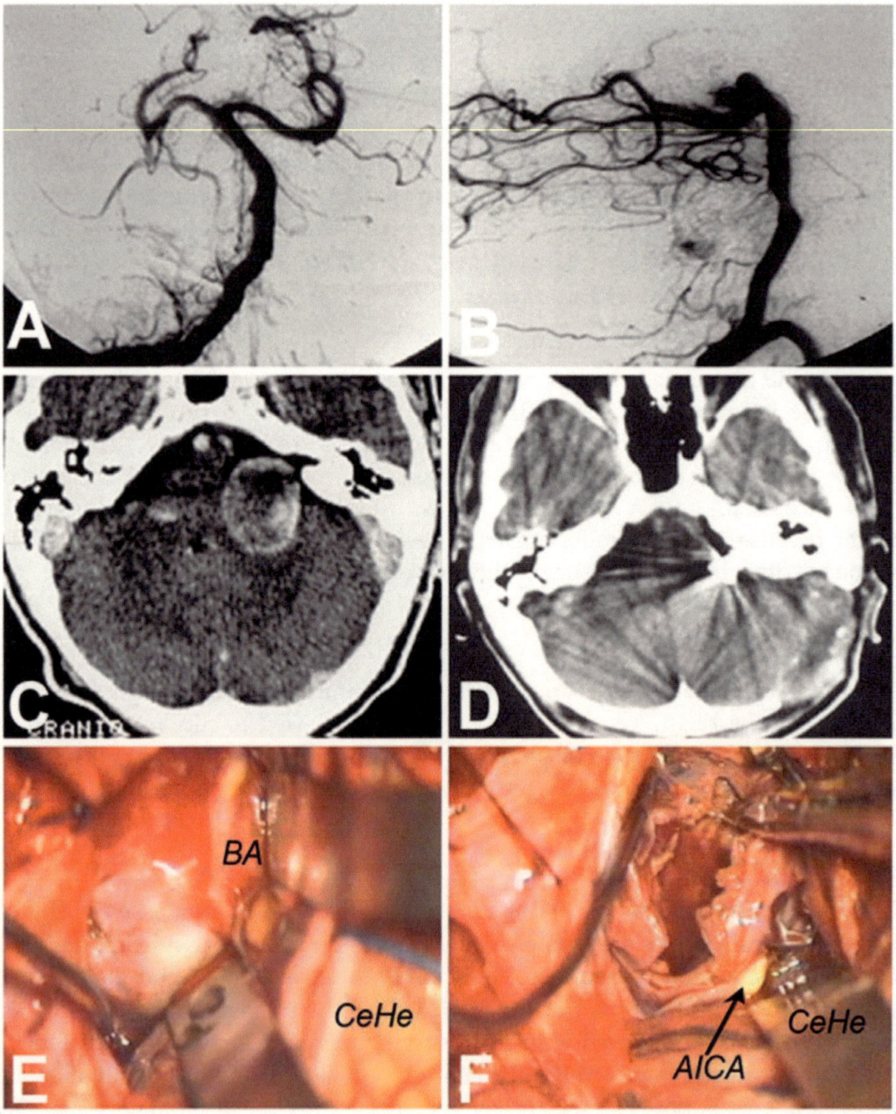


Fig. 24. Preoperative angiography(A,B), preoperative and postoperative CT scan (C,D) and intraoperative images of a giant thrombosed aneurysm of the AICA after its origin from the basilar artery (BA), which was clipped and opened through a left retrosigmoid approach. The aneurysm mimicked, clinically, a vestibular schwannoma and its exposure required a certain degree of retraction of the left cerebellar hemisphere (CeHe).

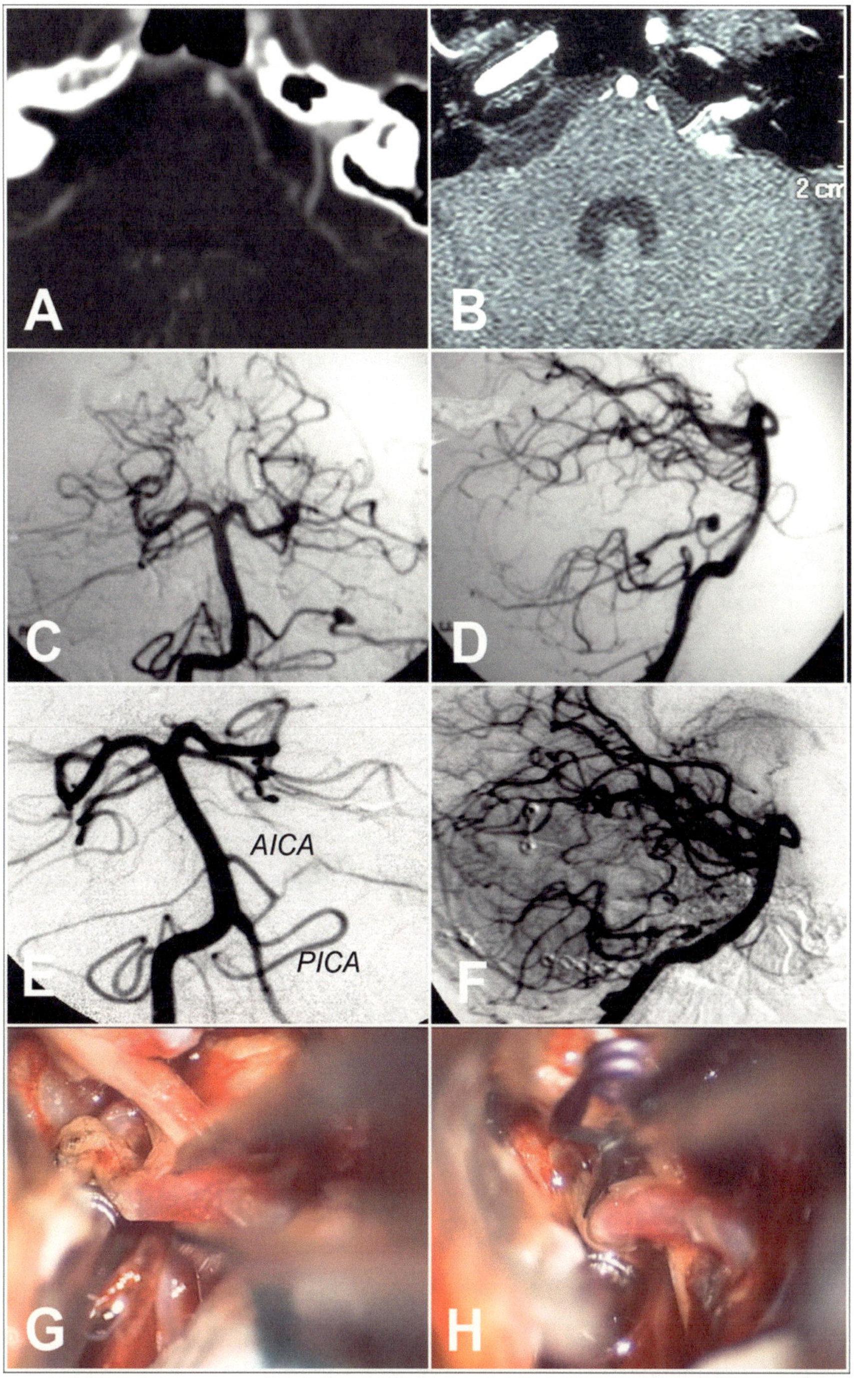


Fig. 25. Preoperative angio-CT (A), preoperative MRI (B), preoperative angiography (C,D), postoperative angiography (E,F) and intraoperative images of a distal AICA aneurysm, located intrameatally, which was treated through a left retrosigmoid approach; exposure of the aneurysmal sac required drilling of the posterior wall of the internal acoustic meatus.

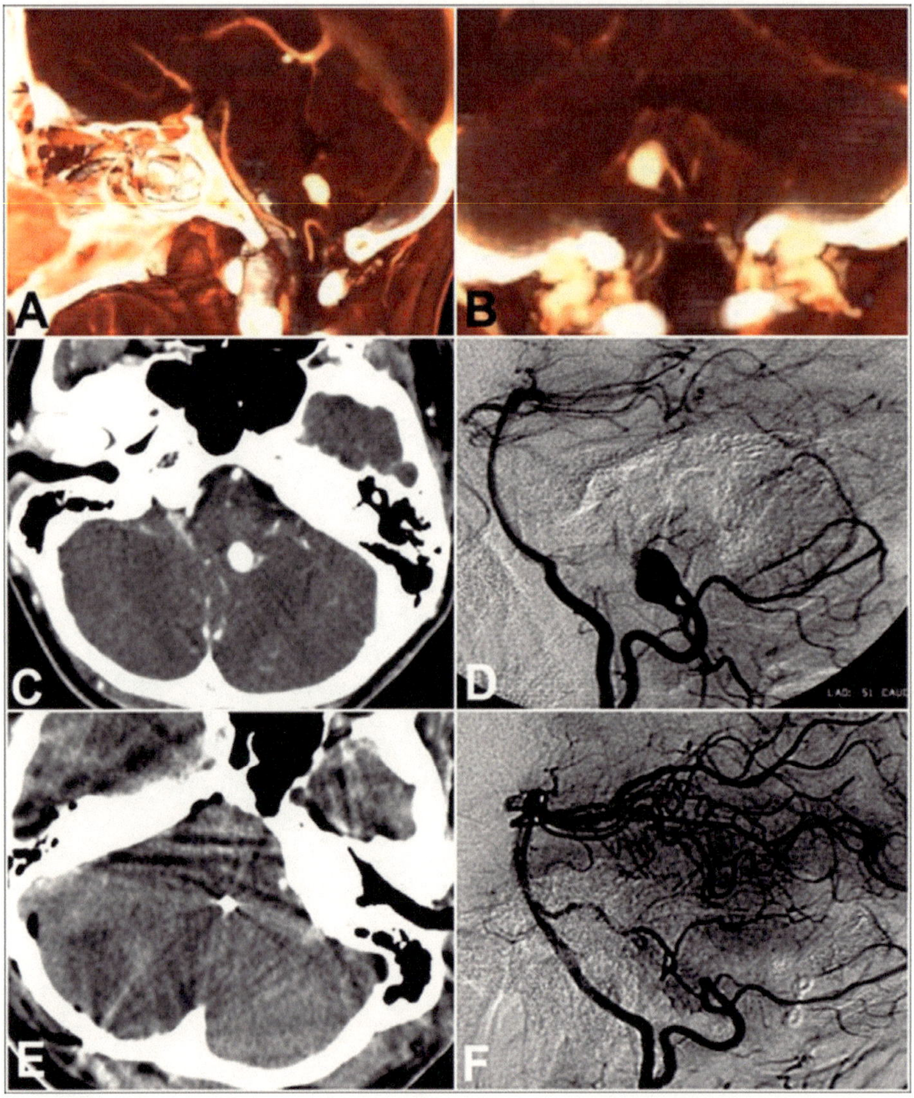


Fig. 26. Preoperative angio-CT sagittal and coronal reconstructions (A,B), preoperative angio-CT scan (C), preoperative angiography (D), postoperative CT scan (E) and postoperative angiography (F) of a large, wide based, aneurysm of the distal portion of the right PICA, deeply embedded into the left lateral recess of the fourth ventricle, which was approached through a suboccipital telovelar approach.

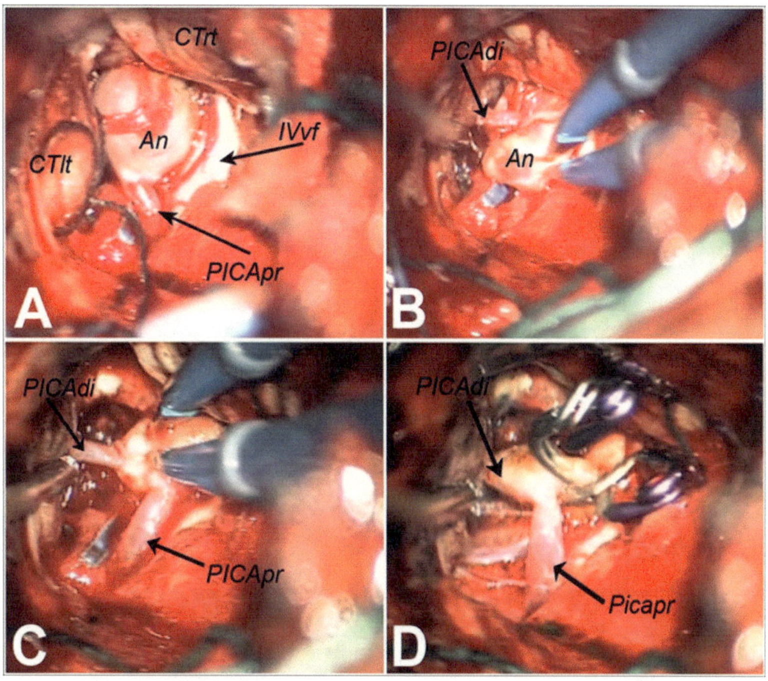


Fig. 27. Intraoperative images of the same case of Fig.26: the left cerebellar tonsil (CTlt) and the right cerebellar tonsil (CTrt) have been upward mobilized and divaricated to expose the floor of the fourth ventricle (IVvf) and the aneurysm (An), which presents an almost fusiform shape, with the proximal portion of the parental branch of the right posterior inferior cerebellar artery (PICApr) entering the lesion in full channel (A); the aneurysm is shrunk using the bipolar coagulator to reconstruct an implant base (B,C), where two embricated clips are definitively apposed, with preservation of flow in the post-aneurismal.

In the last two decades, new endovascular devices and special methodologies for device use have been introduced and reported, thus allowing the treatment of very complex cases. Wide-necked basilar tip aneurysms can be treated using two stents inserted from the basilar artery into each posterior cerebral artery in a Y-configuration to allow stent-assisted coil embolization [Chow 2004, Perez-Arjona 2004, Thorell 2005]; flow-diverting stents allow aneurysm occlusion without the addition of coils also in cases of wide-necked vertebro-basilar lesions [Lylyk 2009, Fischer 2011] (Figure 28). Several advances have been achieved with microsurgery, from the adoption of skull base approaches to the use of intraoperative digital subtraction angiography and indocyanine green angiography; use of intraoperative ultrasonography and neurophysiological monitoring may prevent ischemic complications; endoscopic assistance allows a better control of clipping (Figures 29 and 30). Indirect microsurgical treatment by revascularization and parental vessel occlusion and combined microsurgical and endovascular management allow the treatment of very complex aneurysms with satisfactory outcomes.

Recent papers have shown that microsurgery remains an important and unavoidable method of treatment, especially in cases of particularly located or shaped lesions [Fraser 2011, Sekhar, 2011]. The specific role of microsurgery remains essential and has not be abandoned also for posterior circulation aneurysms [Sanai, 2008].

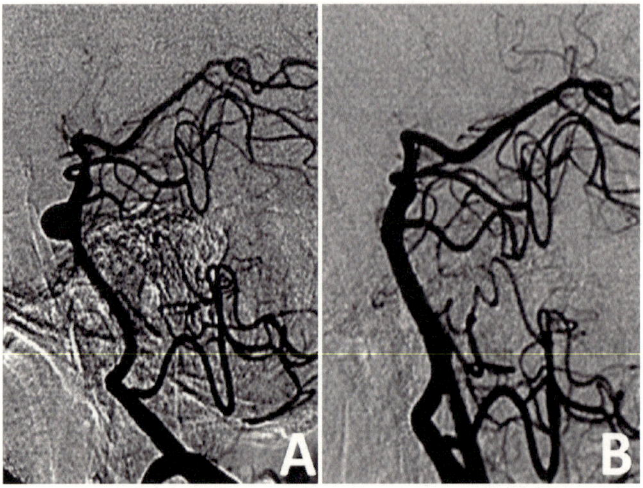


Fig. 28. Preoperative (A) and postoperative (B) angiography of a wide-necked mid-basilar aneurysm treated through flow diverter stenting.

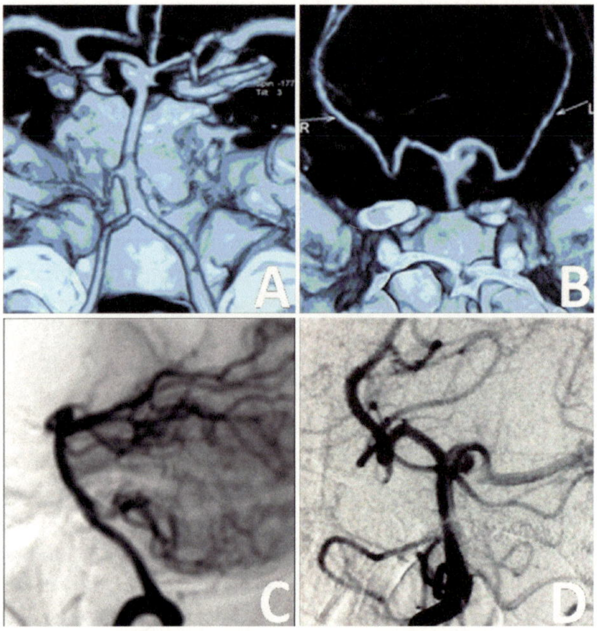


Fig. 29. Preoperative angio-CT reconstructions (A,B) and preoperative angiograms (C,D) of an aneurysm of the left PCA/SCA junctional portion of the basilar artery.

On the other hand, better surgical results can only be achieved in dedicated and specialized centers treating a high volume of cases, with a multidisciplinary cerebrovascular team where microsurgical and endovascular expertise cooperate in an integrated and collaborative way [Peschillo 2011].

In this chapter, the Authors present results and surgical approaches used in 144 patients harbouring 150 aneurysms of the posterior circulation, microsurgically treated over a period of 20 years (January 1990 - December 2010). This report is based on the experience of the Senior Author (RG), who has been involved in neurovascular surgery since 1978. Endovascular therapy was routinely introduced in our Institution at the end of the Nineties and consequentially almost all cases treated before 2000 were managed by direct microsurgical approach, while endovascular therapy has been progressively used more frequently during the second decade, so that the number of surgically treated patients has progressively reduced, while the percentage of surgical procedures for complex aneurysms has relatively increased.

A comparison between endovascular and microsurgical treatment of posterior circulation aneurysms goes beyond the aims of this paper and, because of the long period of time considered, some of the cases of the presented series would not be treated nowadays by direct microsurgery. However, from this experience, we have learned a number of lessons that can be summarized in some helpful suggestions..

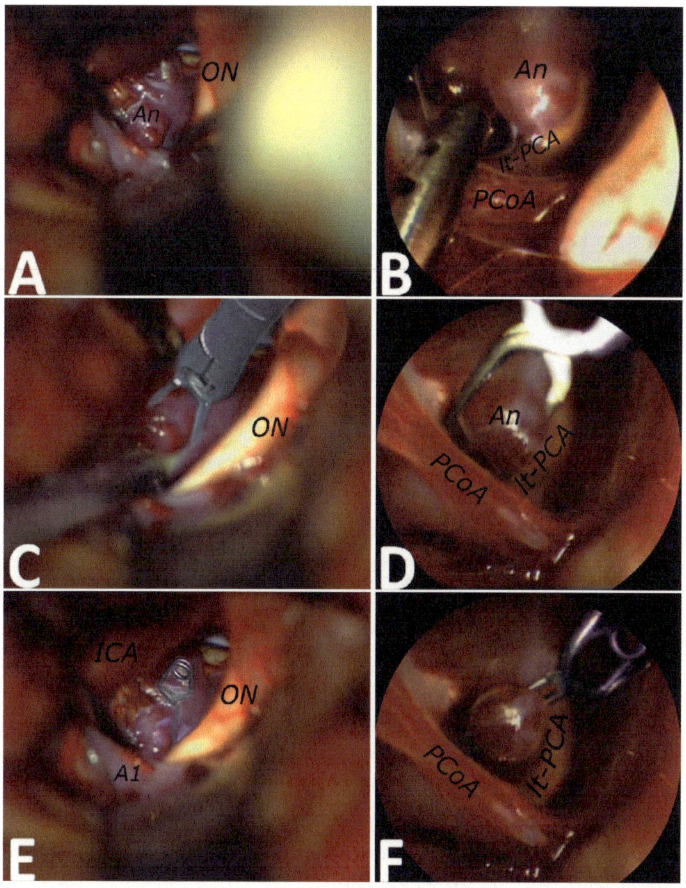


Fig. 30. Intraoperative images of the same case of Fig. 29. The aneurysm has been approached through a left pterional approach (the patient had been operated 1 year before elsewhere for a right ICA bifurcation aneurysm). The aneurysm was exposed under microscopic vision, passing in the corridor between ON and ICA: exposure of the lesion required excessive distortion of the ICA (A). A handheld upward-oriented 30°-scope was

used to explore the anatomical situation of the aneurismal sac and its relationship with the surrounding neurovascular structures (B). The aneurysm was clipped passing the clip applier through the corridor between ON and ICA, with the scope attached to a mechanical holder for control of surgical maneuvers (C,D). The final endoscopic control allowed to confirm patency of the left PCA which was not clearly visible under the microscope (E,F). [An: Aneurysm; ON: optic nerve; ICA: internal carotid artery; PCoA: posterior communicating artery; lt-PCA: left posterior cerebral artery; A1: A1 tract of the left anterior cerebral artery].

## 4. Expert suggestions

Each patient harbouring an intracranial aneurysm, both if located in the anterior or in the posterior circulation, has to be evaluated on individual basis by a cerebral vascular team with multidisciplinary expertise.

Decision making is essentially depending on aneurysms intrinsic features and patient's condition, but also patient's preferences and institutional specific expertise can influence the therapeutic choice. Location, morphology and size of the aneurysm, presence of branches originating from the implant base or from the sac, intraluminal thrombosis, atheromasic changes are all factors to be considered, as it is for patient's symptomatologies and comorbidities.

Treatment considerations are different for ruptured and unruptured aneurysms. There is no doubt that patients with ruptured aneurysms should be treated, because of the high incidence of rebleeding in the first days after the initial haemorrhage; aneurysms with a favorable dome-to-neck ratio (≥2) can be usually treated by coil; stent- or balloon-assisted coiling can be used for aneurysms with a relatively large neck (dome-to-neck ratio: 1.5-2); aneurysms with aberrant arterial branches and very small ones most frequently have to be treated by direct surgery; dissecting and fusiform aneurysms have to be treated by alternative or combined surgical techniques (i.e. diversion by-pass with surgical or endovascular parent vessel occlusion); flow-diverting stents can not be used in haemorrhagic patients because of the need to maintain these patients on dual antiplatelet therapy, which also inhibits other brain related surgeries (i.e. ventriculostomies or decompression). These general rules have especially to be applied to vertebro-basilar aneurysms. For unruptured aneurysms, the decision about to treat or to observe is crucial, also considering that posterior circulation aneurysms are more prone to rupture than their counterpart in the anterior circulation (ISAT). Flow-diverting stents can be used to treat not haemorrhagic aneurysms, also with unfavourable dome-to-neck ratio, when located in non-junctional areas as in the basilar trunk. When aneurysms are equally suitable for clipping or coiling, patient's preference has to be kept into account: patients who are unwilling to have seriated follow-up angiographies are not good candidates for endovascular treatment, as also are patients unable to such follow-up procedures because of contrast medium intolerance. Patient's age and location of the aneurysm represent the main factors to be considered in choosing the most appropriate treatment. Younger patients are preferred surgical candidates, while older ones and subjects with important comorbidities are preferably treated by endovascular technique. In our institution, lesions located in the distal vertebro-basilar branches are mostly treated by direct microsurgery, while basilar trunk, vertebro-basilar junction and vertebral artery aneurysms are mostly managed through an endovascular approach. Distal basilar lesions are treated by direct surgery when efferent branches are incorporated in the sac and when massive tumor-like expansive symptomatology is present. Also small aneurysms, especially if located in the tract between the origin of the superior cerebellar artery and the origin of the posterior cerebral artery are preferentially treated by microsurgery. Blister aneurysms, if occasionally found, are observed.

Nowadays we use dynamic multislice CT angiography (MSCTA) as primary preoperative study for all intracranial aneurysms, because this non invasive procedure provides quick 3D volumetric imaging with comparable sensitivity to rotational digital subtraction angiography (DSA), also allowing the disclosure of calcifications in the walls of the arteries or in the sac. Rotational 3D DSA is sometimes used, in addition, for more complex cases in which dynamic flow assessment is needed.

When the direct microsurgical treatment appears to be the best therapeutic option, the choice of the adequate approach constitutes the key point to get the best access and exposure to posterior circulation aneurysms. The use of the principles of the skull base surgery, which means to electively remove bone structures to minimize manipulation and retraction of critical perilesional neurovascular structures, allows the possibility to work in an adequate working room controlling both the lesion and the parental and efferent arteries from different angles of vision.

Most of distal basilar artery aneurysms can be exposed through a conventional pterional approach; in effect, this approach can be considered the first described skull base approach because the original description by Yasargil [Yasargil 1984] conceived drilling of the sphenoid wing exactly to avoid retraction of the fronto-temporal structures and to reduce manipulation of the neurovascular structures located in the basal cisterns. The cranio-orbital approaches are used only for most complex cases: wide lesions laterally directed require a fronto-temporo-orbital approach, while lesions located high to the biclinoidal line require a fronto-temporo-orbito-zygomatic approach. Aneurysms located in basilar trunk can be, as previously described, exposed through a retrolabyrinthine presigmoid approach or through a combined transpetrosal approach; nowadays we prefer this last approach because the first one provides a very small working room and exposes to higher risks of labyrinthine structures impairment; moreover, most of the small lesions that can be treated through the retrolabyrinthine approach are nowadays better managed endovascularly. On the contrary, the most complex lesions that have to be treated by direct microsurgery require a larger exposition, that only can be provided by the combined transpetrosal approach.

Even though, in the first period of our experience, we have used the combined transpetrosal approach in the treatment of vertebro-basilar junction aneurysms, nowadays we expose this kind of lesions exclusively through the far lateral approach, which is simpler and less challenging for the sigmoid sinus; the combined transpetrosal approach remains an option only in cases of very high located vertebro-basilar junction or of patients with evident platybasia. The far lateral approach remains the ideal approach also for vertebral artery aneurysms; when used for aneurysms, this approach does not require drilling of the condyle and thereafter occipito-cervical stabilization is not required.

Aneurysms located distally to the origin of the PCA and of the SCA are treated through the subtemporal approach, while distal AICA aneurysms are treated through the retrosigmoid approach, which is performed as described by Lawton [Quiñones-Hinojosa, 2006]; the median/paramedian sub-occipital approach is used for the treatment of distal PICA aneurysms [Kellogg, 1997; Mussi, 2000].

Nowadays we routinely use neurophysiological monitoring (BAEPs, SSEPs, MEPs) during posterior circulation aneurysms surgery. EEG monitored burst suppression is employed when temporary trapping or clipping of the parental vessel is performed [Quiñones-Hinojosa, 2004; Isley, 2009]. Monitoring of the facial nerve is performed when AICA's aneurysms are treated.

Neuronavigation is used whenever we perform a transpetrosal or a far lateral approach: it allows a safer localization of the venous structures (sigmoid sinus and jugular vein) that can be endangered during the preparation of the approaches as well as a safer exposition of the parental vessel and of the aneurysms itself.

Post-operative angiography is normally performed in any case, about six month after the surgical procedure.

## 5. Conclusion

The choice of the adequate approach constitutes the key point to get the best access and exposure to VB circulation aneurysms. The use of the principles of skull base surgery, which means to electively remove bony structures to minimize manipulation and retraction of perilesional neurovascular structures, allows the possibility to work in a wide working room thus controlling both the lesion and the parent and the efferent arteries, from different angles of vision. Obviously an adequate planning and a skilful experience with every possible additional technique and methodology are required for better outcomes.

## 6. References

Akdemir H, Oktem IS, Tucer B, Menkü A, Başaslan K & Günaldi O (2006): Intraoperative microvascular Doppler sonography in aneurysm surgery. *Minim Invasive Neurosurg* Vol. 49, No. 5, pp. 312-6;

Baussart B, Aghakhani N & Tadié M (2005): [Temporary vessel occlusion]. *Neurochirurgie* Vol. 51, No. 1, pp. 23-36;

Bowles AP, Kinjo T & Al-Mefty O (1995): Skull base approaches for posterior circulation aneurysms. *Skull Base Surg* Vol. 5, No. 4, pp. 251-60;

Coscarella E, Vishteh AG, Spetzler RF, Seoane E & Zabramski JM (2000): Subfascial and submuscular methods of temporal muscle dissection and their relationship to the frontal branch of the facial nerve. Technical note. *J Neurosurg* Vol. 92, No. 5, pp. 877-80;

Chow MM, Woo HH, Masaryk TJ &Rasmussen PA (2004): A novel endovascular treatment of a wide-necked basilar apex aneurysm by using a Y-configuration, double-stent technique. *Am J Neuroradiol* Vol 25, pp. 509–512;

Dashti R, Laakso A, Niemelä M, Porras M & Hernesniemi J (2009): Microscope-integrated near-infrared indocyanine green videoangiography during surgery of intracranial aneurysms: the Helsinki experience. *Surg Neurol* Vol. 71, No. 5, pp. 543-50;

Day JD, Fukushima T & Giannotta SL (1997): Cranial base approaches to posterior circulation aneurysms. *J Neurosurg* Vol. 87, pp. 544–554;

de Oliveira JG, Borba LAB, Rassi-Neto A, de Moura SM, Sanchez-Júnior SL, Rassi MS, de Holanda CVM, & Giudicissi-Filho M (2009): Intracranial aneurysms presenting with mass effect over the anterior optic pathways: neurosurgical management and outcome. *Neurosurg Focus* Vol. 26, No. 5, E3;

Dolenc VV, Skrap M, Sustersic J, Skrbec M & Morina A (1987): A transcavernous-transsellar approach to the basilar tip aneurysms. *Br J Neurosurg* Vol. 1, No. 2, pp. 251-9;

Fischer S, Vajda Z, Aguilar Perez M, Schmid E, Hopf N, Bäzner H & Henkes H (2011): Pipeline embolization device (PED) for neurovascular reconstruction: initial experience in the treatment of 101 intracranial aneurysms and dissections. *Neuroradiology – In press;*

Fraser JF, Smith MJ, Patsalides A, Riina HA, Gobin YP & Stieg PE (2011): Principles in Case-Based Aneurysm Treatment: Approaching Complex Lesions Excluded by International Subarachnoid Aneurysm Trial (ISAT) Criteria. *World Neurosurg* Vol. 75, No. 3/4, pp. 462-475;

Fujitsu K & Kuwabara T (1985): Zygomatic approach for lesions in the interpeduncular cistern. *J Neurosurg* Vol. 62, No. 3, pp. 340-3;

Fukushima T, Day JD & Hirahara K (1996): Extradural total petrous apex resection with trigeminal translocation for improved exposure of the posterior cavernous sinus and petroclival region. *Skull Base Surg* Vol. 6, No. 2, pp. 95- 103;

Galzio RJ & Tschabitscher M (2010): Endoscope-assisted microneurosurgery: Principles, Methodology and Applications. Karl Storz, Tuttlingen;

Galzio RJ, Ricci A & Tschabitscher M (2010): The orbitozygomatic approach. In Cappabianca (ed): Atlas of cranio-facial and skull base approach. Springer Verlarg, New York;

George B & Laurian C (1980): Surgical approach to the whole lenght of the vertebral artery with special reference to the third portion. *Acta Neurochir* Vol. 51. No. 3, pp. 259-72;

George B (2000): Surgical approaches to the foramen magnum. In Robertson JT, Coakham HB, Robertson JH (eds.): Cranial Base Surgery. London, Churchill-Livingstone, pp 259-281;

Giannotta & Steven L (2002): Ophthalmic Segment Aneurysm Surgery. *Neurosurgery* Vol. 50, No. 3, pp. 558-562;

Harsh GR & Sekhar LN (1992): The subtemporal, transcavernous, anterior transpetrosal approach to the upper brainstem and clivus. *J Neurosurg* Vol. 77, No. 5, pp. 709-17;

Heros RC (1986): Lateral suboccipital approach for vertebral and vertebrobasilar artery lesions. *J Neurosurg* Vol. 64, No. 4, pp. 559-62;

Hosobuchi Y (1979): Direct surgical treatment of giant intracranial aneurysms. *J Neurosurg* Vol. 51, No. 6, pp. 743-56;

Ikeda K, Yamashita J, Hashimoto M & Futami K (1991): Orbitozygomatic temporopolar approach for a high basilar tip aneurysm associated with a short intracranial internal carotid artery: A new surgical approach. *Neurosurgery* Vol. 28, pp. 105–110;

Inao S, Kuchiwaki H, Hirai N, Gonda T & Furuse M (1996): Posterior communicating artery section during surgery for basilar tip aneurysm. *Acta Neurochir (Wien)* Vol. 138, No. 7, pp. 853-61;

Isley MR, Edmonds HL Jr, Stecker M (2009); Guidelines for intraoperative neuromonitoring using raw (analog or digital waveforms) and quantitative electroencephalography: a position statement by the American Society of Neurophysiological Monitoring. *J Clin Monit Comput* Vol. 23, No. 6, pp. 369-390;

ISUIA investigators (1998): Unruptured intracranial aneurysms - risk of rupture and risks of surgical intervention. *N Engl J Med* Vol. 339, pp. 1725-1733;

Jennett B & Bond M (1975): Assessment of outcome after severe brain damage. A practical scale. *Lancet* Vol. 1, pp. 480– 484;

Kalavakonda C, Sekhar LN, Ramachandran P & Hechl P (2002): Endoscope-assisted microsurgery for intracranial aneurysms. *Neurosurgery* Vol. 51, No. 5, pp. 1119-26;

Kapsalaki EZ, Lee GP, Robinson JS 3rd, Grigorian AA & Fountas KN (2008): The role of intraoperative micro-Doppler ultrasound in verifying proper clip placement in intracranial aneurysm surgery. *J Clin Neurosi* Vol. 15, No. 2, pp. 153-7;

Kasdon DL & Stein BM (1979): Combined supratentorial and infratentorial exposure for low-lying basilar aneurysms. *Neurosurgery* Vol. 4, pp. 422–426;

Kato Y, Sano H, Imizu S, Yoneda M, Viral M, Nagata J & Kanno T (2003): Surgical strategies for the treatment of giant or large intracranial aneurysms: our experience with 139 cases. *Min Inv Neurosurg* Vol. 46, No. 6, pp. 339-43;

Kawase T, Toya S, Shiobara R & Mine T (1985): Transpetrosal approach for aneurysms of the lower basilar artery. *J Neurosurg* Vol. 63, pp. 857-861;

Kellogg JX & Piatt JH Jr (1997): Resection of fourth ventricle tumors without splitting the vermis: the cerebellomedullary fissure approach. *Pediatr Neurosurg* Vol. 27, No. 1, pp. 28-33;

Lawton MT, Daspit CP & Spetzler RF (1997): Technical aspects and recent trends in the management of large and giant midbasilar artery aneurysms. *Neurosurgery* Vol. 41, No. 3, pp. 513-20;

Lawton MT & Spetzler RF (1998): Surgical strategies for giant intracranial aneurysms. *Neurosurg Clin N Am* Vol. 9, pp. 725-42;

Lemole GM Jr, Henn JS, Zabramski JM & Spetzler RF (2003): Modifications to the orbitozygomatic approach. A technical note. *J Neurosurg* Vol. 99, No. 5, pp. 924–930;

Levy ML, Day JD & Giannotta SL (1995): Giant aneurysms of the paraclinoid ophthalmic segment of the internal carotid artery: intradural approaches. In Awad IA, Barrow DL (eds): Giant Intracranial Aneurysms. Park Ridge, AANS; pp 131-142;

Lylyk P, Miranda C, Ceratto R, Ferrario A, Scrivano E, Luna HR, Berez AL, Tran Q, Nelson PK & Fiorella D (2009): Curative endovascular reconstruction of cerebral aneurysms with the pipeline embolization device. *Neurosurgery* Vol. 64, pp. 632-643;

Mitchell P, Kerr R, Mendelow AD & Molyneux A (2008): Could late rebleeding overturn the superiority of cranial aneurysm coil embolization over clip ligation seen in the International Subarachnoid Aneurysm Trial? *J Neurosurg* Vol. 108, pp. 437-442;

Molyneux A, Kerr R, Stratton I & Holman R (2001): International Subarachnoid Aneurysm Trial (ISAT) of neurosurgical clipping versus endovascular coiling in 2143 patients with ruptured intracranial aneurysms: a randomised trial. *Lancet* Vol. 360, pp. 1267-1274;

Motoyama Y, Ohnishi H, Koshimae N, Kanemoto Y, Kim YJ, Yamada T & Kobitsu K (2000): Direct clipping of a large basilar trunk aneurysm via the posterior petrosal (extended retrolabyrinthine presigmoid) approach-case report. *Neurol Med Chir (Tokyo)* Vol. 40, No. 12, pp. 632-6;

Mussi A & Rhoton AL Jr (2000): Telovelar approach to the fourth ventricle: microsurgical anatomy. *J Neurosurg* Vol. 92, pp. 812–823;

Noguchi A, Balasingam V, Shiokawa Y, McMenomey SO & Delashaw JB Jr (2005): Extradural anterior clinoidectomy. Technical note. *J Neurosurg* Vol. 102, No. 5, pp. 945-50;

Oikawa S, Mizuno M, Muraoka S, Kobayashi S (1996): Retrograde dissection of the temporalis muscle preventing muscle atrophy for pterional craniotomy. Technical article. *J Neurosurg* Vol. 84, No. 2, pp 297-299;

Perez-Arjona E, Fessler RD (2004): Basilar artery to bilateral posterior cerebral artery'Y stenting' for endovascular reconstruction of wide-necked basilar apex aneurysms: report of three cases. *Neurol Res* Vol. 26, pp. 276-281;

Peschillo S & Delfini R (2011): Endovascular neurosurgery in Europe and in Italy: what is in the future? *World Neurosurg - In press;*

Quiñones-Hinojosa A, Alam M, Lyon R, Yingling CD, Lawton MT (2004): Transcranial motor evoked potentials during basilar artery aneurysm surgery: technique application for 30 consecutive patients. *Neurosurgery* Vol. 54, No. 4; pp. 916-924;

Quiñones-Hinojosa A, Chang EF, Lawton MT (2006): The extended retrosigmoid approach: an alternative to radical cranial base approaches for posterior fossa lesions. *Neurosurgery* Vol. 58, No. 4(2), pp. 208-214;

Raabe A, Nakaji P, Beck J, Kim LJ, Hsu FP, Kamerman JD, Seifert V & Spetzler RF (2005). Prospective evaluation of surgical microscope-integrated intraoperative near-infrared indocyanine green videoangiography during aneurysm surgery. *J Neurosurg* Vol. 103, No. 6, pp. 982-9;

Salas E, Sekhar LN & Ziyal IM (1999): Variations of the extreme lateral craniocervical approach: anatomical study and clinical analysis of 69 patients. *J Neurosurg* Vol. 90, pp. 206–219;

Samii M & Turel KE (1985): Possibility of the excision of aneurysms in the vertebrobasilar system followed by end-to-end anastomosis for the maintenance of circulation. *Neurol Res* Vol. 7, No. 1, pp. 39-45;

Sanai N, Tarapore P, Lee AC & Lawton MT (2008): The current role of microsurgery for posterior circulation aneurysms: a selective approach in the endovascular era. *Neurosurgery* Vol. 62, No 6, pp. 1236-49;

Sato S, Sato M, Oizumi T, Nishizawa M, Ishikawa M, Inamasu G & Kawase T (2001): Removal of anterior clinoid process for basilar tip aneurysm: clinical and cadaveric analysis. *Neurol Res* Vol. 23, No. 4, pp. 298-303;

Sekhar LN, Ramanathan D, Hallam DK, Ghodke BV & Kim LJ (2011): What is the correct approach to aneurysm management in 2011? *World Neurosurg* Vol. 75, No. 3/4, pp. 409-411;

Seifert V, Raabe A & Zimmermann M (2003): Conservative (labyrinth-preserving) transpetrosal approach to the clivus and petroclival region: indications, complications, results and lessons learned. *Acta Neurochir (Wien)* Vol. 145, No. 8, pp. 631-42;

Seifert V & Stolke D (1996): Posterior transpetrosal approach to aneurysms of the basilar trunk and vertebrobasilar junction. *J Neurosurg* Vol. 85, No. 3, pp. 373-9;

Sharma BS, Gupta A, Ahmad FU, Suri A & Mehta VS (2008): Surgical management of giant intracranial aneurysms. *Clin Neurol Neurosurg* Vol. 110, No. 7, pp. 674-81;

Sindou M, Emery E, Acevedo G & Ben David U (2001): Respective indications for orbital rim, zygomatic arch and orbito- zygomatic osteotomies in the surgical approach to central skull base lesions. Critical, retrospective review in 146 cases. *Acta Neurochir (Wien)* Vol. 143, No. 10, pp. 967–975;

Taniguchi M, Takimoto H, Yoshimine T, Shimada M, Miyao Y, Hirata M, Maruno M, Kato A, Kohmura E & Hayakawa T (1999): Application of a rigid endoscope to the microsurgical management of 54 cerebral aneurysms: results in 48 patients. *J Neurosurg* Vol. 91, No. 2, pp. 231-7;

Taylor CL, Selman WR, Kiefer SP & Ratcheson RA (1996): Temporary vessel occlusion during intracranial aneurysm repair. *Neurosurgery* Vol. 39, No. 5, pp. 893-905;

Thorell WE, Chow MM, Woo HH, Masaryk TJ & Rasmussen PA (2005): Y-configured dual intracranial stent assisted coil embolization for the treatment of wide necked basilar tip aneurysms. *Neurosurgery* Vol. 56, pp. 1035-1040;

Yasargil MG, Antic J & Laciga R (1976): Microsurgical pterional approach to aneurysms of the basilar bifurcation. *Surg Neurol* Vol. 3, pp. 7-14;

Yasargil MG (1984): Interfascial pterional (frontotemporosphenoidal) craniotomy. In Yasargil MG (eds): Microneurosurgery. New York, Georg Thieme Verlag, Vol. 1, pp. 217-220;

Zabramski JM, Kiris T, Sankhla SK, Cabiol J & Spetzler RF (1998): Orbitozygomatic craniotomy. Technical note. *J Neurosurg* Vol. 89, No. 2, pp. 336–341;

Zotta DC, Stati G, De Paulis D & Galzio RJ (2011): Intrameatal aneurysm of the anterior inferior cerebellar artery. *J Clin Neurosci* Vol. 18, No. 4, pp. 561-563.

# 13

# Endovascular Approaches to the Carotid Cavernous Sinus for Endovascular Treatment of Carotid Cavernous Fistulas and Hormone Sampling

Akira Kurata
*Kitasato University School of Medicine*
*Japan*

## 1. Introduction

### 1.1 Venous morphology of the cavernous sinus

A precise knowledge of the venous morphology of the carotid cavernous sinus is essential in order to choose the appropriate access routes to the cavernous sinus. The sinus is trabeculated and subdivided in compartments. Newton and Potts 1 mentioned two parts, the anterior and posterior part. The anterior receives blood from the superior ophthalmic vein (SOV), inferior ophthalmic vein (IOV), sphenoparietal sinus and superficial middle cerebral vein (sylvian vein). We prospectively investigated the morphology of the cavernous sinus in recent ten consecutive dural carotid cavernous fistula (CCF) patients treated using three dimensional (3D) coils. All CCFs of our series except two were mainly under the internal carotid artery. According to our findings, we divided all cavernous sinuses into three compartments: the antero-lateral; intermediate; and postero-medial (Fig 1). The antero-lateral compartment combined with the postero-medial compartment make up the anterior part of Newton and Potts 1. The antero-lateral compartment receives blood as mentioned above and sometimes from the olfactory vein and deep middle cerebral veins. The intermediate compartment receives blood from the pterigoid plexus. The postero-medial compartment corresponds to the posterior part of Newton and Potts 1. The postero-medial compartment mainly receives blood from the inferior petrosal sinus (IPS). The two cavernous sinuses communicate with each other by way of coronary (anterior and posterior intercavernous) sinuses anteriorly and occipital transverse sinus posteriorly.

### 1.2 Transvenous approaches to the CS

Transvenous approaches to the carotid cavernous sinus are used for endovascular treatment of carotid cavernous fistulas (CCFs) and venous hormone sampling [2,3]. Various kinds of venous approaches have been reported: the inferior petrosal sinus (IPS) route was the first established and most commonly used [4-6], especially for venous hormone sampling[2,3]. When the ophthalmic vein [7-20], superior petrosal sinus (SPS) [21] and pterigoid plexus (PP) [22] are involved in venous drainages of CCFs, each venous channel may become an appropriate access route.

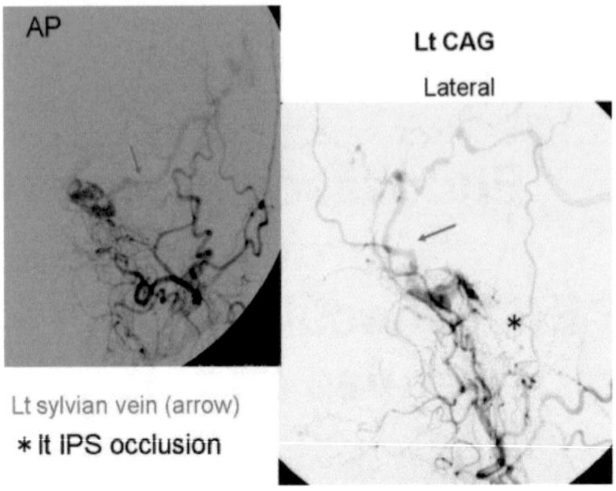


Fig. 1A. Left carotid angiogram (lt CAG) (AP: anteroposterior view, lateral: lateral view) showing a dural CCF draining into the sylvian vein only (arrow) and occlusion of the left inferior petrosal sinus (IPS) (*)

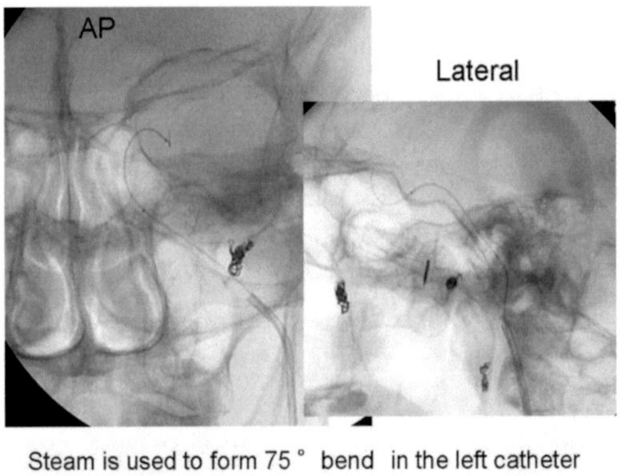


Fig. 1B. Skull radiograph (AP: anteroposterior view, lateral: lateral view) showing the running of the inferior petrosal sinus (IPS) with the aid of a microcatheter and catheter.

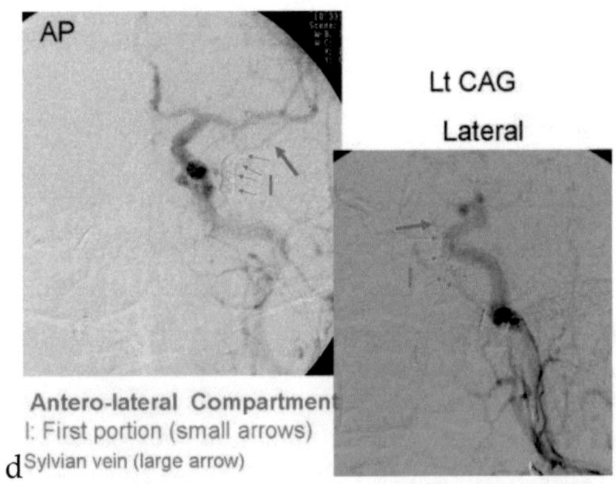


Fig. 1C. Left carotid angiogram (CAG)(AP: anteroposterior view, lateral: lateral view) showing the antero-lateral compartment(I: First portion) of the cavernous sinus (4 small arrows) and sylvian vein (large arrow)

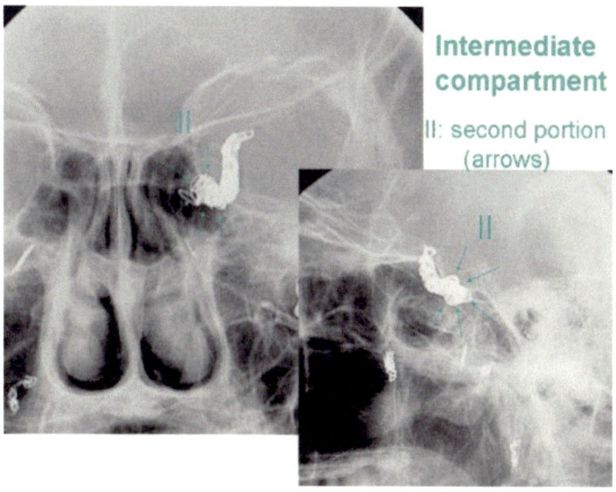


Fig. 1D. Skull radiograph (left: anteroposterior view, right: lateral view) showing the intermediate compartment (II: second portion) (arrows) of the cavernous sinus.

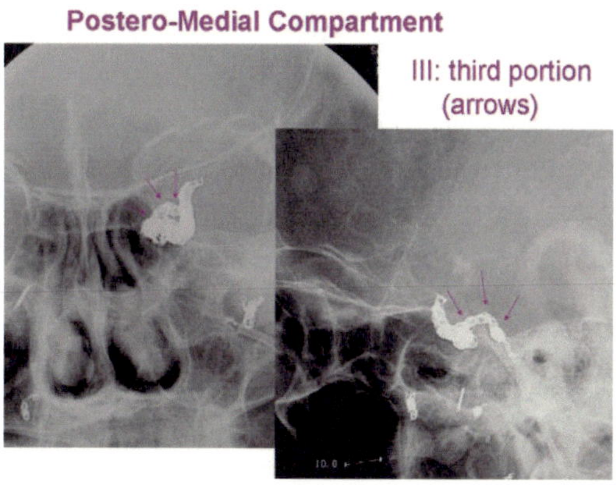


Fig. 1E. Skull radiograph (left: anteroposterior view, right: lateral view) showing the posteromedial compartment (III: third portion) (arrows) of the cavernous sinus

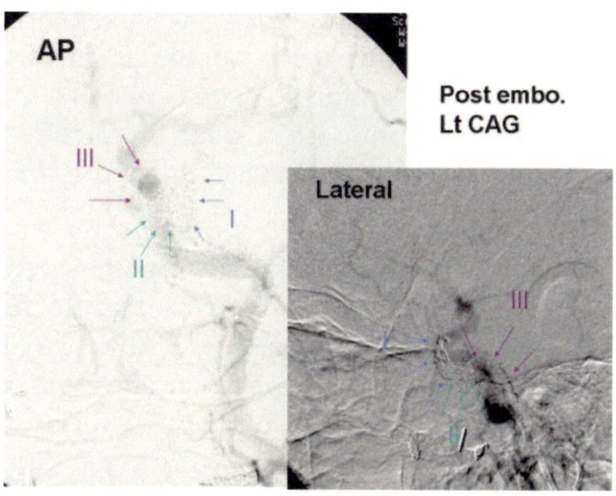


Fig. 1F. Left carotid angiogram (CAG)(AP: anteroposterior view, lateral: lateralview) showing the three compartments of the cavernous sinus(I: first portion=antero-lateral compartment, II: second portion=intermediate compartment, III: third portion=postero-medial compartment)

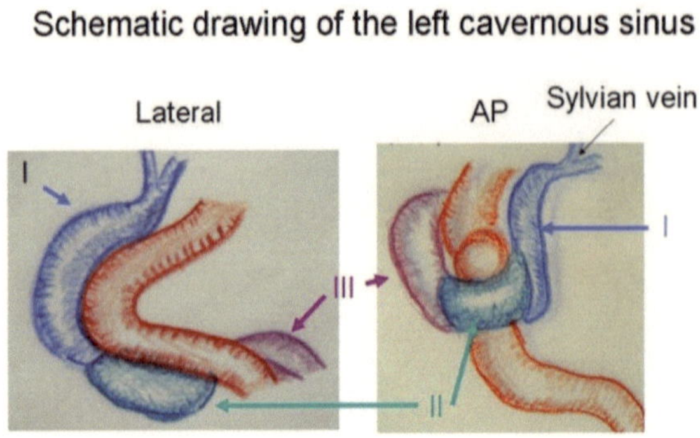


I: first portion(antero-lateral compartment)
II: second portion (intermediate compartment)
III: third portion (postero-medial compartment)

Fig. 1G.

## 2. Alternative approaches

1. Transvenous approach to the carotid-cavernous via the inferior petrooccipital vein
2. Direct puncture approach to the extraconal portion of the superior ophthalmic vein

## 3. Indications and contraindications of each procedure

The transvenous approach via the IPS [4-6] for dural CCF and hormone sampling [2,3] from the cavernous sinus is the standard access route. However, when there is obstruction of the IPS or other problem such as non-communication with the jugular vein, other venous drainage routes should be attempted. Benndorf G, et al [5] described that a thrombosed IPS may also become an alternative transvenous approach route for dural CCFs, reporting four cases and a review of the literature. Obstructions caused by secondarily formed thrombi which are not organized or old may allow introduction of a microcatheter preceded by a guide wire.

However, when the obstruction of the IPS is stiff with an organized old thrombus [11], the another access route to the cavernous sinus is needed. In our series, with two (cases 1 and 2) (11%) of 18 dural CCF patients the conventional venous approach via the IPS failed [23]. These two patients were referred to our institute more than 1 year after development of initial symptoms, which may have contributed to obstruction of the IPS with an organized old thrombus.

Shiu et al.[24] described that the IPS does not join the IJV, sometimes emptying directly into the anterior condylar vein (7%). Mitsuhashi et al. [25] demonstrated the IPS drainage directly into the vertebral plexus with no connection to the IJV in 3/83 sides (3.6%) and the IPS was absent in 14/ 83 sides (16.9%). In our series also, absence of connection with the IJV was noted in one (10%) of 10 venous sampling procedures from the cavernous sinus in five patients [23].

Yamashita et al [6] reported complications occurring in 7 of 16 patients with TVE. One was epidural extravasation from perforation of the inferior petrosal sinus. Major complications especially will occur in cases with cortical venous reflux. Araki et al.[26] reported such a case featuring extravasation from the uncal vein during TVE for SOV and IOV via the IPS. They emphasized that it is important to obliterate the cortical venous drainage as early as possible, even if the reflux is small. Watanabe et al [27] reported a patient with a dural CCF in whom the cavernous sinus received normal cortical venous drainage from the insular vein. Nakamura et al.[28] emphasized preservation of sylvian venous flow because the affected cavernous sinus received not only the shunted flow but also sylvian venous drainage in three cases (12%) of 26 dural CCFs.

Targeting TVE using minimum coils may become an ultimate treatment after being first established by TAE useful to reduce the arterial inflow and the affected lesions. In dural CCF patients, bilateral cavernous sinuses and also ICS are often widely involved [29] which is important to chose the right treatment strategy. In dural CCF patients with wide involvement of the sinuses (bilateral CS and bilateral CS &ICS types), especially with a cortical venous reflux, TAE for initial reduction of inflow has been recommended as a reasonable approach to avoid serious complications because of the comparative non-aggressive nature of the disease. Kupersmith et al [30] reported complications in 5 of 38 cases with dural CCF by TAE, but four of these were due to IBCA treatment. Particles provides safer emboli compared with liquid matertial. In our series of TAE using only particles, no complications were encountered [31]. Repeated provocative testing and care of dangerous anastomoses are also important to avoid untoward outcome.

When the SOV route is accessible it may be the first choice. However, the distal roots of the SOV often show focal narrowing and tortuosity, which make difficulty in the conventional transvenous approach via the SOV difficult. Direct exposure of the SOV roots under general anesthesia is widely used [7-14], but may be complicated. Direct exposure may damage the superior root of the fifth nerve resulting in numbness of the forehead [17]. Furthermore, it may also cause palsy of the superior levator muscle resulting in palpebral ptosis

Direct-puncture approach to the intraconal portion of the SOV has been reported in the literature [13, 15-20]. This method is a useful in cases with a dilated SOV only within the intraconal segment, according to the thrombosed branches of the SOV [17]. However, the possibility of damage to the optic nerve, cranial nerves III-VI and ophthalmic arterial divisions needs to be taken into account. With deep-puncture (the posterior third of the SOV [17], the posterior half of the SOV [18], the superior orbital fissure [19] to the SOV) precise access and prevention of bleeding from the puncture point is usually difficult. Massive retro-orbital bleeding may occur and result in an untoward increase of orbital pressure [13].

It is recommended that dural CCF patients without aggressive symptoms, aged more than 70 years, classified as Barrow type B [32], and/or with slow flow and mild inflow into the cavernous sinus be conservatively treated because spontaneous cure is not rare. In our series, eleven out of 76 dural CCF patients were selected for this option, three being aged more than 70 years old. Five others were classified as Barrow type B and the remaining three demonstrated slow and mild inflow. All lacked aggressive symptoms like decrease of visual acuity, severe retro-orbital pain or cranial nerve palsies. Radiological findings revealed no cortical venous reflux. In 9 of the 11, all except one fistulas were completely occluded on MRA after 1months to 13 years 5 months (average: 5 years 3 months). One patient was still exhibited a residual fistula on follow-up angiography 1 year after the initial symptoms. Another was complicated with central retinal thrombosis during follow-up period and the other 2 patients were lost to follow-up.

Dural CCF patients with aggressive symptoms and or cortical venous reflux on angiography are indicated for reduction of arterial inflow first by TAE followed by TVE.

For the high flow CCF patients with a traumatic and/or aneurysmal nature, urgent treatment with TVE or TAE via the internal carotid artery [33] is recommended because hemorrhage and /or congestive infarction may occur frequently in the early clinical course.

## 4. Key steps for each procedure

### i. IPS approach [4-6]

The IPS enters the anteromedial aspect of the internal jugular vein (IJV), approximately 2mm in diameter, about 6mm inferior to the level of the entrance of the jugular foramen. It courses just lateral to the clivus, along the posterior inferior edge of the petrous ridge. The right IPS runs at an acute angle and left at an obtuse angle. Steam is used to form 95 °bend in a right catheter (Fig 1B) and 75 °bend in a left catheter 2. Shiu et al. 24 described four types of variation of the junction between the IPS and the internal jugular vein (IJV), on the basis of their experience with cavernous sinus venography. In type I, the IPS anastomosis with the IJV and the anterior condylar vein is small or absent (45%). In type II, the anterior condylar vein is large and there is a prominent anastomosis of this vessel with the IPS (24%). In type III, the IPS exists as several small channels, which may form a plexus (24%). In type IV, the IPS does not join the IJV, emptying directly into the anterior condylar vein (7%) (Fig 2). Mitsuhashi et al 25 evaluated morphological aspects of the caudal end of the IPS using 3D rotational venography and described IPS drainage into the jugular bulb in only one /83 sides (1.2%), the remainder draining into the IJV below the jugular bulb. The IPS was found to drain directly into the vertebral plexus with no connection to the IJV in 3/83 sides (3.6%) and the IPS was absent in 14/ 83 sides (16.9%).

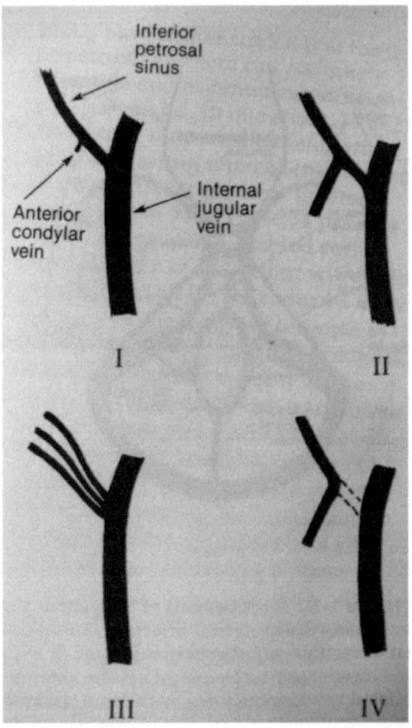


Type I : 45%,
Type II: 24%
Type III: 24%
Type IV: 7%

Fig. 2A. Schematic drawing of the four variation of the junction between the IPS and the IJV (Shiu et al.[7])

ii. **SPS approach** [21]

For the CCF patients mainly draining into the SPS, this approach will become useful. However, the SPS receives the petrosal vein, so that with advancement of the microcatheter attention should be paid not to disturb this fragile vein. In the majority of the cases with hemorrhage in the posterior fossa, cortical venous drainages from the petrosal vein through the SPS is recognized. Coaxial navigation of the microcatheter through a 4F catheter (Cerulean 4F catheter, Medikit Co.ltd., Japan) may be useful for dvancement to the cavernous sinus (mentioned in detail as Explicative case).

**iii. Contralateral cavernous sinus approach**

This is available approach for bilateral or the type of dural CCFs with drainage mainly into the contralateral IPS, SPS or pterigoid plexus [22].

iv. **SOV, IOV approach**[7-20]

Approaches via direct puncture approach to the SOV and IOV and through the SOV from the dilated superficial temporal vein or division of external jugular vein are limited to CCF patients with comparative high flow drainages mainly inflowing into the SOV and/ or the inferior ophthalmic vein (IOV).

Initially the IPS approach should be tried as the most appropriate approach because it is comparative large and stiff with no division of the fragile branches. However, if a venous approach route may also attempted, but if neither of these are successful, our new IPOV approach should be explored as an alternative. If the apparent venous drainage route is SOV, direct puncture of the extraconic portion of the SOV is recommended because the anterior apsidal vein is a good landmark, located in the junction of the first and second segment.of intra-conal portion with a possibility of damage to the eloquent structures of the optic nerve, cranial nerves III-VI and ophthalmic arterial divisions.of the SOV.

v. **Transvenous approach to the carotid-cavernous via the inferior petrooccipital vein** [23]

The transvenous approach via the inferior perusal sinus (IPS) is commonly used as the most appropriate for carotid cavernous fistula (CCF) or cavernous sinus sampling. However, it may be that the IPS is not accessible because of anatomical problems and/or complications, so that an alternative route is needed. In this paper, we have presented and discussed the utility of a transvenous approach to the cavernous sinus via the inferior petrooccipital vein (IPOV) [23].

Trolard [34] initially named this small vein differing from the IPS as the IPOV. San Millan ruiz et al [35] reported venous plexus of Rektorzik, corresponding to Trolard's inferior petrooccipital vein found coursing exracranially along the petrooccipital suture, which regularly contributes in forming the anterior condylar confluent.

Katsuta et al. [36] stressed the utility of the IPOV a small vein running in the extracranial groove (Fig. 3A) of the petrooccipital fissure, pouring into the petrosal confluens (anterior condylar confluent) and acting like a mirror image of the inferior petrosal sinus (Fig 3B). To our knowledge there have been no previous reports of its use as an actual access route to the cavernous sinus through the IPOV. The IPOV might be mistaken as the IPS because their running courses resemble each other.

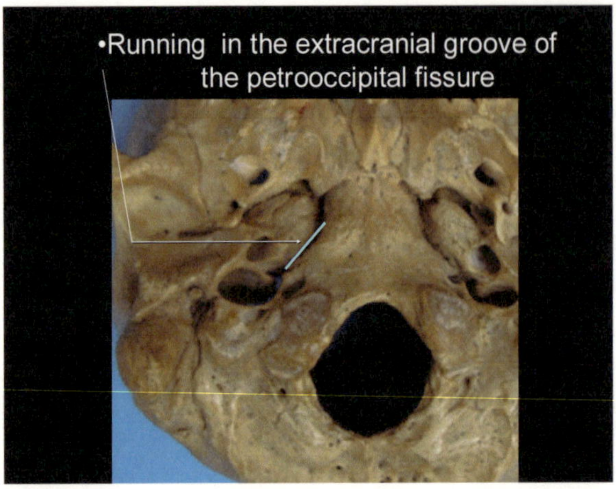


Fig. 3A. Inferior petrooccipital vein

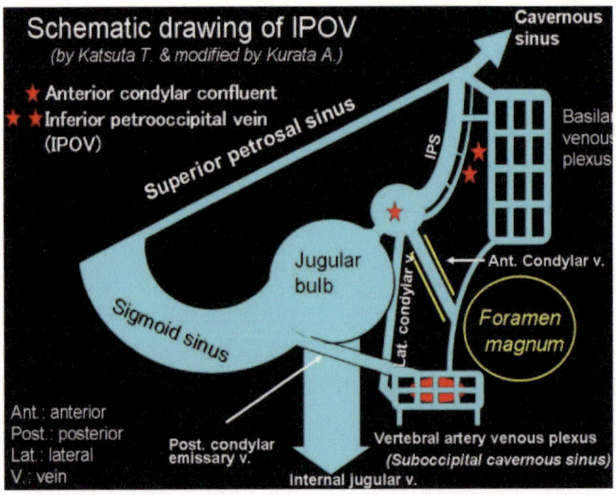


Fig. 3B. Schematic drawing of the inferior petrooccipital vein

**Techniqes to navigate a microcather into the cavernous sinus through the IPOV**

To navigate a small diameter and soft tip microcather into the IPOV, use of a preceding small soft guide wire is essential because of the small size of the vein, even if it is dilated. The microcatheter should be advanced considering the running course. Initially the IPOV originating from the medial part of the petrosal confluence runs in parallel and slightly deeper with the IPS (mirror image), finally changes course to become lateral

vi. Direct puncture approach to the extraconal portion of the superior ophthalmic vein[37]

The transvenous approach via the superior ophthalmic vein (SOV) is available approach for carotid cavernous fistula (CCF), where no other suitable approach route exists. Surgical exposure of the peripheral roots of the SOV is commonly used, but the SOV is often not accessible because the distal roots may show focal narrowing and tortuosity. We therefore here present our original direct-puncture approach to the extraconal portion of the SOV. The efficacy and safety of this approach have already been documented [37].

**Anatomy of the SOV (Fig. 8A -C) 38**

The SOV originates at its superior and inferior tributaries (roots). The junction of these roots is situated approximately 4-5 mm behind the tendon of the superior oblique muscle through the trochlea. The SOV is divided into three segments. The first segment, which courses obliquely upward and laterally, extends from the trochlea to the roof of the orbit (the extraconal portion). The second segment enters the muscle cone to course posterolaterally along the undersurface of the superior rectus muscle (Fig. 4). The anterior (medial) apsidal vein drains the internal rectus muscle and empties into the posterior aspect of the first segment of the SOV near the junction of the first and second segments. This vein is a good marker to distinguish the junction of the segments. The posterior (external) apsidal vein drains the lateral rectal muscle and enters the third segment. The second and third segments (the intraconal portion) are close to the optic nerve and the orbicular motor nerves.

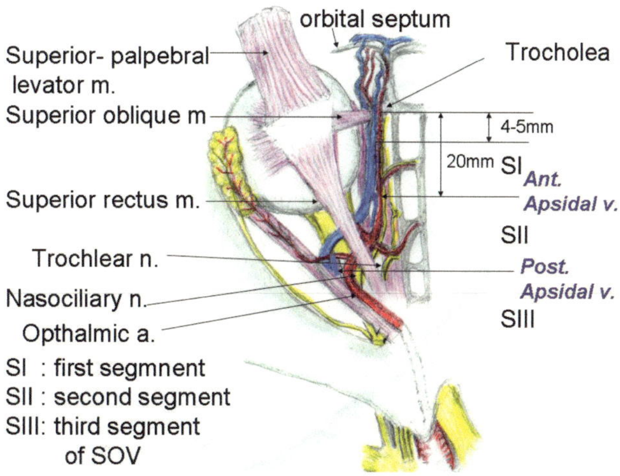


Fig. 4A. Schematic drawing of the upper view of the orbita and SOV.

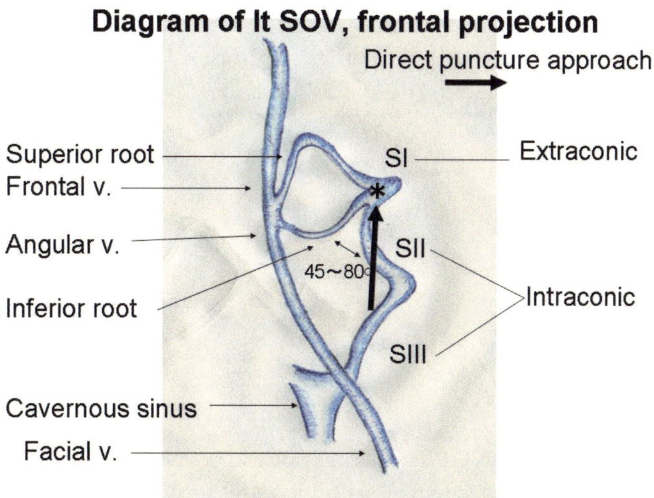


Fig. 4B. Schematic drawing of the SOV (Anterior-posterior view).

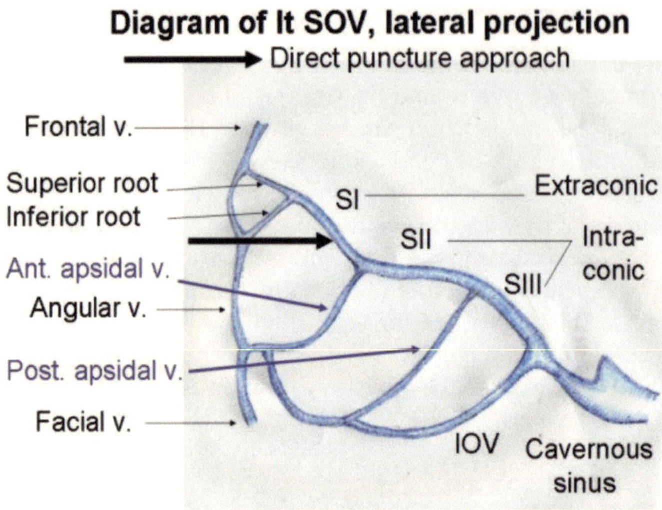


Fig. 4C. Schematic drawing of the SOV (lateral view).

Direct exposure of the SOV roots under general anesthesia is widely used [7-14] (Fig 4D), but may be complicated and damage may occur to the superior root of the fifth nerve resulting in numbness of the forehead [15]. Furtheremore, it may also cause palsy of the superior levator muscle and palpebral ptosis .

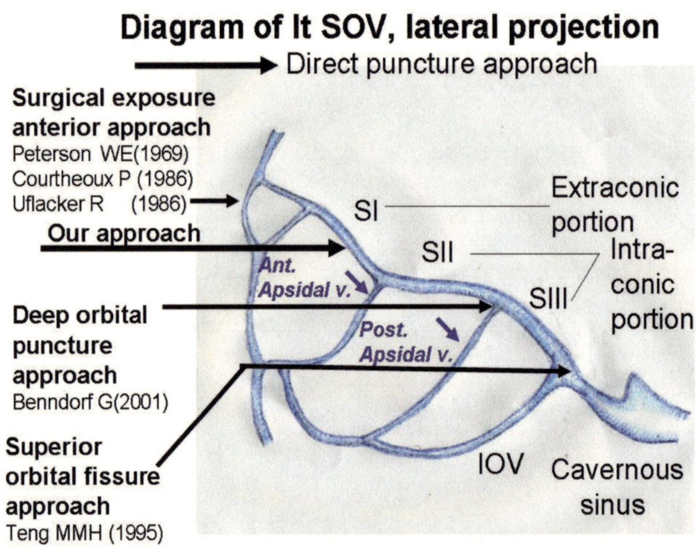


Fig. 4D.

The direct-puncture approach to the intraconal portion of the SOV has been reported in the literature [13,16-20] (Fig 4D). It is particularly useful in cases with a SOV dilated only within the intraconal segment, with thrombosed branches of the SOV [16] . However, there is a possibility of damage to the eloquent structures of the optic nerve, cranial nerves III-VI and ophthalmic arterial divisions. Using the deep-puncture approach (the posterior third of the SOV [17], the posterior half of the SOV [18], the superior orbital fissure [19] to the SOV usually results in difficulty in making an exact access and in preventing bleeding from the puncture point. Massive retro-orbital bleeding may occur and result in an inadequate increase of orbital pressure [13] Recently, the direct percutaneous approach to the cavernous sinus by the way of the inferior ophthalmic vein (IOV) was reported [20]. This method will be of assistance in cases with dilatation of the IOV. However, the IOV is less often found as the main drainage route than the SOV. In the present series as well, the main drainage route was the SOV in all three patients without dilatation of the IOV.

Our direct-puncture approach (Fig 4C,D) has particular advantages. One is that the extra-conal portion of the SOV is anatomically thick and less prone to damage than the intraconal portion. When the SOV is the draining vein of the CCF, the SOV will become dilated more and thicker during the time course, which facilitates easy puncture and makes the technique safer. When bleeding occurs, hematomas can be minimized because the extraconal portion of the SOV is relatively shallow and therefore hemostasis can be achieved by direct compression with a finger. The anterior apsidal vein is a good landmark for this approach because it originates from between the extraconal and the intraconal portions of the SOV.

Initially the IPS approach should be tried as the most apparent approach because it is comparative large and stiff with no division of the fragile branches. However, if the IPS is not successful, our new IPOV approach should be explored as an alternative. If apparent venous drainage route is SOV, direct puncture of the extraconic portion of the SOV is recommended because the anterior apsidal vein is a good landmark, located in the junction of the first and second segment of intra-conal portion and risk of damage to the eloquent structures of the optic nerve, cranial nerves III-VI and ophthalmic arterial divisions is low.

## 5. Postoperative care

In pre- as well as in postoperative care, it is essential to improve the venous outflow and reduce the venous congestion in order to avoid worsening of symptoms and prevent venous infarction and/or hemorrhagic complication, especially in the patients featuring high flow CCF with cortical venous drainage. Patients usually show an aggravation of the symptoms when getting up in the morning. Therefore, the upper part of the body should be elevated up to 30 degrees during sleeping before and immediately after treatment. It is recommended to avoid increase in venous pressure in the day time. Newton et al [39] detailed 5 of 11 dural AVF patients, which fistula onset may have been related to straining or heavy lifting. Especially in patients undergoing TVE, venous pressure may readily become raised, so that they should be guided to avoid straining actions such as with constipation, coughing, head standing and also lifting heavy weights. A posture to keep up the head should be recommended to improve the venous circulation. These precautions should be observed after diagnosis of CCF and until disappearance of CCF. TVE may be an effective treatment for dural AVFs localized in the sinus, particularly with regard to aggressive lesions with cortical venous reflux, but for patient with complete occlusion defined by angiography, insufficient attention may be paid to venous pressure. New development of dural AVF after TVE for dural AVF has been reported [40-47], sometimes in sites distant from the primary lesion [45], with time after sinus packing ranging from 4 months to 30 months (average: 10 months).Tearing of the vessels may be a feature [45]. Terada et al [48] from an experimental study, concluded that chronic venous hypertension of 2 to 3 months' duration, without associated venous or sinus thrombosis, can induce new AVF's affecting the dural sinuses. For dural AVF patients with complete occlusion defined by angiography careful attention should thus be paid to venous pressure as well as radiological and clinical examination over the long term.

During the postoperative course, in our experience [29], 4 of eighteen patients treated by TVE, a VIth cranial nerve palsy developed between two and four days after the treatment. It resolved within one year in two cases and in the other two persisted longer. Aihara et al.[49] reported two patients featuring deterioration of oculo-motor dysfunction out of 9 patients with dural AVF involving the cavernous sinus after treatments of the TVE. Two different mechanisms were put forward: high intra-sinus pressure caused by the obliteration of the drainage pathway resulting in cranial nerve palsy in one and direct compression of the cranial nerve by implanted coils in the other. In our series, the VIth cranial nerve palsy was caused by thrombosis developing around the platinum coils inserted into the postero-medial part of the cavernous sinus appeared to contribute. Minimum insertion of the coils is therefore a point in order to avoid such complications and anticoagulation agents such as warfarin is also indicated. The international ratio of prothrombin time (PT-INR) should be controlled around 2.0~3.0 until disappearance of symptoms.

## 6. Complications

Recently, TVE has been proposed as a more curative treatment for CCFs compared with trans-arterial embolization (TAE). However, it may induce serious complications. Embolic stroke was reported by Halbach et al [4], especially if it is performed at first without previous arterial supply reduction by TAE. Yamashita et al [6] reported complication occurred in 7 of 16 patients by TVE. One was epidural extravasation from perforation of the IPS, and the other 6 were transient aggravation of symptoms (chemosis and VIth/IIIrd cranial nerve palsy in each 3). To navigate a small diameter and soft tip microcather into the cavernous sinus via venous sinus and vein, use of a preceding small soft guide wire is essential because of the fragile nature of venous channels.

Major complication especially will occur in the cases with cortical venous reflux. Araki et al.[24] reported such a case of extravasation from uncal vein during TVE for SOV and IOV via IPS. To avoid such serious complications, reduction of the arterial inflow into the cortical vein by TAE before TVE will is of help.

## 7. Outcomes (including results of the authors' own series)

Time of flight 3D-MRA is useful for long-term clinical follow-up of CCF cases [29]. In 47 dural CCF patients treated with only TAE in our series [34], all except two were followed using this modality. In 43 (90 %) of 45, complete obliteration was established on MRA in periods ranging from 1 month to 13 years 8 months (average: 4 years 6 months). Two patients with residual fistulas were still recognized on follow-up MRA (6 years 2 months, and 2 years) after TAE, but both refused additional treatments because of the lack of any symptoms.

In all of 18 patients undergoing TAE followed by TVE, fistulas were completely occluded on follow-up MRA ranged from 1month to 3 years 6 months (average: 2 years 3 months) after the treatment. In one patient receiving TAE, TVE and SRS, follow-up MRA 10 years and 8 months after the treatment confirmed the disappearance of the fistula.

## 8. Expert suggestions

In dural CCF patients with wide involvement of the sinuses (type of bilateral CS and bilateral CS &ICS: 39%), especially with a cortical venous reflux, TAE for initial reduction of inflow has been recommended as a reasonable treatment strategy to avoid serious complications because of the comparatively non-aggressive nature of the disease. Onyx-is a newly developed liquid embolic agent, effective in the treatment of CCFs but not without hazards [50]. Particles may be safer than liquid emboli and in our series of TAE using only particles, no complications occurred. Repeated provocative testing and care of dangerous anastomosis are also important. Repeated TAE will establish targeting TVE because of diminishing the fistulas point.

A relative long follow-up by MRA (average: 4 years 6 months) showed complete obliteration in 93% [29] . Additional TVE is needed for residual fistulas, especially for the ones with residual cortical venous drainages. TVE can cure the fistulas as evidenced by their complete occlusion of fistulas in all 18 of our patients treated with TAE followed by TVE. Hydro-coil (Terumo Co, Japan) is the ultimate embolic material for TVE because of the small mass effect. Stereotactic radiosurgery (SRS) can be recommended for limited residual lesion after TAE and TVE. One last CCF of our series received stereotactic radiosurgery as reported earlier [51]. Stereotactic radiosurgery is an appropriate treatment for cavernous sinus dural AVFs resistant to endovascular treatment, especially with small, slow flow.

## 9. Explicative cases

### 9.1 Transvenous approach to the cavernous sinus via the inferior petorooccipital vein (case 1-4)

#### Case 1

A 72-year-old man suddenly developed diplopia, and was followed up conservatively in an outpatient clinic because the symptoms caused by left IIIrd cranial nerve palsy gradually improved with time. Six months later, the diplopia disappeared. However, after one year, left pulsating exophthalmos, conjunctival chemosis and pulsatile- tinnitus developed. The patient was examined by magnetic resonance imaging (MRI) in another hospital and referred to our institution. Magnetic resonance angiography (MRA) showed increase of the vascular structure in the left cavernous sinus communicating with a dilated cortical vein. Angiography showed a dural CCF in the left cavernous sinus draining into the cortical veins (the superficial middle cerebral vein and the deep middle cerebral vein), SOV and IOV (Fig 5A). Initially, transarterial embolization using platinum coils for the inflowing external carotid arteries (bilateral middle menigeal arteries and sphenopalatine arteries) was performed to decrease arterial inflow. Next, the transvenous approach via the IPS was tried, but this failed because of an obstruction. The peripheral roots of SOV and IOV showed lack of dilatation. The left inferior petrooccipital vein (IPOV) route was then attempted (Fig. 5B, C), and this proved successful without any complications. Angiography after the endovascular surgery showed no residual fistula and no cortical venous drainage (Fig. 5D).

Although, postoperative new left VIth cranial nerve palsy worsened two days later, this had disappeared by 3 months after the treatment. Follow-up MRA three months after the treatment showed no recurrence of the CCF.

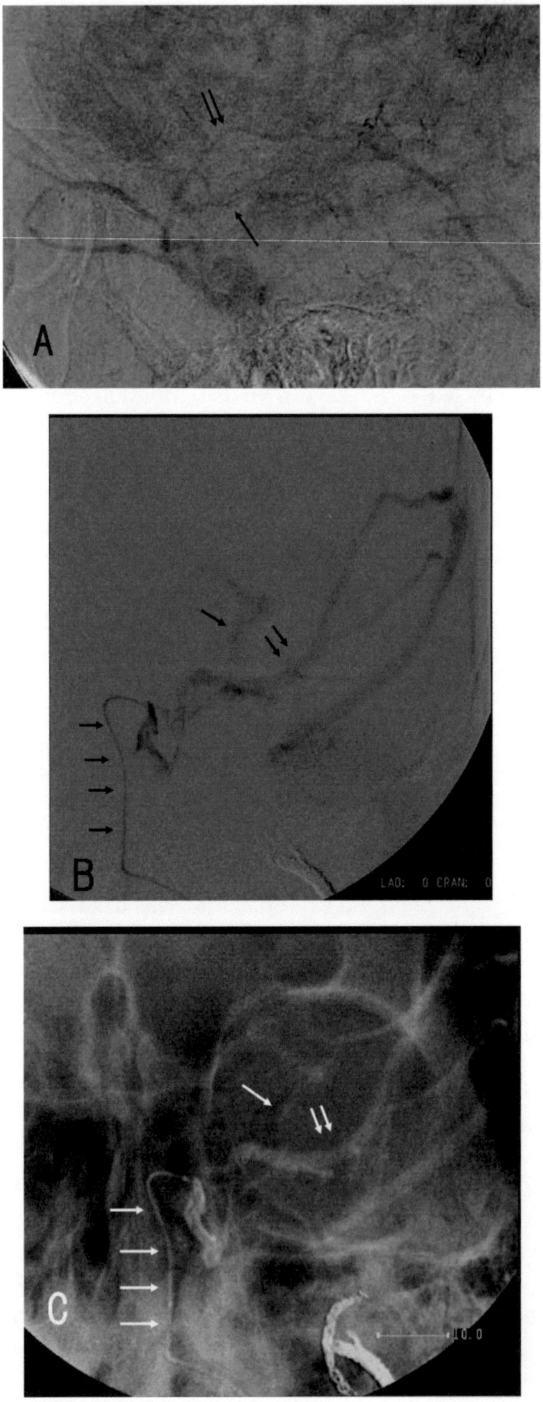

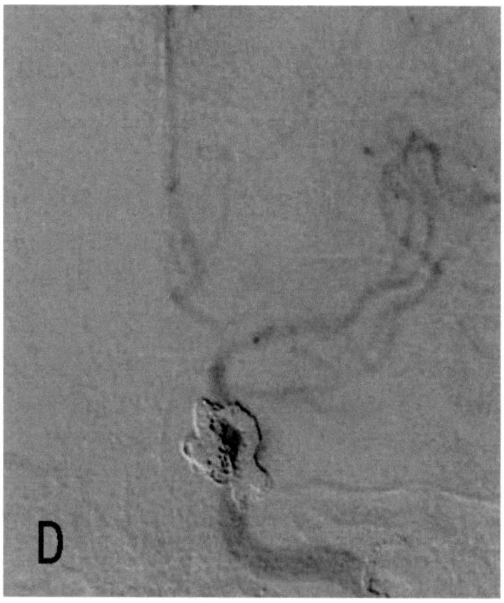

Fig. 5. Left carotid angiogram, lateral view(A) ,showing a carotid cavernous fistula (CCF) supplied by sphenopalatine and middle meningeal arteries with drainage into the superficial middle cerebral vein (SMCV) (double arrows), the deep middle cerebral vein (DMCV) (single arrow), the superior ophthalmic vein (SOV) and the inferior ophthalmic vein (IOV). The peripheral roots of the SOV and IOV lack any dilatation. Digital subtraction angiography, anteroposterior view (B), and skull radiograph, anteroposterior view (C), showing venography from the microcatheter into the left cavernous sinus via the inferior petrooccipital vein (arrows). SMCV: double arrows, DMCV: arrow. Left carotid angiogram, anteroposterior view (D) after endovascular surgery showing complete obliteration of the fistula and no cortical venous reflux.

Case 2

A 76-year-old woman suddenly developed diplopia and was followed up conservatively in an outpatient clinic because the symptoms caused by the left VIth cranial nerve palsy gradually improved with time. Six months later, the diplopia disappeared. However, after two years, the patient developed symptoms and was examined by MRI in another hospital and referred to our institution. MRA showed increase of the vascular structure in the left cavernous sinus communicating with a dilated cortical vein. Angiography showed a dural CCF in the left cavernous sinus draining into the superficial middle cerebral vein and the deep middle cerebral vein only (Fig 6A, B). Initially, transarterial embolization of the inflowing external carotid arteries (left sphenopalatine, accessory menigeal and middle meningeal arteries) was performed to decrease the inflow. Next, the transvenous approach via the IPS was tried, but this failed because of an obstruction of the IPS. The left IPOV route was then attempted (Fig. 6C), and this proved successfully without any complications. Angiography after the endovascular surgery showed no residual fistula and no cortical venous drainage (Fig. 6D). Although left VIth cranial nerve palsy worsened two days later, this had disappeared by 3 months after the treatment. Follow-up MRA two months after the treatment showed no recurrence of the CCF.

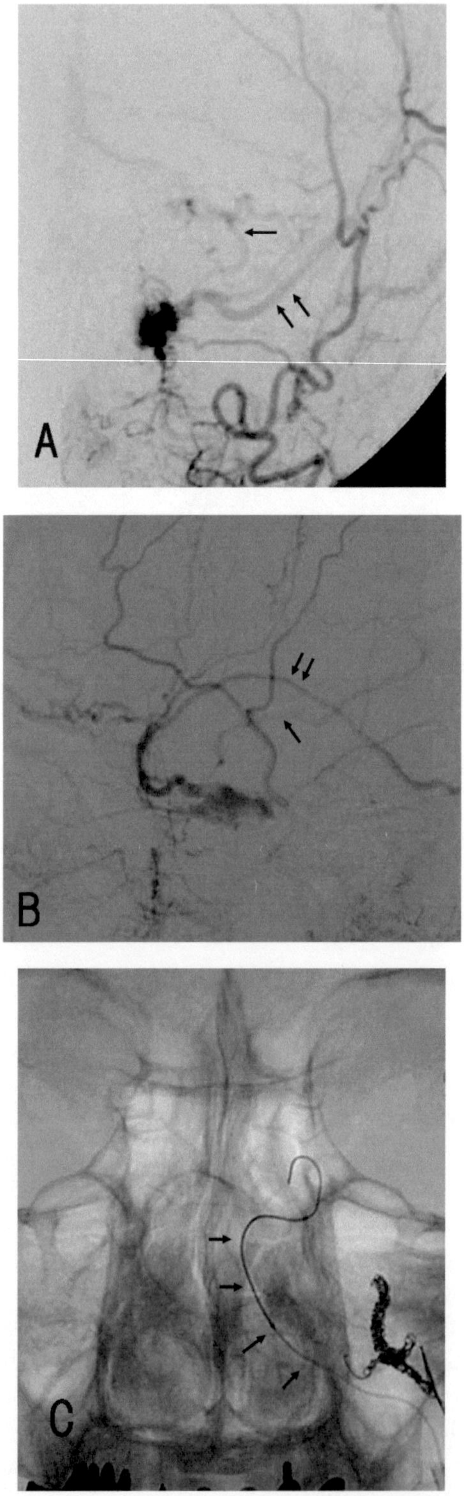
A
B
C

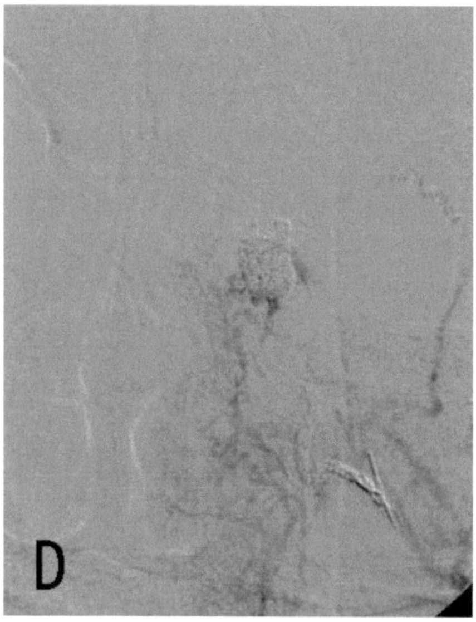


Skull radiograph, anteroposterior view (C) showing the microcatheter with microguide wire introduced into the left cavernous sinus via the inferior petroccpital vein (arrows). Left external carotid angiogram, anteroposterior view (D), after endovascular surgery showing complete obliteration of the fistula and no cortical venous reflux.

Fig. 6. Left carotid angiogram, anteroposterior view (A) and lateral view (B) showing a carotid cavernous fistula (CCF) supplied by sphenopalatine, accessory menigeal and middle meningeal arteries with drainage limited to the superficial middle cerebral vein (double arrows) and the deep middle cerebral vein (single arrow).

Case 3

A 77-year-old woman developed left chemosis and was followed up conservatively in an outpatient clinic. The symptoms worsened with time and proptosis also appeared. One month later, the patient was examined by MRI in another hospital and referred to our institution. MRA showed increase of the vascular structure in the left cavernous sinus. Angiography showed a dural CCF in the left cavernous sinus, supplied by sphenopalatine , middle meningeal and ascending pharyngeal artery, draining into the SOV, the IOV and the IPOV (Fig. 7A, B). Initially, transarterial embolization of the inflowing external carotid arteries was performed to decrease the inflow. Next, the transvenous approach via the left IPOV route was attempted (Fig. 7C, D), and this proved successful without any complications. Angiography after the endovascular surgery showed no residual fistula and no cortical venous drainage (Fig. 7E). Three months after the treatment, the symptoms had completely disappeared and follow-up MRA 8 month after the treatment showed no recurrence of the CCF.

Case 4

A 67-year-old woman was referred to our department for cavernous venous sampling to distinguish between Cushing disease and the ectopic adrenocorticotrophic hormone (ACTH) syndrome because the patient showed no suppression by means of a high -dose dexamethasone suppression test (Liddle test), but a micro-pituitary adenoma was suspected

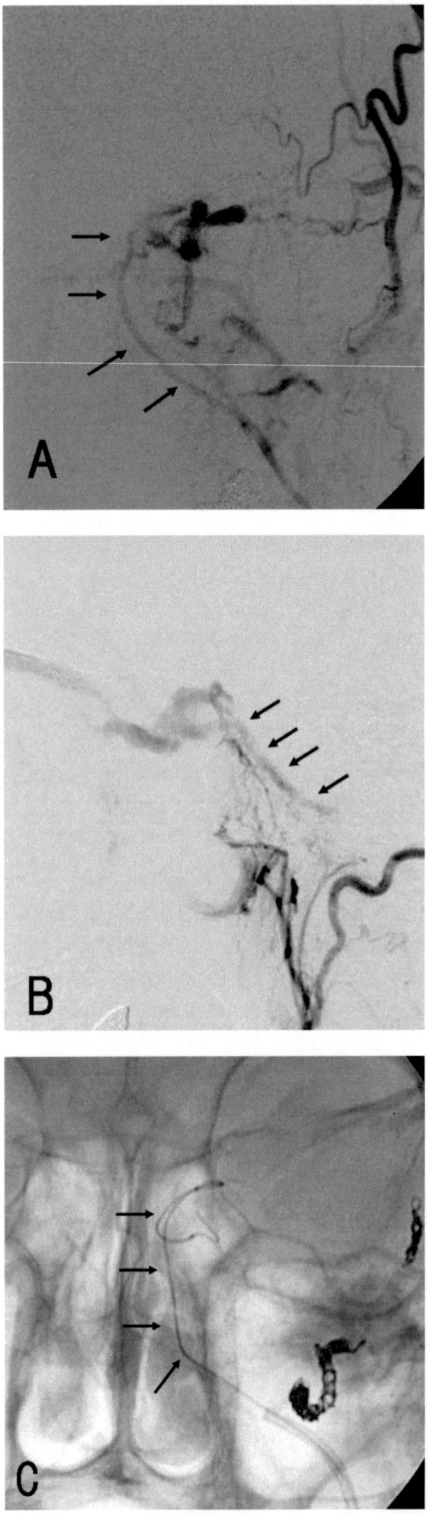
A
B
C

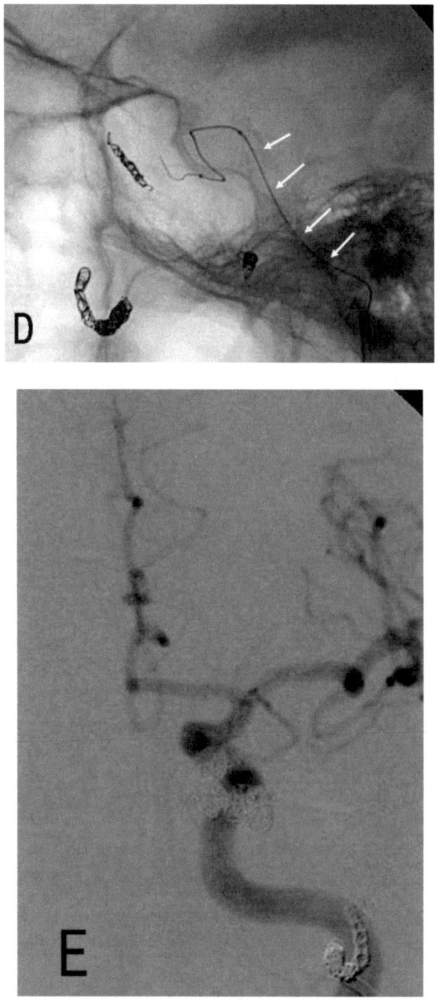


Skull radiograph, anteroposterior view(C) and lateral view (D)showing a microcatheter with a micro-guide wire introduced into the left cavernous sinus via the IPOV (arrows). Left carotid angiogram (E: anteroposterior view) after endovascular surgery showing complete obliteration of the fistula and no cortical venous reflux.

Fig. 7. Left carotid angiogram, anteroposterior view (A) and lateral view ( B), showing a carotid cavernous fistula (CCF) supplied by sphenopalatine , middle meningeal and ascending pharyngeal arteries with drainage into the superior ophthalmic vein, the inferior ophthalmic vein and the inferior petroccipital vein (IPOV) (arrows).

on MRI. A transvenous approach to the right cavernous sinus via the right IPS was initially attempted, but failed because of an obstruction. Next, the right IPOV route was attempted , which was successful. The left transvenous approach to the left cavernous sinus via the left IPS was conventionally performed (Fig 8). Venous sampling from the bilateral cavernous sinuses and femoral veins was possible and resulted in diagnosis of Cushing disease caused by a micro-pituitary adenoma in the left side of the pituitary gland, which was successfully removed by a trans-sphenoidal approach.

The transvenous approach to the cavernous sinus via the OPOV should be considered as an alternate in cases when use of the IPS is precluded by an anatomical problem and there are no other suitable venous approach routes.

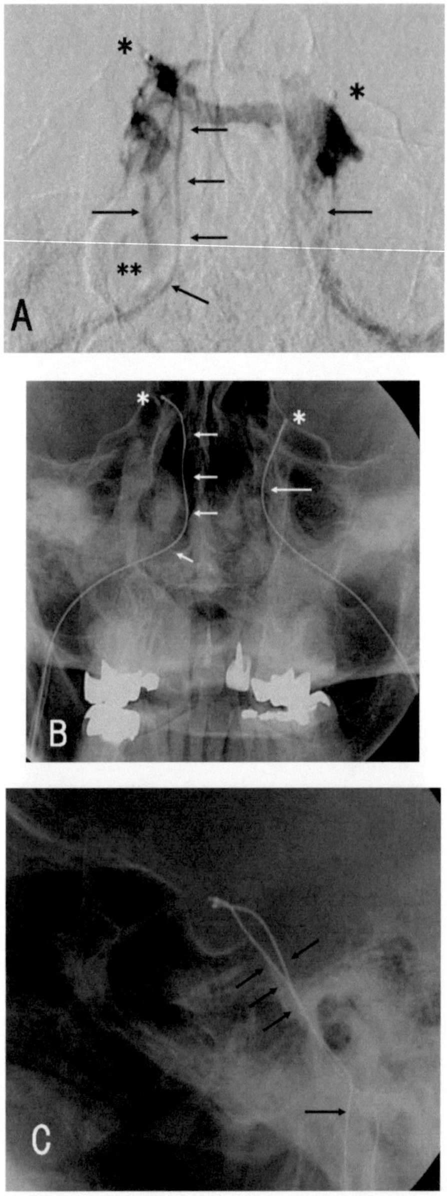


Fig. 8. Venography, anteroposterior view (A) from a microcather in the right cavernous sinusInferior petrosal sinus (IPS)= single arrow, IPOV(inferior petrooccipital vein )=.four arrows. tip of the microcatheters=asterisk, obstruction of the right IPS= double asterisks. Skull radiograph, anteroposterior view (B) and lateral view (C) showing a microcatheter introduced into the left cavernous sinus via the left IPS (single arrow) and a microcatheter introduced into the right cavernous sinus via the IPOV(arrows).

### 9.2 Direct puncture approach to the extraconal portion of the SOV (case 5)

Case 5

A 40-year-old man was injured in a traffic accident resulting in a left cerebellar and frontal contusion, fracture of the left optic canal and skull base. The patient was followed up conservatively. Consciousness gradually improved, but the loss of the left visual acuity unfortunately did not show any improvement. Two months later, left chemosis and pulsatile proptosis developed and worsened with time and after four months the patient was admitted to our hospital. when an angiogram showed a left CCF. Collateral flow from the right carotid system and the vertebro-basilar system were poor. Drainage routes of the left superior petrosal sinus and inferior sinus were obliterated (Fig. 9A). Remarkable cortical venous refluxes to the cerebellar hemisphere were evident. A collateral flow to the affected left internal carotid artery was poor because of hypoplastic left A1portion. The transvenous approach was determined to be a more suitable approach than the transarterial approach because of the occlusion time for the balloon protection so as not to permit migration of embolic material into the internal carotid artery. The transvenous approach via the femoral vein was attempted, but failed because of an obstruction in the left internal jugular vein (Fig. 9B). The only residual drainage route was via the SOV, but its distal divisions were tortuous and narrowed. The direct-puncture approach to the extraconal portion of the SOV was therefore selected as the only available residual transvenous approach route. Transvenous embolization for closure of the fistula using 18 platinum coils through the direct-puncture approach to the extraconal portion using 2D road mapping was successfully performed without any complications (Fig. 9C). Angiography after the endovascular surgery showed no residual fistula and no cortical venous refluxes (Fig. 9D, 9E). The patient's symptoms immediately improved after the procedure and he could be discharged 7 days later without any new neurological deficits. Follow-up MRA 1year after the treatment showed no recurrence of the CCF (Fig. 9F).

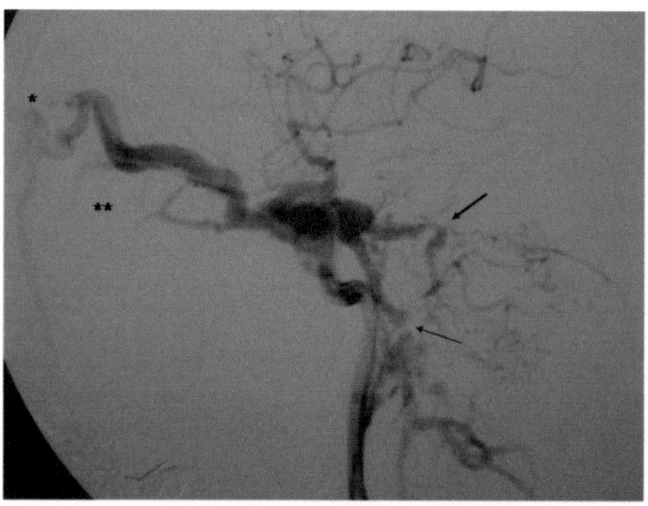


A

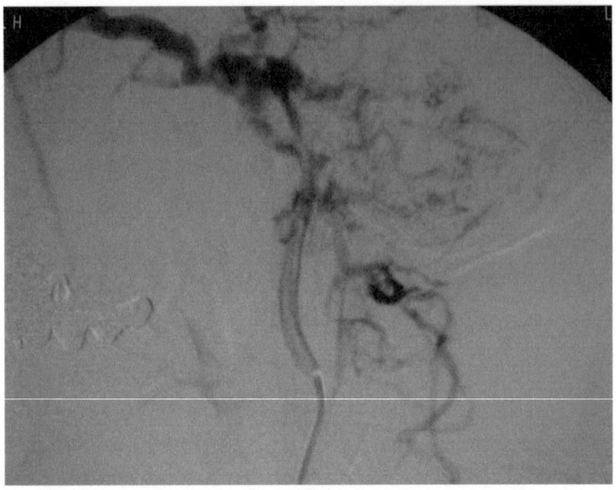

B

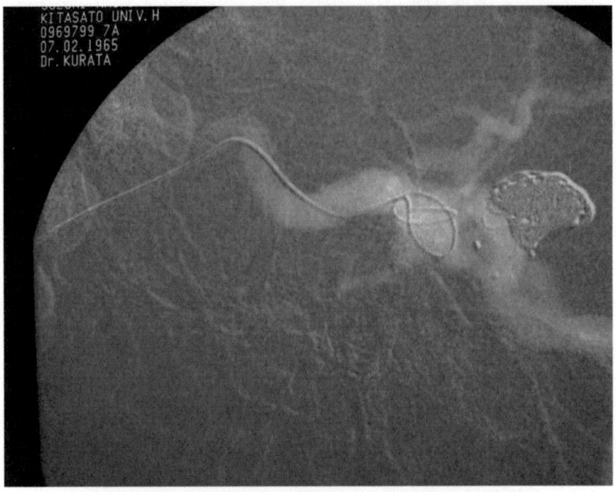


C

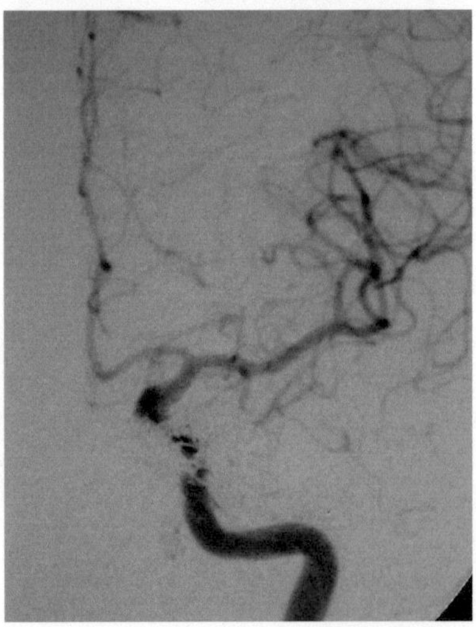

D

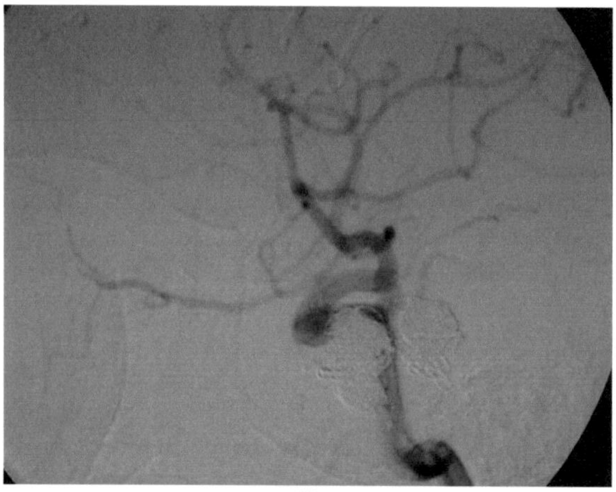

E

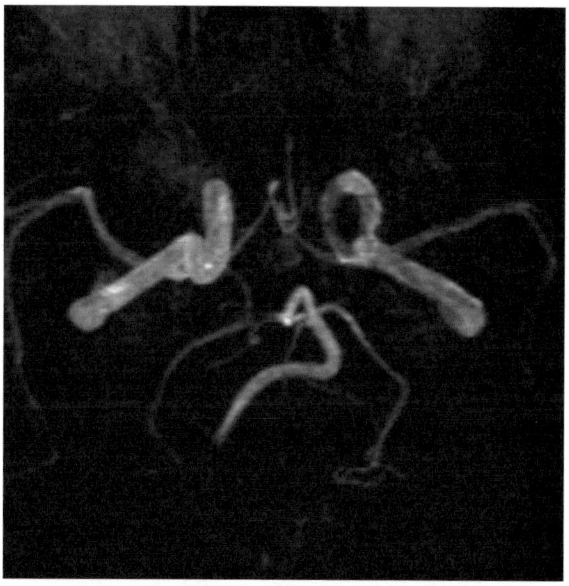

F

Fig. 9. Left carotid angiogram, lateral view (A) showing a carotid cavernous fistula (CCF) and the anterior apsidal vein (double asterisks). Drainage routs were the SOV, the superior petrosal sinus (SPS), and the inferior petrosal sinus (IPS). The SPS and IPS were obstructed (arrows) resulting in remarkable cortical venous reflux into the cerebellar hemisphere. Distal divisions of the SOV were tortuous and narrowed (asterisk). Left carotid angiogram, late arterial phase, lateral view (B) showing obstruction in the left internal jugular vein (arrow). Road mapping image of the magnified left carotid angiogram (C) during endovascular surgery showing a microcatheter (arrow) introduced via the direct-puncture approach into the extraconal portion of the SOV. The left carotid angiogram, left anteroposterior view (D) and lateral view (E) after endovascular surgery showing complete obliteration of the fistula and no cortical venous reflux. Follow-up magnetic resonance angiography (F) 1 year after the endovascular surgery showing no recurrence of the fistula.

## 10. Transvenous approach to the cavernous sinus via SPS (case 6)

Case 6

A 71-year-old women suffered sudden onset of diplopia and three weeks later the patient was admitted to our hospital. Physiological and neurological and examination on admission showed right chemosis, right bruit, bilateral VIth cranial nerve palsies and left IIIrd nerve palsy. Angiography showed a bilateral CCF type D by Barrow's classification. Bilateral middle meningeal , accessory meningeal, sphenoparatine and ascending pharyngeal arteries all extensively supplied a CCF into the bilateral CS and ICS. Drainage routes were the right SPS, SOV and cortical vein (superficial middle cerebral vein) (Fig 10A). Remarkable cortical venous reflux to the right fronto-temporal lobe was evident. Repeated TAEs for reducing bilateral external carotid supply were initially before TVE. After three procedures, the dural fistula was located only in the right cavernous sinus with slight cortical venous reflux (Fig 10B). Initially, the transvenous approach via the IPS route was attempted, but this failed because of obstruction of the left IPS and lack of communication of the right IPS with the CS. The residual drainage route was via the right SPS. TVE via the right SPS was aimed to occlude the antero-lateral compartment of the right CS and reducing cortical venous reflux, but the SPS was partially narrowed (Fig. 10B). A 1.7F microcatheter (Excelsior SL- 10, Stryker, USA) assisted with a 4F catheter (Cerulean 4F catheter, Medikit Co., Japan) was successfully advanced through a 6F catheter (Envoy, Cordis/Johnson&Johnson, USA) into the antero-lateral compartment of the right CS (Fig. 10C) via the SPS. Transvenous embolization using 25 platinum coils was successfully performed without any complications (Fig. 10D). Angiography after the endovascular surgery showed no residual fistula and no cortical venous refluxes (Fig. 10E). The patient's symptoms immediately improved after the procedure, but two days later right VIth cranial nerve palsy once again worsened. However, the patient could be discharged 5 days later and the right VIth cranial nerve palsy gradually improved and completely disappeared within 1 year. Follow-up MRA 1year after the treatment showed no recurrence of the CCF (Fig.10F).

**Anteroposterior view**

Right carotid angiogram Left carotid angiogram

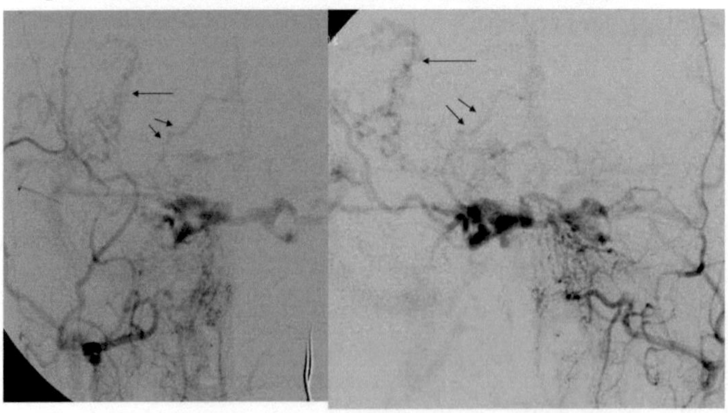

**Superficial middle cerebral vein (single arrow)**
**Deep middle cerebral vein (double small arrows)**

A

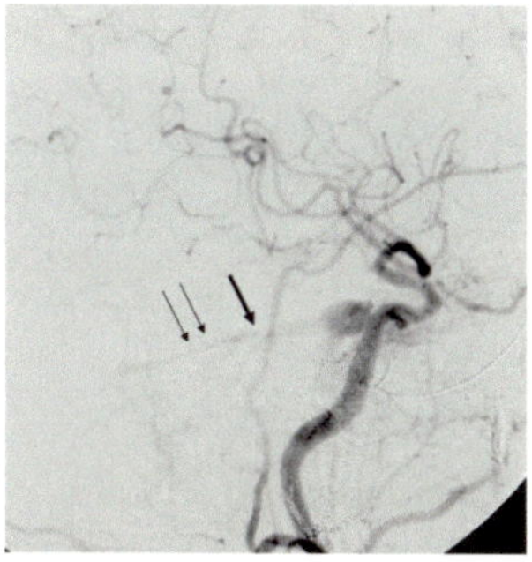


B

Right carotid angiogram, lateral view showing CCF mainly draining into the SPS (single arrow) with stenosis (double small arrows)

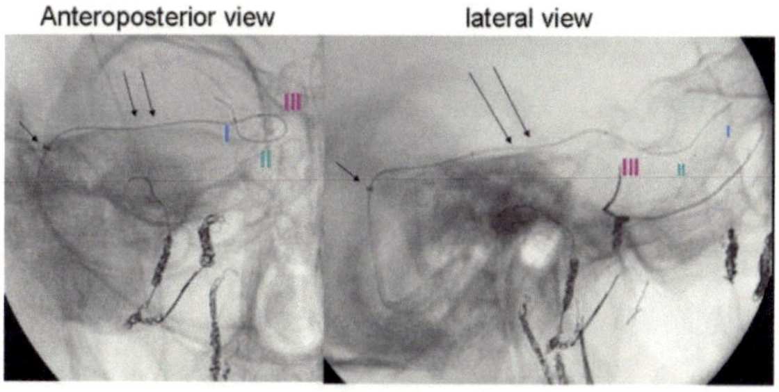


C

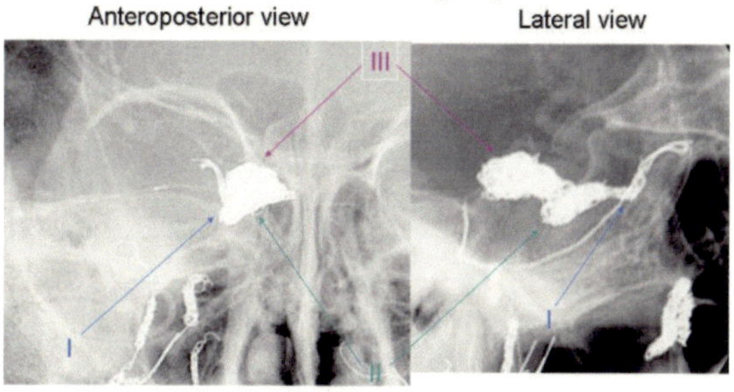


D

Right carotid angiography

Anteroposterior view Lateral view

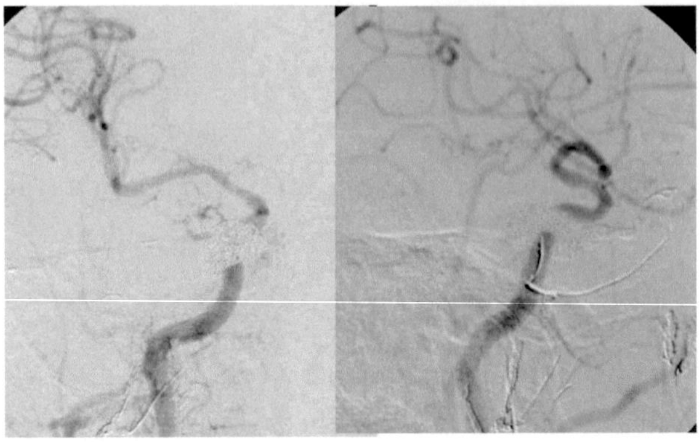

E

Follow-up Magnetic resonance angiogram

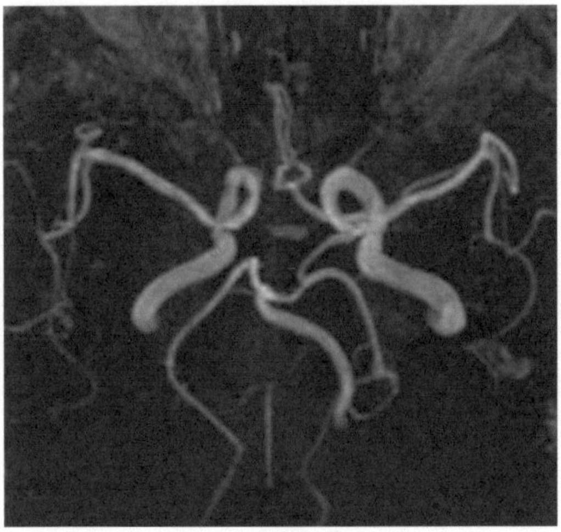

F

Fig. 10. Right carotid angiogram (left) and left carotid angiogram (right) (A)showing CCF supplied by bilateral middle meningeal, accessory meningeal, sphenoparatine and ascending pharyngeal arteries draining into the right SPS, SOV, superficial middle cerebral vein (single arrow) and deep middle cerebral vein (double arrows)Right carotid angiogram, lateral view ( B) showing CCF mainly draining into the SPS (single arrow) with stenosis (double small arrows)

## 11. References

[1] Newton TH, Potts DG. Veins in Radiology of the Brain angiography 1974 chapter 76. Vol.2, book 3

[2] Miller DL, Doppman JL. Petrosal sinus sampling: Technique and rationale. Radiology 1991; 178:37-47

[3] Teramoto A, Yoshida Y, Sanno N, Nemoto S. Cavernous sinus sampling in patients with adrenocorticotrophic hormone-dependent cushing's syndrome with emphasis on inter- and intracavernous adrencortiotrophic hormone gradients. J Neurosurg 1988; 89:762-768

[4] Halbach VV, Higashida RT, Hieshima GB, Harin CW, Yang PJ. Transvenous embolization of direct carotid cavernous fistulas. AJNR Am J Neuroradiol 1988; 9: 741-747

[5] Benndorf G, Bender A, Lehmann R, Lanksch W. Transvenous occlusion of dural cavernous sinus fistulas through the thrombosed inferior petrosal sinus: report of four cases and review of the literature. Surg Neurol 2000; 54: 42-54

[6] Yamashita K, Taki W, Sadato A, Nakahara I, Kikuchi H, Yonekawa Y. Transvenous embolization of dural caroticocavernous fistulae: technical consideration. Neuroradiology 1993; 35: 475-479

[7] Coutheoux P, Labbe D, Hamel C, Lecoq PJ, Jahara M, Theron J. Treatment of bilateral spontaneous dural carotid-cavernous fistulas by coils and sclerotherapy. J Neurosurg 1987; 66: 468-470

[8] Hanneken AM, Miller NR, Debrun GM, Nauta HJ. Treatment of carotid-cavernous sinus fistulas using a detachable balloon catheter through the superior ophthalmic vein. Arch Ophthalmol 1989; 107:87-92

[9] Miller NR, Monsein LH, Debrun GM, Tamargo RJ, Nauta HJW. Treatment of carotid-cavernous sinus fistulas using a superior ophthalmic vein approach. J Neurosurg 1995; 83:838-842

[10] Monsein LH, Debrun GM, Miller NR, Nauta HJW, Chazaly JR. Treatment of dural carotid-cavernous fistulas via the superior ophthalmic vein. AJNR Am J Neuroradiol 1991; 12:435-439

[11] Oishi H, Arai H, Sato K, Iizuka Y. Complications associated with transvenous embolization of cavernous dural arteriovenous fistula. Acta Neurochir (Wien) 1999; 141:1265-1271

[12] Quinones D, Duckwiler G, Gobin PY, Goldberg RA, Vinuela F. Embolization of dural cavernous fistulas via superior ophthalmic vein approach. AJNR Am J Neuroradiol 1997; 18:921-928

[13] Tress BM, Thomson KR, Klug GL, Mee RRB, Crawford B. Management of carotid-cavernous fistulas by surgery combined with interventional radiology. Report of two cases. J Neurosurg 1983; 59:1076-1081

[14] Uflacker R, Lima S, Ribas GC, Piske RL. Carotid-cavernous fistulas: embolization through the superior ophthalmic vein approach. Radiology 1986; 159:175-179

[15] Lee JW, Kim DJ, Jung JY, Kim SH, Huh SK, Suh SH, Kim DI. Embolization of indirect carotid-cavernous sinus dural arterio-venous fistulae using the direct superior ophthalmic vein approach. Acta Neurochir (Wien) 2008; 150: 557-561

[16] Chan CCK, Leung H, O`Donnell B, Assad N, Ng P. Intraconal superior ophthamic vein embolization for carotid cavernous fistula. Orbit 2006; 25: 31-34

[17] Benndorf G, Bender A, Campi A, Menneking H, Lansksch WR. Treatment of a cavernous sinus dural arteriovenous fistula by deep orbital puncture of the superior ophthalmic vein. Neuroradiology 2001; 43:499-502

[18] Teng MM, Guo WY, Huang CI, Wu CC, Chang T. Occlusion of arteriovenous malformations of the cavernous sinus via the superior ophthalmic vein. AJNR Am J Neuroradiol 1988; 9:539-546
[19] Teng MM, Lirng JF, Chang T, Chen SS, Guo WY, Cheng CC, Shen WC, Lee LS. Embolization of carotid cavernous fistula by means of direct puncture through the superior orbital fissure. Radiology 1995; 194:705-711
[20] White JB, Layton KF, Evans AJ, Tong FC, Jensen ME, Kallmes DF, Dion JE, Cloft HJ Transorbital puncture for the treatment of cavernous sinus dural fistulas. AJNR Am J Neuroradiol 2007; 28: 1415-1417
[21] Mounayer C, Piotin M, Spelle L, Moret J. Superior petrosal sinus catheterization for transvenous embolization of a dural carotid cavernous sinus fistula. AJNR Am J Neuroradiol 2002; 23:1153-1155
[22] Jahan R, Gobin YP, Glenn B, Duckwiler GR, Vinuela F. Transvenous embolization of a dural arteriovenous fistula of the cavernous sinus through the contralateral pteriogoid plexus. Neuroradiology 1998 40: 189-193
[23] Kurata A, Suzuki S, Iwamoto K, Kuniaki Nakahara K, Inukai K, Niki, J , Satou K, Yamada M, Fujii, K, Kan S, Katsuta T. A new transvenous approach to the carotid cavernous sinus via the inferior petrooccipital vein. J Nurosurg in press
[24] Shiu PC, Hanafee WN, Wilson GH, Rand RW. Cavernous sinus venography. AJR 1968; 104: 57-62
[25] Mitsuhashi Y, Nishio A, Kawahara S, Ichinose T, Yamauchi S, Naruse H, et al. Morphologic evaluation of the caudal end of the inferior petrosal sinus using 3D rotational venography. AJNR Am J Neuroradiol 2007; 28: 1179-1184
[26] Araki K, Nakahara I, Taki W, Sakai N, Irie K, Isaka F, Ohwaki H, Kikuchi H. A case of cavernous dural arteriovenous fistula resulting in intracerebral extravasation during transvenous embolization. Neurol Surg 1997; 25: 733-737.
[27] Watanabe A, Hirano K, Suzuki Y, Kamada M, Mohri H, Okamura H, Ishii R Venous congestion of the insular cortex after transvenous coil embolization of a dural carotid-cavernous fistula. In Taki W, Picard L, Kikuchi H (eds) Advances in Interventional Neuroradiology and Intravascular Neurosurgery. Amsterdam: Elsevier, 1996；pp 271-274.
[28] Nakamura M, Tamaki N, Kawaguchi T, Fujita S. Selective transvenous embolization of dural carotid-cavernous sinus fistulas with preservation of sylvian venous outflow. J Neurosurg 1998; 89: 825-829.
[29] Kurata A, Suzuki S,Iwamoto K, Nakahara K Sasaki M, Kijima C, Inukai M, Abe K, Niki J, Satou K, Fujii K, Kan S. Dural arteriovenous fistulas in the cavernous sinus: Clinical research and treatments. Neurology 2011; in press
[30] .Kupersmith MJ, Berenstein A, Choi IS, Warren F, Flamm E.Management of nontraumatic vascular shunts involving the cavernous sinus.Ophthalmology 1988; 95: 121-130
[31] Kurata A, Miyasaka Y, Kunii M, Nagai S, Ohmomo T, Morishima H, Fujii K.The value of long-term clinical follow-up for cases of spontaneous carotid cavernous fistula. Acta Neurochir (Wien) 1998; 140: 65-72.
[32] Barrow DL, Spector RH, Braun I, Landman JA, Tindall SC, Tindall GT. Classificication and treatment of spontaneous carotid cavernous fistulas. J Neurosurg 1985；62: 248-256.

[33] Kurata A, Miyasaka Y, Saegusa H, Fujii K, Kan S. Treatment of a small hole post traumatic carotid-cavernous fistula with a non-detachable balloon catheter. Technical note. Intervent Neuroradiol 1997; 3: 87-90

[34] Trolard P. Anatomie du systeme veineux de l'encephale et du crane [in French]. Paris: These de la Faculte de Medecine de Paris 1868, pp1-32

[35] San millan ruiz D, Gailloud P, Rufenacht DA. The craniocervical venous system in relation to cerebral venous drainage. AJNR Am J Neuroradiol 2002; 23:1500-1508

[36] Katsuta T, Matsushima T, Uda K. Surgical anatomy of the skull base venous system:petroclival region. JPN J Neurosurg 2008; 17(10): 738-743

[37] Kurata A, Suzuki S, Iwamoto K, Miyazaki T, Inukai M, Abe K, Niki J, Yamada M, Fujii K, Kan S. Direct Puncture approach of the extraconal portion of the superior ophthalmic vein for carotid cavernous fistulae. Neuroradiology 2009; 51: 755-759

[38] Doyon DL, Aron-Rosa DS, Ramee A. Orbital veins and cavernous sinus. Editor: Newton TH, Potts DG. Radiology of the skull. 1974 Chapter 76 pp 2220-2254

[39] Newton TH, Weidner W, Greitz T. Dural arteriovenous malformation in the posterior fossa. Radiology1968; 90: 27-35

[40] Nakagawa H, Kubo S, Nakajima Y. Shifting of dural arteriovenou malformations from the cavernous sinus to the sigmoid sinus to the transverse sinus after transvenous embolization. Surg Neurol 1992; 37: 30-38

[41] Yamashita k, Taki W, Nishi I, Sadato A, Kikuchi H. Development of sigmoid dural arteriovenous fistulas after transvennous embolization of cavernous dural arteriovenous fistulas. Am J Neuroradiol AJNR 1993; 14 : 1106-1108

[42] Machiuchi T, Takasaki K, Yamagami M, Oda H, Todoroki K, Atsuchi M, Kadota K. A case of sigmoid sinus dural arteriovenous fistula after treated cavernous dural arteriovenous fistula. Intervent Neuroradiol 1998; 4 (Suppl 1): 219-222

[43] Kubota Y, Ueda T, Kaku Y, Sakai Nl. Development of a dural arteriovenous fistula around the jugular valve after transvenous embolization of cavernous dural arteriovenous fistula. Surg Neurol 1999; 51: 174-176

[44] Kawaguchi T, Kawano T, Kaneko Y, Tsutsumi M, Ooigawa H, Kazekawa K. Dural fistula of the transverse sigmoid sinus after transvenous embolization of the carotid cavernous fistula. Brain and Nerve 1999; 51: 1065-1069

[45] Kiyosue H, Tanoue S, Okahara M, Yamashita M, Nagatomi H, Mori H. Recurrence of dural arteriovenou fistula in another location after selective transvenous coil embolization: report of two cases. AJNR Am J Neuroradiol 2002; 23: 689-692

[46] Piske RL, Campos CMS, Chaves JBL, Abicataf R, Dabus G, Batista LL, Baccin C, Lima SS. Dural sinus compartment in dural arteriovenous shunts: a new angioarchitectural feature allowing superselective transvenous dural sinus occlusion treatment. AJNR Am J Neuroradiol 2005; 26: 1715-1722

[47] Kurata A, Suzuki S, Iwamoto K, Yamada M, Fujii K, Kan S: New development of a dural arterio-venous fistula (AVF) of the superior sagittal sinus after transvenous embolization of a left sigmoid sinus dural AVF. Case report and review of the literature. Intervent Neuroradiol 2006; 12: 363-368

[48] Terada T, Higashida RT, et al. Development of acquired arteriovenous fistulas in rats due to hypertension. J Neurosurg 1994; 80: 884-889

[49] Aihara N, Mase M, Yamada K, Banno T, Watanabe K, Kamiya K, Takagi T. Deterioration of ocular motor dysfunction after transvenous embolization of dural

arteriovenous fistula involving the cavernous sinus. Acta Neurochir (Wien) 1999; 141:707-710
[50] Elhammady MS, Quintero S, Wolfe SQ, Farhat H, Moftakhar R, Aziz-Sultan MA. Onyx embolization of carotid-cavernous fistulas. J Neurosurg 2010; 112: 589-594
[51] Kurata A, Miyasaka Y, Irikura K, Fujii K, Kan S. Stereotactic gamma surgery combined with endovascular surgery for treatment of a spontaneous carotid cavernous sinus fistula. Neuro-ophthalmology 2002; 23: 35-41

# Section 4

## Spinal Issues

# 14

# Craniovertebral Junction Chordomas

Pratipal Kalsi and David Choi
*National Hospital for Neurology & Neurosurgery, London*
*United Kingdom*

## 1. Introduction

Chordomas are rare tumours that arise from remnants of the embryonic notochord. They can be located in all places where the notocord existed, such as the nasopharynx, clivus, sella turcica, foramen magnum, cervical spine and sacrococcygeal region. This chapter will focus on chordomas affecting the craniovertebral junction (CV). Chordomas are rare malignant tumours with an incidence of less than 1 per 100,000. The site of origin of skull base chordomas is usually the clivus and from here they can extend into the anterior fossa, middle fossa, the sellar and parasellar regions, and through the foramen magnum into the upper cervical spine. In the majority of cases the typical histological appearances and characteristic location of chordomas render the diagnosis straightforward. The symptoms and signs are highly variable and depend on the exact site of the lesion and the involvement of adjacent structures. These can range from cranial nerve palsies, motor and sensory deficits, to gait disturbance and balance problems. Radiological diagnosis of craniovertebral junction chordomas has improved with the advent of modern CT and MR imaging modalities and tumour location and extent of skull base involvement can be precisely defined. Surgery is the most effective form of treatment for patients with craniovertebral junction chordomas and radical resection augmented with adjuvant therapies such as proton beam therapy have been shown to prolong survival. Although chordomas are usually slow-growing tumours they are locally aggressive with a tendency to infiltrate adjacent tissues and organs. Local recurrence is common and often causes death. Metastasis is well documented but is uncommon. This chapter will aim to give an overview of the diagnosis and management of CV junction chordomas.

## 2. Epidemiology

Chordomas are rare tumours arising from persistent rests of notochordal remnants. They constitute 0.2% of all CNS tumours. Chordomas represent between 1% to 8% of primary malignant bone tumours and 20% of those arising from the spine. (Rosenberg AE, 2003) The age adjusted incidence for chordomas is 0.08 per 100 000.

There is a 2:1 male preponderance for all chordomas. However, CV junction chordomas have a more equal sex distribution. There is a strikingly low incidence in ethnic minorities and the incidence in African Americans is around quarter of that in white populations.

These tumours tend to occur across a wide age range and the peak incidence varies with anatomical location. Chordomas of the CV junction present more commonly during the fourth and fifth decades with the average age at diagnosis being 38 years. They generally present at a younger age than sacral and vertebral chordomas. In comparison, sacral chordomas tend to present at an older age, with the average age of presentation being 56 years.

Small series of childhood chordomas have been reported and these are usually found at the skull base. However, they account for less than 5% of all chordomas. Familial chordoma has been described but is extremely rare and several chromosomal loci have been identified including 7q33 and isochromosome 1q. (Bhadra & Casey, 2006)

## 3. Embryology & genetics

Chordomas arise from remnants of the embryonic notochord and are located in all places where the notocord existed, including the clivus, sella turcica, foramen magnum, upper cervical spine and nasopharynx.

The notochord is a rod-like structure which comprises the embryonic axis of the body. It arises from ectodermal cells and forms during the third week of life. It is known to have an important role in the development of the vertebral column and is thought to play a part in somite differentiation, vertebral chondrogenesis and vertebral column segmentation as well as other possible roles. (Fleming et al., 2001)

During fetal life the notochord regresses but at the site of the intervertebral discs it persists and contributes to the formation of the nucleus pulposus. (Pazzaglia et al., 1989)

There is a large amount of evidence to support the theory that chordomas arise from notochordal cells. Portions of the notochord are known to persist at a number of sites including the skull base, coccyx and spine. These small, well-circumscribed, gelatinous collections of cells were first described by Muller, as ecchordoses physaliphoria. (Muller H, 1858) There is a morphological similarity between the cells of chordomas and ecchordoses physaliphoria. (Ribbert H, 1895) The immunohistological similarity between chordomas and notochord cells has been demonstrated in a number of studies. In addition, a study by Salisbury et al. (1993) demonstrated that although the notochord is a rod-like structure the rostral and caudal ends of the notochord are more complicated structures that demonstrate forking at the ends with fragments of chordal tissue separate from the main bulk of the notochord. This anatomical feature may help explain why regression of the notochord in fetal life may leave behind collections of notochordal cells which may subsequently give rise to chordomas in the common sites such as the skull base and sacrococcygeal region. (Salisbury et al., 1993)

Cytogenetic studies of chordoma show a number of abnormalities including triploidy, marker chromosomes, losses of or from chromosomes 1,3,4,10 and 13, and gains of chromosomes 7 and 20. (DeFrancesco et al., 2006) Microsatellite instability resulting from DNA mismatch repair deficiencies has also been demonstrated. (Klingler et al., 2000) However, no chordoma-specific translocations have yet been identified.

## 4. Pathology

Chordomas are typically found in three locations in the spine, with 50% occurring in the sacrum. The second most common site is the clivus, accounting for 35% of tumours and they are also seen less commonly in any part of the vertebral column. Other intraaxial and extraxial sites have been reported in the literature.

The site of origin of skull base chordomas is the clivus. From here they can extend into the anterior fossa, middle fossa, the sellar and parasellar regions and through the foramen magnum into the upper cervical spine. In the majority of cases the typical histological appearances and characteristic location of chordomas renders the diagnosis straightforward.

Chordomas are typically multilobulated masses. They are soft and gelatinous with a well-defined, greyish surface. The cut surface is usually homogenous but calcifications and occasional haemorrhages may be seen. However, chordomas are not histologially encapsulated and extensions of the fibrous tissue on the surface penetrate the tumour as fibrous septa creating a lobular appearance.

Microscopically chordomas are composed of relatively uniform populations of cells with cytoplasmic vacuoles of varying sizes. This abundant cell type is the pathognomic physaliphorous cells, while some cells have signet ring morphology and others have a more eosinophilic cytoplasm. The tumour cells are embedded in an basophilic and mucinous matrix. The cell nuclei are usually small, round or oval, with a dense chromatin pattern but occasional tumours may contain focal pleomorphism. Mitoses, although present, are usually rare. Mild atypia may be present but necrosis is uncommon. (Figure 1)

The cells of chordomas contain glycogen, and the matrix stains positively with mucicarmine and Alcian blue and metachromatically with toluidine blue. Ultrastructural examination of chordomas shows evidence of epithelial differentiation, with the presence of cell junctions and intracytoplasmic connections. Membrane-bound glycogen, intermediate filaments and rough endoplasmic reticululm are also found.

Chordomas stain positive for a number of immunohistochemial markers including positivity for cytokeratins, EMA, vimentin and occasionally S100 protein and carcinoembryonic antigen. Brachyury expression can also be used to distinguish them from other tumours such as chondrosarcoma. However, actin, demin, CD31, CD34 and collagen are usually negative. (DeFrancesco et al., 2006)

Variations of chordomas containing cartilaginous tissue have been described as chondroid chordomas. These account for a third of clival chordomas, have a slight female preponderance and occur in a younger age group. Those containing areas of sarcoma are described as dedifferentiated chordomas and they have a high risk of metastasis and a poor prognosis. The dedifferentiated component is usually not seen at presentation but occurs after recurrences and sometimes radiotherapy.

A few other lesions can mimic the appearance of chordoma on histology. These include chordoid meningioma, chondroma, chondrosarcoma (Figure 2), melanoma and metastatic adenocarcinoma. However, these lesions can usually be differentiated using further laboratory techniques.

## 5. Symptoms and signs

The craniovertebral region is a vital entry and exit point for a number of important neural pathways and structures. The precise nature of these clinical features and symptom progression depends entirely on the location of the chordoma and the rapidity of growth into the vital adjacent structures. It is therefore imperative that a thorough clinical history and clinical examination are undertaken to elucidate as much clinical information as possible at the time of diagnosis.

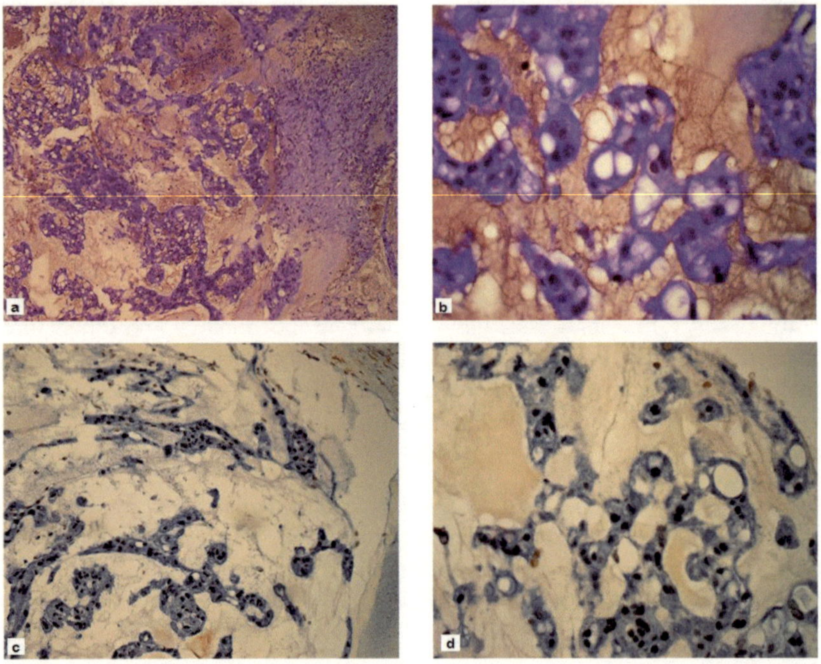


Fig. 1. a&b) H&E staining showing characteristic features of a chordoma (x40 & x100). Typical sheets of cells with cells containing vacuoles of various sizes can be seen. At higher magnification the phylasipharous cell, with it's large vaculole, can be easily made out as the abundant cell type. c&d) Brachyury immunohistochemistry identifying the characteristic chordoma cells.

Patients with chordomas at the CV junction can present in a number of ways including symptoms and signs of central and peripheral nervous system dysfunction. Clinical features can include sensory or motor disturbances, problems with gait, proprioception, coordination and respiratory compromise.

Neck pain is a presenting feature in 86% of patients. (Choi et al., 2010) Pain may occur in a dermatomal distribution, especially if the C2 nerve root is involved, but this is not always the case. Due to the propensity of chordomas to cause bone destruction the neck pain is usually non-specific and can sometimes be attributed to degenerative changes, particularly in older patients who do not have other features suggestive of more sinister disease at this location. Myelopathy is a common presenting feature, present in 18.6% of patients (Choi et al., 2010) and this may lead to weakness of the hands and associated spasticity of the extremities due to compression of the corticospinal tracts. (Crockard et al., 1993) Rarely a syrinx may be a present and these patients may present with atrophy of upper limb muscles and sensory disturbances.

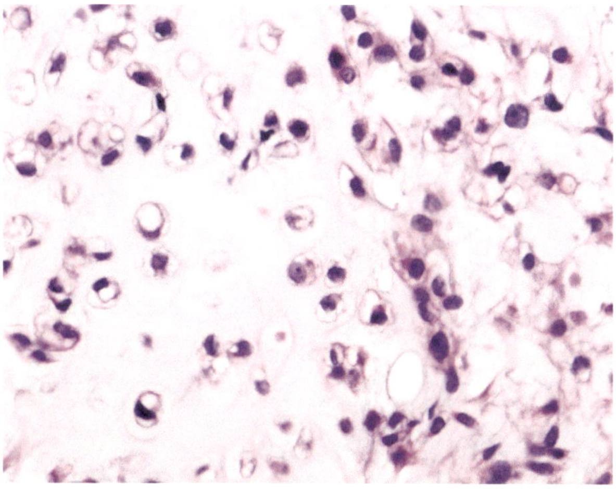

Fig. 2. H&E staining demonstrating chondrosarcoma (x100). The cells are not always arranged in a dense sheet like manner and contain less vacuoles and no phylasipharous cell. However, there are different grades of chondrosarcoma, which can all have slightly different appearances which need to be distinguished from chordoma using immunohistochemistry.

A number of cranial nerve deficits can result from chordomas at this location. Compression of the pons, medulla and rostral cervical region can lead to dysfunction of the trigeminal nucleus. In addition some branches of the facial, glossopharyngeal and vagus nerves supplying sensation to the face and tongue may also be affected as well as the motor supply to the palate. In addition, the accessory nerve may be compressed as it travels through the foramen magnum leading to motor deficits of the sternocleidomastoid and trapezius muscles. Chordomas located at the ventral surface of the foramen magnum may lead to compression of the hypoglossal nerve, which leads to ipsilateral tongue dysfunction and atrophy. If the jugular foramen is involved by the spread of chordoma then a number of distinct neurological syndromes may arise including Vernets, Collet-Sicard amd Villaret Syndromes. (Svien et al., 1969)

## 6. Imaging

Radiological diagnosis of CV junction chordomas has improved with advent of modern imaging modalities. Tumour location and extent of skull base involvement can now be precisely defined. Computed tomography (CT) and Magnetic Resonance Imaging (MRI) provide the mainstay of diagnostic information. However, plain radiographs, especially lateral radiographs of the cervical spine also have an important role to play, particularly in the postoperative assessment of cervical spine instrumentation. (Figures 3 a & b)

High resolution CT of the CV junction with bone and soft-tissue windows is very sensitive for detecting chordomas of the craniocervical junction. Fine cut axial and coronal unenhanced and contrast enhanced CT can evaluate bone involvement. On a CT scan, intracranial chordoma has a characteristic appearance with tumours being centrally located, well-defined, soft tissue masses arising from the clivus and causing lytic bone destruction. (Figure 4) Chordomas are usually hyper attenuating lesions and on administration of intravenous contrast they show a degree of enhancement.

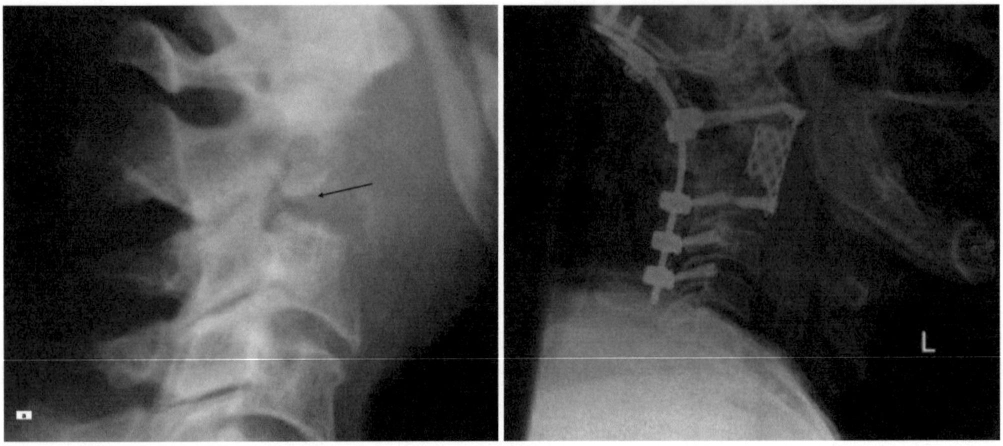


Fig. 3. a) Plain cervical spine lateral radiograph demonstrating osteolytic bone destruction in the region of the odontoid peg (arrow) . The chordoma mass can be seen anterior to the osteolyitc bone destruction, pushing the pharyngeal tissues anteriorly b) Post-operative plain cervical spine radiograph showing C2 corpectomy with insertion of cage and instrumented occipitocervical fusion using screws and rod fixation system.

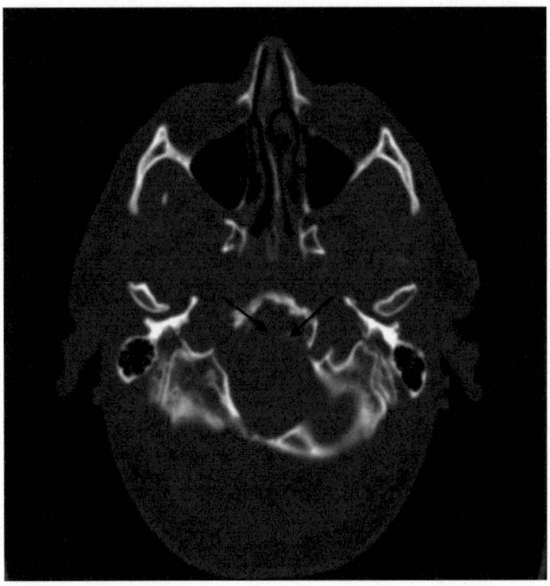

Fig. 4. Non-contrast enhanced axial CT of the craniovertebral junction, showing lytic bone destruction of the anterior clivus (arrows).

MRI of the CV junction is the best modality for evaluation of craniocervical junction chordomas. MR defines the extent of the tumour and it's spread to adjacent structures and is therefore useful both for diagnosis and for preoperative planning. Sagital images are the most useful as they define the posterior margin of the tumour and importantly, the relation to the brainstem and the nasopharyngeal extension of the chordoma. (Figures 5 a & b) Axial and coronal images are useful in detecting extension into surrounding structures.

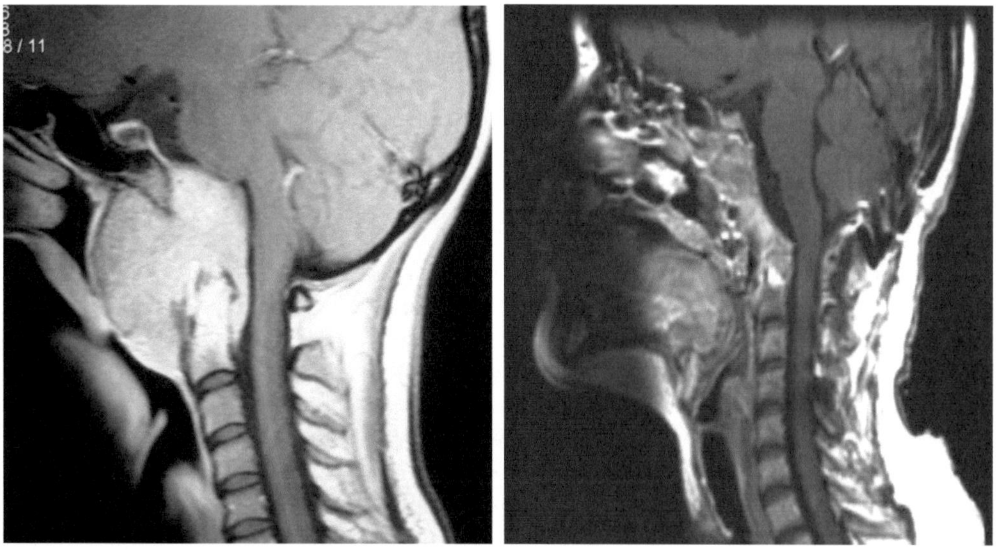


Fig. 5. a) Pre-operative T1 weighted sagital MRI showing extensive chordoma affecting the craniovetebral junction and spreading anteriorly to displace the pharyngeal structures. The tumour has a high signal and tumour expansion into the surrounding structures can be well delineated. b) Post-operative T1 weighted MRI of the craniovertebral junction showing resection of the tumour.

On T1 weighted MR imaging, chordomas usually demonstrate low signal intensity. Areas of high signal may be seen on T1 weighted images and these usually represent areas of focal haemorrhage. Chordomas classically have a high signal on T2-weighted MR scans due to their high fluid content. In addition T2 imaging is excellent for delineating the tumour from adjacent structures.

Craniovertebral junction chordomas demonstrate a degree of enhancement with gadolinium contrast. The enhancement is sometimes described as a 'honeycomb' appearance, which is due to intratumoural areas of low signal intensity. Fat suppression sequences can be used to differentiate tumour margins from adjacent fatty bone marrow. Small intraclival chordomas may be better demonstrated with these sequences.

MR Angiography (MRA) has a role in demonstrating the patency of the basilar artery as well as involvement of other large vessels including the internal carotid artery, which may be involved in large craniovertebral junction chordomas with significant anterior extension. Chordomas in this region often displace or encase vessels in this region and MRA has an advantage over digital subtraction angiography (DSA), which does not allow detection of encasement without luminal narrowing or occlusion. MRA is usually sufficient in pre-operative planning but DSA can demonstrate the collateral circulation and allow balloon occlusion of the internal carotid to help determine whether a patient is at risk if an important vessel is sacrificed.

Local recurrence of these tumours is a common finding and gadolinium enhanced MR is the best mode of assessing the degree of tumour excision and for follow-up. Marked high signal on T2 weighted imaging suggests tumour recurrence rather than post-operative changes.

The lesions most often confused with craniovertebral junction chordomas are chondroscarcomas. Although the majority of these usually occur in or around the sutures of the petrous bone, they can sometimes arise from the midline and mimic the MR appearance of a chordoma. Meningiomas arising from the clival region often do not cause bony destruction and tend to have a characteristic dural attachment.

### 6.1 Illustrative case

A 42-year-old man presented with a two-year history of neck pain, progressive difficulty in swallowing and visual disturbance. He had no significant medical problems and no family history of any illness. On examination he was alert and orientated in time, place and person. The only neurological deficit he had a left occulomotor and abducens nerve palsy. Plain radiographs of his cervical spine were unremarkable. Non-enhanced CT scan showed a lytic destruction of the anterior clivus (Figure 4). MR imaging was subsequently performed. The non-enhanced sagital T1-weighted MRI (Figure 5) demonstrated a large homogenous mass arising from the region of the craniovertebral junction and extending anteriorly compressing the pharyngeal structures. There is also associated lytic change within the odontoid peg. It was decided that the patient should have surgery to debulk the tumour followed by adjuvant radiation treatment. (See below)

## 7. Treatment

Harvey Cushing was the first surgeon to remove a chordoma successfully. (Cushing, 1912) Chordomas are usually extradural tumours that are found in the midline but they often extend into surrounding regions. There is a large body of evidence to suggest that maximal tumour resection is associated with a better outcome.

A number of approaches for the treatment of craniovertebral junction chordomas have been described but the most commonly used surgical approaches for lesions of the lower clivus, foramen magnum and the upper cervical spine is the standard transoral approach. A number of extended anterior midline transoral approaches exist including a transoral approach with a palatotomy, an 'open-door' maxillotomy, transmandibular and midface degloving procedures but the approach used depends on the exact site and extent of the lesion and surgeon experience and preference. More recently, endoscopic trans-nasal approaches have also been used with success.

All of the above approaches are suitable for midline clival chordomas but where there is significant lateral extension the midline approach alone may be insufficient for the removal of the entire tumour and more complex lateral approaches may have to be used as a primary or secondary procedure. A number of these approaches have been described for tumours of the upper clivus and include the subtemporal, transcavernous and the transpetrous approaches. (Gay et al., 1995a) For lateral lesions of the midclivus a subtemporal and infratemporal approach have been described. For lesions of the lower clivus with lateral extension to the occipital condyle and jugular foramen, the extreme lateral transcondylar approach can be used. (Sen & Sekhar, 1990) Larger chordomas involving the entire clival region, the sphenoid and the sellar region with extension anteriorly to the optic nerves may need staged surgery via multiple approaches.

### 7.1 Surgical approaches

The standard transoral approach is the main authors preferred approach to ventral midline craniocervical junction chordomas. It was first described by Kanavel (1908) who used it to remove a bullet between the skull base and atlas. This approach has since been modified and used to treat a number of aetiologies. (Kanavel, 1908) The standard transoral approach is the most frequently used approach for resecting chordomas of the craniocervical junction in the region of the lower clivus down to the level of C2. It may be combined with a soft palate split or an 'open-door' maxillotomy. Upper clival lesions may be excised using endoscopic trans-nasal techniques, which may have a lower complication rate than the 'open-door maxillotomy'.

Prior to performing the transoral procedure it is essential to ensure that the maximal interdental opening is greater than 25mm. A nasotracheal intubation is preferred and a nasogastric tube must be inserted. This ensures that the stomach is decompressed and more importantly, allows the administration of enteral nutrition following the procedure yet allowing the oropharyngeal wounds to heal. The patient's head is placed in a Mayfield head holder with the patient supine in the head-up position. The mouth is then cleaned with antiseptic solution, topical hydrocortisone applied to the mouth and oropharynx to reduce post-operative inflammation and parenteral antibiotics administered preoperatively and a further two doses following surgery.

The transoral retractor is inserted and the tongue blade ensures that the tongue is pushed down and out of the way. Insertion of the palatal retractors ensures that the palate is pulled upwards in the opposite direction and the nasotracheal and nasogastric tubes are pulled clear of the surgical field. The surgical anatomical landmark is the anterior tubercle of C1, to which is attached the anterior longitudinal ligament and the overlying longus colli muscle. A midline vertical incision is made on the tubercle of C1 and the pharyngeal retractors inserted and the longus colli muscle and the anterior longitudinal ligament cut using monopolar diathermy. This reveals the arch of C1 and the odontoid peg. The extent of the chordoma however, will dictate the craniocaudal and lateral extent of the exposure, and care should be taken to avoid damage to the hypoglossal nerve and the vertebral artery laterally. The C1 anterior arch and the peg are drilled out and the inferior clivus can be removed with drill and Kerisson rongeurs. The dural basilar plexus must be carefully dissected off the inferior border of the clivus to prevent vascular injury and bleeding. From here chordoma affecting the clivus can be resected. (Bouramas & Crockard, 2003)

If necessary the soft palate can be split in the midline to extend the superior and lateral exposure and this allows greater visualisation and access to the lower clivus. Another modification of the transoral procedure combines a LeFort I osteotomy with a midline incision in the hard and soft palate, the so-called 'open-door' maxillotomy. This provides excellent exposure to the upper middle clivus and sphenoid and gives good exposure inferiorly and laterally. For unilaterally extending tumours a unilateral LeFort osteotomy can be performed.

The endoscopic transnasal approach was developed to provide access to lesions of the middle and upper clivus and provides excellent visualization craniocervical junction. At the same time it avoids the complications of the traditional transoral approach and significantly reduces the morbidity associated with a LeFort osteotomy with 'open-door' maxillotomy. After the patient has undergone preoperative planning and the nasal anatomy has been assessed, the patient is put in a Mayfield head holder and topical adrenaline is applied to the nasal septum and mucosa of the turbinate bones. The entire procedure is performed under direct visualisation using an endoscope. The posterior aspect of the nasal septum is perforated near the rostrum of the sphenoid sinus to provide access to the nasopharynx. The rostrum of the sphenoid sinus is opened and the vomer and floor of the sphenoid sinus are removed. The mucosa of the nasophrynx is incised and usually reflected downwards into the oropaharynx and can be used as a flap at the end of the procedure. This allows visualisation of the anterior arch of C1 and the odontoid and resection of the tumour can then be performed. (Kassam et al., 2005)

Following an anterior approach to debulk the tumour a posterior occipito-cervical fixation is often required to provide stability to the upper cervical spine.

### 7.2 Surgical complications

A number of series have demonstrated high complication rates from excision of craniocervical junction chordomas. Harbour et al. (1991) reported 3 postoperative deaths in a series of 11 patients. Carpentier et al. (2002) reported 3 perioperative deaths in a series of 36 patients. Gay et al. (1995b) had a CSF leak rate of 30% and Pallini et al. (2003) reported 17 significant complications in 26 patients including 3 CSF fistulae. Choi et al. (2010) had a CSF leak rate of 6.2% and other complication rates included dysphagia (3.1%), nasal regurgitation (3.1%), meningitis (3.1%), sepsis (3.1%), chest infections, cranial nerve deficits and fixation failure. In the study by Choi et al. (2010), there were no differences in sepsis rates when comparing the standard transoral with the more extensive procedures. The study also showed that patients having the more extended surgeries appeared to have a worse prognosis than the standard transoral approach, although this was not statistically significant. It was also noted that patients who had their primary surgery at the specialist centres had a better outcome than those patients who had been initially treated elsewhere and had been referred on recurrence. Nasal regurgitation was more common with open-door maxillotomies than the standard procedure but the incidence of nasal regurgitation was not significantly different following division of the soft palate. Dysphagia was more common with mandibulotomy and glossotomy. (Choi et al., 2010)

It is clear that surgery confers a better survival benefit than with conservative treatment. Erikson et al. (1981) showed that survival rate for 11 patients with untreated chordoma was only 1 year. Radical resection of the tumour appears to confer the best survival outcomes as previously stipulated by Crockard et al. (2001) and also demonstrated by the large series of Choi et al. (2010). Colly & Al-Mefty (2001) achieved complete tumour excision in almost half of their patients with greater than ninety percent in almost 80%. However, they had a complication rate approaching 60%, with predominantly neurologic complications including cranial nerve palsies, cerebrospinal fluid leak, hydrocephalus, meningitis and oronasal fistulae. However, they found that complication rates did not greatly increase with greater extents of resection but there is a correlation of better survival with greater than 90% tumour resection. Gay et al. (1995) also demonstrated that there was no difference in complication rates in those patients receiving complete excision and those receiving partial debulking procedures. Although true oncological resection of these tumours is virtually impossible, aggressive tumour resection, including removal of bone margins where possible to reduce tumour load does appear to confer a survival benefit.

## 8. Radiation therapy

Despite the application of radiotherapy and radiosurgery for the treatment of CV junction chordomas, the importance of maximal surgical resection remains unequivocal. Greater survival has been shown to correlate with radical removal as opposed to partial resection. However, radical resection is not always possible due to the close proximity of these tumours to critical structures and the associated morbidity this entails. Traditionally chordomas have been regarded as relatively radio-resistant tumours but a number of treatment strategies using radiation treatments have been developed to gain control of these locally aggressive tumours. However, the size and precise location of the tumour is the most important factor in considering radiation planning.

Fractionated radiotherapy with high energy photons and radiotherapy with charged particles are the two most common forms of radiotherapy for CV junction chordomas. Fractionated radiotherapy has the benefit of sublethal damage repair of normal tissues in between treatment fractions, and thus the importance of surgery in resecting tumour from critical structures is vital.

### 8.1 Conventional radiation therapy

Conventional radiation therapy has been used for decades to gain local control of skull base chordomas and most patients undergo adjuvant fractionated radiotherapy to reduce the risk of tumour recurrence. However, initial doses of 50 to 55 Gy after resection did not provide successful local control and were associated with poor progression-free and overall survival rates. (Catton et al., 1996; Cummings et al., 1999) Catton et al reported on 13 patients who received a median dose of 50 Gy but only one of these patients remained disease free at 93 months following treatment. In the study by Cummings et al 24 patients diagnosed with chordoma were treated with megavoltage radiation therapy following incomplete tumour resection. The 5 year survival was 62% and at 10 years it was 28%.

Conventional radiotherapy with high energy photons, ranging from 40-70 Gy in different series, has been shown to be of survival benefit compared to surgery alone. However, local recurrence rates after residual incomplete resection followed by photon radiation therapy have been reported between 80% to 100%. (Catton et al., 1996; Cummings et al., 1999; Fuller & Bloom, 2003; Zorlu et al., 2000)

Although higher doses of fractionated radiotherapy have been shown to reduce the rate of tumour recurrence and increase survival rates, administration of higher doses are associated with greater side effects. Subsequently, other forms of radiation therapy have been pursued to greater success.

### 8.2 Proton beam radiation therapy

The largest amount of data in the use of radiation therapy for CV junction chordomas relates to proton beam therapy. Radiotherapy with charged particles has been used with success in the treatment of these tumours and has the advantage that it has a steeper fall-off then conventional therapy. Proton radiation allows improved dose localization than conventional photon therapy. In addition the positive charge of protons allows a energy dependent finite range in tissues, and the energy deposition demonstrates a sudden rise in dose at the end of the range with a subsequent sharp fall-off to zero dose, thereby providing excellent dose localization. This is known as the Bragg peak effect. Protons are assumed to have a slightly higher relative biological effectiveness compared with conventional photon radiotherapy. Proton beam radiation therapy is not restricted to the size of the tumour.

There are three large centres which have reported their outcomes of proton beam therapy in the literature: Loma Linda University Medical Centre (Loma Linda, CA), Harvard Cyclotron Laboratory at Massachusettes General Hospital (MGH/HCL) (Cambridge, MA) and the Institut Curie, Centre Protontherapie d'Orsay (Orsay Cedex, France)

The first patient to undergo proton irradiation for a CV junction chordoma was in 1974 at MGH/HCL. Since then, techniques have been developed to provide high dose, fractionated radiotherapy in doses excess of 70 Gy.

At LLUMC (Hug et al, 1999, 2001) Chordoma patients were treated with fractionated proton beam therapy to a mean dose of 70.7 CGE. The researchers observed a 3-year control rate of 67% with 5-year overall survival of 79%. In 1999 the MGN/HCL published there results of 519 cases of skull base tumours, of which 290 were chordomas. These patients were treated with combined proton and photon technique. The 5- and 10-year local recurrence free survival rates were 64% and 42% respectively. (Muzenrider & Liebsch, 1999) A hundred patients diagnosed with chordomas of the skull base and cervical spine were treated at the Centre de Protontherapie d'Orsay with a combined proton and photon technique. The median dose delivered to the tumour was 67 CGE. The 2- and 4-year local control rates were 86% and 54%.

Another form of charged particle therapy is the use of carbon ions, which also has a steep dose fall off after the Bragg peak. At the Gessellschaft fur Schwerionenforschung Darmstadt center in Heidelberg, Germany 96 patients with skull base chordoma were treated with carbon ion therapy. (Schulz-Ertner et al., 2007) The median dose delivered was 60 CGE with a mean follow-up time of 31 months. At 3 years, the local control rate in this series was 81% and 70% at 5-years. Overall survival rates were 92% and 89% at 3- and 5-years respectively.

The superior local tumour control and overall survival achieved using proton beam over conventional photon radiotherapy are due to the superior dose localisation characteristics of protons that result in a higher dose of radiation being delivered. However, side effects of this radiation therapy are relatively common and include the typical early and late radiation sequelae including nausea, headaches and radiation necrosis of the brain. It is important to note that there have not been any randomised trials comparing proton beam therapy to other types of radiation treatment.

### 8.3 Stereotactic radiosurgery

Stereotactic radiosurgery is a technique which is designed to achieve a greater radiobiological effect than conventional forms of radiotherapy. Due to its precision and steep dose fall off, stereotactic radiosurgery has been used as a minimally invasive primary, adjuvant and palliative management option in patients with CV junction chordomas.

Stereotactic radiosurgery is a potent treatment option for small sized chordomas. The greatest benefit of stereotactic radiosurgery is the steep dose gradient achievable, which minimizes radiation outside the tumour target, thus allowing the delivery of a larger dose to the tumour without exceeding the radiation-related tolerance of normal tissues.

The North American Gamma Knife Consortium (NAGKC) was established to evaluate the outcomes of patient with relatively rare tumours including chordomas. Their collaboration identified 71 patients who underwent stereotactic radiosurgery with Gamma Knife for chordoma. The median age of patients was 45 years and the median SRS target volume was 7.1 cm3 (range 0.9-109 cm3). Their study suggests that SRS is as effective as proton beam therapy for small tumours that have not been treated with prior radiation.

However, more rigorous studies need to be carried out to discover the relative merits of stereotactic radiosurgery over proton beam therapy.

For patients with craniocervical junction chordoma, maximal surgical resection with proton beam therapy remains the mainstay of treatment with stereotactic surgery possibly having a role in selected cases.

## 9. Medical therapies

Medical therapies do not routinely form the mainstay of treatment of chordomas. As with most other low grade malignancies these tumours are not reported to be sensitive to chemotherapy. A number of anecdotal reports of responses to chemotherapy exist (Azzarelli et al., 1988; McSweeney & Sholl, 1959; Razis et al., 1974; Scimeca et al., 1996) but these are limited to case reports. A prospective phase II clinical trial using the chemotherapy agent 9-nitro-camptothecin (9-NC), a topoisomerase inhibitor, has been conducted and although it only showed a 7% objective response rate it did demonstrate 6-month progression-free survival rate of 33% and a median time to progression of 9.9 weeks. (Chugh et al., 2005) No phase III clinical study of systemic therapy of chordomas been reported.

Other groups have attempted to investigate the effects of molecular targeted therapies as potential adjuvant treatments for low-grade chordomas. A phase II study of chordoma response to Imatinib Mesylate, a tyrosine kinase inhibitor, demonstrated a clinical benefit in 32 of 44 patients but reduction in tumour size was only observed in 7 of 44 patients. (Stacchiottis F et al., 2007)

In another study patients with PDGFR B positive inoperable or metastatic chordoma treated with imatinib mesylate, demonstrated stabilisation of the disease as a best response. (Ferraresi V et al., 2010) Other signal transduction pathways that may provide therapeutic targets include EGFR, which has been used in a single patient and showed clinical response. (Signal N et al., 2009)

Possible targets for immunotherapy include high molecular weight-melanoma associated antigen (HMW-MAA). This is expressed in over 60% of chordomas and studies have shown that this may be a useful target to apply immunotherapy to these tumours. (Schwab JH et al., 2009)

As laboratory and clinical investigations have started to reveal the genetic and molecular pathways involved in the pathogenesis of chordoma, future efforts may be focused on finding novel techniques to that can be translated into clinical practice.

## 10. Prognosis

Interpretation of published data on survival rates is difficult because of the heterogeneity of published series, small numbers of patients, short follow-up periods and difficulties in histological diagnoses, which has been common in earlier studies. Colli and Mefty (2001) documented a 5-year survival of 85.9% but this series included lesions, which may actually represent chondrosarcomas, which are known to have a better prognosis. In the large series by Choi et al 2010 the median survival rate was 84-months and the mean survival was 99 months from the date of surgery with 5- and 10-year survival times 55% and 36% respectively. Other studies have shown similar survival rates to this with Carpentier et al. (2002) having 5- and 10-year survival rates of 80% and 65% and Forsyth et al. (1993) showing survival rates of 51% and 35% following surgery.

## 11. Expert suggestions

Craniocervical junction chordomas are unique tumours that pose significant treatment challenges. As these lesions are rare we advocate that they should be treated at the first presentation at specialist centres where patients undergo careful selection and counselling and where specialists can perform a maximal resection of the tumour whilst keeping complications to a minimum.

## 12. Conclusion

Craniovertebral junction tumours are rare tumours that can present in a number of different ways. The majority of these tumours require radical surgery followed by adjuvant radiation therapy to improve outcome. Due to the heterogeneity of published series it is not possible to compare survival outcomes between existing series. However, due to the location of these tumours the prognosis remains poor.

## 13. Acknowledgements

The authors would like to thank the Dr Maria Thom, Consultant Neuropathologist at the National Hospital for Neurology and Neurosurgery, for supplying us with the histopathological images.

## 14. References

Azzarelli A, Quagliuolo V, Cerasoli S, Zucali R, Bignami P, Mazzaferro V, Dossena G & Gennari L. 1988. Chordoma: Natural history and treatment results in 33 cases. *Journal of Surgical Oncology*. 37(3):185-191.

Bhadra AK, Casey AT. 2006. Familial Chordoma. A report of two cases. *The Journal of Bone & Joint Surgery*. 88B:634-66.

Bouramas D & Crockard A. 2003. Anterior Odontoid Resection. In Surgical Techniques for the Spine. Haher TR, Merola AA. Pp 10-15. Thieme Medical Publishers, ISBN 3131247614, New York.

Carpentier A, Polivka M, Blanquet A, Lot G, George B. 2002. Suboccipital and cervical chordomas: The value of aggressive treatment at first presentation of the disease. *Journal of Neurosurgery*. 97:1070-1077.

Catton C, O'Sullivan B, Bell R, Laperriere N, Cummings B, Fornasier V & Wunder J. 1996. Chordoma: Long term follow-up after radical photon irradiation. *Radiotherapy & Oncology*. 41(1):67-72.

Chugh R, Dunn R, Zalupski MM, Bierman JS, Sondak VK, Mace JR, Leu KM, Chandler WF & Baker LH. 2005. Phase II study of 9-nitro-camptothecin in patients with advanced chordoma or soft tissue sarcoma. *Journal of Clinical Oncology*. 23(15):3597-604.

Choi D, Melcher R, Harms J, Crockard A. 2010. Outcome of 132 operations in 97 patients with chordomas of the craniocervical junction and upper cervical spine. *Neurosurgery*. 66(1):59-65.

Colli BO & Al-Mefty O. 2001. Chordomas of the skull base: follow-up review and prognostic factors. *Journal of Neurosurgery*. 95:933-943.

Crockard HA, Heilman AE, Stevens JM. 1993. Progressive myelopathy secondary to odontoid fractures: clinical, radiological and surgical features. *Journal of Neurosurgery*. 78(4)579-586.

Crockard HA, Steel T, Plowman N, Singh A, Crossman J, Revesz T, Holton JL, Cheeseman A. 2002. A multidisciplinary team approach to skull base chordomas. *Journal of Neurosurgery*. 95:175-183.

Cummings BJ, Hodson DI, Bush RS. 1999. Chordoma: The results of megavoltage therapy. *International Journal of Radiation Oncology, Biology, Physics*. 9:633-642.

Cushing H. 1912. The pituitary body and its disorders. Philadelphia: JB Lippincott.

DiFrancesco LM, Cristobal A, Castillo D, Temple WJ. 2006. Extra-Axial Chordoma. *Archives Pathological and Laboratory Medicine*. 130:1871-74.

Eriksson B, Gunterberg B, Kindblom LG. 1981. Chordoma: A clinicopathological and prognostic study of a Swedish national series. *Acta Orthopaedica Scandinavica*. 52:49-58.

Ferraresi V, Nuzzo C, Zoccali C, marandino F, Vidiri A, Salducca N, Zeuli M, Giannarelli D, Cognetti F, Biagini R. 2010. Chordoma: clinical characteristics, management and prognosis of a case series of 25 patients. *BMC Cancer*. 22:1471-2407.

Fleming A, Keynes RJ, Tannahill D. 2001. The role of the notochord in vertebral column formation. *Journal of Anatomy*. 199;177-80.

Forsyth PA, Cascino TL, Shaw EG, Scheithaeur BW, O'Fallon JR, Dozier JC, Piepgras DG. 1993. Intracranial chordomas: A clinicopathological and prognostic study of 51 cases. *Journal of Neurosurgery*. 78:741-747.

Fuller DB & Bloom JG. 2003. Radiotherapy for chordoma. *International Journal of Radiation Oncology, Biology, Physics*. 56:7-13.

Gay E, Sekhar LN, Wright DC. 1995a. Chordomas and chondrosarcomas of the cranial base. In Brain Tumours. Kaye AH, Laws ER Jr. Pp. 777-794. Churchill Livingstone, ISBN 0443048401, Edinburgh.

Gay E, Sekhar LN, Rubinstein E, Wright DC, Sen C, Janecka IP, Snyderman CH. 1995b.Chordomas and chondrosarcomas of the skull base: results and follow-up of 60 patients. *Neurosurgery*. 36:887-897.

Harbour JW, Lawton MT, Criscuolo GR, Holliday MJ, Mattox DE, Long DM. 1991. Clivus chordoma: A report of 12 recent cases and review of the literature. *Skull Base Surgery*. 1:200-206.

Kanavel AB. 1908. Bullet located between the atlas and the base of the skull: technique of removal through the mouth. *Surgical Clinics of Chicago*. 1:361-366.

Kassam AB, Gardner P, Snyderman C, Mintz A, Carrau R. 2005. Expanded endonasal approach: fully endoscopic, completely transnasal approach to the middle third of the clivus, petrous bone, middle cranial fossa and infratemporal fossa. *Neurosurgery Focus*. 15;19(1):E6.

Klingler L, Shooks J, Fiedler PN, Marney A, Butler MG. 2000. Microsatellite instability in sacral chordoma. *Journal of Surgical Oncology*. 73:100-3.

McSweeney AJ & Sholl PR. 1959. Metastatic chordoma use of mechlorethamine (nitrogen mustard) in chordoam therapy. *AMA Archives of Surgery*. 79:152-155.

Muzenrider JE & Liebsch NJ. 1999. Proton beam therapy for tumours of the skull base. *Strahlentherapie und Onkologie*. 175(Suppl 2):57-63.

Pallini R, Maira G, Pierconti F, Falchetti ML, Alvino E, Cimino-Reale G, Fernandez E, D'Ambrosio E, Larocca LM. 2003. Chordoma of the skull base: predictors of tumour recurrence. *Journal of Neurosurgery*. 98(4):812-822.

Pazzaglia UE, Salisbury JR, Byers PD. 1989. Development and involution of the notochord in the human spine. *Journal of the Royal Society of Medicine*. 82:413-415.

Muller H. 1858. Ueber das Vorkommen von resten der chorda dorsalis bei menschen nach der geburt und uber ihr verhaltniss zu den gallertgeschwulsten am clivus. *Z Ration Medic*. 2:202-229.

Razis DV, Tsatsaronis A, Kyriazides I et al. 1974. Chordoma of the cervical spine treated with vincristine sulfate. *Journal of Medicine*. 5:274-277.

Ribbert H. 1895. Uber die experementelle Erzuegung einer Ecchondrosis physalifora. *Verh Dtsch Kong Inn Med*. 13:455-464.

Rosenberg AE. 2003. Pathology of chordoma and chondrosarcoma of the axial skeleton. In: Chondromas and Chondrosarcomas of the Skull Base and Spine. Harsh GD, Janecka IP, Mankin HJ, Ojemann RG, Suit H, pp.8-15. Thieme Medical Publishers, ISBN 9783131247711, New York.

Salisbury JR, Deverell MH, Cookson JH & Whimster WF. 1993. Three dimensional reconstruction of human embryonic notochords: clue to the pathogenesis of chordoma. *Journal of Pathology*. 171:59-62.

Scimeca PG, James-Herry AG, Black KS, Kahn E & Weinblatt ME. 1996. Chemotherapeutic treatment of malignant chordoma in children. *Journal of Pediatric Hematology & Oncology*. 18:237-240.

Scwab JH, Boland PJ, Agaram NP, Socci ND, Guo T et al. 2009. Chordoma and chondrosarcoma gene profile: implications for immunotherapy. Cancer Immunology & Immunotherapy. 58:339-349.

Sculz-Ertner D, Karger CP, Feuerhake A, Nikoghosyan A, Combs SE, Jakel O, Elder L, Scholz M & Debus J. 2007. Effectiveness of carbon ion therapy in the treatment of skull base chordomas. *International Journal of Radiation Oncology, Biology, Physics*. 68:449-457.

Sen CS, Sekhar LN. 1990. An extreme lateral approach to intradural lesions of the cervical spine and foramen magnum. *Neurosurgery*. 27:197-204.

Singhal N, Kotasek D, Parnis FX. 2009. Response to erlotinib in a patient with treatment refractory chordoma. *Anticancer Drugs*. 20:953-955.

Stacchiottis FV, Ferraresi G, Grignani F, Crippa A, Messina E, Tamborini CS, Gronchi A, Casali PG. 2007. Imatinib mesylate in advanced chordoma: a multicenter phase II study. *Journal of Clinical* Oncology. 25:1000-1003.

Svien HJ, Baker HL, Rivers MH. 1969. Jugular foramen syndrome and allied syndromes. *Neurology*. 13:797-809.

Zorlu F, Gurkaynak M, Yildiz F, Oge K & Atahan IL. 2000. Conventional external radiotherapy in the management of clival chordomas with overt residual disease. *Neurological Science*. 21:203-207.

# 15

# Anatomical and Surgical Perspective to Approach Degenerative Disc Hernias

H. Selim Karabekir[1], Nuket Gocmen-Mas[2] and Mete Edizer[3]
[1]*Department of Neurosurgery, Kocatepe University School of Medicine, Afyonkarahisar,*
[2]*Department of Anatomy, Faculty of Medicine, Kocatepe University, Afyonkarahisar,*
[3]*Department of Anatomy, Faculty of Medicine, Dokuz Eylul University, Izmir,*
*Turkey*

## 1. Introduction

The anatomy of the vertebral colomn is very important for neurosurgeons, orthopedists, traumatologists, neurologists, radiologists, anestesiologists and pathologists to aid in diagnosis, treatment, planning surgery, and the application of anesthesia or surgery (Winn, 2004).

Intervertebral discs are placed on between adjacent surfaces of vertebral bodies from axis to sacrum. There is no intervertebral disc between atlas and axis. The lowest functional intervertebral disc is located between fifth lumbar (L5) and sacrum. Thicknesses of the discs show variations in different regions and part of the same disc. They are thicker anteriorly and the anterior convexity is obvious in lumbar and cervical regions, but they are nearly uniform and the anterior concavity is large due to vertebral bodies in the thoracic region. In the upper thoracic region, discs are thinnest, but they thickest in the lumbar region. Intervertebral discs are avascular. They supplied by diffusion through the trabecular bone of nearby vertebrae. In brief, discs supplied from neighborhood blood vessels, except for their periphers. Vascular and avascular parts of discs show different reaction to injury.

Radicular damages related with degenerative disc hernias negatively affect innervation area of the spinal nerves, sensibility and ability of the patients to translate patterns of altered nerves activity into meaningful motor behaviors. The sensory or motor alterations can be attributed to functional or anatomical changes within the nerve roots after resolution of inflammation and edema and also surrounding of the nerves (Chaichana et al., 2011; Van Zundert et al., 2010; Lipetz, 2002).

## 2. Anatomy of vertebral column

### 2.1 Embriology

Vertebrae develop from the sclerotome parts of the somites, which are undergone, a change from the paraaxial mesoderm. A typical vertebra forms a vertebral arch and foramen, a body, transverse process, and usually a spinous process. Sclerotome cells move around the spinal cord and notochord to merge with cells from the opposing somite on the opposite side of the neural tube during the fourth week. As development continues, the sclerotome part of each somite also transposes a resegmentation. Resegmentation means as growing and blending of the caudal half of each sclerotome with the cephalic half of each subjacent sclerotome. So, each vertebra is combined between the caudal half of one somite and the cranial half of its neighbor. Modeling of the shapes of the different vertebrae is modulated by HOX genes (Sadler, 2006). Hox genes were defined to be involved in the manufacture of vertebrae with individual properties (Krumlauf 1994; Wellik 2007; Mallo et al., 2009). Mesenchymal cells which placed between two caudal parts of the sclerotome segment and fill the space between two precartilaginous vertebral bodies. In this way, they form the intervertebral discs. Although the notochord regresses entirely in the region of the vertebral bodies, it asserts and expands in the disc space. It supports the nucleus pulposus, which is covered loop shaped fibers of the annulus fibrosus. These two structures compose the intervertebral disc together (Sadler, 2006; Moore, 1992; Williams et al, 1995; Snell, 1997; April, 1990)

Resegmentation of sclerotomes into descriptive vertebrae cause the myotomes to bridge the intervertebral discs. This differentiation gains the discs spine motion capacity. Due to this development, intersegmental arteries, at first placed between the sclerotomes, to come to pass midway over the vertebral bodies (Sadler, 2006). Spinal nerves go to near the intervertebral discs and exit from the intervertebral foramina to leave vertebral column at that level (Moore, 1992; Williams et al, 1995; Snell, 1997; April, 1990).

### 2.2 Vertebral morphology

The vertebral column compose 33-34 number of vertebrae which are seven cervical, twelve thoracic, five lumbar vertebrae, a sacrum and three to five coccygeal vertebrae (Standrings et al, 2005; Williams et al, 1995). Each typical vertebra has a ventral body (except atlas) and dorsal vertebral arch, together enclosing a vertebral foramen. The adjacent bodies are attached together by intervertebral discs. The foramina form a vertebral canal for spinal cord. Intervertebral foramina which are located between adjoining vertebral arches, allow transmit spinal nerves, blood and lymphatic vessels. The vertebral body varies in size according to its level on vertebral column. The vertebral arch has one each side anteriorly the *pedicle,* and posteriorly the *lamina.* It also has paired transverse, superior and inferior articular processes and posteriorly a median spinous process. The pedicles are thick, short vertically narrower parts. Adjacent vertebral notches assist to an intervertebral foramen when vertebrae are articulated by the intervertebral discs. The laminae which directly continuous with pedicles are vertically broader flattened parts. The articular processes which are named as zygoapophyses joint compose paired superior and inferior articular processes. The superior ones locate on cranially, and the inferior ones caudally. Articular processes of adjoining vertebrae thus form synovial zygoapophyses joints together. These joints permit limited movement between vertebrae. The transverse processes project laterally. Only the thoracic transverse processes articulate with the ribs via their articular faces. The spinous process projects posteriorly and often caudally from the laminal junction. The spines vary in size, shape and directions according to vertebral level.

There are some regional features and differences of vertebrae. Vertebrae in different regions of the vertebral column show some modified characteristics from the typical pattern. There are conspicuous varieties in the size of the vertebral foramina in the same regions of different persons. There are also differences in the size and shape of the vertebral canal. These variations occur because of the spinal cord enlargements in the cervical and lumbosacral regions for the innervations of the limbs via plexuses (Moore, 1992).

Distinctive characterization of the cervical vertebrae is the oval shaped foramen transversarium. The vertebral arteries pass through the foramina in the transverse process, except those in prominent vertebra (C7) which lie only small accessory vertebral veins. Each of the processes has anterior and posterior tubercles on their upper surfaces. The groove for the spinal nerves locates between the tubercles from third cervical vertebra (C3) to C7 vertebrae, bilaterally. The anterior tubercle of sixth cervical vertebra (C6) which is named as carotic tubercle is bigger than the others. Due to large size of the tubercle, it may compress the common carotic artery. The spinous processes of C3 to C6 vertebrae are short and bifid. The spinous process of C7 is very long, so it is also important as an anatomical landmark for clinicians.

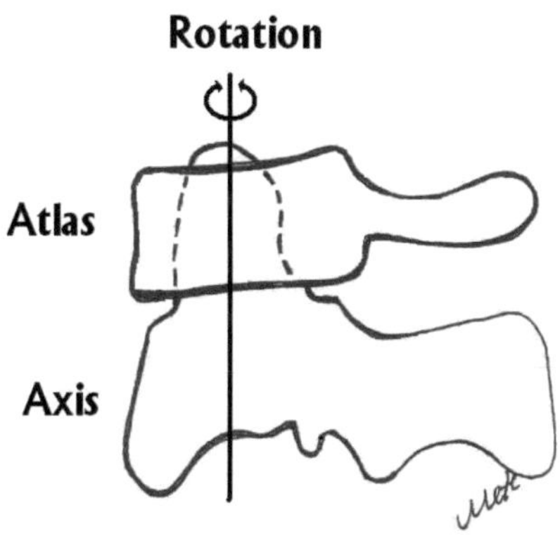


Fig. 1. The relationship between atlas and axis were shown while rotation (Illustrated by Edizer).

Atlas (C1) and axis (C2) are atypical vertebrae. C1 is a ring-shaped bone. The kidney-shaped, concave superior articular surfaces of C1 have the occipital condyles. The atlas has no spinous process or body; it has anterior and posterior arches. Each of the arch consists a tubercle and a lateral mass which is named as massa lateralis atlantis. C2 is named as axis and the skull rotates on it. The axis consists two large flat bearing the superior articular facets upon which the atlas rotates (Figure 1). Its distinguishing characteristic, however, is the blunt tooth-like dens which are called as odontoid process; place on superiorly from its body. The transverse ligament of the atlas supports dens for its position and prevents horizontal displacement of the atlas (Moore, 1992).

Distinctive features of the thoracic vertebrae are existance of the fovea costalis to articulate with the ribs (Figure 2). Adjoining upper and lower costal fovea and also intervertebral disc together articulate with fovea costalis of a rib. The thoracic vertebra has a small nearly oval foramen vertebra. The spinous processes of the thoracic vertebrae are long and slender. The middle ones are directed inferiorly over the vertebral arches of the inferior vertebrae to them. But the laminae are short, broad and thick. The spinous process is long and oblique shaped and lies inferiorly. The transverse processes which are large, strong and club-like, project from the vertebral arch at pediculolaminar junctions. They point dorsolaterally, near their apex, ventral oval facets articulating with tubercles of corresponding ribs. The eleventh and the twelfth thoracic vertebrae have not the costal tubercles.

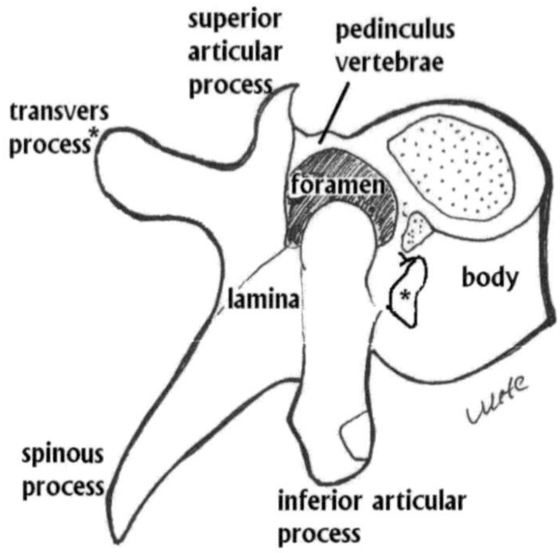


Fig. 2. Typical thoracic vertebra was shown (Illustrated by Edizer)

Differences of the lumbal vertebrae are their large size, absence of costal facets and transverse foramina (Moore, 1992). The body is big, thick and kidney shaped. The vertebral foramen is triangular shaped. The pedicles are short and the spinous process is nearly horizontal, quadrangular shaped and thick. L5 is distinct to its stout transverse processes. It is mostly amenable for the lumbosacral angle between the lumbar region and sacrum.

The sacrum which is fused by five vertebrae is a large, triangular shaped bone. It locates behind the pelvis and between two of the coxae. Its blunted, caudal tip articulates with the coccyx and its upper wide base articulates with the fifth lumbar vertebra. It consists dorsal, pelvic and lateral surfaces and a sacral canal between the apex and the base. Anterior projecting edge of the base is the sacral promontory. Four pairs of anterior sacral foramina place on the pelvic (anterior) surface. The ventral rami of the upper four sacral spinal nerves transmit through intervertebral foramina with the sacral canal via the pelvic sacral foramina. Similarly, four pairs of dorsal sacral foramina locate on the dorsal surface. The lateral surface projects as a broad articular part. Its upper parts have auricular surfaces, bilaterally. The sacral canal forms by sacral vertebral foramina. Its caudal opening is called as sacral hiatus. The canal contains the cauda equina including its flum terminale and spinal meninges. The coccyx is a small triangle bone. It usually consists of three to five fused rudimentary vertebrae (Williams et al, 1995; Moore, 1992).

As a conclusion the vertebral architecture is significant as it combine stability, load-bearing capacity and motor function and also covers contained neurovascular structures such as vessels, spinal nerves, irrespective of its position (Williams et al, 1995). Regional variants can see in mobility of the verterbrae on the geometry, position, placement and properties of both zygoapophysial joints and related ligaments around the column. The ligament flava, interspinous, supraspinous and posterior longitudinal ligaments and posterior margin of intervertebral disc are tensed, interlaminar intervals wider, inferior facet glide on superior facet of subjacent vertebrae and their capsules become taut.

## 2.3 Intervertebral disc morphology

The discs are composed of circular anuli fibrosi covering gelatinous nuclei pulposi. The anuli fibrosi insert into compact bony edges on articular face of the vertebral bodies. It has a narrow outer collagen zone and a wider inner fibrocartiloginous zone. The annulus fibrosus consists of concentric lamellae of collagenous fibers which lie obliquely from one vertebra to the other (Figure 3). The lamellae are less numerous posteriorly and thinner than they are anteriorly and laterally. The nuclei pulposi contact the hyaline articular cartilages, which are attached to endplates of the bodies. It is large, soft and gelatinous and mucoid materials with a multinucleated notochordal cell at birth. The cells disappeare in the first decade followed by gradual replacement of mucoid material by fibrocartilage derivated principally from the annulus fibrosus and the hyaline cartilaginous plates adjoining vertebral bodies. The nucleus pulposus is better developed in cervical and lumbar regions. It behaves toward like shock absorber for axial forces and like water bed bearing during flexion, extension and lateral bending of the vertebral column. The water content of nucleus pulposus is about 88% and its turgor and also fullness is great in the young adults. Discs are more often damaged by twisting and flexing the vertebral column. The intervertebral discs are so strong that violence first damages the neighborhood bone in young adults. It is possible to damage a healthy disc by forcible flexion as well as extension. Degenerative changes on discs may result in necrosis, sequestration of the nucleus pulposus, weakening or softening of annulus fibrosus after second decade. Then minor strains may cause internal disharmony with eccentric displacement of the nucleus pulposus. The minor strains may also cause external disharmony. In this case, the nucleus pulposus than bulges through annulus fibrosus may occur usually posterolaterally. The discs are also show pathological changes that may result in protrusion of nucleus pulposus through the annulus fibrosus known as a herniated or prolapsed disc. As people getting older, the nuclei pulposi lose their turgor and become thinner due to degeneration and dehydration. Symptom producing disc herniations happen in the cervical region almost as in the lumbar region. In geriatric ages, degenerative changes may occur in the discs because of relatively minor stress.

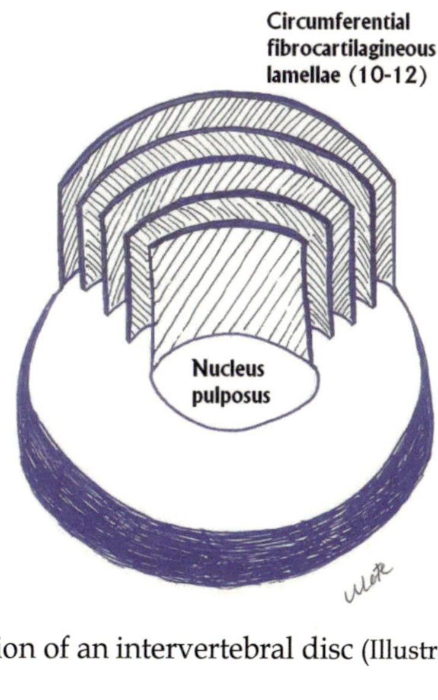


Fig. 3. Structural demonstration of an intervertebral disc (Illustrated by Edizer).

The discs support by anterior and posterior longitudinal ligaments. These ligaments lie throughout vertebral column. The anterior longitudinal ligament holds on the vertebral bodies strongly, but it adheres to the intervertebral disc tenderly. It originates from occipital bone and lies to sacral canal. Despite to anterior longitudinal ligament, the posterior longitudinal ligament which is the principal, but narrow ligament of intervertebral discs to each other adheres to the intervertebral discs strongly. The posterior surface of the vertebral bodies have a little concave shape, so while the posterior longitudinal ligament lies from one body to the other adhere with loose connective tissue in the canal (Figure 4) (Moore, 1992; Williams et al,1995 ; Snell, 1997; April, 1990).

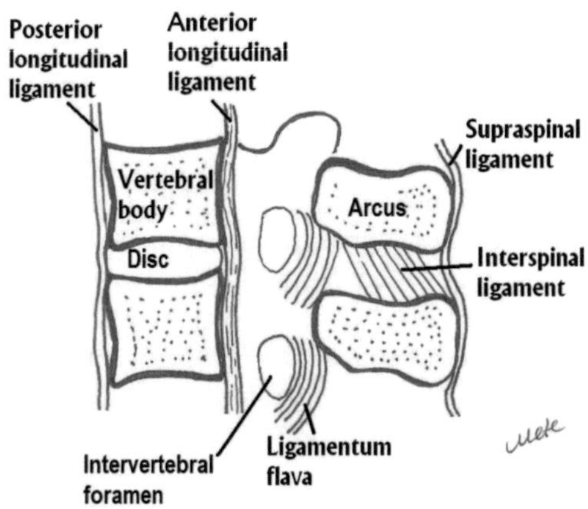


Fig. 4. Vertebral column and related ligaments were shown (Illustrated by Edizer).

### 2.4 Spinal nerve morphology

There are 31 pairs of the spinal nerves as eight cervical, twelve thoracic, five lumbar, five sacral and a coccygeal, bilaterally. They originate through intervertebral foramina for each level. However, the first spinal nerve leaves the vertebral canal between atlas and the occipital bone, bilaterally. So, the nerve is named as the suboccipital nerve. Each of the nerve is continous with the spinal cord by the anterior (ventral) and posterior (dorsal) roots, the latter each bearing a spinal ganglion (Taner D, 2004; Van de Graaf, 1998; Williams et al, 1995; Moore, 1992 ). The anterior roots compose axons of neurons in the anterior and lateral spinal grey columns. The posterior roots also contain centripedal process of neurons sited in the spinal ganglia. The spinal nerves have clinically significant relations in the vertebral foramina. The relations are anteriorly, with the intervertebral discs and adjacent vertebral bodies. Posterior are the zygapophysial joints. Superior and inferior are vertebral notches of the pedicles of adjoining vertebrae. Each of the spinal nerve accompanied by a spinal artery, a small venous plexus and its meningeal branch or branches together traverse a foramen (Williams et al, 1995). Dorsal (posterior) rami of spinal nerves, usually smaller than the ventral (anterior) and directed posteriorly divide into medial and lateral branches (except for the first cervical, fourth and fifth sacral and coccygeal nerves) to innervate the muscles and skin of the posterior regions of the neck and trunk. The ventral rami of spinal nerves innervate the limbs and the anterolateral aspect of the trunk, they are mostly larger than the dorsal rami. The thoracic nerves are independent and retain, like all dorsal rami, mostly segmental distirubition. The cervical, lumbar and sacral spinal nerves connect near their origins to form plexuses like cervical plexus in cervical region, brachial plexus in lower cervical and thoracic region and lumbosacral plexus in lumbosacral region, which are called as the peripheric nerves. Dorsal rami do not join these plexuses (Williams et al, 1995).

The spinal nerves might be compressed by herniated discs. Because of the protrusion and compression, the patients suffer from chronic pain symptom. All symptoms and signs occure usually on the same side as the herniation but sometimes the cases have contralateral side pain symptom, which leads to the fact that operators are in doubt about the decision to perform disc surgery. In the literature the possible mechanism of contralateral pain symptoms may occure due to hyperthrophy of ligamenta flava (Karabekir et al 2010). So, surgeons should take care for anatomical landmarks releated with ligamentous complex during surgery.

## 3. Degenerative disc hernias

### 3.1 Description and scope

Degenerative disc disease (DDD) occurs when the outer ring, annulus fibrosus, damaged of worn. The contents of the disc may then protrude or impinge on a spinal root. This will cause pain in the lower back and that radiates to the hips and down the back of the legs. Backpain is an unpleasent and noxius sensation of varying severity localized in different regions of the back. The simplified etiologic or pathogenetic classification of back pain includes myofascial, articular (including degenerative disc changes), and neurogenic components. Because of increased incidance of low back pain (LBP) or lumbosacral radicular syndrome, low back pain becomes a serious problem for healthy and active individuals between the ages 30-50.

If a degenerative disc hernia is obtained then simple discectomy is offered to the individuals. Neverthless there are some problems followed by degenerative disc disease operations such as recurrence, loss of height and instability. The most effective treatment of discogenic pain to unresponsive to conservative care is interbody fusion in the literature (Karabekir et al, 2008).

The development of molecular biology enabled a better understanding of the processes that caused the degenerative disease of intervertebral discs. Many studies aiming to clarify the causes and risk factors for this degenerative disorder have been performed (Patel et al, 2007). It is now known that degenerative disc disease is strongly correlated to genetic factors, investigations indicating that heredity has a major role for degeneration of disc and implies approximately 74% in adult populations, as a variation. Since 1998 there were many genes associated with degenerative disc hernias declarated such as MMP-3, VDR, collagen I, collagen IX (COL9A2 and COL9A3), collagen XI (COL11A2), vitamin D receptor, IL-1, IL-6, CILP, and aggrecan (Cevei et al 2011).

When the outer ring, annulus fibrosus, damage because of aging and/or degeneration, the degenerative disc disease occure (Figure 5). Then, the contents of the disc may protrude or impinge on a spinal root, unilaterally or sometimes bilaterally. This process will cause pain in the lower back and that radiates to the hips and down the back of the legs. At the same time degenerative disc disease may cause to segmental instability due to following ligamentous laxity, fall in the amount of the nucleus pulposus, and loss of disc height.

Segmental instability which appears as aberrant vertebral motion may be accountable for the pain. Low back pain may arise from the facet joints, but various clinical outcomes have not verified this theory (Marks et al, 1992; Schwarzerger et al, 1994; 1994).

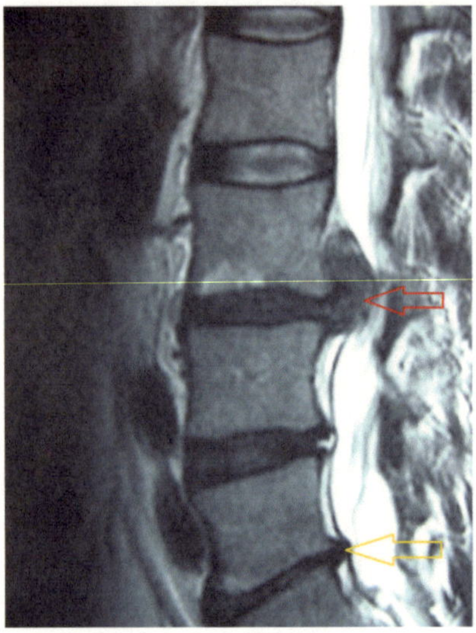

Fig. 5. An extrude disc hernia was shown by the red arrow and degenerative disc hernia was shown by the yellow one

Low back pain can unpleasantly appear in different regions of the back. The pathogenetic classification of low back pain divides into three types as myofascial, articular (including degenerative disc changes), and neurogenic. Back pain can cause several problems. It can effect healthy, active individuals between 30 and 50 years old. Invasive treatment options for chronic LBP are mostly tried after conservative cures have failed to obtain the desired results (Buric et al, 2011). Fusion and total disc arthroplasty are the most frequent surgical procedure to treat LBP caused by DDD with or without segmental instability. Nonetheless, the clinical achievement of fusion varies widely (16–95%) and to relate principally with the indication value being used (Turner et al, 1992; 1993; Waddel et al, 2000). Cases who undergo spinal fusions or total disc replacement mostly have more complications, longer stay in hospital and higher charges from hospital than cases undergoing other types of operation. LBP is usually resulting from mechanical reasons like load, which may initiate internal disc degeneration and trigger loss of water from the nucleus pulposus. The consecutive step of degenerative episode gives rise to a decline in disc height, narrowing of the intervertebral space, and non-organized facet joints. These episodes disturb anatomical and physiological motion between two neighborhood vertebrae and increase instability due to laxity of the ligaments and the annulus fibrosus (Buric et al, 2011).

Modic firstly delineated classifications of lumbar spine degeneration via imaging technique (Hutton et al, 2011). The author classified the cases as grade I, II or III using MRI. According to his follow up results, MRI changes compose of vertebral bodies parallel with the vertebral plateau of degenerated disc which indicates hyposignal on the slices in T1 and hyperintensity in T2 for Type I. The changes of MRI composed of rised intensity of the signal on the images in T1 and an isointense signal or lightly hyperintense in T2 and represent the imagistic expression of disc lesions consisting of annular protrusion and comparatively recent initial beginning disc hernia for Type II. Both Type I and II have not a radiological correspondent. MRI investigations revealing type III changes, represent decreasing intensity of the signal on the slices both in T1 and T2, being related on regular planar radiographic slices with extensive bone sclerosis. Those changes are related with disc extrusion, disc hernia, free disc fragment, problems of the posterior vertebral ligament (Gocmen-Mas, 2010; Karabekir et al, 2010). The composition of the disc changes during development, growth, ageing and degeneration and this impress the response of the disc to changes in mechanical stress (Cevei et al 2011; Modic, 2007).

Diagnosis of degenerative disc disease is confirmed by MRI scans (West et al, 2010). Direct x-rays, especially planar flexion-extension radiographies may help to recognize instability which develops because of degenerative disc disease. Discography is also important for diagnostic survey of the degenerative disc disease.

## 4. Treatment modalities of degenerative disc hernias

### 4.1 Surgical procedures

In biomechanical respect posterior lumbar interbody fusion (PLIF), introduced by Dr.Ralph Cloward in the 1940.s, is an optimal fusion. A succesful PLIF carries the advantages of immobilizing the unstable degenerated intervertebral disc area, decompressing the dural sac and nerve roots, restoring disc height and load bearing to anterior structures. In spite of a lot of fusion techniques, such as autologous iliac crest bone graft, allograft bone, dowelshaped graft, key stone graft, tricortical graft, and bone chips, interbody cages preferred. There is various types of cages, carbon-titanium-polyetherether keton etc., are used for interbody fusion (Figure 2-5). In our daily practice we prefered polyetherether keton (PEEK) cages because of their safety usage and wide graft space contains (Karabekir et al, 2009).

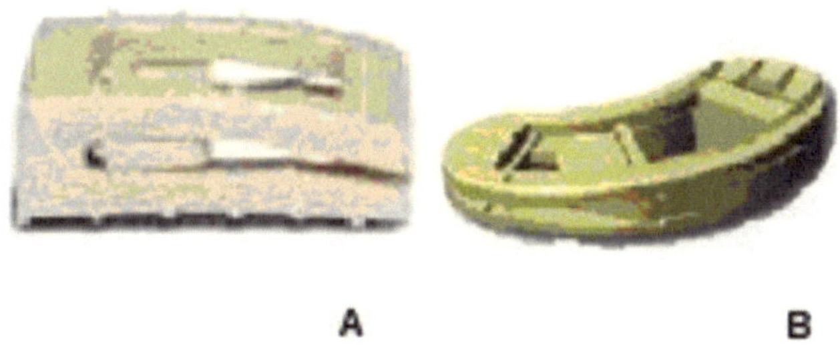


Fig. 6. Samples of expandable PEEK cages; A. Cervical, B. Lumbal

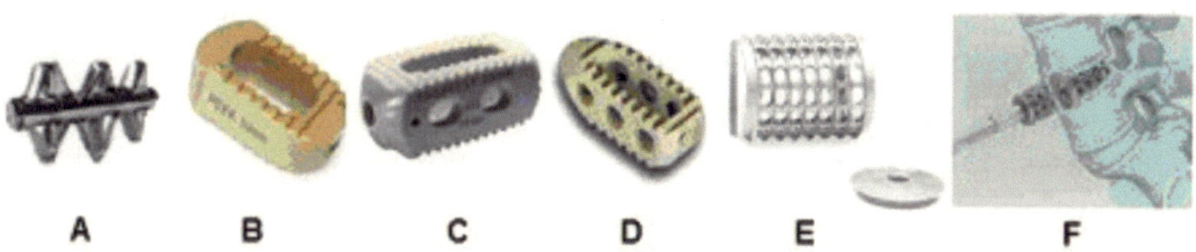


Fig. 7. Samples of the intervertebral cages; A. B-twin, B. B-D PEEK cages, E-F. Cylendiric titanium cages.

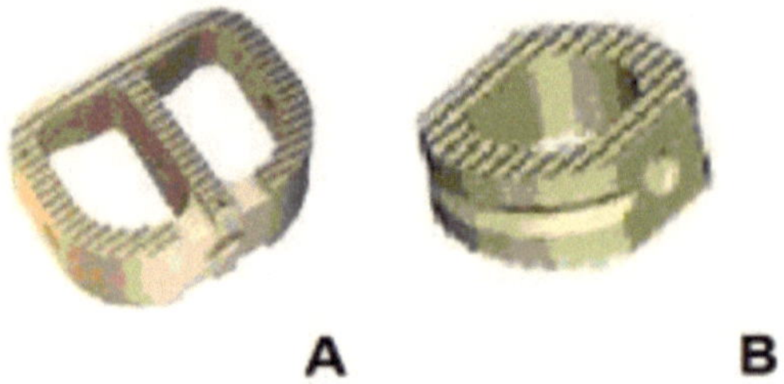


Fig. 8. Samples of the cervical PEEK cages (A and B)

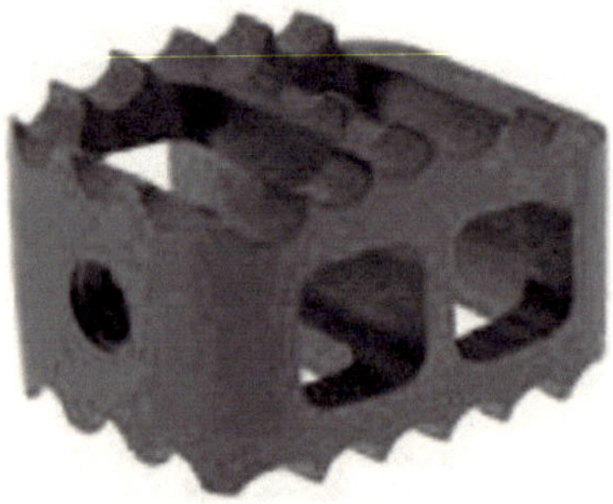

Fig. 9. A sample of the carbon intervertebral cage

PLIF usually has been accomplished with implantation of two threaded cages (Bagby, 1988). The rate of fusion of bone grafts alone have ranged from 46% to 90% at the literature. Because of difficulty in maintaining spinal stabilization and achieving fusion, spinal instrumentation has become an important and popular adjunct to bone grafting in lumbar arthrodesis, further increasing the fusion rates, 80-90% (Karabekir et al, 2009).

More recently, interbody fusion techniques have also shown high fusion rates with distinct advantages (Lin et al, 1983; Ray, 1997). Some of these advantages include immediate anterior column load sharing, a large surface area for fusion, bone graft subjected to compressive loads that is advantegous in achieving fusion and the ability to restore normal sagittal contour while indirectly decompressing the intervertebral foramen (Lin et al, 1983). Interbody fusion technique also appear to be the most effective cure of discogenic back pain unresponsive to conservative care (Weatherly et al, 1986).

Blume, in 1981, described a unilateral approach for posterior lumbar interbody fusion to address some of the potential complications of the standart PLIF such as spinal nerves' roots injuries, and instabilization. The unilateral posterior lumbar interbody fusion (UPLIF) popularized by Harms et al (1997) is a surgical technique in which bilateral anterior column support can be achieved through a unilateral posterior approach.

Weatherly et al (1986) reported on five cases during a 10-year period who had solid posterolateral fusions, but still had positive discography under the fusion and had their back pain relieved by anterior interbody fusion.

Recently, Derby et al (1999) noted that cases with highly sensitive discs as determined by pressure controlled discography achieved significantly better long-term outcomes with combined anterior and posterior fusion.

Nevertheless, there are some problems followed by degenerative disc disease operations such as recurrence, lost of height and instability. Many authors develop some different surgical approaches for preventing the recurrence of disc herniation and to protect the disc height. Of these modified techniques, we prefer, in our daily practice consists of unilateral and bilateral polyetheretherketon (PEEK) posterior lumbar cages by using demineralized bone matrix (DBM) putty graft (Karabekir et al, 2008).

UPLIF is indicated for chronic mechanical pain associated with degenerative disc disease, recurrent disc herniation. With this concept recurrence of disc and the possibility of foraminal narrowing and loss of height can also be reduced. The most advantage of the PEEK cage is to preserve the disc space height and prevent the recurrence. Unilateral posterior PEEK cage application and fusion is a safe and reproducible technique to provide unilateral posterior column support (Karabekir et al, 2009). With this method, recurrence of the disc and the possibility of foraminal narrowing and loss of height can also be reduced (Karabekir et al 2008).

Although PLIF has shown satisfactory clinical outcomes in treatment of degenerative disc diseases, many studies have reported that accelerated adjacent segment degeneration (ASD) may occur after PLIF management, particularly at the rostral level (Kumar et al., 2001; Okuda et al., 2008; Park et al., 2004; Zencica et al., 2010; Chen et al., 2011).

There is controversial relationship between fusion surgery and adjacent segment degeneration. Battie et al (2004) declared that adjacent segment degeneration after fusion was a natural status that was not associated to the fusion surgery. However, some other investigators implied in vitro mechanical studies and found that lumbar fusion may increase abnormal intradiscal pressure and too much movement at the adjacent spinal levels, resulting in adjacent segment degeneration (Lee et al, 2009). Therefore, it appears that adjacent segment disease may be especially caused by the abnormal discal stresses distribution that occurred by lumbar fusion and fixation. The other serious complication of posterior fixation and fusion operations is damaging of the nerve roots because of the placement of pedicular implants from the posterior (Ebrahaim et al, 1997). And also neuropathic pain associated with implant placement is not rare in literature. In the implantology literature, complications related to nerve are mentioned as 'sensory disturbances', focusing on the occurrence of paresthesia and dysesthesia, eventually accompanied by transitory pain sensations during implant placement (Ebrahaim et al, 1997; Butt et al, 2007).

DDD and its related symptoms have classically been cured with spinal fusion where the affected vertebrae are immobilized with mechanical fasteners or cages. This method stabilizes the impressed segments and achieved pain recipe (Balsano et al, 2011; Gornet et al, 2011).

A modified PLIF method named as transforaminal lumbar interbody fusion (TLIF), was first definated in 1982. Because the bone graft can be inserted far laterally, the TLIF technique can be safely indicated for interbody fusion of the upper lumbar spine. Moreover, TLIF can be performed at any lumbar level below first lumbar vertebra (L1), because it avoids significant retraction of the dura and conus medullaris (Hioki et al, 2011).

The minimally invasive lateral transpsoas method to the lumbar spine such as extreme lateral interbody fusion (XLIF) and direct lateral interbody fusion (DLIF) occurs as an alternative to interbody placement at levels L1 to L5 in the setting of spondylolisthesis, degenerative disc disease, and scoliotic or kyphotic anomalies (Benglis et al, 2008; Bergey et al, 2004; Cox et al, 2008; Dezawa et al, 2000; Mayer, 1997; Mc Afee et al 1998; Benglis et al, 2009).

But all of these approaches are not without complications. Outcomes of spinal fusion in a decreased range of movement and might caused a degenerative series in adjacent vertebral segments (Rahms, 1996). There have been many efforts to substitute the disc via various equipments for avoiding this and treating cases leaving its usual anatomic and physiologic movement (Balsano et al, 2011).

Recently, spinal movement preservation has so important in spine surgery as a potential planning to arrange a more normal spinal motion and providing against the biomechanical stress and a kinematic strain on nearby segments (Junjie et al, 2011). For protecting spinal motion an alternative to spinal fusion, total disc replacement (TDR) intervention is more and more becoming an adopted alternative for cases with degenerative disc disease. Theorically, the surgery carries on various benefits over spinal fusion, as it is desired to preserve mobilization and may diminish adjacent level degeneration. But, failures can make revision surgery a necessity for all kind of implant surgeries. McAfee et al (2009) report 8.8% revision procedures at the index level. Retrification of artificial discs is candidate to complications, because of revision surgery carries individual major risks for cases. McAfee et al (2009) claimed that a 3.6% incidence of vascular injury in primary TDR and 16.7% in anterior revision surgery. Revision surgery is usually applied to the cases with persistent severe low back pain or leg pain. This pain may releate with implant as malpositioning, prosthesis migration, subluxation, subsidence, and breakage of the metal ring of the core or wear.

Owing to adhesions, vascular structures are more vulnerable and adherent to the spine. Major vascular structures are placed on front to the discs at levels above L5 to S1. The vena cava and the aortic bifurcation mainly lie superior to the L5 to S1 disc levels, so the vascular complications give rise to anxiety. Other potential various complications are ureteral damage of the neural prevertebral plexus.

However, no definite proof of its biomechanical and clinical efficacy has yet been provided stand-alone devices are threaded cages designed for anterior lumbar interbody fusion (ALIF). Therefore all the instrument sets are designed for a wide approach to the disc. Moreover, additional space is required for to keep a regular distance between the vertebral endplates throughout the entire procedure by the working tube. The outer diameter of the smallest cage is 12 milimeters; the additional 2–3 mm of the working tube diameter would require about 15 mm of minimal working space on either side (Costa et al, 2011). Using these stand-alone cages is limited because they can be used only for discs which do not exceed 10 mm in height. Furthermore, these cages are suitable for any interbody fusion associated with pedicle screw fixation.

Nuclear replacement began with implantation of devices into the intervertebral disc space following discectomy. Pioneer prostheses contain stainless steel balls, self-curing silicone, silicone-Dacron composite, and polymethylmethacrylate. Other unsuccessful mechanical implants including springs and pistons have been developed. Most of these implants have been unsuccessful because of some complications such as extrusion, subsidence, and reactive endplate changes. Edeland (1981) implied that a nuclear implant should have viscoelastic features and permit influx and egress of water, thereby mimicking normal disc behaviors. The prosthetetic disc nucleus (PDN) prosthesis consist a capsule of woven polyethylene enclosing a hydroscopic thixotropic gel. Various similar products, which have including sheaths with elastic elements, have been tested but none are accepted. Another concept has been to directly inject hydrogel polymers such as polyvinyl alcohol into the intervertebral disc space. Water absorption and subsequent material expansion prevent protrusion. Nuclear replacement theorically restores degenerative disc biomechanics by changing height and at the same time effect the anular tension.

Symptomatic cases with soft disc hernia or moderate degenerative disc disease may be reckoned for TDR. Few investigations on the intervention of TDR in cervical spondylosis have been declared in literature (Byran VE, 2002; Lafuente et al, 2005; Pimenta et al, 2007; Sekhon LHS 2004), but concern remains on reasonable, efficacy, suitable and safety of disc prostheses in cases with multilevel spondylotic status of the cervical spine, due to accompanied facet joints differency and segmental bony degenerative alterations. The anterior cervical discectomy and fusion (ACDF) is the most largely accepted intervention for the cases with single or double level spondylotic disease. It has acceptable clinical outcomes and radiological fusion ranging from 90 to 100% are frequently cured either by anterior decompression and fusion (Matz et al, 2007), with (Mummaneni et al, 2007; Kaiser et al, 2002) cases with multilevel, symptomatic, spondylotic myeloradiculopathy or without plating (Ashkenazi et al, 2005) or by posterior decompression with or without lateral mass screw fixation (Wiggins et al, 2007). ACDF, a suitable and reliable method, is accepted as the gold standard intervention for single or multilevel cervical spondylosis to cause radiculopathy or myelopathy. It is not absolute whether or not anterior cervical discectomy is due to the physiological senescence of the spine or changes on the ground that previous fusion (Hilibrand et al, 2004). Fusion may be related with other causes such as pseudoarthrosis (Albert et al, 2004), donor site complications and factors of the neighborhood motion segments' biomechanics. The hybrid, single stage, fusion-nonfusion technique appears to be a promising and viable alternation in the treatment of symptomatic multilevel cervical DDD with prevalent anterior myeloradicular compression and different severity per single level, particularly in younger patients. It allows protecting or healing motion in some segments without defining iatrogenic spine instability or painful secondary to severely degenerated levels. Long-term follow-up on larger series of cases are need to approve all of the results (Barbagallo et al, 2009).

Presently there are two types of disc prosthesis as total disc and nucleus disc equipments (Bao et al, 2002; Bao et al, 2007; Bertagloni et al, 2003, Hedman et al 1991). Contrary to total disc replacement, nucleus disc prosthesis protects the existing constitutions, where include the ligaments, annulus, and endplates (Enker et al, 1993; Fernstrom 1966; Kostuik 1997). Nowadays, there are several types and designs of nucleus disc equipments, and surgical applications such as Nubactm which is the first articulating nucleus disc. Given that the mainly avascular intervertebral disc bears some of the highest loads in the human body and it is not surprising that DDD is a common phenomenon in middle age and a universal condition of the inevitable consequences of aging (Rothman et al 1982). The broad majority of cases achieve acceptable clinical outcomes without surgery (Weinstein, 1992). However, some cases do not respond to nonsurgical treatments. Chronically malformated cases population surgery may be useful. DDD and its related signs have classically been cured with spinal fusion. This method results in a diminished range of movement and may caused a degenerative process in adjacent vertebral segments (Lee CK, 1998; Ray, 1997; Lee CK et al, 1991; Nachemson, 1992; Kuslisch et al 1998). For a long time, fusion was reckoned as the gold standard of surgical procedure. However, clinical outcomes have yielded the acceptance of disc arthroplasty as the cure option (Balsano et al, 2011).

Several types of prosthesis have been planned with frequent improvements. The polyethylene core of the Charite´ prosthesis is sensitive to wear and hurts with breakage of the metal wire marker whether or not associated with impingement. This polyethylene wear gives rise to third-body debris in the intervertebral space near the spinal canal, which may lead to vertebral osteolysis. Retrieval surgery of Charite´ TDRs is convenient and relatively relaible, it has major risks due to adjacent vessels and scar tissue. Removal of keeled TDRs like Prodisc and Maverick implants is more hard and more bone removal is a necessity when above L5-S1 levels so, a lateral approach is preffered to avoid damage the major vascular structures (Gerardus et al, 2009). In our series we generally used porus coated motion (PCM) type cervical prosthesis and recently M-6 cervical disc prosthesis at cervical levels, and Nubac at lumbar regions.

The significant cause of recurrent low back pain after TDR may be facet degeneration or adjacent degeneration. The features of intervertebral disc prosthesis with articulating properties like long endurance are so important (Gerardus et al, 2009). The artificial disc or prosthesis is composed of critical importance to prevent premature disintegration; the artificial disc should generate a normal or near-normal movement compared with the pattern of healthy human spinal motion segment, so that corresponding facet joints and adjacent level or levels are not overloaded; and long-term fixation is necessary to avoid subsidence or migration. It seems almost impossible to provide a disc prosthesis that possesses all these features.

Disc arthroplasty provides a new concept not only in the cure of DDD but also in researching its biomechanics on anatomical changes and pathologies of the spine. Disc arthroplasty may fill the gap between simple discectomy and fusion concepts (Fekete et al, 2010).

A less invasive procedure, which is nowadays proposed for the management of chronic lumbar pain due to degenerative discopathy, involves the implantation of dynamic interspinous fixation devices (Bono et al 2007).

Lumbar interspinous spacers (ISPs) have recently become popular as an alternative treatment for lumbar DDD. Several spacers X-STOP, Coflex, Wallis, and DIAM are currently available and there have been various proposed indications (Figure 6). In the literature largest number of studies has been with the X-STOP device. The biomechanical studies with all the devices showed that ISPs have a beneficial effect on the kinematics of the degenerative spine. Apart from two randomized controlled trials, the other studies with the X-STOP device were not of high methodological quality (Kabir et al, 2011). Nevertheless, analysis of those studies showed that X-STOP may improve outcome when compared to non-operative cure in selected cases whose aged 50 or over, with radiologically confirmed lumbar canal stenosis and neurogenic claudication, who have improvement of their symptoms in flexion. Studies on the other interspinous devices show satisfactory outcome to varying degrees. However, due to small number and poor design of the studies, it is difficult to clearly define indications for ISP's use in lumbar degenerative disease. Lumbar ISPs may have a potential beneficial effect in selective cases with degenerative disease of the lumbar spine. However, further evidence based and good quality trials are needed to clearly outline the indications for ISP's use.

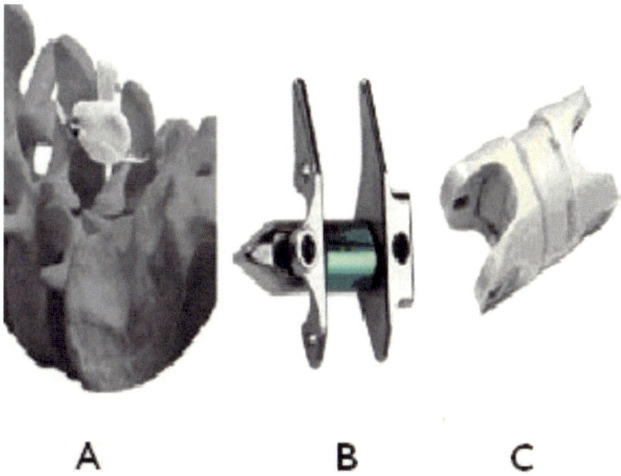


Fig. 10. Samples of the interspinous devices; A.Diam, B.X-Stop, C.PEEK interspinous devices

Nowadays advances in minimally invasive spine surgery (MISS) have allowed spinal surgeons to treat a broader range of degenerative spinal disorders. This is due to the development of advanced technology and new ways of approaching the spine. Some of the many factors that have driven these developments are the request of patients and spinal surgeons to lessen the morbidity and improve the outcome associated. Percutaneous axial anterior lumbar spine surgery is a possible and safe technique (Aryan et al, 2008). This technique is made feasible by a union of established spine surgery principles and the new technology of minimally invasive spinal surgery. The technique is important because it permits the implantation of biomechanically sound implants without the morbidity encountered in open surgery or other types of minimally invasive posterolateral spinal surgery (Aryan et al, 2007). The access orientation makes disc surgery with minimally invasive instruments more intuitive and accomplish. This technique will permit a routine percutaneous fusion from a single access site without paraspinal dissection and will lend itself to the development of new minimally invasive implant. This annulus fibrosus preserving and muscle-sparing approach will moderate postoperative pain, avoid postoperative scarring, speed healing, and eliminate problems encountered with annulus removal. This technique lends itself to spicing biomechanical solutions for motion preservation. Also, therapeutic interbody implants that can be replaced, expanded and revised easily will satisfy the patient and spine surgeon with a novel range of treatment options. The percutaneous paracoccygeal approach to the L5-S1 and L4-L5 interspaces provide a minimally invasive corridor through which discectomy and interbody fusion can safely be actualized. This approach can be used alone or in combination with minimally invasive or classical open fusion procedures. The technique may provide a disjunctive route of access to the L5-S1 or L4-L5 interspaces or both in those patients who may have aberrant anatomy for or contraindications to classical open anterior approach to this level (Aryan et al, 2008). Still this study does not provide Class 1 data, and is subject to the bias of any retrospective series, and further investigation beyond retrospective analysis is warranted before recommending the routine use of this technique.

Another technique can use after simple discectomy for preventing disc height. It also provides to replace a new injectable synthetic nucleus pulposus material instead of degenerative nucleus pulposus. Nucleus pulposus replacement is a non-fusion technique currently being investigated to treat painful disc degeneration. Replacement of nucleus pulposus with an injectable implant or tissue engineered construct, in patients with healthy annulus fibrosus, may reduce pain while simultaneously restoring spinal mobility and delaying disc degeneration (Boyd et al, 2006; Di Martino et al, 2005; Joshi et al, 2005; Klara et al, 2002; Larson et al, 2006; Cloyd et al, 2007). The challenge for any synthetic nucleus replacement material is to mimic the function of native nucleus pulposus. This bio-adhesive hydrogel material is one of the samples of these kinds of surgical materials (Cloyd et al, 2007; Gloria et al, 2010). After using these materials there's adhesions around the application site could observed. And a question related with application of these materials is the amount of these materials. This can be measured as weight at the operating room after discectomy by measuring the weight of the excising disc material.

Surgeons can measure the cages dimension preoperatively, but there's an easy and unbiased method that can be used before surgery. With this simple volume analysis technique surgeons can calculate how many cc disc material take place at intervertebral space and after discectomy the surgeons can calculate how many cc graft or bioglue substance can be necessary to put this space and what will be the dimensions of the cage or cages to put intervertebral disc space (Karabekir et al, 2011).

The stereological volume analysis is simple, reliable, unbiased and inexpensive. Intervertebral space volumes can evaluate using stereological method. A uniform point-grid with a point-associated area of 0.156 $cm^2$ is randomly superimposed on each MRI using the "Grid". Points hitting the lumbar intervertebral space are manually counted for area estimation of the profiles. Automated area estimation by manual perimeter tracing is generally take too much time and hence, more rapid point counting method is preferred. Volume estimation is accomplished by the Cavalieri's principle as described previously using the formula given below:

$$V = t \times [((SU \times d)/ SL]^2 \times \Sigma P$$

where t is the section thickness, SU is the scale unit, d is the distance between two points in the point grid, SL is the scale length and $\sum P$ is the number of points counted. SU and SL are used to include the linear magnification in the final estimate. All data have been entered to a previously prepared Microsoft Excel spread sheet for automatic calculation of both the results of the above formula and the statistical evaluation parameters including the nugget variance and the coefficient of error (CE). All measurements are performed blinded to subject details and the results of any other measurements, and are done three times in each trial for inter-observer analysis by different researchers.

The surgeons can calculate the intervertebral space volume and discectomy material amount before surgery using this unbiased and inexpensive method (Karabekir et al, 2011). So while operating the cases the surgeons can use the correct amounts of materials and the materials which have correct dimensions.

### 4.2 Illustrative cases

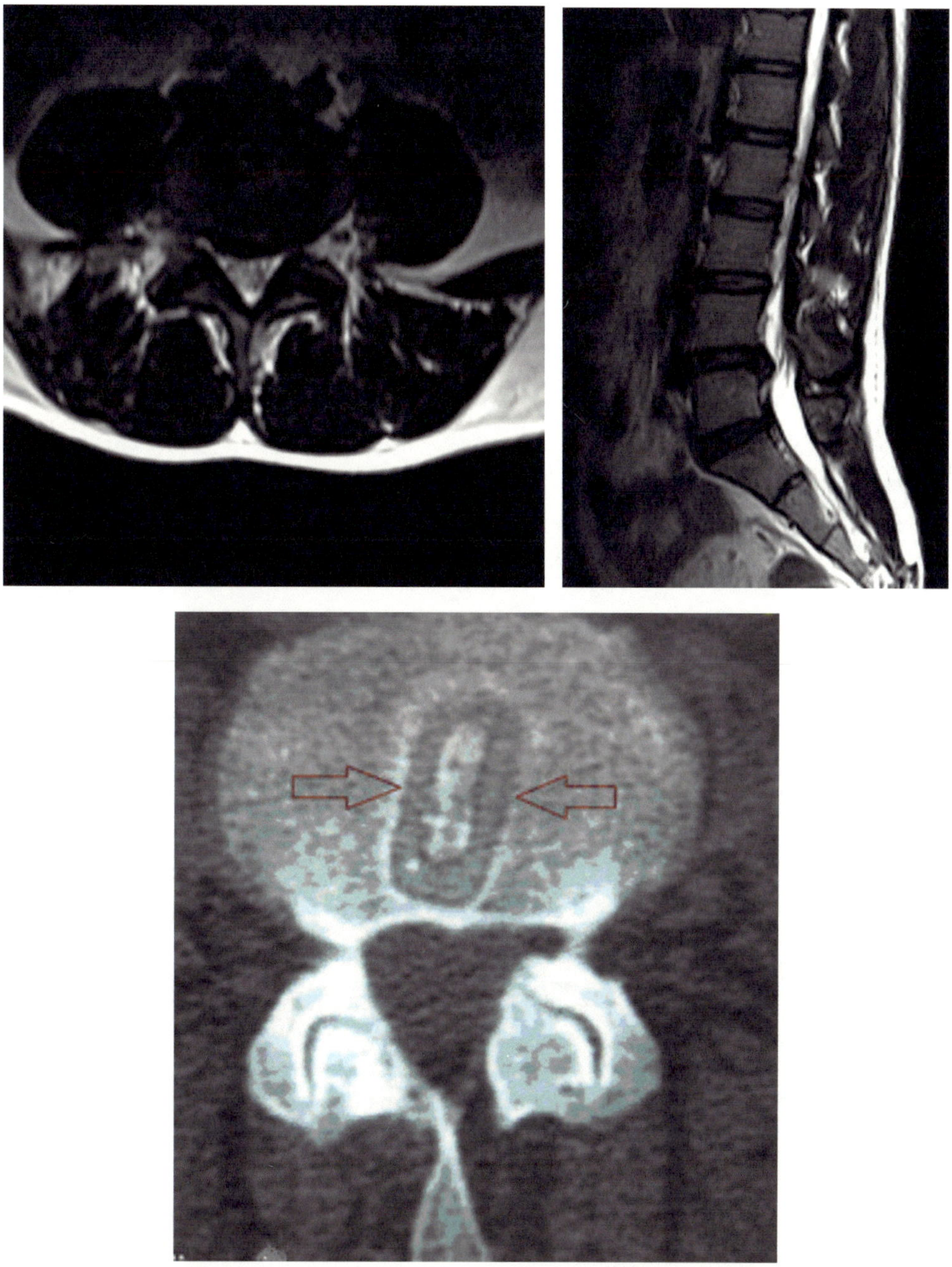

Fig. 11. Preoperative MRI and postoperative CT of 52-year old female case with degenerative disc disease were shown: The patient was admitted with left radicular leg pain and numbness. At physical examination loss of left L5 sensation and left dorsoflexion deficit were obtained. She was operated from left side and after discectomy unilateral PEEK cage was placed on L4-L5 levels (Karabekir, 2006). She had no complaint at 5 years follow-up.

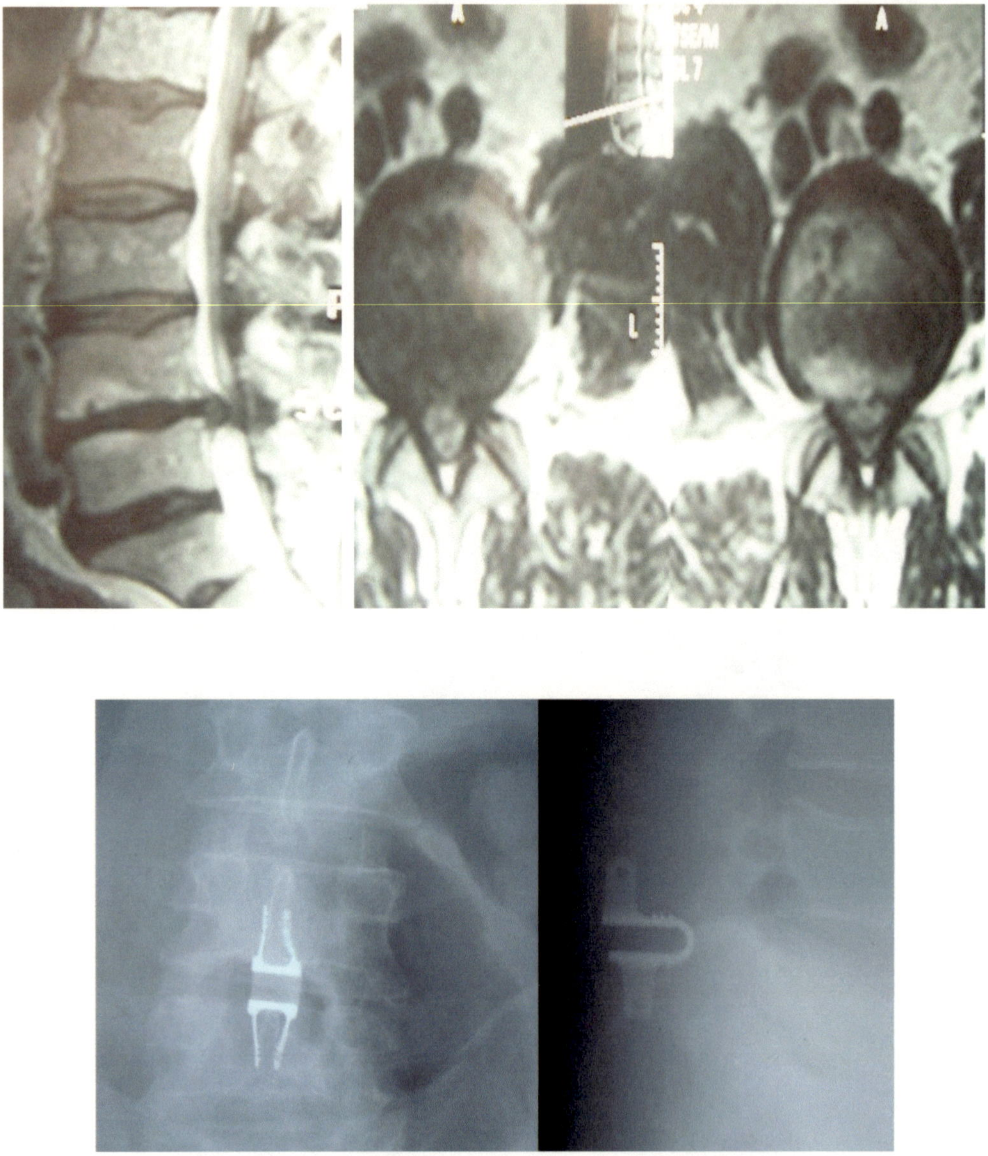

Fig. 12. L4-L5 diffuse protrusion and bilateral foraminal stenosis on preoperative MRI of a 55 year old men, whom had low back and bilateral leg pain which dominate at right side with numbness and causalgia during last 6 months, was shown. At physical examination bilateral muscle weakness at ankle dosoflexion and L4-S1 hypoesthesia were obtained. Postoperative anteroposterior and lateral X-rays of the case was shown. The interspinous device (Coflex) was applied at L4-L5 level after discectomy posteriorly to preserve the height of the interspinal foramens (Karabekir, 2005).

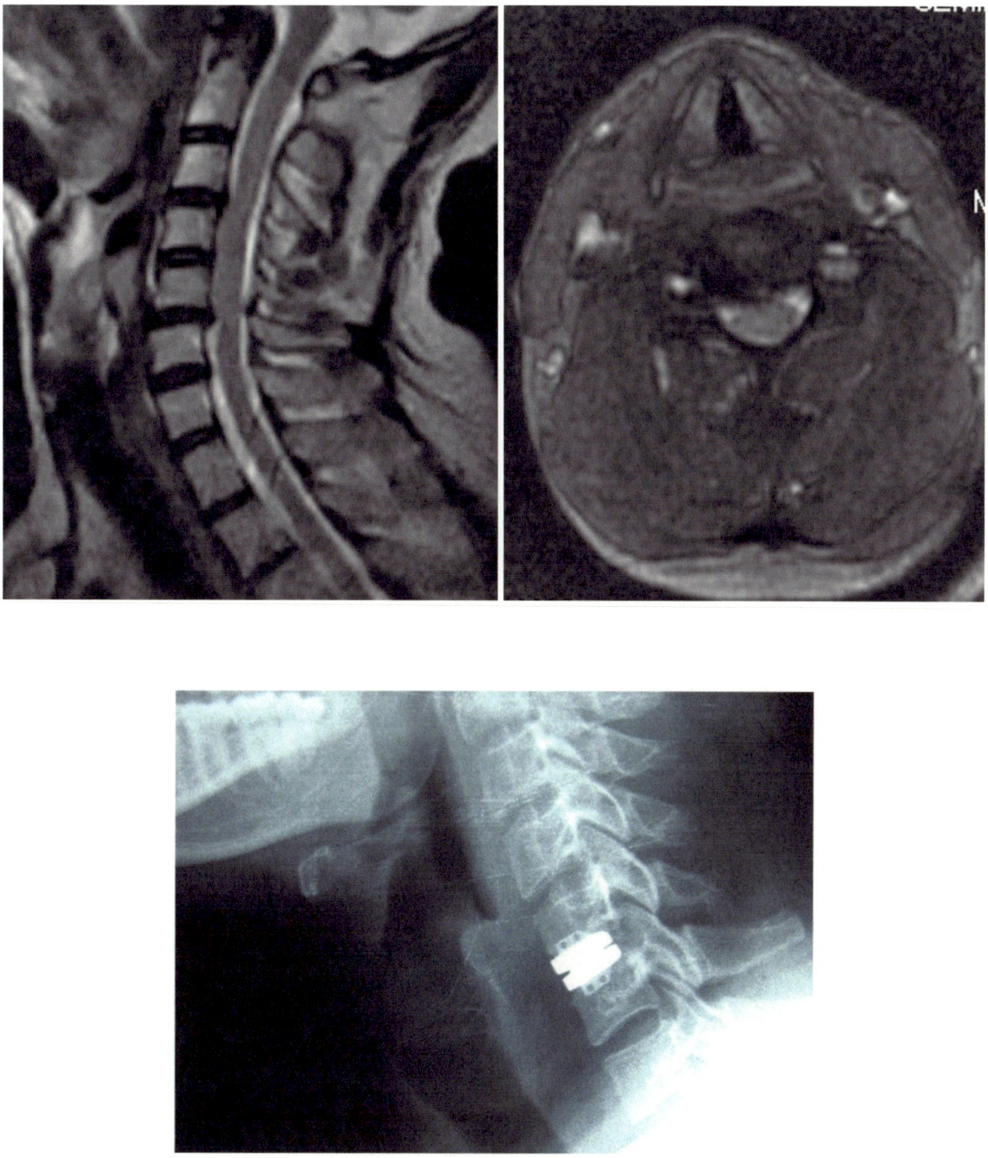

Fig. 13. Preoperative servical MRI was shown with C5-C6 servical degenerative disc hernia. 39 year-old male subject was admitted with right arm pain and numbness for three months period. At physical examination left C5-6-7 sensation lost, muscle weakness and biceps reflex hipoactivity were observed. Patient was operated and applicated Maverick artificial disc prosthesis at C5-C6 level (Karabekir, 2010). Artficial disk was shown at postoperative direct x-ray.

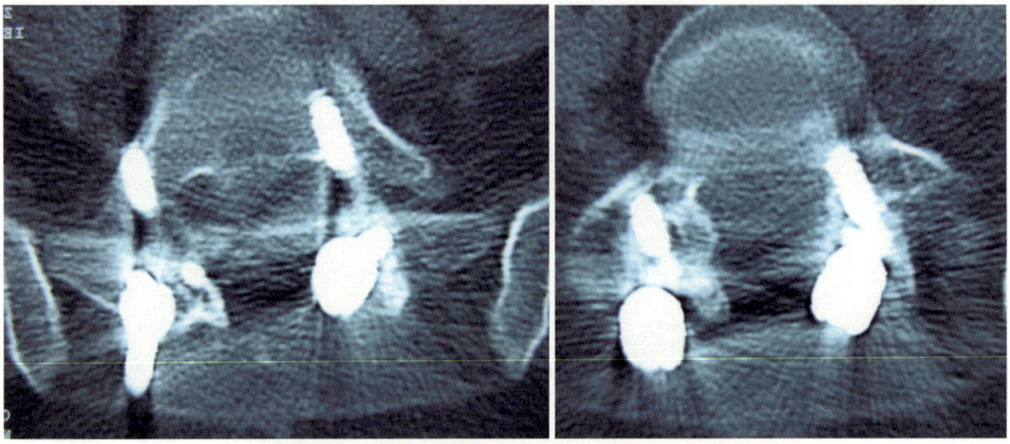

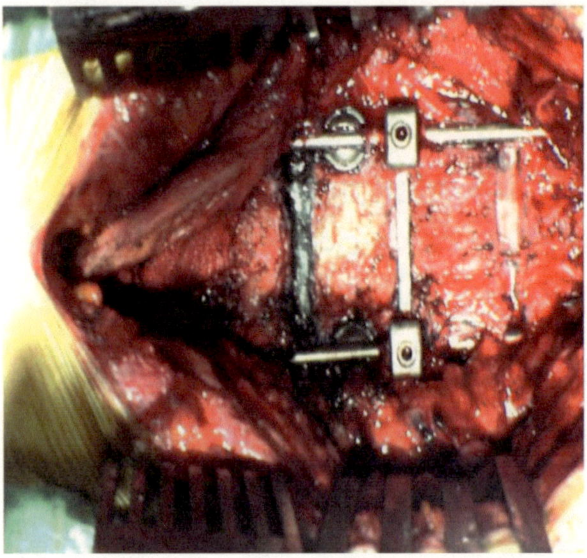

Fig. 14. Peroperative image of 64-year old female revision case; 3rd operation of the case, first simple discectomy and interbody fusion, the second posterior pedicle screws implantation because of chronic lowback pain and the third was performed because of broken screws. Broken screws were shown at W-B pictures (Karabekir, 2008).

## 5. Expert suggestions

The cases of degenerative disc disease should be evaluated carefully preoperatively and at operative period. The surgeon should know topographic and clinic anatomical knowledge of the region in detailed. Critical important anatomical landmarks should be defined before surgical approach such as lateral border of ligamentum flava and posterior longitudinal ligament, medial margin of superior articular process (superior facet). At the time of preoperative planning and during surgery; surgeon should aim to perform limited invasive procedure for preserving neighbourhood tissue and neurovascular structures of the region. Meticulous dissection should be performed and minimally invasive techniques must be selected to avoid major complications such as bleeding, iatrojenic neurovascular damage etc. Particularly, resection of the posterior longitudinal ligament must be a little wider then standart discectomy procedure for placing intervertebral implants or grafts. During this procedure, retraction of the dura and roots must be gentle and care. While replacing the implant, surgeon should use scopy for right and exact position and level of it.

## 6. Conclusion

As a conclusion, anatomical knowledge of the vertebral column and/or spinal cord and also careful preoperative evaluation of the cases as both clinically and radiologically are of importance for realizing successful approach on the degenerative disc diseases.

## 7. References

Albert T.J., Eichenbaum M.D. (2004) Goals of cervical disc replacement. *Spine J* 4:292S–293S

Aldskogius, H., Arvidsson, J. & Grant, G. (1985) The reaction of primary sensory neurons to peripheral nerve injury with particular emphasis on transganglionic changes. *Brain Res* 357(1): 27-46.

April, E.W. (1990) Clinical anatomy. *The National Medical Series for Independent Study*. 2nd ed. Harwal Publishing Company, USA.

Aryan H.E., Newman C.B., Gold J.J., Acosta Jr F.L., Coover C, Ames C.P. (2008) Percutaneous Axial Lumbar Interbody Fusion (AxiaLIF) of the L5-S1 Segment: Initial Clinical and Radiographic Experience. Minim Invas Neurosurg 51: 225- 230)

Ashkenazi E., Smorgick Y., Rand N., Millgram M.A., Mirovsky Y., Floman Y. (2005) Anterior decompression combined with corpectomies and discectomies in the management of multilevel cervical myelopathy: a hybrid decompression and fixation technique. *J Neurosurg Spine* 3: 205–209

Bao Q.B., Yuan H.A. (2002) New technologies in spine: nucleus replacement. *Spine* 27: 1245–1247

Bao Q.B., Yuan H.A. (2002) Prosthetic disc replacement: the future? *Clin Orthop* 394:139–145

Bao Q.B., Songer M., Pimenta L., Werner D., Reyes-Sanchez A.,Balsano M., Agrillo U., Coric D., Davenport K., Yuan H. (2007) Nubac disc artyhroplasty: preclinical studies and preliminary safety and efficacy evaluations. *SAS J* 1: 36–45

Battie M.G., Videman T., Parent E. (2004) Lumbar disc degeneration: epidemiology and genetics influences. *Spine* 29: 2679–2690

Benglis D.M., Vanni S., Levi A.D. (2009) An anatomical study of the lumbosacral plexus as related to thr minimally invasive transpsoas approach to the lumbar spine. *Neurosurg Spine*. 10(2):139-44.

Benglis D., Elhammady S., Levi A., Vanni S.(2008) Minimally invasive anterolateral approaches for the treatment of back pain and adult degenerative deformity. *Neurosurgery* 68: 191–196

Bergey D.L., Villavicencio A.T., Goldstein T., Regan J.J.(2004) Endoscopic lateral transpsoas approach to the lumbar spine. *Spine* 29: 1681–1688

Bertagnoli R., Vazquez R.J. (2003) The anterolateral transpsoatic approach (ALPA). A new technique for implanting prosthetic disc nucleus devices. *J Spinal Disord* 16: 398–404

Blume H.G., Rojas C.H. (1981) Unilateral lumbar interbody fusion (posterior approach)utilizing dowel graft. *J Neurol Orthop Surg* 2: 171-175.

Bono C.M., Vaccaro A.R. (2007) Interspinous process devices in the lumbar spine. *J Spinal Disord Tech.* 20(3): 255–261

Boyd L.M., Carter A.J. (2006) Injectable biomaterials and vertebral endplate treatment for repair and regeneration of the intervertebral disc. *Eur Spine J* 15(Suppl 3): 414–421

Bryan V.E. (2002) Cervical motion segment replacement. *Eur Spine J* 11(Suppl 2): 92–97

Buric J.,Pulidori M. (2011) Long-term reduction in pain and disability after surgery with the interspinous device for intervertebral assisted motion (DIAM) spinal stabilization system in patients with low back pain: 4-year follow-up from a longitudinal prospective case series. Josip Buric *Eur Spine J* DOI 10.1007/s00586-011-1697-6)

Butt M.F., Farooq M., Dhar S.A., Mir M.R., Mir B.A., Kangoo K.A. (2007) Retrospective analysis of the occurrence of radiologically detectable surgical error in cases of failed pedicle screw implants. *Acta Orthop Belg.* 73(4): 500-6.

Chaichana K.L., Mukherjee D., Adogwa O., Cheng J.S., McGirt M.J. (2011) Correlation of preoperative depression and somatic perception scales with postoperative disability and quality of life after lumbar discectomy. J Neurosurg Spine. Feb;14(2): 261-7.

Chen B.L.,Wei F.X., Ueyama K., Xie D.H., Sannohe A., Liu S.Y.(2011) Adjacent segment degeneration after single-segment PLIF: the risk factor for degeneration and its impact on clinical outcomes. *Eur Spine J* DOI 10.1007/s00586-011-1888-1

Cevei M., Roşca E., Liviu L., Muțiu G., Stoicănescu D., Vasile L. (2011) Imagistic and histopathologic concordances in degenerative lesions of intervertebral disks. *Rom J Morphol Embryol.* 52(1 Suppl):327-32.

Cloward R.B. (1953)The treatment of ruptured lumbar intervertebral discs by vertebral body fusion: indications, operating technique, after care. *J Neurosurg* 10: 154-168.

Cloyd J.M., Malhotra N.R., Weng L., Chen W., Mauck R.L., Elliott D.M. (2007) Material properties in unconfined compression of human nucleus pulposus, injectable hyaluronic acid-base hydrogels and tissue engineering scaffolds. *Eur Spine J* 16(11):1892-8. Epub 2007 Jul 28.

Costa F.,Sassi M., Ortolina A.,Cardia A., Assietti R., Zerbi A., Lorenzetti M.,Galbusera F., Fornari M. (2011) Stand-alone cage for posterior lumbar interbody fusion in the treatment of high-degree degenerative disc disease: design of a new device for an "old" technique. A prospective study on a series of 116 patients. *Eur Spine J* (2011) 20 (Suppl 1):S46–S56

Cox C.S., Rodgers W.B., Gerber E.J. (2008) XLIF in the treatment of single-level lumbar spondylolisthesis: 6 month and 1 year follow up. *J Neurosurg* 108:A853, 2008 (Abstract)

Cummings, C.W., Fredrickson, J.M., Harker, L.A., Krause, C.J., & Schuller, D.E. (1993). *Otolaryngology-Head and Neck Surgery.* 2nd ed. Vol I, Mosby Year Book.

de Maat G.,PuntI.M., van Rhijn L.W., Schurink G.H.,van Ooij A. (2009) Removal of the Charite´ Lumbar Artificial Disc Prosthesis Surgical Technique. *J Spinal Disord Tech* 22; 5:334-339

Derby R., Howard M.W., Grant J.M., Lettice J.J., Van Peteghem P.K., Ryan D.P. (1999) The ability of pressurecontrolled discography to predict surgical and nonsurgical outcomes. *Spine* 24: 364-372.

Dezawa A., Yamane T., Mikami H., Miki H. (2000) Retroperitoneal laparoscopic lateral approach to the lumbar spine. *J Spinal Disord* 13: 138–143

Di Martino A., Vaccaro A.R., Lee J.Y., Denaro V., Lim M.R. (2005) Nucleus pulposus replacement: basic science and indications for clinical use. *Spine* 30: 16– 22

Ebraheim N.A., Xu R., Darwich M., Yeasting R.A. (1997) Anatomic relations between the lumbar pedicle and the adjacent neural structures. *Spine* (Phila Pa 1976). 15; 22(20):2338-41.

Edeland H.G. (1981) Suggestions for a total elasto-dynamic intervertebral disc prosthesis. *Biomater Med Devices Artif Organs.* 9(1):65-72.

Enker P., Steffee A., Mcmillan C., Keppler L., Biscup R., Miller S. (1993) Artificial disc replacement. Preliminary report with a 3-year minimum follow-up. *Spine* 18:1061–1070

Fekete T.F., Porchet F. (2010) Overview of disc arthroplasty-past, present and future. *Acta Neurochir (Wien).* 152(3):393-404. Review.

Fernstrom U. (1966) Arthroplasty with intercorporal endoprothesis in herniated disc and in painful disc. *Acta Chir Scand* (Suppl) 357:154–159

Ferrera, P.C., & Chandler, R. (1994) Anesthesia in the emergency setting: Part II. Head and neck, eye and rib injuries. *Am Fam Physician* 15; 50(4):797-800.

Gloria A., Borzacchiello A., Causa F., Ambrosio L. (2010) Rheological Characterization of Hyaluronic Acid Derivatives as Injectable Materials Toward Nucleus Pulposus Regeneration. *J Biomater Appl.* [Epub ahead of print]

Gocmen-Mas N., Karabekir H., Ertekin T., Senan S., Edizer M., Yazici C., Duyar I. (2010) Evaluation of Lumbar Vertebral Body and Disc: A Stereological Morphometric Study. *Int. J. Morphol.,* 28(3):841-847.

Gornet M.F., Burkus J.K., Dryer R.F., Peloza J.H. (2011) Lumbar Disc Arthroplasty with MAVERICK™ Disc Versus Stand-Alone Interbody Fusion: A Prospective,Randomized, Controlled, Multicenter Investigational Device Exemption Trial. *Spine (Phila Pa 1976).* [Epub ahead of print]

Haghighat, K. (2007). "Bone augmentation techniques." *J Periodontol* 78(3): 377-96.

Harms J.(1997) True spondylolisthesis reduction and more segmental fusion in spondylolisthesis. In: Bridwell KH, DeWald RL (Eds.). *The Textbook of Spinal Surgery.* 2nd Ed. Philadelphia, Lippincott-Raven.

Hedman T.P., Kostuik J.P., Fernie G.R., Hellier W.G. (1991) Design of an intervertebral disc prosthesis. *Spine* 16(Suppl 6):256–260

Hilibrand A.S., Robbins M. (2004) Adjacent segment degeneration and adjacent segment disease: the consequences of spinal fusion? *Spine J* 4: 190–194

Hioki A., Miyamoto K., Hosoe H., Sugiyama S., Suzuki N., Shimizu K. (2011) Cantilever transforaminal lumbar interbody fusion for upper lumbar degenerative diseases (minimum 2 years follow up). *Yonsei Med J.* 52(2): 314-21.

Hutton M.J., Bayer J.H., Powell J., Sharp D.J. (2011) Modic vertebral body changes: The natural history as assessed by consecutive magnetic resonance imaging. *Spine* (Phila Pa 1976). Feb 25. [Epub ahead of print]

Joshi A., Mehta S., Vresilovic E., Karduna A., Marcolongo M. (2005) Nucleus implant parameters significantly change the compressive stiffness of the human lumbar intervertebral disc. *J Biomech Eng* 127: 536–540

Junjie D., Mo L., Hao L., Hao M., Qizhen H., Zhuojing L. (2011) Early follow-up outcomes after treatment of degenerative disc disease with the discover cervical disc prosthesis *The Spine Journal* 11: 281–289

Kabir S.M., Gupta S.R., Casey A.T. (2010) Lumbar interspinous spacers: a systematic review of clinical and biomechanical evidence. *Spine* (Phila Pa 1976). 1; 35(25): 1499-506.

Kaiser M.G., Haid R.W.Jr., Subach B.R., Barnes B., Rodts G.E.Jr. (2002) Anterior cervical plating enhances arthrodesis after discectomy and fusion with cortical allograft. *Neurosurgery* 50: 229–238

Karabekir H.S., Atar E.K., Yaycioglu S., Yildizhan A.(2008) Comparison of unilateral posterior lumbar interbody fusion and bilateral posterior lumbar interbody fusion with simple discectomy at degenerative disc herniations. *Neurosciences* 13 (3): 248-252

Karabekir H.S., Korkmaz S., Ozturk U. (2009) Comparison of unilateral posterior lumbar interbody fusion with simple discectomy at degenerative disc disease. *The J Turkish Spinal Surgery* 20 (1): 47- 52.

Karabekir H.S., Yildizhan A.,Atar K.E., Yaycioglu S., Gocmen-Mas N., Yazici C. (2010) Effect of ligamenta flava hypertrophy on lumbar disc herniation with contralateral symptoms and signs: a clinical and morphometric study. *Arch Med Sci* 6(4): 617-622

Karabekir H.S.,Mas N.G., Edizer M.,Ertekin T., Yazici C, Atamturk D (2011). Lumbar Vertebra Morphometry and Stereological Assesment of Intervertebral Space Volumetry: A Methodological Study *Ann Anatomy* 193(3): 231-6. Epub 2011 Apr 2.

Klara P.M., Ray C.D. (2002) Artificial nucleus replacement: clinical experience. *Spine* 27:1374–1377

Kostuik J.P. (1997) Intervertebral disc replacement. In: Bridwell KH, DeWald RL (eds) *The textbook of spinal surgery*, 2nd edn. Lippincott-Raven, Philadelphia.

Krumlauf R. (1994) Hox genes in vertebrate development. *Cell.* 29; 78(2): 191-201. Review.

Kumar M.N., Jacquot F., Hall H. (2001) Long-term follow-up of functional outcomes and radiographic changes at adjacent levels following lumbar spine fusion for degenerative disc disease. *Eur Spine J* 10: 309–313

Kuslich S.D., Ulstrom C.L., Griffith S.L., Ahern J.W., Dowdle J.D. (1998) The Bagby and

Kuslich method of lumbar interbody fusion. History, techniques, and 2-year follow-up results of a United States prospective, multicenter trial. *Spine* 23: 1267–1279

Lafuente J., Casey A.T., Petzold A., Brew S. (2005) The Bryan cervical disc prosthesis a san alternative to arthrodesis in the treatment of cervical spondylosis. *J Bone Joint Surg Br* 87(4): 508–512

Larson J.W., Chadderon R.C., Georgescu H., Lee D., Hubert M., Werkmeister-Lewis L.,

Irrang J.,Gilbertson L.G., Kang J.D. (2006) Prevention of intervertebral disc degeneration after surgical discectomy using an injectable nucleus pulposus prosthesis. In: *Proceedings of the 52nd annual meeting of the orthopaedic research society, Chicago*, USA.

Lee C.K. (1988) Accelerated degeneration of the segment adjacent to a lumbar fusion. *Spine* 13: 375–377

Lee C.K., Langrana N.A., Parsons J.R., Zimmerman M.C. (1991) Development of a prosthetic intervertebral disc. *Spine* 16(Suppl 6): 253–255

Lee C.S., Hwang C.J., Lee S.W., Ahn Y.J., Kim Y.T., Lee D.H., Lee M.Y. (2009) Risk factors for adjacent segment disease after lumbar fusion. *Eur Spine J* 11: 1637–1643

Lin P., Cautilli R., Joyce M. (1983) Posterior lumbar interbody fusion. *Clin Orthop* 180: 154-167.

Lipetz J.S. (2002) Pathophysiology of inflammatory, degenerative, and compressive radiculopathies. *Phys Med Rehabil Clin N Am.* 13(3): 439-49. Review.

Lundborg, G. (1988) Intraneural microcirculation. *Orthop Clin North Am* 19(1): 1-12.Review.
Mallo M., Vinagre T., Carapuço M. (2009) The road to the vertebral formula. *Int J Dev Biol.* 53(8-10): 1469-81. Review.
Marks R.C., Houston T., Thulbourne T. (1992) Facet joint injection and facet nerve block: a randomised comparison in 86 patients with chronic low back pain. *Pain* 49: 325–328
Matz P.G., Pritchard P.R., Hadley M.N. (2007) Anterior cervical approach for the treatment of cervical myelopathy. *Neurosurgery* 60(Suppl): 64–70
Mayer H.M. (1997) A new microsurgical technique for minimally invasive anterior lumbar interbody fusion. *Spine* 22: 691–699
McAfee P.C., Regan J.J., Geis W.P., Fedder I.L. (1998) Minimally invasive anterior retroperitoneal approach to the lumbar spine Emphasis on the lateral BAK. *Spine* 23: 1476–1484
McAfee P.C., Phillips F.M., Allen T.R., Regan J.J., Albert T.J., Cappuccino A., Devine J.G.,
Ahrens J.E., Hipp J.A. (2009) Cervical disc replacement in patients with and without previous adjacent level fusion surgery: a prospective study. *Spine* (Phila Pa 1976). 15; 34(6): 556-65.
Moore, K.L. (1992) *Clinically orianted anatomy*. The Williams and Wilkind Company USA.
Mummaneni P.V., Burkus J.K., Haid R.W.,Traynelis V.C., Zdeblick T.A. (2007) Clinical and radiographic analysis of cervical disc arthroplasty compared with allograft fusion: a randomized controlled clinical trial. *J Neurosurg Spine* 6(3): 198–209
Nachemson A.L. (1992) Challenge of the artificial disc. In: Weinstein JN (ed) *Clinical efficacy and outcome in the diagnosis and treatment of low back pain.* Raven Press, New York,USA
Okuda S., Oda T., Miyauchi A., Tamura S., Hashimoto Y., Yamasaki S., Haku T., Kanematsu F., Ariga K., Ohwada T., Aono H., Hosono N., Fuji T., Iwasaki M. (2008) Lamina horizontalization and facet tropism as the risk factors for adjacent segment degeneration after PLIF. *Spine* 33: 2754–2758
Park P., Garton H.J., Gala V.C., Hoff J.T., McGillicuddy J.E. (2004) Adjacent segment disease after lumbar or lumbosacral fusion: review of the literature. *Spine* 29: 1938–1944
Patel K.P.,Sandy J.D., Akeda K., Miyamoto K., Chujo T., An H.S., Masuda K. (2007) Aggrecanases and aggrecanasegenerated fragments in the human intervertebral disc at early and advanced stages of disc degeneration, *Spine* (Phil Pa 1976) 32 (23) : 2596–2603.
Pimenta L., McAfee .PC., Cappuccino A., Bellera F.P., Link H.D. (2007) Superiority of multilevel cervical arthroplasty outcomes versus single-level outcomes: 229 consecutive PCM prostheses. *Spine* 32(12): 1337–1344
Ray C.D. (1997) Threaded titanium cages for lumbar intebody fusions. *Spine* 22(6): 67-80.
Rahm M.D., Hall B.H. (1996) Adjacent-segment degeneration after lumbar fusion with instrumentation: a retrospective study. *J Spinal Disord* 9: 392–400
Rothman R.H., Simeone F.A., Bernini P.M. (1982) Lumbar disc disease. In: Rothman RH,
Simeone FA (eds) The spine, 2nd edn. WB Saunders, Philadelphia, USA
Schwarzer A.C., Aprill C.N., Derby R., Fortin J., Kine G., Bogduk N. (1994) Clinical features of patients with pain stemming from the lumbar zygapophysial joints. Is the lumbar facet syndrome a clinical entity? *Spine* (Phila Pa 1976) 19:1132–1137

Schwarzer A.C., Aprill C.N., Derby R., Fortin J., Kine G., Bogduk N. (1994) The false-positive rate of uncontrolled diagnostic blocks of the lumbar zygapophysial joints. *Pain* 58:195–200

Sekhon L.H.S. (2004) Cervical arthroplasty in the management of spondylotic myelopathy: 18-month results. *Neurosurg Focus* 17(3): 55–61

Sekhon L.H.S. (2004) Two-level artificial disc placement for spondylotic cervical myelopathy. *J Clin Neurosci* 11(4): 412–415

Snell R.S. (2011) *Clinical Anatomy*. Williams and Wilkins 8th ed.Walters Kluwer, USA.

Standring S., Ellis H., Healy J.C., Johnson D., Williams A., Collins P. (2005) *Gray's Anatomy* (ed 39). London, Churchill Livingstone.

Steffee A., Sitkowski D.(1988) Posterior lumbar interbody fusion and plates. *Clin Orthop* 227: 99-102.

Sunderland S., (1951) A Classification of Peripheral Nerve Injuries Producing Loss of Function *Brain* 74(4): 491-516.

Taner D. (2004) Functional Neuroanatomy. 4th ed. ODTU Press, Ankara, Turkey.

Turner J.A., Ersek M., Herron L., Haselkorn J., Kent D., Ciol M.A., Deyo R. (1992) Patientoutcomes after lumbar spinal fusions. *JAMA* 268: 907–911.

Turner J.A., Herron L., Deyo R.A. (1993) Meta-analysis of the results of lumbar spine fusion. *Acta Orthop Scand Suppl* 251: 120–122

Van de Graaff. (1998). *Human Anatomy 5th ed.* WBC McGraw-Hill Companies, USA.

Van Zundert J., Huntoon M., Patijn J., Lataster A., Mekhail N., van Kleef M. (2010) Cervical radicular pain. *Pain Practice.Pain Pract.* 10(1): 1-17. Review.

Waddell G., Gibson J.N.A., Grant I. (2000) Surgical treatment of lumbar disc prolapse and degenerative lumbar disc disease. In: Nachemson AL, Jonssom E (eds) *Neck and back pain.* Lippincott Williams & Wilkins, Philadelphia.

Weatherly C.R., Prickett C.F., O.Brien J.P.(1986) Discogenic pain persisting despite solid posterior fusion. *J Bone Joint Surg* 68-B:142-143.

Weinstein J.N. (ed) (1992) *Clinical efficacy and outcome in the diagnosis and treatment of low back pain.* Raven Press, New York

Wellik D.M. (2007) Hox patterning of the vertebrate axial skeleton. *Dev Dyn.* 236(9): 2454-2463 Review.

West W., West K.P., Younger E.N., Cornwall D. (2010) Degenerative disc disease of the lumbar spine on MRI. *West Indian Med J.* 59(2): 192-5.

Wiggins G.C., Shaffrey C.I. (2007) Dorsal surgery for myelopathy and myeloradiculopathy. *Neurosurgery* 60(Suppl): 71–81

Williams P.L., Bannister L.H., Berry M.M., Patricia C.,Dyson M., Dussek J.E., Ferguson M.W.J. (1995) *Gray's Anatomy*. 38th ed. Churchill-Livingstone, UK.

Winn H.R. (2004) *Youmans Neurological Surgery*. 5th ed. Saunders, Philadelphia,PA., USA.

Woodburne R.T., Burkel W.E. (1994) *Essentials of Human Anatomy* 9th ed New York, Oxford University Press.

Zencica P., Chaloupka R., Hladı´kova´ J., Krbec M. (2010) Adjacent segment degeneration after lumbosacral fusion in spondylolisthesis: a retrospective radiological and clinical analysis. *Acta Chir Orthop Traumatol Cech* 77: 124–130

# 16

# Balloon-Kyphoplasty for Vertebral Compression Fractures

Luca Arpino and Pierpaolo Nina
*Department of Neurosurgery, San Giovanni Bosco Hospital, Naples*
*Italy*

## 1. Introduction

### 1.1 Overview

A Vertebral Compression Fracture (VCF) is a collapse of one or more vertebrae. This usually results from a combination of bending forward and downward pressure on the spine. These fractures happen most commonly in the thoraco-lumbar spine, particularly in the lower vertebrae of the thoracic spine.

### 1.2 Causes

In relation to etiopathogenesis, VCFs may be divided into:

- pathologic fractures, as for:
  - *osteoporosis* (the most common cause: about 750,000 people per year in United States): in people with severe osteoporosis, a VCF may be caused by simple daily activities, such as stepping out of the shower, sneezing vigorously or lifting a light object;
  - *metastatic tumors;*
  - *multiple myeloma;*
  - *vertebral hemangiomas;*
- traumatic fractures, which can occur with a fall on the feet or buttocks, a forceful jump, a car accident or any event that stresses the spine past its breaking point.

### 1.3 Symptoms

VCFs may occur suddenly, causing severe back pain, generally referred to mid or lower part of the spine; this pain is most commonly described as "knifelike" and usually disabling. Clinical examination usually shows tenderness to the touch over the affected vertebra/vertebrae.

If the VCF is severe, the nerves and spinal cord can be affected, which can lead to nerve irritation and inflammation.

### 1.4 Imaging

While a diagnosis can usually be made through history and a clinical examination, X-ray and CT-scan (as first-step diagnosis in Emergency Room) or MRI and bone densitometry can help in confirming diagnosis, predicting prognosis, and determining the best treatment option for this patient.

### 1.5 Balloon-kyphoplasty (BKP) technique

BKP is a percutaneous vertebral augmentation technique initially developed to treat osteoporotic VCFs. It is a minimally invasive procedure: a small incision is made in the back through which the surgeon places a hollow tube called *trocar*. Using fluoroscopy to guide it to the correct position, the trocar creates a path into the fractured area through the pedicle of the involved vertebrae (*fig1*):

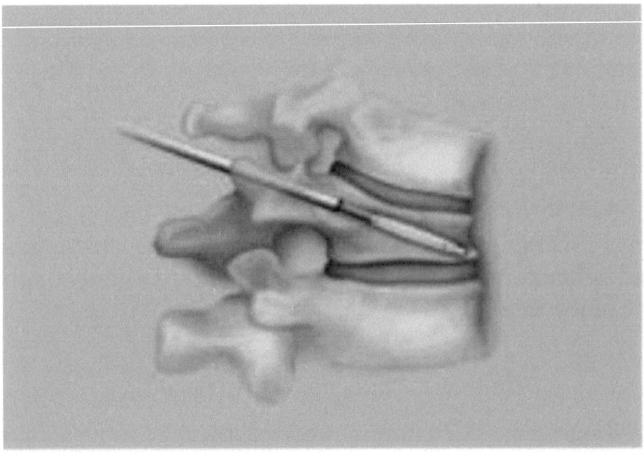

Fig. 1. Trocar insertion

Then a special balloon is inserted through the trocar into the vertebra and it is gently inflated by the surgeon (*fig2*):

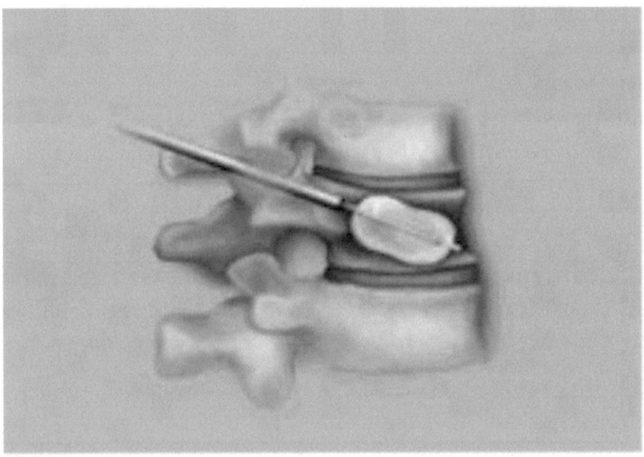

Fig. 2. Balloon inflation

As the balloon inflates, fractured vertebra is elevated while its inner cortical bone is compacted: so a cavity into the vertebra is created (*fig3*):

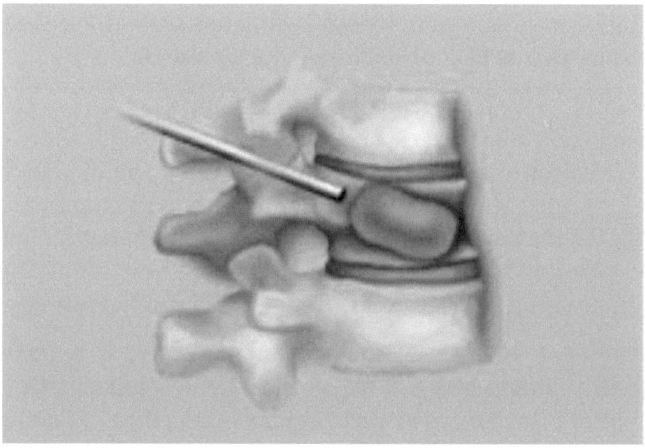

Fig. 3. Void filling by bone cement

Finally, the balloon is removed and the surgeon fills the cavity with bone cement in order to achieve fracture stabilization and body height restoration (*fig4*):

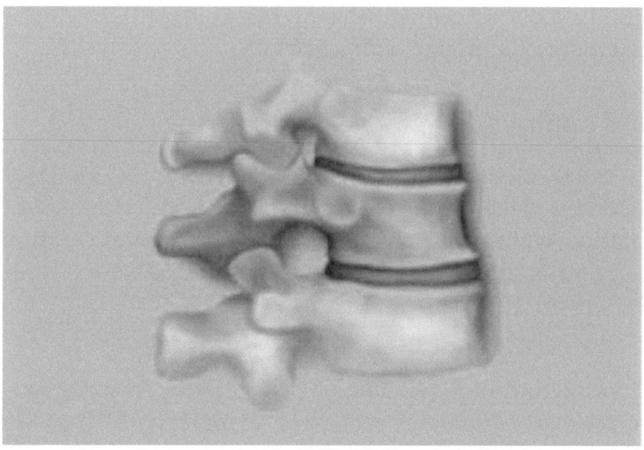

Fig. 4. Fracture stabilization

## 2. Alternative procedures

According to kind of VCF, related symptoms and health conditions, there are many ways to treat these fractures.

When permitted by a doctor, self-care at home, taking rest, with a back brace and/or using medications (nonsteroidal anti-inflammatories, narcotics or muscle relaxants) may be enough in case where pain is not so severe, neurological examination is negative and radiological tests show minor VCF.

On the other hand, admission to the hospital is necessary when pain or symptoms are severe. Surgery (major or mini-invasive spinal surgery depending on VCF degree) may be required to prevent the spine from pressing on the spinal cord or to stabilize the vertebra adjacent to the fracture site. When spinal cord compression is not a risk and neurological examination is negative instead, percutaneous techniques such as vertebroplasty or *vertebral augmentation techniques* such as BKP or stentoplasty are enough.

Unlike BKP, in **vertebroplasty** bone cement is injected into the vertebra at high pressure and *free*: so cement-leakage rate is higher, especially if there are many fracture cracks, such as for traumatic VCFs [Schmelzer et al, 2009]. In his meta-analysis on 69 clinical studies, Hulme [Hulme et al, 2006] reported leakage rates in 41% of cases during vertebroplasty and in 9% of cases during BKP. While most leaks were clinically asymptomatic, clinical complications (i.e. major complications) occurred in 3.9% and 2.2% of the vertebroplasty and kyphoplasty cases, of which pulmonary emboli accounted for 0.6% and 0.01%, respectively.

Vertebral body stenting (VBS), also known as **stentoplasty,** is a further adaptation of vertebroplasty and BKP. It is a new technique, recently developed, that involves placing a metal stent (cage) within the collapsed vertebral body and then expanding this to try and enable some height restoration before filling that cavity created with cement. The main advantage of VBS over BKP is that the height gain after balloon inflation can be maintained whereas with BKP alone it is well-known that in many cases significant height loss occurs during balloon deflation. However, after this procedure, stent remains into the vertebral body to keep vertebral body height restoration; furthermore the stent does not represent a *closed system* like the balloon: so cement-leakage rate is most likely higher than BKP, even though there are not longer follow-up studies for VBS.

## 3. Indications and contraindications of BKP

BKP is a broadly used method for the management of VCFs [Molina et al, 2011]. Originally introduced for osteoporotic fractures, surgical indications for this percutaneous vertebral augmentation technique were extended to vertebral fractures resulting from multiple myeloma [Zou et al, 2010], spinal metastases [Dalbayrak et al, 2010], vertebral hemangiomas [Jones et al, 2009] and trauma [Doria et al, 2010; Costa et al, 2009; de Falco et al, 2005].

In a recent study, Rollinghof et al. [Rollinghof et al, 2010] reported on a multiple choice questionnaire submitted to 580 clinics registered to practice BKP in Germany. For most participante (95,4% of the users), the main clinical indication was permanent back pain at the fractured level with an average VAS of 5. Although there is no common agreement about the etiopathogenetic and neuroradiological types of VCF to treat with kyphoplasty [Movrin et al, 2010, Bula et al, 2010, Dashti et al, 2005], over 80% of the users regarded A1.1, A1.2, and A3.1 fractures as main indications for kyphoplasty while for more than 60%, osteoporotic A1.1 fracture constituted the main indication for vertebroplasty [Rollinghof et al, 2010]. Although gradual pain resolution following these fractures is the expected natural history, pain can persist and or resolve slowly with conservative management. While patients may be not responsive to non-surgical therapies [Nairn et al, 2011]. Furthermore - especially in osteoporotic patients - VCFs can be complicated by deformity, loss of stature, impairment of pulmonary function and (considering that most VCFs will heal in 8 - 10 weeks with rest, bracing, and pain medications[Klazen et al, 2010]) the attendant risks of poor mobility/immobilisation in the elderly, such as venous thrombo-embolism or discomfort. Whereas BKP could allow rapid pain relief, as well as improved physical function and quality of life [Ledlie et al, 2006].

Obvious contrainticatons to BKP are pregnancy, congenital or aquired coagulopathies (warfarin, ASA), pain unrelated to vertebral collapse, fractured pedicles, solid tumors, osteomyelitis, contrast allergy (balloons are filled with contrast that can extravasate if they rupture), complete loss of vertebral height (vertebra plana).

## 4. Preoperative planning

A plain X-ray of the spine is generally enough to make the radiographic diagnosis of VCF (*fig5*):

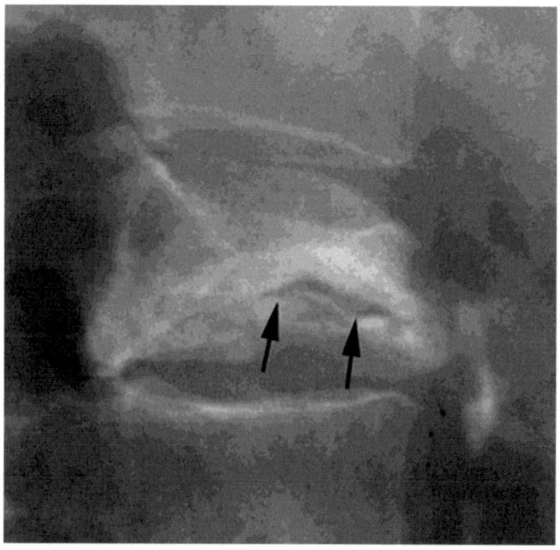

Fig. 5. 71-year-old woman with traumatic VCF. Lateral radiographs of lumbar spine show loss of vertebral body height and linear well-demarcated radiolucency characteristic of intravertebral fracture cleft (arrows).

CT is the most sensitive means to evaluate the location, severity, and extension of the collapsed vertebra, as well as to ascertain the visibility of the vertebral pedicles and the integrity of the posterior wall [Masala et al, 2004] (*fig6*):

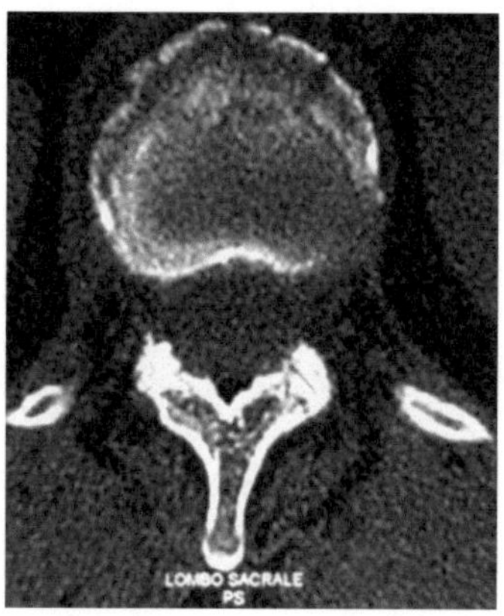


Fig. 6. 52-year-old woman with traumatic VCF of L1. Axial CT scan showing Magerl A1.2 type fracture of the vertebra.

Furthermore, CT scan of the spine allows multi-planar reconstructions, very useful to classify a traumatic VCF according to AO-Magerl classification (*fig7-8*) [Magerl et al, 1994]:

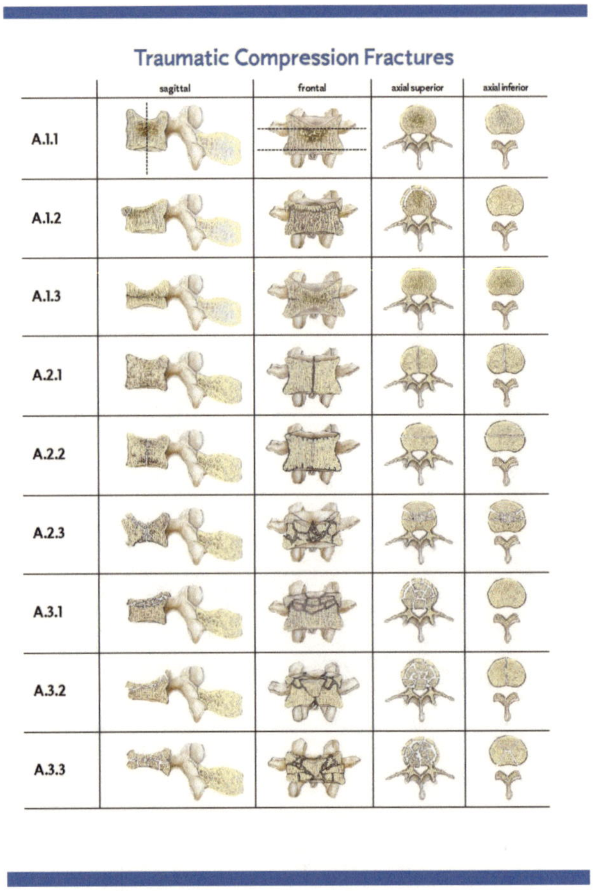


Fig. 7. AO-Magerl classification for type-A fractures

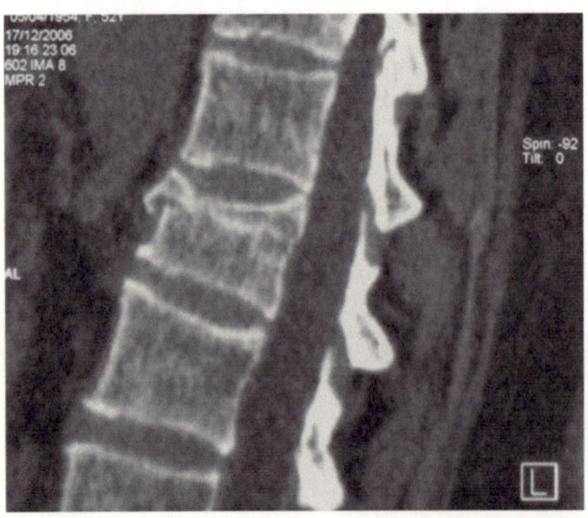

Fig. 8. 52-year-old woman with traumatic VCF of L1. Sagittal CT reconstruction of the previous fracture.

MRI is essential in identifying cord compression as consequence of a posteriorly displaced bone fragment, especially at levels where spinal cord is present (e.g. from the cervical spine to second lumbar vertebra) (*fig9*):

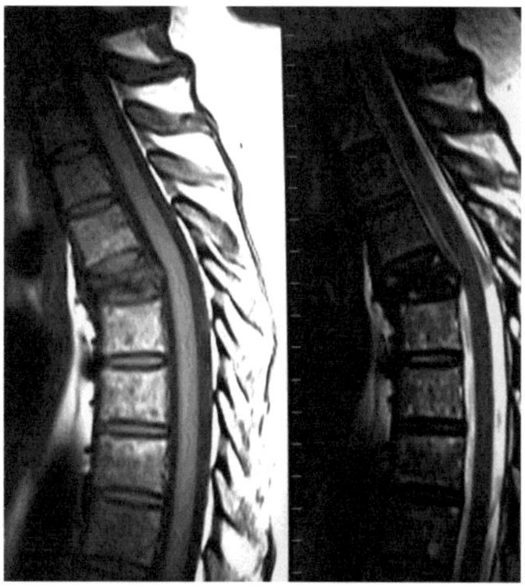

Fig. 9. 49-year-old woman with pathologic (myeloma) VCF. Sagittal MRI of the spine showing mild cord compression at T6 level by a displaced bone fragment.

When there is no data about the timing of fracture, it is important to perform a specific sequence MRI (e.g. STIR, *Short Tau Inversion Recovery*) scan before a kyphoplasty or vertebroplasty procedure is carried out, since it is impossible to distinguish between an old, healed fracture and a new fracture on X-rays or a CT scan. STIR MRI, in fact, is an inversion recovery pulse sequence with specific timing so as to suppress the signal from fat; in this way, the focal hyperintensity (bone marrow edema) that lasts for 2-4 months after fracture can be distinguished from fat signal, suggesting an acute or subacute VCF [Masala et al, 2004].

Finally, bone scintigraphy is helpful in assessing metastatic disease and when pain is elicited on palpation at levels other than where a fracture is radiographically identified (*fig10*):

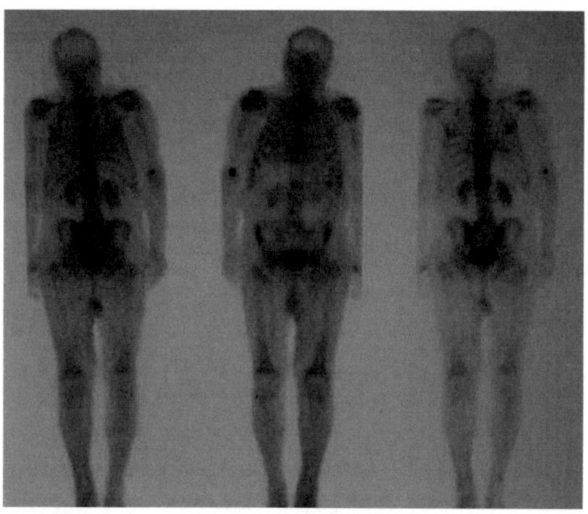

Fig. 10. Bone scan showing an acute vertebral fracture.

## 5. Key steps of the procedure

As is done in many surgical procedures, prophylactic antibiotics are administered to the patient approximately 30 minutes before the actual procedure; however, the efficacy of this practice in preventing infection has never been affirmed by controlled study [Mathis et al, 2001].

BKP is usually not painful and requires only intravenous mild sedation and local anesthesia. The local anesthetic is injected in to the skin, subcutaneous tissues, and periosteum of the vertebra. General anesthesia is another possible choice, especially for lengthy cases involving numerous levels of vertebral fractures; but local anesthesia with sedation is generally enough, especially when general anesthesia is contraindicated by patient's health conditions (e.g. pathologic VCFs in tumors, myeloma, etc.) [Lavelle et al, 2007].

Prone positioning is achieved and a C-arm is provided; biplane fluoroscopy will allow simultaneous visualization in two projections during injection of bone cement. It allows the procedure to be performed more rapidly [Wehrli et al, 1995] and is often chosen when the procedure is performed in a radiology department because of equipment availability and familiarity.

After fluoroscopic localization, a small incision is made and a thin cannulated trocar with bone biopsy needle is advanced to the antero-posterior radiographic projection of the pedicle. Then the cannula is passed through the pedicle into the vertebral body being treated. Both lateral and antero-posterior projections provide necessary visualization of the path of the needle. An alternative approach is the extrapedicular. This is most often used to access the upper thoracic spine, where pedicles are smaller then in the lumbar tract. The extrapedicular approach involves inserting the cannula between the lateral margin of the pedicle of thoracic vertebrae and the rib head [Hide et al, 2004]. When fracture fragments are reached, the needle is removed and a drill bit is inserted into the cannula; so a passage to the anterior part of the vertebral body is created. Then a void is created within the cancellous bone by an inflatable bone tamp prior to cement delivery (*fig1 and 2*): in this way, bone cement is not *free*, cement-leakage rate is considerably lower than vertebroplasty and a lower pressure is needed to inject bone cement into the vertebra (*fig3*). Occasionally patients report pain when a tool is removed too quickly from the cannula, reasonably due to the sudden negative pressure. This procedure takes about one hour or less for each vertebra involved.

Sometimes kyphoplasty allows achieving height restoration of the fractured vertebral body, thus preventing kyphosis – therefore *kyphoplasty* (*fig4*).

## 6. Postoperative care

Recovery from a kyphoplasty is relatively quick. In our experience, patients feel almost immediate pain relief after the surgery. Most patients can go home on the day of the procedure; however we prefer to discharge the patient the day after, so he/she may obtain adequate information from our staff about post operative care at home. During hospitalization, in fact, the nurse staff will provide the patient with medication for pain and will encourage him/her to get up, and move around, as soon as possible after the surgery. Bending or sitting should be avoided for an hour or more. Most patients are very satisfied with the procedure and are able to gradually resume activity once discharged from the hospital. Once at home, patients may resume their activities of daily living as soon as they are able. The bandages may be removed two or three days after they return home from the hospital; the incision on the back should require very little care: keeping it clean and dry is the best. Showering is allowed after only one day, but the patient should not take a bath or go swimming for three weeks. Driving or lifting of heavy objects is forbidden until after about two weeks.

Postoperative bracing is unnecessary, because bone cement hardens during the procedure (PMMA) or within one hour after it (CPC): in fact, the resistance to compressive forces of CPC has been demonstrated not to differ significantly from PMMA after in vitro vertebroplasty in human cadavers [Bai et al, 1999] while another in vitro study reported that CPC can attain compressive strength comparable to that of an intact vertebral body within 15-20 minutes after implantation: thus, the biomaterial is sufficiently strong for safe transfer of the patient within a reasonable time, following setting (bed-rest for 24h after BKP with CPC is suggested by this study: that's what we do) [Schwardt et al, 2006].

An appointment for radiological and clinical follow-up is scheduled a month after discharge: patients will come to hospital with a plain X-ray of the spine and blood tests (looking for indicators of an acute phase response).

## 7. Complications

The most commonly described complication is an extravertebral leakage of bone cement [Groen et al, 2004], more likely in traumatic VCFs compared to pathologic VCFs due to more fracture cracks in traumatic fracture [Schmelzer-Schmied et al, 2009]. The systematic review of the literature by Hulme found rates of cement leakage in vertebroplasty of 41% (n = 2283 levels) and in kyphoplasty of 9% (n = 1486 levels) of treated vertebrae. This can lead to spinal stenosis or to pulmonary cement embolism [Choe et al, 2004]. But most leaks were clinically asymptomatic: consider that leaks-distribution is mainly paraspinal (48%) and intradiscal (38%), then epidural (11%) and finally pulmonary (1.5%) and foraminal (1.5%) [Hulme et al, 2009]. In our series, there is a 33% of asymptomatic cement-leakage rate.

In addition, systemic allergic or toxic reactions to bone cement have been described [Kalteis et al, 2004]. New fractures of adjacent vertebrae occurred for both procedures at rates that are higher than the general osteoporotic population but approximately equivalent to the general osteoporotic population that had a previous vertebral fracture [Hulme et al, 2009].

## 8. Clinical series and outcome

In his systematic review of 69 clinical studies, Hulme compared outcomes from vertebroplasty and kyphoplasty [Hulme et al, 2009]: in both case a large proportion of subjects had some pain relief independent of the type of procedure (87% vertebroplasty, 92% kyphoplasty). Visual analog pain scores (VAS) (normalized to 10-point scale) were reduced from an average of 7.15 to 3.4 for BKP while only two kyphoplasty studies reported on improvement in physical function [Ghros et al, 2006; Gaitains et al, 2005]: this suggests that reporting improvements in physical function appears to be of secondary importance to the investigators; therefore, measurement scales used are inconsistent and scores cannot be pooled [Hulme et al, 2009]. The pain relief experienced by patients appears to be promising for both BKP and vertebroplasty in the short-term (<1 year) whereas it appears that pain relief is durable: in fact, little change was noted between postoperative scores and long-term. [Hulme et al, 2009, Zoarski et al, 2002]. However, note that long-term follow-up results were not as frequently reported [Hulme et al, 2009]

A qualitative examination of the data collected by Hulme indicates that vertebral height restoration is similar both for vertebroplasty and BKP (mean 6.6°). However, interstudy comparisons are further complicated by the use of different methods for percentage height restoration and reduction of kyphosis angle calculation [Hulme et al, 2009, McKiernan et al, 2003]. As described in the section above, cement leaks occurred for 41% and 9% of treated vertebrae for vertebroplasty and kyphoplasty respectively, while adjacent level fracture rates are similar between both procedures and approximately equivalent to the general osteoporotic population that had a previous vertebral fracture. Furthermore, the stabilization of a specific fracture level by kyphoplasty may lead to secondary fractures of adjacent vertebrae due to the changed biomechanics of the spine [Baroud et al, 2006, Berlemann et al, 2002]. However, these studies refer to osteoporotic VCFs, so the adjacent vertebral fractures are related to a low bone density [Tseng et al, 2009].

### 8.1 Our series

From March 2005 to March 2011, 137 hospitalized patients underwent BKP for VCF at our Department. Among these, 76 patients (55,5%) fulfilled the criteria set at our Institution to be offered BKP after having suffered traumatic VCF (*tab1*):

| **Parameters** | **N = 76** |
|---|---|
| Gender (M) | 40 (52.6%) |
| Level (>=2) | 2 (2.6%) |
| Magerl | |
| A 1.2 | 31 (43.0%) |
| A 1.3 | 14 (19.4%) |
| A 3.1 | 27 (37.5%) |
| Age | 53±15 |
| VAS pre | 8.8±1.1 |
| VAS post | 3.0±2.0 |
| DeltaVAS | 67±21 |

Table 1. Demographic and clinical charatteristics; DeltaVAS = (VAS pre-VAS post)/VAS pre)*100

Inclusion criteria were:

1. no neurological deficits;
2. one or, at most, two vertebral body injuries involving the spine from T5 through L4 or, when feasible, L5;
3. no radiological evidence of mechanical instability;
4. Magerl nonsurgical and stable fractures, that are – in our opinion – A1.2 (wedge impaction) (N=31), A1.3 (vertebral body collapse) (N=14) and A3.1 (incomplete burst

fracture) types without retro-pulsed fragment. We exclude A2.1 to A2.3 types because there is always a split of the vertebral body that could allow cement leakage.

Mean age was 53±15 years and 53% males. Mean preoperative VAS was 8.7±1.1 while Post-operative VAS was 3.0±2.0 significantly lower with p-value<0.0001. As reported in *graph1:*

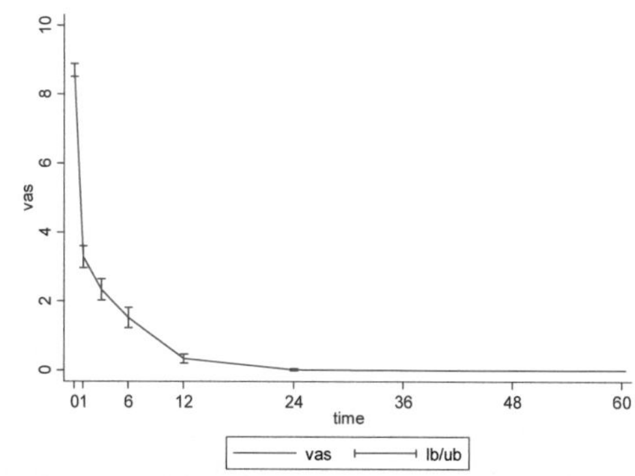


Graph. 1. Outcome: pain-relief during follow-ups; lb = lower bund, ub = upper bund

VAS decreased significantly after surgery while complete pain releif was obtained at 2-year follow-up for 42 patients; this result is durable for 8 patients with 6-year follow-up. We believe that, unlike patients with pathologic VCFs, in traumatic patients healthy conditions are good (no osteoporosis, tumors or myeloma): so a complete pain relief is a possible goal after BKP.

Early mobilization (i.e., within 24-48h from BKP) was obtained in all cases. Because our philosophy is to not overfill traumatic fractured vertebra, height restoration is not our target for this kind of VCFs. So we didn't take any measurement of Cobb angle. In 23 subjects (30%) asymptomatic cement leakages occurred.

## 9. Traumatic VCFs: Tips and tricks

Because we work closely with our Emergency Department, more than 50% of our cases are traumatic VCFs

One of the most controversial issues millitating against BKP in traumatic VCFs relates to the main bone cement used in this procedure (i.e. poly-methlyl-metacrylate, PMMA), which cannot integrate into bone and can not allow for bone-healing.

On the contrary, we prefer to use PMMA because the potential local reaction to PMMA (incidental to the exothermic reaction that occurs while the PMMA bone cement is hardening *in situ*) brings fibrous tissue formation at the interface between bone and bone cement [Kalteis et al, 2004], which may be a serious disadvantage for a joint (e.g. hip) but seems not to be significant for a non-articulating bone such as the vertebral body.

However, we suggest some care in performing BKP in traumatic VCF:

1. In traumatic factures there is much higher rate of cement leakage compared to non-traumatic VCF; this is due to the nature of these traumatic fractures: the cement can leak

through the many fracture cracks [Schmezler-Schmied et al, 2009]. So we prefer to not overfill the fractured vertebra with cement because an excessive amount of bone cement could lead to a higher rate of leakage. This also explains why we mainly prefer kyphoplasty over vertebroplasty, which needs a much higher pressure.

2. Unlike osteoporotic VCFs, it's very difficult to achieve height restoration in traumatic fractures because these patients have a normal bone density [Schmezler-Schmied et al, 2009]: so over-inflating the balloon seems to be unnecessary. Higher rates of cement leakage and/or balloon burst are present.
3. Because a low risk of adjacent vertebral fractures is described for vertebral augmentation techniques (generally for vertebroplasty) with PMMA cement [Gerztbein et al, 1994; Kalteis et al, 2004; Tseng et al, 2009], we prefer to not overfill the fractured vertebra keeping this risk to the minimum: reported clinical studies have shown that even "insufficient" filling of vertebral bodies during a vertebroplasty can lead to a successful outcomes in pain reduction, and stiffening and stabilizing of the fractured vertebrae [Luo et al, 2007; Furtado et al, 2007; Oakland et al, 2009]. The mechanism for adjacent vertebral fractures is still unclear, but from experimental and computational studies, it appears that vertebroplasty changes the mechanical loading in adjacent vertebrae because of excessive cement rigidity of treated vertebra [Baroud et al, 2006; Berlemann et al, 2002]. However, it is noted that these studies refer to VCF from osteoporosis, so the adjacent vertebral fractures are related to a low bone density. In fact, Tseng concluded that older patient ages, lower baseline BMD, and more pre-existing vertebral fractures were found to be risk factors for multiple vertebral compression fractures [Tseng et al, 2009].
4. Inflammatory response to PMMA exothermic reaction could lead to bone resorption all around this cement. Although this is a serious disadvantage for prostheses integration into the bone (a common technique to aid in implant fixation into surrounding bone is to inject bone cement into the space between the implant and surrounding bone [Kuhn et al, 2000]), this seems not to be very significant for a non-articulating bone, as represented by a vertebral body, especially if we consider that some authors successful treated intravertebral pseudarthroses (whose neuroradiological findings is are the rare and, so-called, *intravertebral vacuum fenomenon* [Van Eenenaan et al, 1993]) by BKP with PMMA [Ghros et al, 2006]. Furthermore, Aebli has shown that temperature levels after usage of intravertebral PMMA cement may be sufficient to cause intravertebral thermal necrosis, but that heat levels outside the vertebral body (e.g. at the intervertebral discs and vertebral endplates) are unlikely to cause thermal injury [Aebli et al, 2006]. However, we prefer to keep to a minimum the amount of cement in order to avoid local bone resorption.
5. Finally, we agree with de Falco [de Falco et al, 2005] about the opportunity to use bioactive cement in patients under 50 years. In fact, although the use of PMMA cement in vertebroplasty is widespread, no data on the long-term behaviour of the material for spinal applications has been published. So, because the majority of patients with traumatic vertebral fractures are aged less than 50 years and the PMMA material remains inside the vertebral body for life, the use of more biocompatible bone cement is preferred [Verlaan et al, 2002]. Thus, the usage of calcium phosphate cement (CPC), which hardens by crystallization at body temperature, avoids thermal injury, whereby it is unclear whether thermal necrosis actually contributes to the fibrous tissue layer around PMMA implants [Libicher et al, 2006]. However, we have to take into

consideration the fact that bioactive cements are much more expensive than PMMA. Therefore, it may be that the use of very expensive bone cement is deemed innaproriate for elderly patients.

## 10. Explicative cases

We present two illustrative cases about among our procedures.

### 10.1 Case 1

52-year-old female, L1 traumatic A1.2 vertebral compression fracture (*fig. 11*):

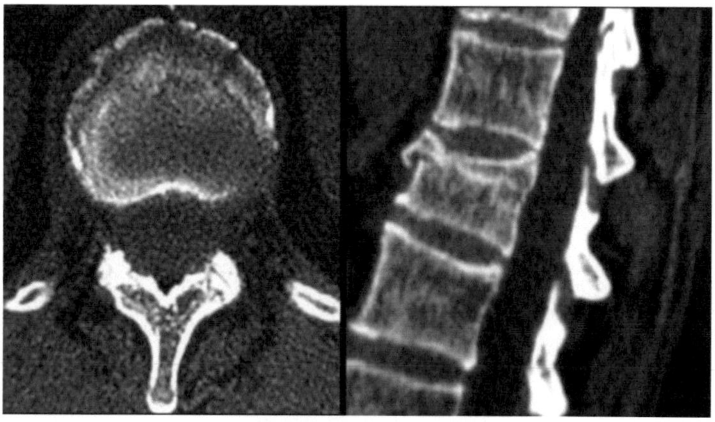

Fig. 11. Case 1. Axial (right) and sagittal MPR (left) CT scan of L1 traumatic A1.2 VCF. Posterior vertebral wall is untouched.

As you can see in the postoperative CT scan (*fig. 12*):

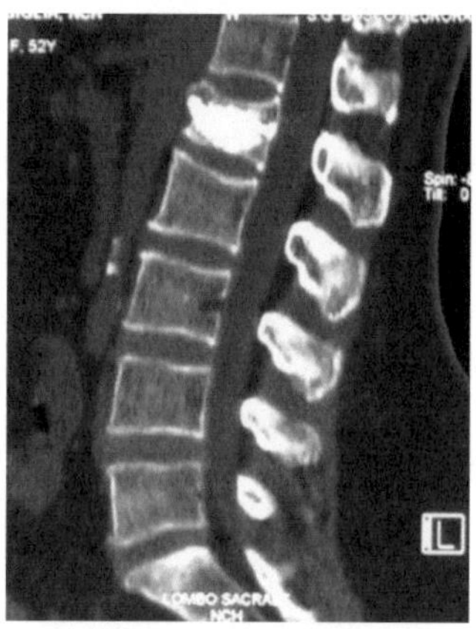

Fig. 12. Case 1. Postoperative CT scan (sagittal MPR)

L1 body was not overfilled by bone cement (PMMA), because our target for traumatic VCFs is stabilization *not* augmentation. X-ray follow-up at 2 (*fig. 13*) and 5 years (*fig. 14*) are showed:

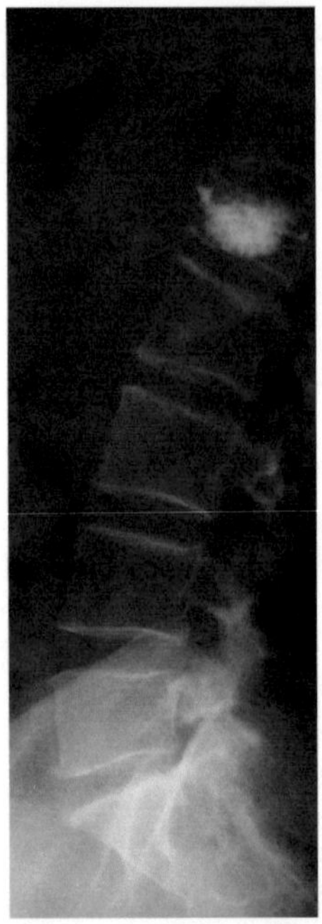

Fig. 13. Case 1. X-ray follow-up (2 years)

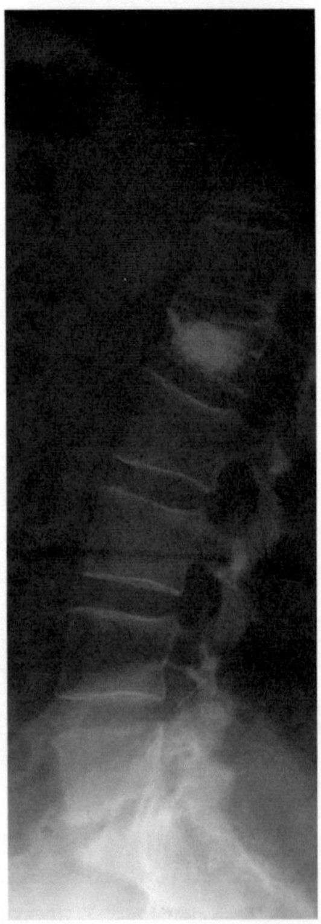

Fig. 14. Case 1. X-ray follow-up (5 years)

Stabilization was held, no further collapse of the kyphoplastied vertebra or adjacent fractures were seen at long-term follow-up. Preoperative VAS was 7 while postoperative VAS became 0 since three months after BKP; this clinical goal was kept at 5 years follow-up.

### 10.2 Case 2

This is one of first case of our series. 53-year-old male, T12 traumatic A3.1 vertebral compression fracture (*fig. 15*):

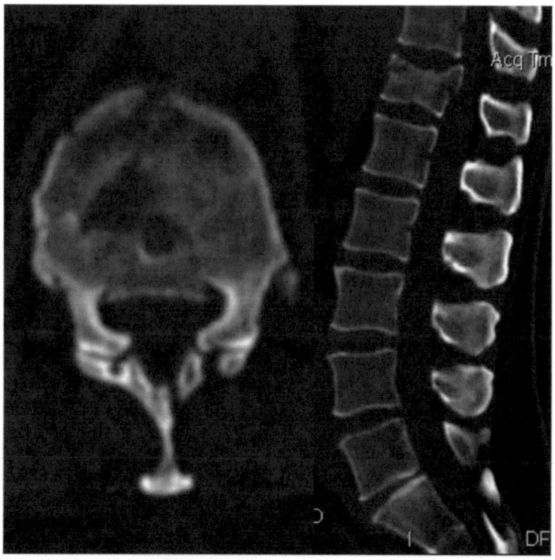

Fig. 15. Case 2. Axial (right) and sagittal MPR (left) CT scan of T12 traumatic A3.1 VCF. Intact pedicles are clearly visible in axial scan. Non-significant retropulsed fragment is present.

As you can see in post-operative CT-scan (fig16):

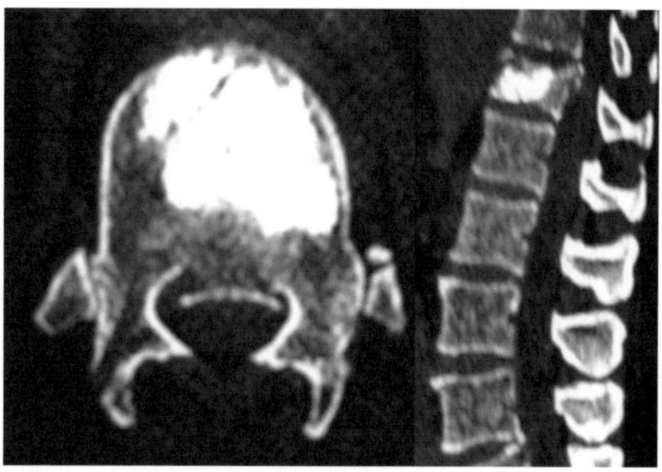

Fig. 16. Case 2. Axial (right) and sagittal MPR (left) CT scan of D12 traumatic A3.1 VCF after BKP. Vertebral body was not overfilled while retropulsed fragment wasn't touched.

we used a little amount of bone cement to fill the vertebral body: stabilization was achieved while vertebral body augmentation was poor; this "undercharging" philosophy was also useful in not touching the retropulsed fragment.

This radiographic result was held after 6-years follow-up (fig17):

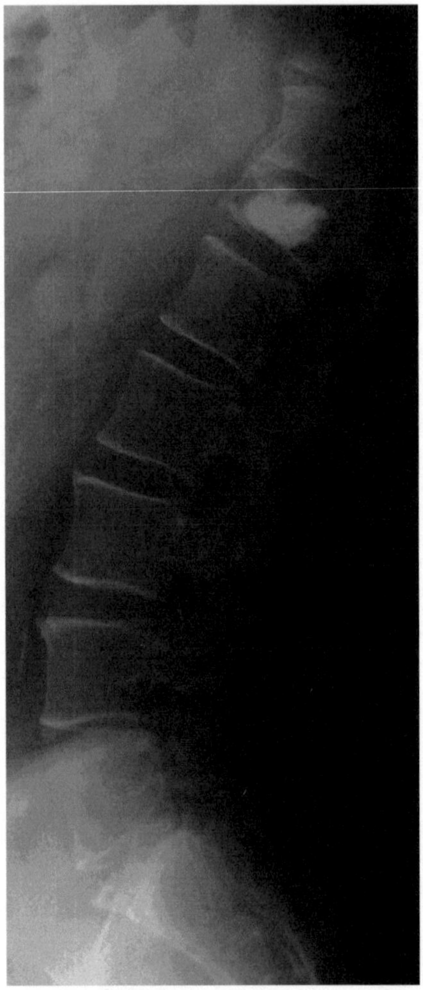

Fig. 17. Case 2. X-ray follow-up (6 years)

Pre-operative VAS was 8 while post-operative VAS significantly improved to 2; complete absence of pain was achieved 6 months after BKP, and this score was held at 6-years follow-up-

## 11. Conclusion

In our experience, BKP is a safe and effective procedure to treat nonsurgical and stable traumatic VCF compared to conservative therapy and to other percutaneous augmentation technique such as vertebroplasty.

Although long-term studies about effectiveness of BKP for traumatic VCFs are unsatisfactory, our 6-years follow-up suggests that this vertebral-augmentation technique represent a very attractive, easy and fully adequate solution to treat this kind of traumatic fractures.

## 12. Acknowledgments

Special thanks to Chris Johnson for correcting English usage in my paper

## 13. References

Aebli N, Goss BG, Thorpe P, Williams R, Krebs J. In vivo temperature profile of intervertebral discs and vertebral endplates during vertebroplasty: an experimental study in sheep. Spine (Phila Pa 1976). 2006 Jul 1;31(15):1674-8; discussion 1679.

Bai B, Jazrawi LM, Kummer FJ, Spivak JM. The use of an injectable, biodegradable calcium phosphate bone substitute for the prophylactic augmentation of osteoporotic vertebrae and the management of vertebral compression fractures. Spine (Phila Pa 1976). 1999 Aug 1;24(15):1521-6.

Baroud G, Vant C, Wilcox R. Long-term effects of vertebroplasty: adjacent vertebral fractures. J Long Term Eff Med Implants. 2006;16(4):265-80.

Berlemann U, Ferguson SJ, Nolte LP, Heini PF. Adjacent vertebral failure after vertebroplasty. A biomechanical investigation. J Bone Joint Surg Br. 2002 Jul;84(5):748-52.

Bula P, Lein T, Straßberger C, Bonnaire F. Balloon Kyphoplasty in the Treatment of Osteoporotic Vertebral Fractures: Indications - Treatment Strategy - Complications. Z Orthop Unfall. 2010 Nov 15. [Epub ahead of print]

Choe DH, Marom EM, Ahrar K, Truong MT, Madewell JE. Pulmonary embolism of polymethyl methacrylate during percutaneous vertebroplasty and kyphoplasty. AJR Am J Roentgenol. 2004 Oct;183(4):1097-102.

Costa F, Ortolina A, Cardia A, Sassi M, De Santis A, Borroni M, Savoia G, Fornari M. Efficacy of treatment with percutaneous vertebroplasty and kyphoplasty for traumatic fracture of thoracolumbar junction. J Neurosurg Sci. 2009 Mar;53(1):13-7.

Costa F, Ortolina A, Cardia A, Sassi M, De Santis A, Borroni M, Savoia G, Fornari M. Efficacy of treatment with percutaneous vertebroplasty and kyphoplasty for traumatic fracture of thoracolumbar junction. J Neurosurg Sci. 2009 Mar;53(1):13-7.

Dalbayrak S, Onen MR, Yilmaz M, Naderi S. Clinical and radiographic results of balloon kyphoplasty for treatment of vertebral body metastases and multiple myelomas. J Clin Neurosci. 2010 Feb;17(2):219-24. Epub 2009 Dec 5.

Dashti H, Lee HC, Karaikovic EE, Gaines Jr RW. Decision making in thoracolumbar fractures. Neurol India 2005;53:534-41.

de Falco R, Scarano E, Di Celmo D, Grasso U, Guarnieri L. Balloon kyphoplasty in traumatic fractures of the thoracolumbar junction. Preliminary experience in 12 cases. J Neurosurg Sci. 2005 Dec;49(4):147-53.

Doria C, Tranquilli Leali P. Percutaneous techniques in the treatment of osteoporotic, traumatic and neoplastic fractures of thoraco-lumbar spine: our institutional experience. Injury. 2010 Nov;41(11):1136-9. Epub 2010 Oct 16

Furtado N, Oakland RJ, Wilcox RK, Hall RM. A biomechanical investigation of vertebroplasty in osteoporotic compression fractures and in prophylactic vertebral reinforcement. Spine (Phila Pa 1976). 2007 Aug 1;32(17):E480-7.

Gaitanis IN, Hadjipavlou AG, Katonis PG, Tzermiadianos MN, Pasku DS, Patwardhan AG. Balloon kyphoplasty for the treatment of pathological vertebral compressive fractures. Eur Spine J. 2005 Apr;14(3):250-60. Epub 2004 Oct 8.

Gaitanis IN, Hadjipavlou AG, Katonis PG, Tzermiadianos MN, Pasku DS, Patwardhan AG. Balloon kyphoplasty for the treatment of pathological vertebral compressive fractures. Eur Spine J. 2005 Apr;14(3):250-60. Epub 2004 Oct 8.

Gertzbein SD. Neurologic deterioration in patients with thoracic and lumbar fractures after admission to the hospital. Spine 1994;19:1723-5.

Greene DL, Isaac R, Neuwirth M, Bitan FD. The eggshell technique for prevention of cement leakage during kyphoplasty. J Spinal Disord Tech. 2007 May;20(3):229-32.

Groen RJ, du Toit DF, Phillips FM, Hoogland PV, Kuizenga K, Coppes MH, Muller CJ, Grobbelaar M, Mattyssen J. Anatomical and pathological considerations in percutaneous vertebroplasty and kyphoplasty: a reappraisal of the vertebral venous system. Spine (Phila Pa 1976). 2004 Jul 1;29(13):1465-71.

Grohs JG, Matzner M, Trieb K, Krepler P. Treatment of intravertebral pseudarthroses by balloon kyphoplasty. J Spinal Disord Tech. 2006 Dec;19(8):560-5.

Hide IG, Gangi A. Percutaneous vertebroplasty: history, technique and current perspectives. Clin Radiol 2004;59:461–7.

Hulme PA, Krebs J, Ferguson SJ, Berlemann U. Vertebroplasty and kyphoplasty: a systematic review of 69 clinical studies. Spine (Phila Pa 1976). 2006 Aug 1;31(17):1983-2001.

Jones JO, Bruel BM, Vattam SR. Management of painful vertebral hemangiomas with kyphoplasty: a report of two cases and a literature review. Pain Physician. 2009 Jul-Aug;12(4):E297-303.

Kalteis T, Lüring C, Gugler G, Zysk S, Caro W, Handel M, Grifka J. Acute tissue toxicity of PMMA bone cements. Z Orthop Ihre Grenzgeb. 2004 Nov-Dec;142(6):666-72.

Kalteis T, Lüring C, Gugler G, Zysk S, Caro W, Handel M, Grifka J. Acute tissue toxicity of PMMA bone cements. Z Orthop Ihre Grenzgeb. 2004 Nov-Dec;142(6):666-72.

Klazen CA, Lohle PN, de Vries J, Jansen FH, Tielbeek AV, Blonk MC, Venmans A, van Rooij WJ, Schoemaker MC, Juttmann JR, Lo TH, Verhaar HJ, van der Graaf Y, van Everdingen KJ, Muller AF, Elgersma OE, Halkema DR, Fransen H, Janssens X, Buskens E, Mali WP. Vertebroplasty versus conservative treatment in acute osteoporotic vertebral compression fractures (Vertos II): an open-label randomised trial. Lancet. 2010 Sep 25;376(9746):1085-92.

Kühn K-D. Bone Cements, Up-to-Date Comparison of Physicaland Chemical Properties of Commercial Materials. 2000 Springer Verlag: Berlin, pp. 12–20.

Lavelle W, Carl A, Lavelle ED, Khaleel MA. Vertebroplasty and kyphoplasty. Anesthesiol Clin. 2007 Dec;25(4):913-28.

Ledlie JT, Renfro MB. Kyphoplasty treatment of vertebral fractures: 2-year outcomes show sustained benefits. Spine (Phila Pa 1976). 2006 Jan 1;31(1):57-64.

Libicher M, Hillmeier J, Liegibel U, Sommer U, Pyerin W, Vetter M, Meinzer HP, Grafe I, Meeder P, Nöldge G, Nawroth P, Kasperk C. Osseous integration of calcium phosphate in osteoporotic vertebral fractures after kyphoplasty: initial results from a clinical and experimental pilot study. Osteoporos Int. 2006;17(8):1208-15. Epub 2006 Jun 8.

Luo J, Skrzypiec DM, Pollintine P, Adams MA, Annesley-Williams DJ, Dolan P. Mechanical efficacy of vertebroplasty: influence of cement type, BMD, fracture severity, and disc degeneration. Bone. 2007 Apr;40(4):1110-9. Epub 2007 Jan 16.

Magerl F, Aebi M, Gertzbein SD, Harms J, Nazarian S. A comprehensive classification of thoracic and lumbar injuries. Eur Spine J. 1994; 3(4):184-201.

Masala S, Fiori R, Massari F, Cantonetti M, Postorino M, Simonetti G. Percutaneous kyphoplasty: indications and technique in the treatment of vertebral fractures from myeloma. Tumori. 2004 Jan-Feb;90(1):22-6.

Mathis JM, Barr JD, Belkoff SM, et al. Percutaneous vertebroplasty: a developing standard of care for vertebral compression fractures. AJNR Am J Neuroradiol 2001;22(2):373–81

McKiernan F, Faciszewski T, Jensen R. Reporting height restoration in vertebral compression fractures. Spine (Phila Pa 1976). 2003 Nov 15;28(22):2517-21; discussion 3.

Molina GS, Campero A, Feito R, Pombo S. Kyphoplasty in the Treatment of Osteoporotic Vertebral Compression Fractures (VCF) : Procedure Description and Analysis of the Outcomes in 128 Patients. Acta Neurochir Suppl. 2011;108:163-170.

Movrin I, Vengust R, Komadina R. Adjacent vertebral fractures after percutaneous vertebral augmentation of osteoporotic vertebral compression fracture: a comparison of balloon kyphoplasty and vertebroplasty. Arch Orthop Trauma Surg. 2010 Sep;130(9):1157-66. Epub 2010 May 7.

Nairn RJ, Binkhamis S, Sheikh A. Current Perspectives on Percutaneous Vertebroplasty: Current Evidence/Controversies, Patient Selection and Assessment, and Technique and Complications. Radiology Research and Practice, vol. 2011, Article ID 175079, 10 pages, 2011. doi:10.1155/2011/175079

Oakland RJ, Furtado NR, Wilcox RK, Timothy J, Hall RM. Preliminary biomechanical evaluation of prophylactic vertebral reinforcement adjacent to vertebroplasty under cyclic loading. Spine J. 2009 Feb;9(2):174-81. Epub 2008 Jul 21.

Röllinghoff M, Zarghooni K, Schlüter-Brust K, Sobottke R, Schlegel U, Eysel P, Delank KS. Indications and contraindications for vertebroplasty and kyphoplasty. Arch Orthop Trauma Surg. 2010 Jun;130(6):765-74. Epub 2010 Mar 11.

Schmelzer-Schmied N, Cartens C, Meeder PJ, Dafonseca K. Comparison of kyphoplasty with use of a calcium phosphate cement and non-operative therapy in patients with traumatic non-osteoporotic vertebral fractures. Eur Spine J. 2009 May;18(5):624-9. Epub 2009 Jan 23.

Schwardt J, Slater T, Lee S, Meyer J, Wenz R. KyphOs FS™ Calcium Phosphate for Balloon Kyphoplasty: Verification of Compressive Strength and Instructions for Use. European Cells and Materials Vol. 11. Suppl. 1, 2006 (page 28).

Tseng YY, Yang TC, Tu PH, Lo YL, Yang ST. Repeated and multiple new vertebral compression fractures after percutaneous transpedicular vertebroplasty. Spine (Phila Pa 1976). 2009 Aug 15;34(18):1917-22.

Van Eenenaam DP, el-Khoury GY. Delayed post-traumatic vertebral collapse (Kummell's disease): case report with serial radiographs, computed tomographic scans, and bone scans. Spine (Phila Pa 1976). 1993 Jul;18(9):1236-41.

Verlaan JJ, van Helden WH, Oner FC, Verbout AJ, Dhert WJ. Balloon vertebroplasty with calcium phosphate cement augmentation for direct restoration of traumatic thoracolumbar vertebral fractures. Spine (Phila Pa 1976). 2002 Mar 1;27(5):543-8.

Wehrli FW, Ford JC, Haddad JG. Osteoporosis: clinical assessment with quantitative MR imaging in diagnosis. Radiology 1995;196(3):631–41.

Zoarski GH, Snow P, Olan WJ, Stallmeyer MJ, Dick BW, Hebel JR, De Deyne M. Percutaneous vertebroplasty for osteoporotic compression fractures: quantitative prospective evaluation of long-term outcomes. J Vasc Interv Radiol. 2002 Feb;13(2 Pt 1):139-48.

Zou J, Mei X, Gan M, Yang H. Kyphoplasty for spinal fractures from multiple myeloma. J Surg Oncol. 2010 Jul 1;102(1):43-7.

# Section 5

## Functional Neurosurgery

# 17

# Cognitive and Behavioural Changes After Deep Brain Stimulation of the Subthalamic Nucleus in Parkinson's Disease

Antonio Daniele, Pietro Spinelli and Chiara Piccininni
*Istituto di Neurologia,*
*Università Cattolica, Rome,*
*Italy*

## 1. Introduction

In patients with Parkinson's disease, cognitive impairment is common, may be detectable in early disease stages, even in young patients, and may progress to overt dementia. In addition, a variety of psychiatric and behavioural symptoms may occur in Parkinsonian patients, including depression, apathy, anxiety, visual hallucinations, sleep disorders, impulse control disorders, punding and the dopamine dysregulation syndrome. The cognitive and behavioural symptoms observed in these patients may be part of the non-motor symptoms of Parkinson's disease, which can appear in various phases of the disease course.

Various mechanisms might be involved in the pathogenesis of cognitive and behavioral symptoms in Parkinson's disease. Cognitive and behavioural symptoms observed in Parkinsonian patients might be related to disruption of various circuits involving dopaminergic, noradrenergic, cholinergic, and serotonergic systems (Candy et al., 1983; Mayeux et al., 1984; Cash et al., 1987; Mattay et al., 2002). Moreover, in patients with Parkinson's disease and dementia, neuropathological examination (Xuereb et al., 1990; Hughes et al., 1993) may show in several cortical areas the presence of Lewy Bodies (the histopathological hallmark of Parkinson's disease) or neurodegenerative lesions typical of Alzheimer's disease (amyloid plaques and neurofibrillary tangles). Furthermore, in patients with Parkinson's disease pharmacological treatment with anti-Parkinsonian dopaminergic drugs may have beneficial or detrimental effects on distinct cognitive functions (Malapani et al., 1994; Kulisevsky et al., 1996; Mattay et al., 2002) and may also play a role in the development of some behavioural disorders.

Among the cognitive deficits which may be detected in patients with Parkinson's disease, deficits of executive functions (planning, problem solving, set-shifting), mediated by disruption of neural circuits involving the frontal lobes and the basal ganglia, are the most common in both early disease phases and in patients with advanced Parkinson's disease (Morris et al., 1988; Cooper et al., 1991; Robbins et al., 1994; Taylor et al., 1986; Cools et al., 2001; Green et al., 2002).

In addition, memory deficits (Taylor et al., 1986; Harrington et al., 1990; Cooper et al., 1991; Robbins et al., 1994; Dubois and Pillon, 1997), deficits of visuo-spatial cognitive functions

(Boller et al., 1984; Hovestadt et al., 1987; Ransmayr et al., 1987), impairment on language tasks of verbal fluency (Matison et al., 1982; Cooper et al., 1991) and tasks of oral naming (Peran et al., 2003) may occur in individual Parkinsonian patients since early phases and become more frequent in advanced Parkinson's disease (Green et al., 2002).

As to memory deficits, different studies reported in Parkinsonian patients an impairment of episodic memory (Taylor et al., 1986), verbal short-term memory (Cooper et al., 1991), spatial short-term memory (Robbins et al., 1994), and procedural memory (Harrington et al., 1990). In patients with Parkinson's disease and dementia, the pattern of neuropsychological impairment may differ in distinct patient subgroups.

A subgroup of Parkinsonian patients, in which neurodegenerative lesions in the cerebral cortex seem to be less remarkable (Xuereb et al., 1990), may show a pattern of subcortical dementia, mainly characterized by remarkable deficits of executive functions (Litvan et al., 1991), associated with mild to moderate deficits of episodic long-term memory (Helkala et al., 1988) and, in some patients, deficits of visuo-spatial cognitive functions (Mohr et al., 1995), with relative sparing of linguistic and praxic functions (Dubois and Pillon, 1997). In another subgroup of patients with Parkinson's disease and dementia, in which neurodegenerative lesions in the cerebral cortex are more remarkable, in addition to the previously described neuropsychological pattern of subcortical dementia, it is possible to observe a an impairment of other cognitive functions mediated by various cortical areas, namely an impairment of linguistic and praxic functions and severe deficits of episodic long-term memory (Mohr et al., 1990; Mohr et al., 1995; Marsh, 2000).

As to psychiatric and behavioural symptoms which may be observed in patients with Parkinson's disease, depression, apathy, anxiety and visual hallucinations are the most common manifestations. Depressive syndromes (major depression and dysthymic disorder) may occur in up to 45% of Parkinsonian patients (Burn, 2002). Both psychosocial and neurobiological factors might be involved in the pathogenesis of depressive syndromes in Parkinson's disease. The role of psychosocial factors (such as a psychological reaction to motor disability) is suggested by studies reporting a significant correlation between severity of depressive symptoms and severity of motor symptoms (Gotham et al., 1986), while other investigations support the role of neurobiological factors such as a disruption of dopaminergic (Torack e Morris, 1988; Mayberg e Solomon, 1995), noradrenergic (Cubo et al., 2000; Menza et al., 2009) and serotonergic (Paulus e Jellinger, 1991) systems, which may occur in early phases of Parkinson's disease (Braak et al., 2004) and might result in the appearance of depressive symptoms. In some Parkinsonian patients, depressive symptoms may occur some years before the appearance of Parkinsonian motor symptoms, in agreement with the hypothesis of a critical role of neurobiological factors (Aarsland et al., 2009).

Apathy, which is characterised by a reduction in interest, motivation and initiative in daily living activities, is common in patients with Parkinson's disease and was detected in 17% to 70% of Parkinsonian patients in different studies (Leentjens et al., 2008; Pedersen et al., 2009). Although the pathogenic mechanisms involved in apathy in Parkinson's disease need to be further clarified, a dysfunction of the "limbic" circuit (Alexander et al., 1986) of the basal ganglia (which involve the ventral striatum, the anterior part of the cingulate gyrus and the mesial orbitofrontal cortex) might play a critical role.

Psychotic symptoms such as delusions and hallucinations are common in patients with Parkinson's disease and may occur in up to 26% of patients (Sanchez-Ramoz et al., 1996). In patients with Parkinson's disease, hallucinations and delusions may result from multiple pathogenic factors. Although these psychotic symptoms may be induced by the administration of dopaminergic anti-Parkinsonian drugs (Factor et al., 1995; Valldeoriola et al., 1997), they may occur also in Parkinsonian patients who do not receive any pharmacological treatment (Factor et al., 1995). The prevalence of hallucinations and delusions does increase with disease progression. Moreover, cognitive impairment is usually more marked in Parkinsonian patients with hallucinations as compared with Parkinsonian patients without hallucinations (Katzen et al., 2010). Visual hallucinations are the most frequent, are characterised by visions of people or animals, and are usually perceived as unpleasant.

Anxiety is also common in patients with Parkinson's disease, although epidemiological studies focussed on the prevalence of anxiety in these patients are still needed. In a recent study carried out in patients with Parkinson's disease in early stages, the prevalence of anxiety was about 27% (Bugalho et al., 2012).

Impulse control disorders (Ambermoon et al., 2011), punding and the dopamine dysregulation syndrome (Lim et al., 2009) have been increasingly recognized in recent years in patients with Parkinson's disease.

It has been reported that up to 13.6% of Parkinsonian patients (Weintraub et al, 2010) may develop behavioural changes due to a reduced impulse control (pathological gambling, hypersexuality, compulsive eating and buying/shopping). Such impulse control disorders may have dramatic implications for the personal life of the patient and for the patient's family.

In Parkinsonian patients, dopamine replacement therapy might play a role in the pathophysiology of impulse control disorders, by inducing an overstimulation of the mesolimbic dopaminergic system, which is critically involved in response to reward and motivation (Demetriades et al, 2011).

It has been suggested that in patients with Parkinson's disease the risk to develop impulse control disorders (Demetriades et al, 2011) may be increased by several demographic and clinical variables (younger age of onset of Parkinson's disease, treatment with dopamine agonists, male gender, pre-existing psychiatric disorders).

In Parkinsonian patients, the dopamine dysregulation syndrome is characterized by an overuse of dopaminergic anti-Parkinsonian drugs, resulting in the compulsive assumption of higher daily doses than those required to treat motor symptoms (Giovannoni et al., 2000).

Punding is a behavioural disorder in which the patient is frequently engaged in repetitive, stereotyped, non-goal-oriented activities. In patients with Parkinson's disease, punding may be triggered by dopaminergic anti-Parkinsonian drugs.

Deep brain stimulation of the subthalamic nucleus is an established neurosurgical procedure in the treatment of Parkinson's disease, which may remarkably improve the motor symptoms and quality of life in Parkinsonian patients (Hamani et al., 2005).

Deep brain stimulation of the subthalamic nucleus is more effective than best medical therapy in improving Parkinsonian motor symptoms and dyskinesias (Hamani et al., 2005) and allows to obtain a long-lasting decrease of the daily doses of anti-Parkinsonian medications. However, a worsening of axial motor symptoms (postural instability, freezing of gait, difficulties in articulation of speech) may be frequently observed at long-term follow-up, as reported in a 8-year follow-up study carried out in 20 Parkinsonian patients who underwent bilateral deep brain stimulation of the subthalamic nucleus (Fasano et al., 2010).

While the beneficial effects of bilateral deep brain stimulation of the subthalamic nucleus on motor symptoms in patients with advanced PD have been clearly analyzed by several studies, the effects of deep brain stimulation of the subthalamic nucleus on cognition and behaviour may at least partially differ among different studies and need to be further investigated.

## 2. Cognitive performance in Parkinsonian patients treated by deep brain stimulation of the subthalamic nucleus

Several investigations have assessed cognitive functioning in patients with Parkinson's disease treated by deep brain stimulation of the subthalamic nucleus, with variable duration of postoperative follow-up in different studies. In these investigations, statistical comparisons were made between preoperative (baseline) performance of Parkinsonian patients on neuropsychological tasks and postoperative performance on the same tasks.

Across all neuropsychological studies assessing cognitive functioning in patients with Parkinson's disease treated by deep brain stimulation of the subthalamic nucleus, a consistently reported finding is a postoperative decline on tasks of phonological and semantic verbal fluency (Ardouin et al. 1999; Pillon et al. 2000, Daniele et al. 2003; Funkiewiez et al. 2004; Parsons et al., 2006), which was detected already few months after surgery in some studies and gradually increased over time in studies with long-term follow-up (Contarino et al., 2007; Fasano et al., 2010).

On the other hand, different studies reported less consistent findings on other cognitive tasks, including tasks of episodic memory and working memory and tasks assessing frontal cognitive functions (Parson et al., 2006).

### 2.1 Performance of Parkinsonian patients treated by deep brain stimulation of the subthalamic nucleus on tasks of verbal fluency

In patients affected by Parkinson's disease who underwent deep brain stimulation of the subthalamic nucleus, a postoperative decline on tasks of phonological and semantic verbal fluency has been consistently reported by all neuropsychological investigations. Such decline on performance on verbal fluency tasks has been usually detected few months after the surgical intervention and has been observed in patients with 1-year (Pillon et al., 2000; Daniele et al., 2003), 3-year (Funkiewiz et al., 2004), 5-year (Contarino et al., 2007; Fasano et al., 2010), and 8-year follow-up (Fasano et al., 2010). A recent study aimed at assessing long-term motor and cognitive outcome 8 years after implants for deep brain stimulation of the subthalamic nucleus in 20 patients with Parkinson's disease (Fasano et al., 2010) detected a decline on phonological verbal fluency task, which was slightly more pronounced 8 years than 5 years after surgery.

In this study, 8 years after surgery performance on a phonological verbal fluency task could be assessed in 16 Parkinsonian patients. Interestingly, the analysis of raw scores (adjusted for age and educational level) obtained by individual Parkinsonian patients on the letter verbal fluency task at 8-year follow-up showed that only 2 out of 16 patients (12.5%) performed below the normal range and 1 patient (6.2%) scored around the cut-off score, while 13 out 16 patients (81.2%) performed in the normal range (Fasano et al., 2010). These latter findings suggest that in selected cohorts of Parkinsonian patients treated by deep brain stimulation of the subthalamic nucleus the statistically significant decline on verbal fluency tasks observed as a group effect is associated with large interindividual variability (Contarino et al., 2007) and in some individual Parkinsonian patients might be not remarkable.

It should be pointed out that a poor performance on tasks of verbal fluency is frequently observed also in patients with Parkinson's disease patients treated by pallidotomy, especially after left-sided pallidotomy (Troster et al., 2003) and even in patients with Parkinson's disease who are not treated by neurosurgical procedures (Matison et al., 1982).

Recently, some investigations have attempted to compare performance on verbal fluency tasks in two different groups of patients with Parkinson's disease, namely patients treated by deep brain stimulation of the subthalamic nucleus versus Parkinsonian patients treated only by anti-Parkinsonian drugs (Zangaglia et al., 2009; Castelli et al., 2010; Williams et al., 2011). Such comparative studies consistently found that performance on verbal fluency tasks was significantly better in Parkinsonian patients treated only by anti-Parkinsonian drugs, as compared to patients who underwent deep brain stimulation of the subthalamic nucleus and were followed-up for 6 months (Witt et al., 2008), 1 year (Castelli et al., 2010), 2 years (Williams et al. 2011) and 3 years (Zangaglia et al., 2009).

In a randomized multicentre study (Witt et al., 2008), 123 patients with advanced Parkinson's disease and motor fluctuations were randomly assigned to have deep brain stimulation of the subthalamic nucleus or the best medical treatment for Parkinson's disease (according to the German Society of Neurology guidelines) and underwent neuropsychological and psychiatric examinations to detect possible changes 6 months after surgery, as compared to baseline. Sixty patients were randomly assigned to receive deep brain stimulation of the subthalamic nucleus and 63 patients to have best medical treatment.

After 6 months, the group of Parkinsonian patients treated by deep brain stimulation of the subthalamic nucleus showed a significantly greater decline on tasks of phonological and semantic verbal fluency, as compared to the group of patients treated with the best medical treatment. These findings suggest that the impairment on verbal fluency tasks observed in patients who underwent subthalamic implants is not simply due to disease progression, but might be rather due to the neurosurgical intervention.

In a prospective 3-year follow-up study (Zangaglia et al., 2009), 32 Parkinsonian patients underwent deep brain stimulation of the subthalamic nucleus, while 33 Parkinsonian patients, even though eligible for this surgical procedure, declined surgery and were treated only by anti-Parkinsonian drugs. In this latter study, as compared to the group of patients treated with the best medical treatment, the group of Parkinsonian patients treated by deep brain stimulation of the subthalamic nucleus showed at 1-month and 3-year follow-up a significantly greater decline on a task of phonological verbal fluency.

In conclusion, the postoperative decline on verbal fluency tasks in patients with Parkinson's disease treated by deep brain stimulation of the subthalamic nucleus does not seem to have clinically meaningful effects on daily living activities, even in patients with long-term follow-up (Contarino et al., 2007).

Various hypotheses have been proposed to account for the postoperative decline on tasks of verbal fluency observed in patients with Parkinson's disease treated by deep brain stimulation of the subthalamic nucleus. On one hand, it has been suggested that the postoperative decline on such fluency tasks might be due to the neurosurgical procedure, namely to surgical microlesions affecting cortical-basal ganglionic circuits involved in word retrieval processes (Troster et al., 2003). This hypothesis is supported by the observation that the decline on verbal fluency tasks in Parkinsonian patients has been usually detected in very early phases after the subthalamic implant. An alternative hypothesis suggests that is the stimulation of the subthalamic nucleus which might lead to a decreased activity of various cortical areas in the left cerebral hemisphere (inferior frontal, insular and temporal areas), giving rise to a decreased performance on verbal fluency tasks (Schroeder et al. 2003).

### 2.2 Performance of Parkinsonian patients treated by deep brain stimulation of the subthalamic nucleus on tasks of episodic memory and abstract reasoning

As suggested by a meta-analysis on neuropsychological studies in patients with Parkinson's disease treated by deep brain stimulation of the subthalamic nucleus (Parsons et al., 2006), a statistically significant but small decline of postoperative performance on tasks of episodic verbal memory has been reported in some investigations (Alegret et al., 2001; Daniele et al., 2003; Dujardin et al., 2001; Jahanshahi et al., 2000; Pillon et al., 2000; Saint-Cyr et al., 2000; Trepanier et al., 2000), but not in others. Such postoperative decline on episodic verbal memory tasks was detectable already 3 months after surgery in some studies (Alegret et al., 2001; Daniele et al., 2003), while in one cohort became not statistically significant at 1-year follow-up (Daniele et al., 2003).

In a recent study which attempted to compare performance on various neuropsychological tasks in two different groups of patients with Parkinson's disease followed-up for 12 months, namely 105 patients treated by deep brain stimulation of the subthalamic nucleus versus 40 Parkinsonian patients treated only by anti-Parkinsonian drugs (Smedding et al., 2011), performance at 6 and 12 months of postoperative follow-up on tasks of episodic verbal memory (immediate and delayed recall of the Rey's Auditory Verbal Learning Test) was significantly poorer in Parkinsonian patients who underwent subthalamic implants, as compared to patients treated only by anti-Parkinsonian drugs.

As to studies with long-term follow-up, a statistically significant but slight decline on episodic verbal memory tasks (immediate and delayed recall of the Rey's Auditory Verbal Learning Test) as compared to preoperative baseline was detected 8 years after subthalamic implants (Fasano et al., 2010).

However, in the cohort of 16 Parkinsonian patients followed up in such long-term study (Fasano et al., 2010), the analysis of individual raw scores (adjusted for age and educational level) showed that at 8-year follow-up on the immediate recall subtest of the Rey's Auditory Verbal Learning Test only 3 out of 16 Parkinsonian patients (18.7%) performed below the normal range and 1 out of 16 patients (6.2%) scored around the cut-off score discriminating between normal and pathological performance, while 12 out of 16 patients (75%) performed in the normal range.

In the same cohort, on the delayed recall subtest of the Rey's Auditory Verbal Learning Test, only 3 out of 16 Parkinsonian patients (18.7%) at 8-year follow-up performed below the normal range, while 13 out of 16 Parkinsonian patients (81.2%) performed in the normal range (Fasano et al., 2010).

These latter individual data suggest that in selected cohorts of Parkinsonian patients treated by deep brain stimulation of the subthalamic nucleus the statistically significant decline on episodic verbal memory tasks observed as a group effect is associated with a large interindividual variability and might be not remarkable in some individual Parkinsonian patients.

A statistically significant but slight decline on a task of abstract reasoning (Raven's Progressive Matrices '47) was reported in neuropsychological studies in the same cohort of Parkinsonian patients treated by deep brain stimulation of the subthalamic nucleus, which were assessed 5 years (Contarino et al., 2007) and 8 years after surgery (Fasano et al., 2010).

However, at 5-year follow-up the analysis of individual raw scores (adjusted for age and educational level) obtained by 11 individual Parkinsonian patients showed that on such task of abstract reasoning (Raven's Progressive Matrices '47) only 2 out of 11 Parkinsonian patients performed slightly below the normal range, while the remaining 9 patients performed in the normal range (Contarino et al., 2007).

Similarly, at 8-year follow-up the analysis of the raw scores (adjusted for age and educational level) obtained by 16 individual Parkinsonian patients on Raven's Progressive Matrices '47 showed that only 1 out of 16 patients scored around the cut-off score, while the remaining 15 patients performed in the normal range (Fasano et al., 2010).

These individual data suggest that in selected cohorts of Parkinsonian patients treated by deep brain stimulation of the subthalamic nucleus the statistically significant decline on tasks of abstract reasoning observed as a group effect at long-term follow-up might be not remarkable in individual Parkinsonian patients.

### 2.3 Performance of Parkinsonian patients treated by deep brain stimulation of the subthalamic nucleus on tasks assessing cognitive functions mediated by the frontal lobes

In patients with Parkinson's disease treated by deep brain stimulation of the subthalamic nucleus, different effects have been described on neuropsychological tasks assessing distinct cognitive functions mediated by the frontal lobes.

On one hand, various studies reported after subthalamic implants an impaired performance on frontal tasks assessing response inhibition, such as the interference subtest of the Stroop test (Jahanshahi et al., 2000; Schroeder et al., 2002; Witt et al., 2004), in ON-stimulation condition as compared to the OFF-stimulation condition.

A positron emission tomography study showed that such impaired performance on the interference subtest of the Stroop test in the on-stimulation condition was associated with decreased activation in both the right anterior cingulate cortex and the right ventral striatum (Schroeder et al., 2002).

In a previously mentioned randomized multicentre study (Witt et al. , 2008) carried out in 123 Parkinsonian patients who were randomly assigned to receive deep brain stimulation of the subthalamic nucleus (n =60) or to have best medical treatment (n=63), as compared to the best medical treatment group the group of patients treated by deep brain stimulation showed 6 months after surgery a significantly greater decline on several variables of the Stroop test. This finding might be accounted for by a dysfunction of neural circuits involving the basal ganglia and the frontal lobes, which might play a critical role in response selection (Witt et al., 2008) and response inhibition.

On the other hand, in patients with Parkinson's disease treated by deep brain stimulation of the subthalamic nucleus an improved postoperative performance has been reported in early phases of follow-up (6 six months after surgery) up to 26 months on neuropsychological frontal tasks assessing cognitive flexibility, such as the Modified Wisconsin Card Sorting Test (Jahanshahi et al., 2000; Daniele et al., 2003) and tasks of random number generation (Witt et al., 2004).

In a neuropsychological study carried out in 20 Parkinsonian patients who underwent bilateral deep brain stimulation of the subthalamic nucleus (Daniele et al., 2003), patients were tested 3 months after surgery with stimulators switched off, while 6 and 12 months after surgery they were tested with stimulators switched on. In this study, an improved performance on a task of cognitive flexibility (Modified Wisconsin Card Sorting Test) was detected 6 and 12 months after surgery, when stimulators were switched on. It was hypothesised that such improved performance on the Modified Wisconsin Card Sorting Test could arise either from a genuine improvement of a specific frontal executive function such as cognitive flexibility (i.e. set-shifting ability) due to subthalamic implants or, alternatively, from a practice effect resulting from the repeated administration of the same cognitive task over time (Daniele et al., 2003).

In a study carried out in 23 Parkinsonian patients who underwent bilateral deep brain stimulation of the subthalamic nucleus and were tested 6 to 12 months after surgery with stimulators switched on or off in random order (Witt et al., 2004), in the ON-stimulation condition there was a poorer performance on a task of response inhibition (interference subtest of the Stroop test) and an improved performance on a task of cognitive flexibility (random number generation), as compared to the OFF-stimulation condition.

These findings are at least partially consistent with the results of a preliminary study carried out in 7 Parkinsonian patients treated by bilateral deep brain stimulation of the subthalamic nucleus (Jahanshahi et al., 2000), who were tested at variable intervals after surgery (4 to 26 months after surgery, with a mean of 11.7 months) with stimulators switched ON or OFF in random order. In this latter study, in the ON-stimulation condition there was a better performance on tasks of cognitive flexibility (random number generation, Modified Wisconsin Card Sorting Test), as compared to the OFF-stimulation condition.

On the whole, these studies suggest that stimulation of the subthalamic nucleus might have different effects on distinct neural circuits involving the basal ganglia and the frontal lobes, resulting in a potential improvement of performance on neuropsychological tasks assessing cognitive flexibility (set-shifting ability) and a potential impairment of performance on neuropsychological tasks assessing response inhibition.

As to studies with long-term follow-up, a statistically significant but slight decline on a task of cognitive flexibility (number of correct criteria discovered on the Modified Wisconsin Card Sorting Test) was detected 8 years after subthalamic implants, as compared to preoperative baseline (Fasano et al., 2010). In this study, as to the number of correct criteria on the Modified Wisconsin Card Sorting Test, the analysis of individual raw scores of a cohort of 15 Parkinsonian patients showed that at 8-year postoperative follow-up 6 out of 15 patients (40%) performed below the normal range, while the remaining 9 patients (60%) performed in the normal range (Fasano et al., 2010).

Eight years after surgery, Parkinsonian patients with a worsening of postoperative performance (increased number of total errors as compared to baseline) on the Modified Wisconsin Card Sorting Test showed significantly higher scores on items assessing postural stability (namely, a poorer postural stability), as compared to patients in which postoperative performance on the Modified Wisconsin Card Sorting Test (number of total errors as compared to baseline) was improved or unchanged (Fasano et al., 2010).

As to decision-making processes, in which the subthalamic nucleus and prefrontal cortical areas might play a critical role, some studies reported after deep brain stimulation of the subthalamic nucleus (Frank et al., 2007) a reduced ability of Parkinsonian patients to slow down their decisions in high-conflict conditions (namely, an increased impulsivity), while other studies detected an improved performance on tasks of reward-based decision learning (VanWouve et al, 2011).

### 2.4 Long-term cognitive follow-up in patients treated by deep brain stimulation of the subthalamic nucleus

To summarise the results of the previously mentioned study which assessed motor and cognitive outcome in Parkinsonian patients 8 years after subthalamic implants (Fasano et al., 2010), this investigation reported a statistically significant decline on a phonological verbal fluency task and a statistically significant but slight decline on tasks of abstract reasoning (Raven's Progressive Matrices '47), episodic verbal memory (immediate and delayed recall of the Rey's Auditory Verbal Learning Test), executive functioning (number of correct criteria on the Modified Wisconsin Card Sorting Test).

### 2.5 Prevalence of dementia in patients treated by deep brain stimulation of the subthalamic nucleus

In studies implementing strict selection criteria in recruiting Parkinsonian patients for deep brain stimulation of the subthalamic nucleus, the prevalence of dementia was relatively low, even at long-term follow-up (Krack et al., 2003; Fasano et al., 2010).

In a 5-year follow-up study, the prevalence of dementia was 6%, as 3 out of 49 patients developed dementia 5 years after surgery (Krack et al., 2003).

In the cohort of Parkinsonian patients with 8-year follow-up mentioned above (Fasano et al., 2010), there was a 5% prevalence of dementia. In this latter study, 5 years after surgery only one out of 20 patients developed dementia, which had progressed at 8 years (Fasano et al., 2010). Such prevalence rates are lower than those reported in other studies investigating less strictly selected Parkinsonian patients, such as one study reporting in Parkinsonian patients a 38% prevalence of dementia after 10 years of follow-up (Hughes et al., 2000).

However, in one 3-year follow-up study carried out in 57 Parkinsonian patients treated by deep brain stimulation of the subthalamic nucleus (Aybek at al., 2007), dementia appeared in 5 out of 57 patients (8.7%) 6 months post surgery and in 24.5% of the patients 3 years post surgery, while the rest of the cohort remained cognitively stable over the whole follow-up. These Authors pointed out that in their cohort the prevalence of dementia over 3 years after deep brain stimulation of the subthalamic nucleus is similar to the prevalence reported in medically treated patients (Aybek at al., 2007). Moreover, in this cohort of patients treated by deep brain stimulation of the subthalamic nucleus some demographic and clinical variables (older age, presence of hallucinations, poorer performance on executive tasks) were preoperative risk factors of developing dementia (Aybek at al., 2007).

The observation of a relatively high prevalence (8.7%) of dementia 6 months post surgery may suggest the hypothesis that less strict selection criteria were employed in this study (Aybek at al., 2007), as compared with other studies with long-term follow-up reporting a lower incidence of dementia (Krack et al., 2003; Fasano et al., 2010).

### 2.6 Conclusive remarks on the effects deep brain stimulation of the subthalamic nucleus on cognition

Most neuropsychological studies in Parkinsonian patients treated by deep brain stimulation of the subthalamic nucleus share a methodological limitation, namely the lack of a control group of medically-treated Parkinsonian patients, which should be matched at baseline to patients who undergo deep brain stimulation of the subthalamic nucleus as to various clinical and demographic variables (age, educational level, overall cognitive status, severity of motor impairment).

Comparisons between Parkinsonian patients treated by deep brain stimulation of the subthalamic nucleus and medically treated Parkinsonian patients may allow to take into account cognitive decline due to aging and disease progression, particularly in patients with long-term follow-up.

However, in most studies which recruited a control group of medically-treated Parkinsonian patients the follow-up was relatively short, with follow-up periods of 6 months (Witt et al., 2008), 1 year (Castelli et al., 2010), 2 years (Williams et al., 2011) and 3 years (Zangaglia et al., 2009). Studies recruiting a control group of medically-treated Parkinsonian patients with a longer follow-up period are currently needed.

Only some neuropsychological investigations have attempted to discriminate between the effects on cognitive performance of the surgical intervention and the effects on cognitive performance of deep brain stimulation of the subthalamic nucleus itself (Jahanshahi et al., 2000; Pillon et al., 2000; Daniele et al., 2003), by comparing cognitive performance on neuropsychological tasks in different stimulation condition, namely with stimulators turned "ON" versus with stimulators turned "OFF".

In one study (Jahanshahi et al., 2000), performance on neuropsychological tasks of executive functions was investigated in 7 patients with Parkinson's disease treated by deep brain stimulation of the subthalamic nucleus and 6 patients treated by deep brain stimulation of the internal globus pallidus. Patients were assessed three times: with stimulators OFF, with stimulators ON, with stimulators OFF gain. With stimulators ON, in both groups of patients (Jahanshahi et al., 2000) there was a decline in a conditional associative learning task and an improved performance on several tasks assessing executive functions (Trail Making test part A and B, missing digit test, paced visual serial addition test, colour naming subtest of the Stroop Test). Moreover, with stimulators ON, only the subthalamic group showed a significant improvement on some additional tasks assessing executive functions (random number generation, Modified Wisconsin Card Sorting Test).

In another study (Pillon et al., 2000), cognitive performance of Parkinsonian patients treated by deep brain stimulation of either the subthalamic nucleus or the internal globus pallidus was assessed postoperatively at 3 months and 12 months, in different stimulation conditions. In this study, the group of patients treated by subthalamic implants showed in ON-stimulation condition an improved cognitive performance on neuropsychological tasks of psychomotor speed and spatial working memory (Pillon et al., 2000).

In patients with Parkinson's disease, the investigation of the effects on cognition of deep brain stimulation of the subthalamic nucleus as compared to the internal globus pallidus is of remarkable importance, in order to establish the potential beneficial and detrimental effects of both procedures.

In patients with Parkinson's disease who were treated by unilateral (Vingerhoets et al., 1999) or bilateral (Field et al., 1999) deep brain stimulation of the internal globus pallidus, preliminary short-term studies with a 3-month follow-up did not detect significant postoperative changes in cognitive performance.

By contrast, some investigations detected a mild decline on tasks of semantic verbal fluency (Volkmann et al., 2004) or executive dysfunction (Dujardin et al., 2000) in patients treated by bilateral deep brain stimulation of the internal globus pallidus and a mild decline on visuoconstructional tasks and on tasks of semantic verbal fluency in patients who underwent unilateral deep brain stimulation of the internal globus pallidus (Tröster et al., 1997).

A prospective randomized trial assessed cognition and mood in 23 patients treated by unilateral deep brain stimulation of the internal globus pallidus, as compared to 22 patients treated by unilateral deep brain stimulation of the subthalamic nucleus (Okun et al., 2009).

In this study, a significantly greater decline on a task of phonological verbal fluency was detected 7 months after surgery in the group who underwent subthalamic implants, as compared to the group treated by deep brain stimulation of the internal globus pallidus.

Moreover, in a multicenter long-term study carried out in 35 Parkinsonian patients treated by bilateral deep brain stimulation of the subthalamic nucleus and in 16 patients treated by bilateral deep brain stimulation of the internal globus pallidus (Moro et al., 2010), 5 to 6 years after surgery the occurrence of cognitive decline was higher in the group with subthalamic implants (23% of patients), as compared to the group with implants in the internal globus pallidus (12% of the patients).

In conclusion, although cognitive morbidity after deep brain stimulation of the subthalamic nucleus is relatively low, deep brain stimulation of the internal globus pallidus seems to have even a lower cognitive morbidity and might be a safer option in Parkinsonian patients who are more at risk for cognitive impairment.

## 3. Effects of deep brain stimulation of the subthalamic nucleus on behavioural symptoms

In Parkinsonian patients treated by deep brain stimulation of the subthalamic nucleus, both transient behavioural symptoms (apathy, manic symptoms, hypersexuality) and persistent behavioural symptoms (apathy, impulse control disorders, punding, depression with increased suicidal tendencies in some patients) have been described. On the other hand, some studies reported in Parkinsonian patients treated by subthalamic implants a postoperative improvement of behavioural symptoms (depression, anxiety, hallucinations, impulse control disorders).

### 3.1 Effects of deep brain stimulation of the subthalamic nucleus on mood

#### 3.1.1 Depressive symptoms: Clinical presentation, evolution, and pathophysiology

After implants for deep brain stimulation of the subthalamic nucleus, some studies detected a postoperative improvement of depression (Daniele et al., 2003; Houeto et al., 2006; Kalteis et al., 2006) or no change in depressive symptoms (Drapier et al., 2006; York et al., 2008), while other studies reported the appearance or the worsening of depressive symptoms (Takeshita et al. 2005, Castelli et al., 2006; Temel et al. 2006).

In patients with Parkinson's disease treated by deep brain stimulation of the subthalamic nucleus, the proportion of subjects in which depressive symptoms appear or worsen after surgery as a persistent behavioural change varies between 2% up to 33%, according to different studies (Takeshita et al., 2005, Temel et al., 2006). Such appearance or worsening of depressive symptoms may be detected also in Parkinsonian patients who show a satisfactory postoperative improvement of motor symptoms.

A previously mentioned long-term follow-up study in 20 consecutive Parkinsonian patients who received by deep brain stimulation of the subthalamic nucleus (Fasano et al., 2010) did not detect any significant postoperative change on scales assessing depression 8 years after surgery, as compared with preoperative baseline.

In a previously mentioned prospective randomized study aimed at comparing mood in 22 patients treated by unilateral deep brain stimulation of the subthalamic nucleus and 23 patients treated by unilateral deep brain stimulation of the internal globus pallidus, 7 months after surgery changes in mood did not significantly differ between the two groups of patients (Okun et al., 2009).

In those Parkinsonian patients who show a postoperative improvement of depressive symptoms, such improvement has been interpreted as resulting either from a psychological response to the amelioration of Parkinsonian motor symptoms (Jahanshahi et al., 2000) or to the effects of deep brain stimulation of the subthalamic nucleus on neural systems which play a role in mood (Romito et al., 2002).

It has been hypothesized that in Parkinsonian patients treated with subthalamic implants postoperative depression might result either from the reduction of daily doses of dopaminergic drugs (Giovannoni et al, 2000) or from an indirect inhibition of the activity of serotonergic neurons in the dorsal raphe nuclei induced by deep brain stimulation of the subthalamic nucleus (Temel et al., 2007), possibly through various structures (ventral pallidum, substantia nigra pars reticulata, medial prefrontal cortex) which directly project to dorsal raphe nuclei (Tan et al., 2001).

### 3.1.2 Depressive symptoms: Treatment and prognosis

After deep brain stimulation of the subthalamic nucleus, suicidal tendencies have been reported in some Parkinsonian patients (Soulas et al., 2008; Voon et al., 2008).

In a retrospective survey carried out in 5311 Parkinsonian patients treated with subthalamic implants (Voon et al., 2008) the rate of completed suicide was 0.45%, while the rate of attempted suicide was 0.90%. In this study, an increased risk of attempted suicide was associated with a number of factors (postoperative depression, previous history of impulse control disorders or compulsive medication use, being single) and the highest rate of suicides was detected in the first postoperative year.

In another retrospective survey carried out in a smaller sample (n = 200) of Parkinsonian patients who underwent subthalamic implants (Soulas et al., 2008), despite a remarkable motor improvement, there was a higher than expected frequency of suicide (1% of completed suicide, 2% of attempted suicide) and suicidal behaviour was associated with postoperative depression and altered impulse control.

These latter studies (Soulas et al., 2008; Voon et al., 2008) show that there might be an increased risk of suicidal behaviour in Parkinsonian patients treated with subthalamic implants, suggesting that the main risk factor for attempted and completed suicide is postsurgical depression, which on postoperative follow-up should be adequately diagnosed and treated with anti-depressant drugs.

### 3.1.3 Manic symptoms: Clinical presentation, evolution, and pathophysiology

A systematic review of a large sample (n = 1398) of Parkinsonian patients who underwent bilateral brain stimulation of the subthalamic nucleus showed that the occurrence of manic symptoms was reported in about 4% of PD patients (Temel et al., 2006), more frequently early after surgery (Romito et al., 2002; Schupbach et al., 2005; Visser-Vandewalle et al., 2005; Contarino et al., 2007).

Manic symptoms in patients treated by subthalamic implants mostly last few hours or few days and are usually observed after stimulation of contacts in the ventral part of the substantia nigra, probably in the substantia nigra pars reticulata (Ulla et al., 2006; Ulla et al., 2011).

In some patients, however, manic symptoms might be induced by stimulation of contacts within the subthalamic nucleus (Ulla et al., 2011; Mallet et al., 2007), especially by stimulation of a ventral contact of the electrode within the subthalamic nucleus. In these cases, manic symptoms may disappear by switching off this ventral contact (Mallet et al. 2007). It has been also suggested that stimulation of axons projecting from medial (limbic) subthalamic nucleus to the medial forebrain bundle might give rise to transient reversible hypomania (Coenen et al., 2009).

In Parkinsonian patients who show stimulation-induced manic symptoms after subthalamic implants (Ulla et al., 2011), positron emission tomography showed during the manic state an increase of regional cerebral blood flow in various structures (anterior cingulate cortex, the medial prefrontal cortex, primary motor cortex, globus pallidus), mainly in the right cerebral hemisphere.

These findings support the hypothesis that a dysfunction of limbic structures (particularly, the anterior cingulate cortex and the medial prefrontal cortex) in the right cerebral hemisphere, induced by stimulation of the substantia nigra or the subthalamic nucleus, might play a critical role in the pathophysiology of manic states induced by subthalamic implants in Parkinsonian patients.

#### 3.1.4 Manic symptoms: Treatment and prognosis

In Parkinsonian patients, manic symptoms may disappear after switching to other targets to be stimulated (Raucher-Chene et al., 2008) or readjusting the parameters of stimulation (Mandat et al., 2006).

### 3.2 Effects of deep brain stimulation of the subthalamic nucleus on apathy

#### 3.2.1 Apathy: Clinical presentation, evolution, and pathophysiology

Apathy, which may be defined as loss of motivation (Marin, 1991), is a common behavioural symptom in patients with Parkinson's disease.

Most studies assessing apathy before and after surgery in Parkinsonian patients treated by subthalamic implants found a postoperative worsening of apathy (Funkiewiez et al., 2004; Schupbach et al., 2005; Drapier et al., 2006; Contarino et al., 2007; Le Jeune et al., 2009; Porat et al., 2009; Thobois et al., 2010), while two studies found no postoperative change in apathy (Castelli et al., 2006; Castelli et al., 2007). By contrast, in Parkinsonian patients who underwent bilateral deep brain stimulation of the subthalamic nucleus a transient improvement of apathy was detected after acute subthalamic stimulation, namely in ON stimulation as compared to OFF stimulation condition (Czernecki et al., 2005). To our knowledge, no study reported in Parkinsonian patients a significant improvement of chronic apathy following subthalamic implants.

It has been reported that after subthalamic implants a postoperative worsening of apathy may occur in the absence of significant postoperative changes of depression or anxiety (Drapier et al., 2006).

In a recent study (Kirsh-Darrow et al., 2011), apathy was assessed in Parkinsonian patients who underwent either unilateral deep brain stimulation of the internal globus pallidus (n = 15) or unilateral deep brain stimulation of the subthalamic nucleus (n = 33) and in a control group of medically treated Parkinsonian patients (n = 48). The results of this study show that apathy progressively increased up to 6 months after both subthalamic and pallidal unilateral implants, while it was unchanged in the non-surgical group of Parkinsonian patients (Kirsh-Darrow et al., 2011). In this study, the degree of apathy in patients who underwent deep brain stimulation was not related to postsurgical changes in levodopa equivalent daily doses (Kirsh-Darrow et al., 2011).

In a prospective study focused on the occurrence of apathy and associated symptoms in 63 patients with Parkinson's disease treated with deep brain stimulation of the subthalamic nucleus (Thobois et al., 2010), apathy appeared in 34 patients after a mean of 4.7 months and was reversible in 17 patients by the 12-month follow-up.

In this study, [11C]-raclopride positron emission tomography showed that binding values were greater in apathetic Parkinsonian patients in various structures (orbitofrontal, dorsolateral prefrontal, posterior cingulate and temporal cortices, left striatum and right amygdala) bilaterally, suggesting a greater dopamine D2/D3 receptor density or reduced synaptic dopamine level in such structures.

### 3.2.2 Apathy: Treatment and prognosis

The effects of a 6-week treatment with the dopamine D2-D3 agonist ropinirole was investigated in 8 Parkinsonian patients who developed apathy after complete withdrawal from dopaminergic medication, following successful subthalamic implants (Czernecki et al., 2008). In 7 out of 8 Parkinsonian patients (in which the stimulation contacts were located within the subthalamic nucleus), ropinirole induced an improvement of apathy, while only one patient (in whom the stimulation contacts were located within the zona incerta) remained apathetic. This study suggests that in Parkinsonian patients treated by subthalamic implants apathy may result from a dopaminergic deficiency in associative limbic areas and can be effectively treated in most patients by dopaminergic agonists administered postoperatively (Czernecki et al., 2008).

## 3.3 Effects of deep brain stimulation of the subthalamic nucleus on anxiety

### 3.3.1 Anxiety: Clinical presentation, evolution, and pathophysiology

After subthalamic implants, a number of studies showed in Parkinsonian patients a postoperative improvement of anxiety (Daniele et al., 2003; Houeto et al., 2006; Kalteis et al., 2006; Schupbach et al., 2007) or no change in anxiety symptoms (Drapier et al. , 2006; York et al., 2008), while other studies reported the appearance or the worsening of anxiety (Rodriguez-Oroz et al. 2005; Castelli et al., 2006).

The postoperative improvement of anxiety observed in some studies might result from the beneficial effects of subthalamic implants on the motor symptoms of Parkinson'disease (Daniele et al., 2003).

On the other hand, in Parkinsonian patients treated by subthalamic implants, in which a marked reduction of daily doses of dopaminergic drugs is usually obtained postoperatively, it has been hypothesized that a postoperative worsening of anxiety might result from a delayed dopamine withdrawal syndrome (Thobois et al., 2010).

In Parkinsonian patients, individual differences in both dopaminergic treatment and in the extent of denervation of dopaminergic mesolimbic systems might explain the variable effects of deep brain stimulation of the subthalamic nucleus on anxiety, mood and motivation/apathy (Thobois et al., 2010).

### 3.3.2 Anxiety: Treatment and prognosis

So far, the issue of treatment of anxiety symptoms in Parkinsonian patients who undergo subthalamic implants has been poorly investigated.

In a study with a 6-month follow-up period in which patients were randomly assigned to have subthalamic implants (n = 63) or the best medical treatment for Parkinson's disease (n = 60), anxiety was reduced in the subthalamic implant group, as compared with the medically-treated group (Witt et al., 2008). In a long-term follow-up study in 20 Parkinsonian patients who received subthalamic implants, 8 years after surgery no significant change was observed on a scale assessing anxiety, as compared with baseline (Fasano et al., 2010).

## 3.4 Effects of deep brain stimulation of the subthalamic nucleus on psychotic symptoms

### 3.4.1 Psychotic symptoms: Clinical presentation, evolution, and pathophysiology

In Parkinsonian patients treated by bilateral subthalamic implants, hallucinations and delusions may appear as transient behavioural symptoms shortly after surgery (Romito et al., 2002).

It is still matter of debate whether Parkinsonian patients with history of hallucination may be good candidates for subthalamic implants.

A retrospective review of 10 Parkinsonian patients who suffered from severe medication-induced hallucinations or delusions and underwent bilateral subthalamic implants (Umemura et al., 2011) showed that such psychotic symptoms disappeared in 8 out of 10 patients after postoperative reduction of dopaminergic medication. By contrast, in 2 out of 10 patients hallucinations and delusions worsened immediately after surgery (despite complete withdrawal of dopaminergic medication), but disappeared after treatment with anti-psychotic drugs for some months (Umemura et al., 2011). On the whole, such retrospective review suggests that deep brain stimulation of the subthalamic nucleus is a good treatment option in Parkinsonian patients with medication-induced hallucinations or delusions, provided that the possible worsening of psychotic symptoms which may be observed in a subgroup of patients is carefully monitored and treated.

In a further study aimed at assessing the effects of subthalamic implants on preexisting hallucinations in 18 patients with advanced Parkinson's disease (Yoshida et al., 2009), six months after the implant there was a significant postoperative improvement of severity of hallucinations, as compared with baseline.

These latter studies (Umemura et al., 2011; Yoshida et al., 2009) suggest that in patients with advanced Parkinson's disease a history of hallucinations is not a contraindication to subthalamic implants.

In conclusion, it might be hypothesized that in most Parkinsonian patients with medication-induced hallucinations a postoperative reduction of dopaminergic anti-Parkinsonian drugs might play a critical role in the postoperative improvement of hallucinations.

### 3.4.2 Psychotic symptoms: Treatment and prognosis

As mentioned above, treatment with anti-psychotic drugs is indicated in Parkinsonian patients in whom hallucinations and delusions worsen immediately after surgery (Umemura et al., 2011). In a group of Parkinsonian patients followed up for 3 years after deep brain stimulation of the subthalamic nucleus, the use of antipsychotic drugs was stable until 1 year, while there was a subsequent increase in the use of antipsychotic drugs at 3 years (Zibetti et al., 2009).

## 3.5 Effects of deep brain stimulation of the subthalamic nucleus on impulse control disorders

### 3.5.1 Impulse control disorders: Clinical presentation, evolution, and pathophysiology

In Parkinsonian patients treated by deep brain stimulation of the subthalamic nucleus, impulse control disorders (pathological gambling, hypersexuality, compulsive eating and buying/shopping) may occasionally appear after surgery, while in most cases preexisting impulse control disorders may improve or disappear after subthalamic implants (Broen et al., 2011; Witjas et al., 2005; Bandini et al., 2007; Ardouin et al., 2006; Lim et al., 2009).

As to pathological gambling (Lim et al., 2009) and hypersexuality (Doshi & Bargava, 2008), these disorders may be occasionally be observed in some Parkinsonian patients after subthalamic implants, while Parkinsonian patients may rarely develop compulsive eating after subthalamic implants (Zahodne et al., 2011). A weight gain, which may result from multiple pathogenic factors besides compulsive eating, may be detected in up 48% of Parkinsonian patients after deep brain stimulation of the subthalamic nucleus (Piboolnurak et al., 2007).

In Parkinsonian patients who show a postoperative improvement of preexisting impulse control disorders, such improvement might be due to at least two mechanisms. The most plausible mechanism is a reduction of dopaminergic medication after the subthalamic implants, which leads to decreased stimulation of mesolimbic dopaminergic circuits (Ardouin et al., 2006). Alternatively, it has been proposed that deep brain stimulation of the subthalamic nucleus may induce inhibitory effects on dopaminergic and serotoninergic pathways ascending to limbic circuits involved in reward (Witjas et al., 2005).

On the other hand, in some Parkinsonian patients, impulse control disorders appear after subthalamic implants, notwithstanding with a postoperative reduction of doses of dopaminergic drugs (Romito et al., 2002; Doshi and Bargava, 2008; Smeding et al., 2007; Sensi et al., 2004; Lim et al., 2009). In these latter patients, it might be hypothesised that deep brain stimulation of the subthalamic nucleus may induce changes in the activity of limbic circuits involving the subthalamic nucleus or involving fibres adjacent to this nucleus, giving rise to a tendency to impulsivity (Demetriades et al, 2011). A neurophysiological study aimed at recording local field potentials in the subthalamic nucleus of Parkinsonian patients patients treated by deep brain stimulation of the subthalamic nucleus (Rodriguez-Oroz et al., 2011) showed an oscillatory theta-alpha activity in the ventral subthalamic nucleus, which was associated with impulse control disorders, suggesting that such limbic ventral subthalamic area might be involved in the development of impulse control disorders in these Parkinsonian patients.

It has been previously mentioned that the subthalamic nucleus and prefrontal cortical areas might play a critical role in decision-making processes and that patients with Parkinson's disease may show after deep brain stimulation of the subthalamic nucleus a reduced ability to slow down their decisions in high-conflict conditions, resulting in increased impulsivity (Frank et al., 2007).

### 3.5.2 Impulse control disorders: Treatment and prognosis

In a cross-sectional study aimed at comparing Parkinsonian patients treated by subthalamic implants versus Parkinsonian patients treated by anti-Parkinsonian drugs but eligible for deep brain stimulation (Halbig et al. , 2009), impulsivity was assessed by the Barratt Impulsiveness Scale and was higher in patients with subthalamic implants. In this study, the prevalence of impulse control disorders was higher (3 out of 16 subjects, namely 19%) in patients treated by subthalamic implants than in medically treated Parkinsonian patients (3 out of 37 subjects, namely 8%). The Authors suggest that screening for impulsivity and impulse control disorders should be performed prior to deep brain stimulation (Halbig et al. , 2009).

In conclusion, since the effects of brain stimulation of the subthalamic nucleus on impulse control disorders in Parkinsonian patients are variable, the prognosis of such disorders may vary from patient to patient, although in most Parkinsonian patients preexisting impulse control disorders may improve or disappear after subthalamic implants. Further studies are needed in order to clarify the issue of treatment strategies in those patients in whom impulse control disorders do appear or worsen after surgery.

## 3.6 Long-term behavioural follow-up in patients treated by deep brain stimulation of the subthalamic nucleus

In the previously mentioned study assessing motor and cognitive outcome in patients with Parkinson's disease 8 years after subthalamic implants (Fasano et al., 2010), in the overall group of patients there was no significant change 8 years after surgery on behavioural scales assessing depression and anxiety, as compared to preoperative baseline. In the cohort of 20 Parkinsonian patients who completed the 8-year follow-up (Fasano et al., 2010), a number of persistent behavioral adverse events were reported, such as depressive symptoms (in 25% of the patients), apathy (in 20% of the patients), psychotic symptoms (in 20% of the patients), hypersexuality (in 5% of the patients).

## 3.7 An explicative case of a Parkinsonian patient with manic symptoms after bilateral subthalamic implants

A 52-year-old right-handed man presented a 11-year history of severe rigid–akinetic Parkinson's disease, which became poorly responsive to anti-Parkinsonian medication (Romito et al., 2002). This patient, who had a family history of major depression, at the age of 26 years suffered from a major depressive episode, during his father's terminal illness.

The patient received a implant of quadripolar leads bilaterally in the subthalamic nucleus under stereotactic guidance. Compared to preoperative assessment, he showed a marked improvement of Parkinsonian motor symptoms and activities of daily living, while wearing-off phenomena and on-state dyskinesias (reported before the implantation) disappeared.

Two days after the implant, the patient developed a manic syndrome (Romito et al., 2002), characterized by inflated self-esteem and grandiosity, marked increase in goal-directed activities, need to purchase unneeded items, decreased need for sleep, planning of hazardous business investments, flights of ideas. His appetite decreased and the patient lost 5 to 6 kg. Sexual desire and sexual activity increased and the patient had frequent spontaneous erections, although he was not on dopamine agonists. Despite a lack of interest in religion, he started to spend much time in writing poems on religious themes. Moreover, the patient became irritable, litigious, and over-reactive. A diagnosis of manic episode was made.

When the stimulator was turned off, there was a rapid worsening of Parkinsonian motor symptoms but manic symptoms did not improve (Romito et al., 2002).

In this patient, all antiparkinsonian medication was discontinued 1 month after surgery. Stimulation settings remained unchanged from the second month on. During postoperative follow-up up to 12 months after surgery, he showed no significant change in cognitive performance on neuropsychological tasks, as compared to preoperative performance.

In agreement with his wife, the patient was followed up very carefully, but no pharmacological treatment for manic symptoms was prescribed. Three months after their onset, manic symptoms gradually decreased and then disappeared completely. Twelve months after the subthalamic implant, the patient showed a slight reduction of initiative, in the absence of any significant impairment in daily living activities (Romito et al., 2002).

## 4. Conclusions

Cognitive and behavioural disturbances in patients with Parkinson's disease seem to be relatively more frequent after deep brain stimulation of the subthalamic nucleus, as compared with deep brain stimulation of the internal globus pallidus. This finding might be at least partially due to the fact that the subthalamic nucleus is a smaller target, with different neural circuits (motor, associative, and limbic circuits) in close proximity to each other. Thus, electrode misplacements or current spreading to non-motor circuits involving the subthalamic nucleus may give rise to cognitive and behavioural disturbances after subthalamic implants.

On the whole, nonetheless, most studies agree about the view that the cognitive and behavioural morbidity of deep brain stimulation of the subthalamic nucleus in patients with Parkinson's disease can be considered relatively low, even in the long term, provided that appropriate criteria are used to select candidates for neurosurgery,

Further studies are certainly needed to elucidate the pathophysiological mechanisms underlying the postoperative cognitive and behavioural changes which may be observed in Parkinsonian patients treated by deep brain stimulation of the subthalamic nucleus.

## 5. References

Aarsland D., Brønnick K., Alves G. et al. (2009). The spectrum of neuropsychiatric symptoms in patients with early untreated Parkinson's disease. *Journal of Neurology, Neurosurgery and Psychiatry*, Vol.80, pp. 928-930

Alegret M., Junque C., Valldeoriola F. et al. (2001). Effects of bilateral subthalamic stimulation on cognitive function in Parkinson disease. *Archives of Neurology*, Vol.58, pp. 1223–7

Alexander G.E., De Long M.R.& Strick P.L. (1986). Parallel organization of functionally segregated circuits linking basal ganglia and cortex. *Annual Review of Neuroscience*, Vol.9, pp. 357-381

Ambermoon P., Carter A., Hall W. et al. (2011). Compulsive use of dopamine replacement therapy: a model for stimulant drug addiction? *Addiction*. Vol.106, pp. 283-293

Ardouin C., Pillon B., Peiffer E. et al. (1999). Bilateral subthalamic or pallidal stimulationfor Parkinson's disease affects neither memory nor executive functions: a consecutive series of 62 patients. *Annals of Neurology*, Vol.46, pp 217–23

Ardouin C., Voon V., Worbe Y. et al. (2006). Pathological gambling in Parkinson's disease improves on chronic subthalamic nucleus stimulation. *Movement Disorders* Vol.2, No.11, pp. 1941-6

Aybek S., Gronchi-Perrin A., Berney A. et al. (2009). Long-term cognitive profile and incidence of dementia after STN-DBS in Parkinson's disease. *Movement Disorders*, Vol.15, No.22(7), pp. 974-81

Bandini F., Primavera A., Pizzorno M., & Cocito L. (2007). Using STN DBS and medication reduction as a strategy to treat pathological gambling in Parkinson's disease. *Parkinsonism Related Disorders*, Vol.13, No.6, pp. 369-71

Boller F, Passafiume D, Keefe NC et al. (1984). Visuospatial impairment in Parkinson's disease. Role of perceptual and motor factors. *Archives of Neurology*, Vol.41, pp. 485-490

Braak H., Ghebremedhin E., Rub U. et al. (2004). Stages in the development of Parkinson's disease-related pathology. *Cell Tissue Research*, Vol.318, pp. 121-134

Broen M., Duits A., Visser-Vandewalle V. et al. (2011). Impulse control and related disorders in Parkinson's disease patients treated with bilateral subthalamic nucleus stimulation: A review. *Parkinsonism Related Disorders*. Vol.17, No.6, pp. 413-7

Bugalho P., da Silva J.A., Cargaleiro I. et al. (2012, in press). Psychiatric symptoms screening in the early stages of Parkinson's disease. *Journal of Neurology*. DOI 10.1007/s00415-011-6140-8

Burn D.J. (2002). Beyond the Iron mask: towards better recognition and treatment of depression associated with Parkinson's disease. *Movement Disorders*, Vol.17, pp. 445-454

Candy J.M., Perry R.H., Perry E.K. et al. (1983). Pathological changes in the nucleus of Meynert in Alzheimer's and Parkinson's disease. *Journal of Neurological Sciences* Vol.59, pp. 277-289

Cash R., Dennis T., L'Hereux R. et al (1987). Parkinson's disease and dementia: norepinephrine and dopamine in locus coeruleus. *Neurology* Vol.37, pp. 42-46

Castelli L., Perozzo P., Zibetti M. et al. (2006). Chronic deep brain stimulation of the subthalamic nucleus for Parkinson's disease: effects on cognition, mood, anxiety and personality traits.*European Neurology* Vol.55, No.3, pp. 136-144

Castelli L., Lanotte M., Zibetti M. et al. (2007). Apathy and verbal fluency in STN-stimulated PD patients. An observational follow-up study. *Journal of Neurology,* Vol. 254, No.9, pp. 1238-1243

Castelli L., Rizzi L., Zibetti M. et al. (2010). Neuropsychological changes 1-year after subthalamic DBS in PD patients: A prospective controlled study. *Parkinsonism Related Disord*ers, Vol.16, No2, pp. 115-8

Coenen, V.A., Honey C.R., Hurwitz T. et al. (2009). Medial forebrain bundle stimulation as a pathophysiological mechanism for hypomania in subthalamic nucleus deep brain stimulation for Parkinson's disease. *Neurosurgery,* Vol.64, No.6, pp. 1106-1114; discussion 1114-1105

Contarino M. F., Daniele A., Sibilia A.H. et al. (2007). Cognitive outcome 5 years after bilateral chronic stimulation of subthalamic nucleus in patients with Parkinson's disease. *Journal of Neurology, Neurosurgery and Psychiatry,* Vol.78, No.3, pp. 248-252

Cools R., Barker R.A., Sahakian B.J. & Robbins T.W. (2001). Mechanism of cognitive set flexibility in Parkinson's disease. *Brain,* Vol.124, pp. 2503-2512

Cooper J.A., Sagar H.J., Jordan N. et al. (1991). Cognitive impairment in early untreated Parkinson's disease and its relationship to motor disability. *Brain,* Vol.114, pp. 2095-2122

Cubo E., Bernard B., Leurgans S. et al. (2000). Cognitive and motor functions in patients with Parkinson's disease with and without depression. *Clinical Neuropharmacology,* Vol.23, No.6, pp. 331-334

Czernecki V., Pillon B., Houeto J.L. et al. (2005). Does bilateral stimulation of the subthalamic nucleus aggravate apathy in Parkinson's disease?, *Journal of Neurology, Neurosurgery and Psychiatry,* Vol.76, No.6, pp. 775-779

Czernecki V., Schüpbach M., Yaici S. et al. (2008). Apathy following subthalamic stimulation in Parkinson disease: a dopamine responsive symptom. *Movement Disorders,* Vol.23, No.7, pp. 964-969

Daniele A., Albanese A., Contarino M.F. et al. (2003). Cognitive and behavioural effects of chronic stimulation of the subthalamic nucleus in patients with Parkinson's disease. *Journal of Neurology, Neurosurgery and Psychiatry,* Vol.74, pp. 175–82

Demetriades P., Rickards H. & Cavanna A.E. (2011). Impulse control disorders following deep brain stimulation of the subthalamic nucleus in Parkinson's disease: clinical aspects. *Parkinson's disease.* doi:10.4061/2011/658415

Doshi P. & Bhargava P. (2008). Hypersexuality following subthalamic nucleus stimulation for Parkinson's disease. *Neurology India,* Vol.56, No.4, pp. 474-476

Drapier D., Drapier S., Sauleau P. et al. (2006). Does subthalamic nucleus stimulation induce apathy in Parkinson's disease? *Journal of Neurology* Vol.253, No. 8, pp. 1083-1091

Dubois & Pillon (1997). Cognitive deficits in Parkinson's disease. *Journal of Neurology,* Vol.244, pp. 2-8.

Dujardin K., Krystkowiak P., Defebvre L. et al. (2000). A case of severe dysexecutive syndrome consecutive to chronic bilateral pallidal stimulation. *Neuropsychologia.,* Vol. 38, No.9, pp. 1305-15

Dujardin K. Krystkowiak P., Defebvre L. et al (2001). Memory and executive function in sporadic and familial Parkinson's disease. *Brain.* Vol.124(Pt 2), pp. 389-98

Factor S.A., Mohlo E.S., Podskalny G.D. & Brown D. (1995). Parkinson's disease drug-induced psychiatric states. *Advances in Neurology,* Vol. 65, pp. 115-138

Fasano A., Romito L.M., Daniele A. et al. (2010). Motor and cognitive outcome in patients with Parkinson's disease 8 years after subthalamic implants. *Brain,* Vol.133, No.9, pp. 2664-76

Fields J.A., Tröster A.I., Wilkinson S.B. et al. (1999). Cognitive outcome following staged bilateral pallidal stimulation for the treatment of Parkinson's disease. *Clinical Neurology and Neurosurgery,* Vol. 101, No3, pp. 182-8

Frank M.J., Samanta J., Moustafa A.A. et al. (2007). Hold your horses: impulsivity, deep brain stimulation, and medication in parkinsonism. *Science.* Vol. 23, No.318, pp. 1309-12

Funkiewiez A., Ardouin C., Caputo E. et al. (2004). Long term effects of bilateral subthalamic nucleus stimulation on cognitive function, mood, and behaviour in Parkinson's disease. *Journal of Neurology, Neurosurgery and Psychiatry,* Vol.75, pp. 834–9

Giovannoni G., O' Sullivan J.D., Turner K., et al. (2000). Hedonistic homeostatic dysregulation in patients with Parkinson's disease on dopamine replacement therapies. *Journal of Neurology, Neurosurgery and Psychiatry,* Vol.68, No.4, pp. 423-8

Gotham A.M., Brown R.G. & Marsden C.D.(1986). Depression in Parkinson's Disease: a quantitative and qualitative analysis. *Journal of Neurology, Neurosurgery and Psychiatry,* Vol.49, No.4, pp. 381-389

Green J., McDonald W.M., Vitek J.L. et al. (2002). Cognitive impairment in advanced PD without dementia. *Neurology,* Vol. 59, pp. 1320-1324

Hälbig T.D., Tse W., Frisina P.G. et al. (2009). Subthalamic deep brain stimulation and impulse control in Parkinson's disease. *European Journal of Neurology,* Vol.16, No.4, pp. 493-7

Hamani C., Richter E., Schwalb J.M. et al. (2005). Bilateral subthalamic nucleus stimulation for Parkinson's disease: a systematic review of the clinical literature. *Neurosurgery,* Vol.56, No.6, pp.1313-21

Harrington D.L., Haaland K.Y., Yeo R.A. & Marder E. (1990). Procedural memory in Parkinson's disease. Impaired motor but not visuoperceptual learning. *Journal of Clinical and Experimental Neuropsychology,* Vol.12, pp. 223-239

Helkala E.L., Laulumaa V., Soininen H. & Riekkinen P.J. (1988). Recall and recognition memory in patients with Alzheimer's and Parkinson's diseases. *Annals of Neurology,* Vol.24, pp. 214-217

Houeto J.L., Mallet L., Mesnage V. et al. (2006). Subthalamic stimulation in Parkinson disease: behavior and social adaptation. *Archives of Neurology,* Vol.63, No.8, pp. 1090-5

Hoverstadt A., de Jong G.J., Meerwaldt J.D. et al. (1987). Spatial disorientation as an early symptom of Parkinson's disease. *Neurology,* Vol. 37, pp. 485-487

Hughes A.J., Daniel S.E. & Lees A.J. (1993). The clinical features of Parkinson's disease in 100 histologically proven cases. *Advances in Neurology,* Vol.60, pp. 595-9

Hughes T.A., Ross H.F., Musa S. et al. (2000). A 10-year study of the incidence of and factors predicting dementia in Parkinson's disease. *Neurology,* Vol.25, No.54(8), pp. 1596-1602

Jahanshahi M., Ardouin C.M., Brown R.G. et al. (2000). The impact of deep brain stimulation on executive function in Parkinson's disease. *Brain,* Vol.123 ( Pt 6), pp. 1142-54

Kalteis K.H., Standhardt H., Kryspin-Exner I. et al. (2006). Influence of bilateral STN-stimulation on psychiatric symptoms and psychosocial functioning in patients with Parkinson's disease. *Journal of Neural Transmission,* Vol.113, No.9, pp. 1191-1206

Katzen, H., Myerson C., Papapetropoulos S., et al. (2010). Multi-modal hallucinations and cognitive function in Parkinson's disease.*Dementia and Geriatric Cognitive Disorders,* Vol. 30, No.1, pp. 51-56

Kirsch-Darrow L., Zahodne L.B., Marsiske M. et al. (2011). The trajectory of apathy after deep brain stimulation: from pre-surgery to 6 months post-surgery in Parkinson's disease. *Parkinsonism Related Disorders,* Vol.17, No.3, pp. 182-188

Krack P., Batir A., Van Blercom N. et al. (2003). Five-year follow-up of bilateral stimulation of the subthalamic nucleus in advanced Parkinson's disease. *New England Journal of Medicine,* Vol.349, pp. 1925–34

Kulisesky J., Avila A., Barbanoj M. et al. (1996). Acute effects of levodopa on neuropsychological performance in stable and fluctuating Parkinson's disease patients at different levodopa plasma levels. *Brain,* Vol.119, pp. 2121-2132

Leentjens A.F., Dujardin K., Marsh L., et al. (2008). Apathy and anhedonia rating scales in Parkinson's disease: critique and recommendation. *Movement Disorders,* Vol.23, pp. 2004-2014

Le Jeune F., Drapier D., Bourguignon A. et al. (2009). Subthalamic nucleus stimulation in Parkinson disease induces apathy: a PET study. *Neurology,* Vol.73, No.21, pp. 1746-1751

Lim S.Y., O'Sullivan S.S., Kotschet K. et al. (2009). Dopamine dysregulation syndrome, impulse control disorders and punding after deep brain stimulation surgery for Parkinson's disease. *Journal of Clinical Neuroscience,* Vol.16, No.9, pp. 1148-52

Litvan I., Mohr E., Williams J. et al. (1991). Differential memory and executive functions in demented patients with Parkinson's disease and Alzheimer's disease. *Journal of Neurology, Neurosurgery and Psychiatry,* Vol. 54, pp. 25-29

Malapani C., Pillon B., Dubois B. & Agid Y. (1994). Impaired simultaneous cognitive task performance in Parkinson's disease: a dopamine-related dysfunction. *Neurology,* Vol. 44, pp. 319-326

Mallet L., Schüpbach M., N'Diaye K. et al. (2007). Stimulation of subterritories of the subthalamic nucleus reveals its role in the integration of the emotional and motor aspects of behavior. *Proceedings of the National Academy of Sciences of the United States of America,* Vol.104, No25, pp. 10661-10666

Mandat, T. S., Hurwitz T. & Honey C.R. (2006). Hypomania as an adverse effect of subthalamic nucleus stimulation: report of two cases. *Acta Neurochirurgica (Wien),* Vol.148, No.8, pp. 895-897

Marin R.S. (1991). Apathy: a neuropsychiatric syndrome. *Journal of Neuropsychiatry and Clinical Neurosciences.* Vol.3, No.3, pp.243-54

Marsh L. (2000). Neuropsychiatric aspects of Parkinson's disease. *Psychosomatics*, Vol.41, pp. 15-23

Matison R., Mayeux R., Rosen J. & Fahn S.(1982). "Tip-of-the-tongue" phenomenon in Parkinson's disease. *Neurology*, Vol. 32, pp. 567-570.

Mattay V.S., Tessitore A., Callicot J.H. et al. (2002). Dopaminergic modulation of cortical function in patients with Parkinson's disease. *Annals of Neurology* Vol.51, pp. 156-164

Mayberg H.S. & Solomon D.H. (1995). Depression in Parkinson's disease: a biochemical and organic viewpoint. In: *Behavioral neurology of movement disorders*, Weiner WJ, Lang AE (eds ), Advances in Neurology Vol. 65. Raven Press Ltd, New York

Mayeux R., Stern Y., Sano M. et al. (1988). An estimate of the the prevalence of dementia in idiopathic Parkinson's disease. *Archives of Neurology*, Vol.45, pp. 260-262

Menza M., Dobkin R.D., Marin H. et al. (2009). The impact of treatment of depression on quality of life, disability and relapse in patients with Parkinson's disease. *Movement disorders* Vol.24, pp. 1325-1332

Mohr E., Litvan I., Williams J. et al. (1990). Selective deficits in Alzheimer and Parkinsonian dementia: visuospatial function. *Canadian Journal of neurological Sciences*, Vol.17, pp. 292-297

Mohr E., Mendis T. & Grimes J.D. (1995). Late cognitive changes in Parkinson's disease with an emphasis on dementia. In: *Behavioral neurology of movement disorders*, Weiner WJ, Lang AE (eds ), Advances in Neurology Vol. 65. Raven Press Ltd, New York

Moro E., Lozano A.M., Pollak P. et al. (2010). Long-term results of a multicenter study on subthalamic and pallidal stimulation in Parkinson's disease. *Movement Disorders*, Vol.25, No5, pp.578-86

Morris R.G., Downes J.J., Sahakian B.J. et al. (1988). Planning and spatial working memory in Parkinson's disease. *Journal of Neurology, Neurosurgery and Psychiatry*, Vol. 135, pp. 669-675

Okun M.S., Fernandez H.H., Wu S.S. et al. (2009). Cognition and mood in Parkinson's disease in subthalamic nucleus versus globus pallidus interna deep brain stimulation: the COMPARE trial. *Annals of Neurology*, Vol.65, No.5, pp. 586-9

Parsons T.D., Rogers S.A., Braaten A.J. et al. (2006). Cognitive sequelae of subthalamic nucleus deep brain stimulation in Parkinson's disease: a meta-analysis. *Lancet Neurology*, Vol.5, No.7, pp. 578-88

Paulus W. & Jellinger K. (1991). The neuropathologic basis of different clinical subgroups of Parkinson's disease. *Journal of Neuropathology and Experimental Neurology*, Vol.50, pp. 743-755

Pedersen K.F., Larsen J.P., Alves G. et al. (2009). Prevalence and clinical correlates of apathy in Parkinson's disease: a community-based study. *Parkinsonism and Related Disorders*, Vol.15, pp. 295-299

Péran P., Rascol O., Démonet J.F. et al. (2003). Deficit of verb generation in nondemented patients with Parkinson's disease. *Movement Disorders*, Vol.18, No.2, pp. 150-6.

Piboolnurak P., Lang A.E., Lozano A.M. et al. (2007). Levodopa response in long-term bilateral subthalamic stimulation for Parkinson's disease. *Movement Disorders*, Vol.22, No.7, pp. 990-7

Pillon B., Ardouin C., Damier P. et al. (2000). Neuropsychological changes between "off"and "on" STN or GPi stimulation in Parkinson's disease. *Neurology*, Vol. 55, pp. 411-18

Porat O., Cohen O.S., Schwartz R. et al. (2009). Association of preoperative symptom profile with psychiatric symptoms following subthalamic nucleus stimulation in patients with Parkinson's disease. *Journal of Neuropsychiatry and Clinical Neurosciences*, Vol. 21, No.4, pp. 398-405

Ransmayr G., Schmidhuber-Eiler B., Karamat E. et al. (1987). Visuoperception and visuospatial and visuorotational performance in Parkinson's disease. *Journal of Neurology*, Vol. 235, pp. 99-101

Raucher-Chene D., Charrel C. L., de Maindreville A.D. et al. (2008). Manic episode with psychotic symptoms in a patient with Parkinson's disease treated by subthalamic nucleus stimulation: improvement on switching the target. *Journal of Neurological Sciences*, Vol. 273(1-2), pp. 116-117

Robbins T.W., James M., Owen A.M. et al. (1994). Cognitive deficits in progressive sopranuclear palsy. Parkinson's disease and multiple system atrophy in tests sensitive to frontal lobe dysfunction. *Journal of Neurology, Neurosurgery and Psychiatry*, Vol. 57, pp. 79-88

Rodriguez-Oroz M.C., Obeso J.A., Lang A.E. et al. (2005). Bilateral deep brain stimulation in Parkinson's disease: a multicentre study with 4 years follow-up. *Brain*, Vol. 128 (Pt 10), pp. 2240-9

Rodriguez-Oroz M. C., Lopez-Azcarate J., Garcia-Garcia D. et al. (2011). Involvement of the subthalamic nucleus in impulse control disorders associated with Parkinson's disease. *Brain*, Vol.134 (Pt 1), pp. 36-49

Romito L.M., Raja M., Daniele A. et al. (2002). Transient mania with hypersexuality after surgery for high frequency stimulation of the subthalamic nucleus in Parkinson's disease. *Movement Disorders*, Vol. 17, No.6, pp. 1371-4

Saint-Cyr J.A., Trépanier L.L., Kumar R. et al. (2000). Neuropsychological consequences of chronic bilateral stimulation of the subthalamic nucleus in Parkinson's disease. *Brain*, Vol.123 ( Pt 10), pp. 2091-2108

Sanchez-Ramos J.R., Ortoll R. & Paulson G.W. (1996).Visual hallucinations associated with Parkinson's disease. *Archives of Neurology*, Vol.53, pp. 1265-1268

Schroeder U., Kuehler A., Haslinger B. et al. (2002). Subthalamic nucleus stimulation affects striato-anterior cingulate cortex circuit in a response conflict task: a PET study. *Brain*, Vol.125, pp. 1995–2004

Schroeder U., Kuehler A., Lange K.W. et al. (2003). Subthalamic nucleus stimulation affects a frontotemporal network: a PET study. *Annals of Neurology*, Vol.54, pp. 445–50

Schupbach W. M., Chastan N., Welter M.L. et al. (2005). Stimulation of the subthalamic nucleus in Parkinson's disease: a 5 year follow up. *Journal of Neurology, Neurosurgery and Psychiatry*, Vol. 76, No.12, pp. 1640-1644

Schupbach W. M., Maltete D., Houeto J.L. et al. (2007). Neurosurgery at an earlier stage of Parkinson disease: a randomized, controlled trial. *Neurology*, Vol.68, No.4, pp. 267-271

Sensi M., Eleopra R., Cavallo M.A. et al. (2004). Explosive-aggressive behavior related to bilateral subthalamic stimulation. *Parkinsonism and Related Disorders*, Vol.10, No.4, pp. 247-51

Smeding H.M., Goudriaan A.E., Foncke E.M. et al. (2007). Pathological gambling after bilateral subthalamic nucleus stimulation in Parkinson disease. *Journal of Neurology, Neurosurgery and Psychiatry*, Vol. 78, No.5, pp. 517-9

Smeding H.M., Speelman J.D., Huizenga H.M. et al. (2011). Predictors of cognitive and psychosocial outcome after STN DBS in Parkinson's Disease. *Journal of Neurology, Neurosurgery and Psychiatry*, Vol. 82, No.7, pp. 754-60

Soulas T., Gurruchaga J.M., Palfi S. et al. (2008). Attempted and completed suicides after subthalamic nucleus stimulation for Parkinson's disease. *Journal of Neurology, Neurosurgery and Psychiatry*, Vol.79, No.8, pp. 952-954

Takeshita S., Kurisu K., Trop L. et al. (2005). Effect of subthalamic stimulation on mood state in Parkinson's disease: evaluation of previous facts and problems. *Neurosurgery Review, Vol.* 28, No.3, pp. 179-186

Taylor A.E., Saint-Cyr J.A. & Lang A.E. (1986). Frontal lobe dysfunction in Parkinson's disease: evidence for a "frontal lobe syndrome". *Brain and cognition*, Vol. 13, pp. 211-232

Tan, S.K.H., Hartung H., Sharp T., et al. (2011). Serotonin-dependent depression in Parkinson's disease: a role for the subthalamic nucleus? *Neuropharmacology* Vol. 61, No. 3, pp. 387-399

Temel Y., Kessels A., Tan S. et al. (2006). Behavioural changes after bilateral subthalamic stimulation in advanced Parkinson disease: a systematic review. *Parkinsonism Related Disorders* Vol.12, No.5, pp. 265-272

Temel Y., Boothman L.J., Blokland A. et al. (2007). Inhibition of 5-HT neuron activity and induction of depressive-like behavior by high-frequency stimulation of the subthalamic nucleus. *Proceedings of the National Academy of Sciences of the United States of America* , Vol.23, No.104(43), pp. 17087-92

Thobois S., Ardouin C., Lhommée E. et al. (2010). Non-motor dopamine withdrawal syndrome after surgery for Parkinson's disease: predictors and underlying mesolimbic denervation. *Brain*, Vol. 133(Pt 4), pp. 1111-1127

Torack R.M. & Morris J.C. (1988). The association of ventral tegmental area histopathology with adult dementia. *Archives of Neurology*, Vol.45, No.5, pp. 497-501

Trepanier L.L., Kumar R., Lozano A.M. et al. (2000). Neuropsychological outcome of GPi pallidotomy and GPi or STN deep brain stimulation in Parkinson's disease. *Brain and Cognition, Vol.*42, pp. 324–47

Tröster A.I., Fields J.A., Wilkinson S.B. et al. (1997). Unilateral pallidal stimulation for Parkinson's disease: neurobehavioral functioning before and 3 months after electrode implantation. *Neurology*, Vol.49, No.4, pp. 1078-83

Tröster AI, Woods SP & Fields JA (2003). Verbal fluency declines after pallidotomy: an interaction between task and lesion laterality. *Applied Neuropsychology*, Vol.10, pp. 69–75.

Ulla M., Thobois S., Lemaire J.J. et al. (2006). Manic behaviour induced by deep brain stimulation in Parkinson's disease: evidence of substantia nigra implication? *Journal of Neurology, Neurosurgery and Psychiatry*, Vol.77, No.12, pp. 1363-1366

Ulla M., Thobois S. & Llorca P.M. (2011). Contact dependent reproducible hypomania induced by deep brain stimulation in Parkinson's disease: clinical, anatomical and functional imaging study. *Journal of Neurology, Neurosurgery and Psychiatry*, Vol.82, No.6, pp. 607-14

Umemura A., Oka Y., Okita K. et al. (2011). Subthalamic nucleus stimulation for Parkinson disease with severe medication-induced hallucinations or delusions. *Journal of Neurosurgery*, Vol.114, No.6, pp. 1701-5

Valldeoriola F., Nobbe F.A. & Tolosa E. (1997). Treatment of behavioral disturbances in Parkinson's disease. *Journal of Neural Trasmission (Suppl.)* Vol. 51, pp. 175-204

Van Wouwe N.C., Ridderinkhof K.R., van den Wildenberg W.P. et al. (2011). Deep brain stimulation of the subthalamic nucleus improves reward-based decision-learning in Parkinson's disease. *Frontiers in Human Neurosciences*, Vol.4, pp.5-30

Vingerhoets G., van der Linden C. & Lannoo E. (1999). Cognitive outcome after unilateral pallidal stimulation in Parkinson's disease. *Journal of Neurology, Neurosurgery and Psychiatry*, Vol.66, No.3, pp. 297-304

Visser-Vandewalle V., van der Linden C., Temel Y. et al. (2005). Long-term effects of bilateral subthalamic nucleus stimulation in advanced Parkinson disease: a four year follow-up study. *Parkinsonism Related Disorders*, Vol. 11, No.3, pp. 157-165

Volkmann J., Allert N., Voges J. et al. (2004). Long-term results of bilateral pallidal stimulation in Parkinson's disease. *Annals of Neurology*, Vol. 55, No.6, pp. 871-5

Voon V., Krack P., Lang A.E. et al. (2008). A multicentre study on suicide outcomes following subthalamic stimulation for Parkinson's disease. *Brain*, Vol. 131(Pt 10), pp. 2720-2728.

York M.K., Dulay M., Macias A. et al. (2008). Cognitive declines following bilateral subthalamic nucleus deep brain stimulation for the treatment of Parkinson's disease. *Journal of Neurology, Neurosurgery and Psychiatry*. Vol. 79, No.7, pp. 789-95

Yoshida F., Miyagi J., Kishimoto J. et al. (2009). Subthalamic nucleus stimulation does not cause deterioration of preexisting hallucinations in Parkinson's disease patients. *Stereotactic Functional Neurosurgery*, Vol. 87, No.1, pp. 45-49

Weintraub D., Koester J., Potenza M.N. et al. (2010). Impulse control disorders in Parkinson disease: a cross-sectional study of 3090 patients. *Archives of Neurology.*, Vol.67, No.5, pp. 589-95

Williams A.E., Arzola G.M. & Strutt A.M. (2011). Cognitive outcome and reliable change indices two years following bilateral subthalamic nucleus deep brain stimulation. *Parkinsonism Related Disorders.* 2011, Vol.17, No.5, pp. 321-7

Witt K., Pulkowski U., Herzog J. et al. (2004). Deep brain stimulation of the subthalamic nucleus improves cognitive flexibility but impairs response inhibition in Parkinson disease. *Archives of Neurology*, Vol.61, pp. 697–700

Witt K., Daniels C., Reiff J. et al. (2008). Neuropsychological and psychiatric changes after deep brain stimulation for Parkinson's disease: a randomised, multicentre study. *Lancet Neurology*, Vol. 7, No.7, pp. 605-614

Witjas T., Baunez C., Henry J.M. et al. (2005). Addiction in Parkinson's disease: impact of subthalamic nucleus deep brain stimulation. *Movement Disorders*, Vol. 20, No.8, pp. 1052-1055

Xuereb J.H., Tomlison B.E., Irving D. et al. (1990). Cortical and subcortical pathology in Parkinson's disease: relationship to parkinsonian dementia. In: *Parkinson's disease: anatomy, pathology and therapy*, M.B. Streiffler M.B., Korczyn A.D., Melamed E., Youdim M.B. 35-40, Advances in Neurology, vol. 53. , Raven Press Ltd , New York

Zahodne L.B., Susatia F., Bowers D. et al. (2011) Binge eating in Parkinson's disease: prevalence, correlates and the contribution of deep brain stimulation. *Journal of Neuropsychiatry and Clinical Neurosciences*, Vol. 23, No.1, pp. 56-62

Zangaglia R., Pacchetti C., Pasotti C. et al. (2009) Deep brain stimulation and cognitive functions in Parkinson's disease: A three-year controlled study. *Movement Disorders*, Vol. 15, No.24(11), pp. 1621-8

Zibetti M., Pesare M., Cinquepalmi A. et al. (2009). Neuro-psychiatric therapy during chronic subthalamic stimulation in Parkinson's disease. *Parkinsonism Related Disorders*, Vol. 15, No.2, pp. 128-133

18

# Targeting the Subthalamic Nucleus for Deep Brain Stimulation in Parkinson Disease: The Impact of High Field Strength MRI

Dirk Winkler, Marc Tittgemeyer, Karl Strecker, Axel Goldammer, Jochen Helm, Johannes Schwarz and Jürgen Meixensberger
*Department of Neurosurgery, University of Leipzig, Leipzig Germany*

## 1. Introduction

Functional neurosurgery is the only surgical alternative treatment for patients with Parkinson's disease (PD) (Agid, 1999; Benzzouz & Hallett, 2000; Beric et al., 2001; DeLong & Wichmann, 2001; Dowsey-Limousin et al., 2001; Hariz & Fodstad, 2002; Kopper et al., 2003; Krause et al., 2001; Vesper et al., 2002). Dopamine deficiency in Parkinson's disease leads to increased neuronal activity. Regulation of this overactivity using electrical stimulation of the basal ganglia (deep brain stimulation - DBS) has become an attractive neurosurgical option of alternative treatment strategy (Limousin et al., 1998; Kupsch & Earl, 1999). The subthalamic nucleus (STN) is the key structure for motor control through the basal ganglia and is mostly used as stimulation target since here, all cardinal symptoms of PD can be effectively ameliorated (Anderson et al., 2005; Benabid et al., 1998; Dujardin et al, 2001; Limousin et al., 1998; Martinez-Martin et al., 2002; Koller et al., 2001; Krack et al., 1998; Lopiano et al., 2001; Volkmann et al., 2001). Possible mechanisms of DBS include depolarization blockade, release of local inhibitory neurotransmitters, antidromic activation of inhibitory neurons, and jamming of abnormal neuronal firing patterns. The clinical experiences and practice confirm the beneficial effect of chronic bilateral STN-DBS.

Especially the definition of the target area as well as positioning of test and permanent electrodes are subjects of ongoing debates, reflecting the different possibilities, including ventriculography, CT-guidance, MR-imaging and combined techniques (Hariz & Bergenheim, 1990, 1993). Advances in image acquisition, image postprocessing as well as potentials of multimodality including image supported surgery, microelectrode-recording (MER) and macrostimulation technologies have been the driving forces behind the resurgence in the use of functional stereotaxic surgery. Besides the precise selection of Parkinson patients, which are ideal candidates for deep brain stimulation, correct preoperative target definition and intraoperative target localization are the most important factors for surgical success and good clinical outcome (Lopiano et al., 2002).

This is the first comparative study, which evaluates the value of 3 Tesla MRI data for the definition of the STN as the target region for deep brain stimulation in patients with PD. This study shows the results of DBS-electrode placement using different MR-imaging (T1w,

T2w; 1,5T, 3T), which were used for preoperative visualization of the target region and anatomical landmarks as the precondition for the definition of target coordinates. In the next step, we systematically investigated the effects of bilateral STN-DBS on motor functions and medication in both groups in a twelve-month follow up.

## 2. Methods

The described prospective study included 27 patients (20 male, 7 female) with idiopathic PD in whom STN-DBS surgery was realized. Patient age ranges from 39-75 years. The mean age of males and females was 62.9 years. The mean duration of the disease was 12.3 years, ranging from 4 to 17 years.

Patients qualified for stereotaxic and functional neurosurgery, showed no evidence for psychiatric illness, cognitive impairment, severe brain atrophy, or other substantial medical problems of laboratory abnormalities, dementia, major focal or severe diffuse brain abnormalities, extensive brain atrophy nor any severe systemic internal disease, which could exclude stimulation therapy.

For targeting procedure image fusion of preoperative acquired 3D T1w and T2w 1.5T MR-image series ("Intera", Philips, Germany, 13 patients, group I) and 3D T1w 1.5 T and T2w 3 T MR-image series (Bruker, Germany, 14 patients, group II) was used and the possible benefit of 3 T MRI was evaluated, analyzing surgical and clinical data. In all cases with PD we preferred a bilateral electrode insertion in a single session, beginning with the more symptomatic side. Direct magnetic resonance imaging-based anatomic targeting was used.

### 2.1 Image acquisition and planning procedure

At present time a wide variety of target localization and implantation techniques exists (Limousin et al., 1998; Kupsch & Earl, 1999). Traditional stereotaxic algorithm has been based on an externally fixed stereotaxic frame that encompasses the patient´s head and upon which the micromanipulating equipment can be mounted and maneuvered with highest accuracy (Dujardin et al., 2001; Martinez-Martin, 2002). Corresponding to the existing stereotactic frames and their refinements, all stereotaxic frames have been optimized to allow nearly artefact-free image data sets and to guarantee a precise and reproducible definition of target and entry points. Typically, these frames are mounted on the day of surgery, just before acquisition of planning image data sets.

Beginning this step of functional neurosurgery the patient is free of any L-Dopa medication as a precondition for macrostimulation and awake-neurological examination. Consequently, tremor-related motion artefacts during image acquisition are encountered, despite of the patient´s head fixation using headholders (CT) and headcoils (MRI), which reduce the accuracy of image co-registration theoretically and possible practically. Nevertheless, the delay involved with frame fixation, image acquisition, planning and three dimensional checking can take several hours depending on personal and institutional experiences and the patient´s properties as a kind of stress just before surgery.

In our study on the day of surgery the patient's head was fixed in an MR-compatible ceramic head holder (Zamorano-Dujovny, ZD, Fa. Stryker, Howmedica, Leibinger, Germany) in local anaesthesia. Position of the head ring was chosen in such a way that pin placement and expected metal artefacts of the screw tips were away from the axial plane of the target point (STN) and any structures of interest.

For functional and surgical planning it is necessary to map points and regions of interest from one patient image to another that has been taken at a different time or/and with a different image method. In this study the combination of T1w and T2w image series seemed to be the most practical way. The rational behind this procedure is that T2w image data allow an excellent visualization of target structures (STN) and neighbouring anatomical landmarks (Nc. ruber). The T1w images are used for stereotaxic planning and realization of surgery.

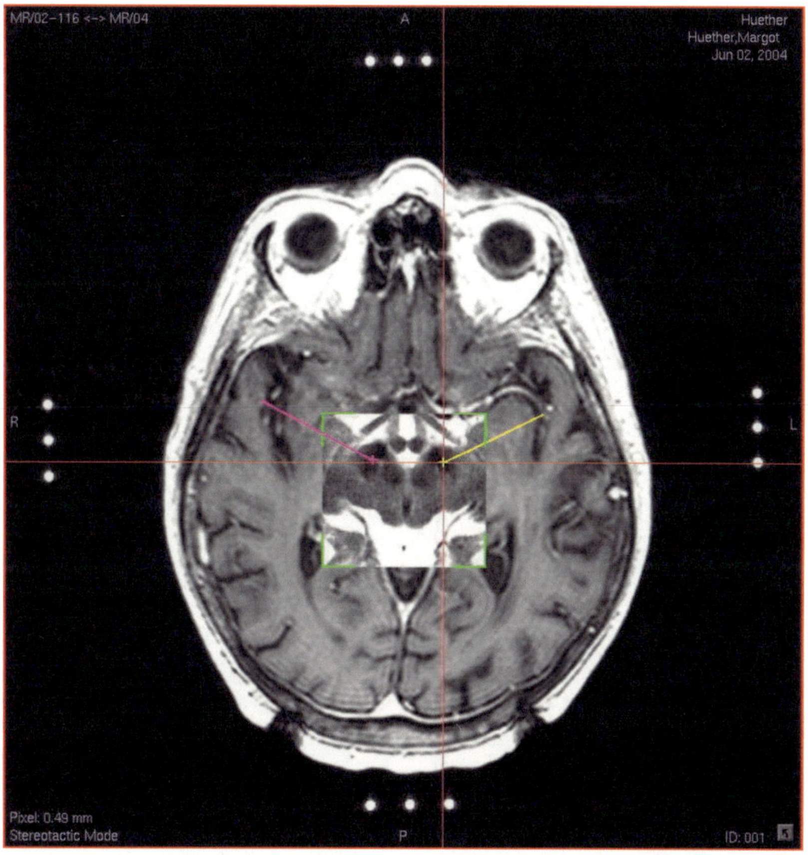


Fig. 1. Postprocessing result (image fusion) for following definition of target coordinates basing of 3D T1w and T2w MR image data of the region of interest (T1w 1.5 T MRI and T2w 3 T MRI)

Corresponding to the different possibilities we analysed two patient cohorts: in the first group (group I) 1.5 Tesla T1w (3D-magnetization-prepared rapid gradient echo-TE 4,6 msec, TR 25 msec) and T2w (Turbo spin echo-TE 120 msec, TR 4389 msec) image series with the following parameters: matrix 256 x 256, slice thickness: 1 mm ("Intera", Philips, Germany, 1.5 Tesla) were acquired and fused together slice identically (Fig. 1). In group II the 1.5 Tesla T1w image series ( "Intera", Philips, Germany, 1.5 Tesla) was combined and fused with the

T2w image series, acquired in the 3 Tesla Bruker MRI (matrix 256 x 256, slice thickness: 1 mm, Turbo spin echo-TE 355 msec, TR 3500 msec), Max-Planck-Institute of Cognition and Neuroscience, Leipzig, Germany. Just before magnetic resonance image acquisition (T1w MRI) contrast media was given in both groups in a standard dose (0.1 mmol/kg bodyweight Gd-DTPA, Magnevist, Schering, Germany) to improve detail informations as well as to identify passing vessels.

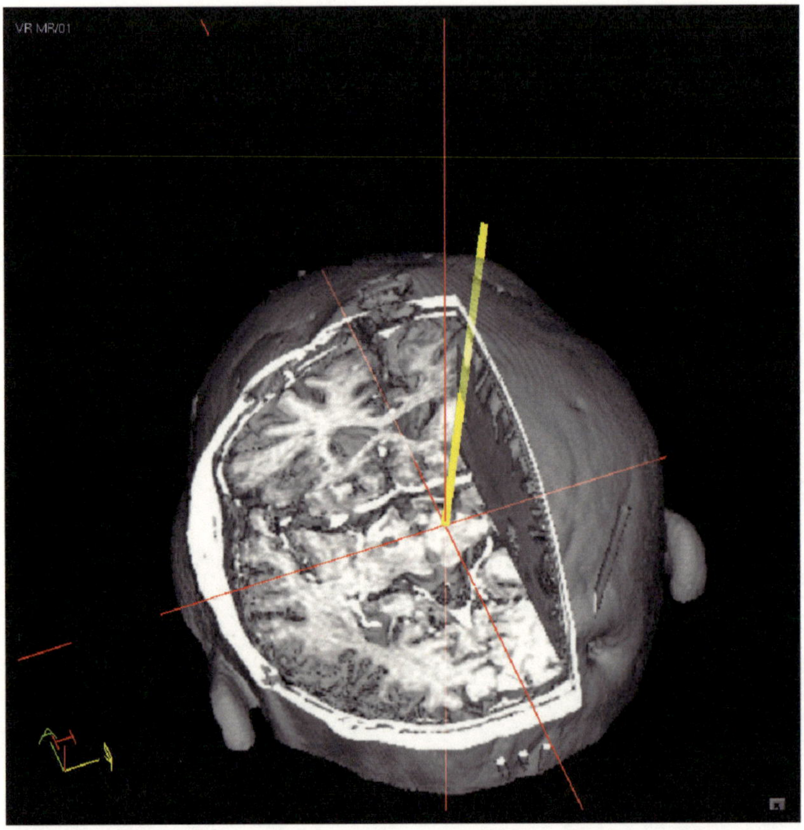


Fig. 2. Virtual 3D reconstruction of planned electrode trajectory

Stereotaxic coordinates were calculated with the "Remote surgical planning software" (RSPS, Fa. Stryker, Howmedica, Leibinger, Germany) or with the VoXim® / microTargeting™ , IVS Technology, Germany, FHC, USA. In the following steps, image postprocessing, definition of functional, entry and target coordinates and visualization of planed trajectories take place. In general, the final stage in the presurgical planning process involves reviewing the proposed trajectory interactively in the sagittal, axial and coronal plane and checking the coordinates verified that the cannula passes exactly to the defined target point. The surgical planning process involved the identification and adaptation of the target using the typical appearance of the STN and the Nc. ruber in T2w image series and reviewing the proposed trajectory interactively in the sagittal, axial and coronal plane. Any field inhomogeneities of the used MRI could be ruled out in previous studies (Figure 3).

Entry and target points were chosen and the coordinates of the space were calculated automatically by the special „frame-based stereotaxy" software program, including the A, B, C, D and E values for the target device of the stereotaxic system. These coordinates were the base for the intraoperative used target arc system, which was connected with the stereotaxic head ring (Zamorano-Dujovny, ZD, Leibinger, Germany). A phantom system called target point simulator was used for intraoperative control of coordinates. Checking the coordinates verified that the cannula passes exactly to the defined target point.

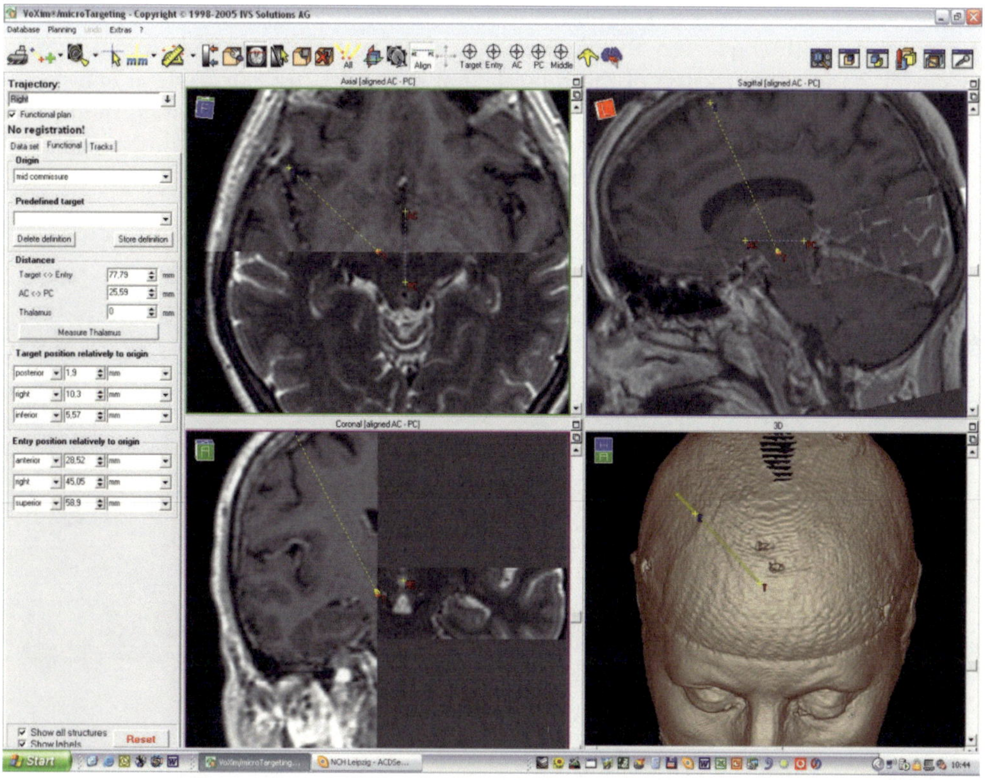


Fig. 3. Identification and adaptation of the target-coordinates using the sagital, axial and coronal plane.

### 2.2 Functional neurosurgery

In the surgical part, the mild sedated patient was transferred to the operating theatre without a possibility of frame dislocation and was fixed normally using a special adapter unit. In the operating theatre patients was lying in a 45° upright position and was mild sedated with intermittend injections of midazolam to allow motor and verbal testing during intraoperative testing stimulation.

Head was cleaned and draped with the entry site in view. Under local anaesthesia and mild sedation, a burr hole craniotomy was made at the desirable entry point and the target arch was installed. The burr hole was placed in the standard location near the coronal suture and approximately 3 to 5 cm from the midline. Five stainless-steel microelectrodes were inserted stereotaxically using multi-channel microelectrodes (Leadpoint 4, medtronic, USA).

Microrecording was performed to identify the STN signature (frequency, pattern, amplitude) as a reliable criterion for the correct electrode position. Target signals were analysed for defining STN target, including frequency, firing rates and interspike intervals (Hutchison et al., 1998, Raeva et al., 1991, 1993).

Recording was started 10 mm above the target and was continued to 4 mm below the supposed STN. The target for the final placement of the electrode was confirmed by macrostimulation using the microelectrode housing cannula. The target was confirmed by the responses of the patient to stimuli (130 Hz frequency, 0-5.0 mA stimulation amplitude, 60 sec pulse width) delivered through the macroelectrode. During test stimulation eye movement, speech, contraction of the contralateral face, neck, tongue, skeletal muscle, and the suppression of tremor and rigidity were checked. Mostly, clinical testing indicating a dramatic improvement of tremor, akinesis and rigidity of the contralateral limb and showed a disappearance of drug-induced dyskinesia postoperatively (Figure 4)

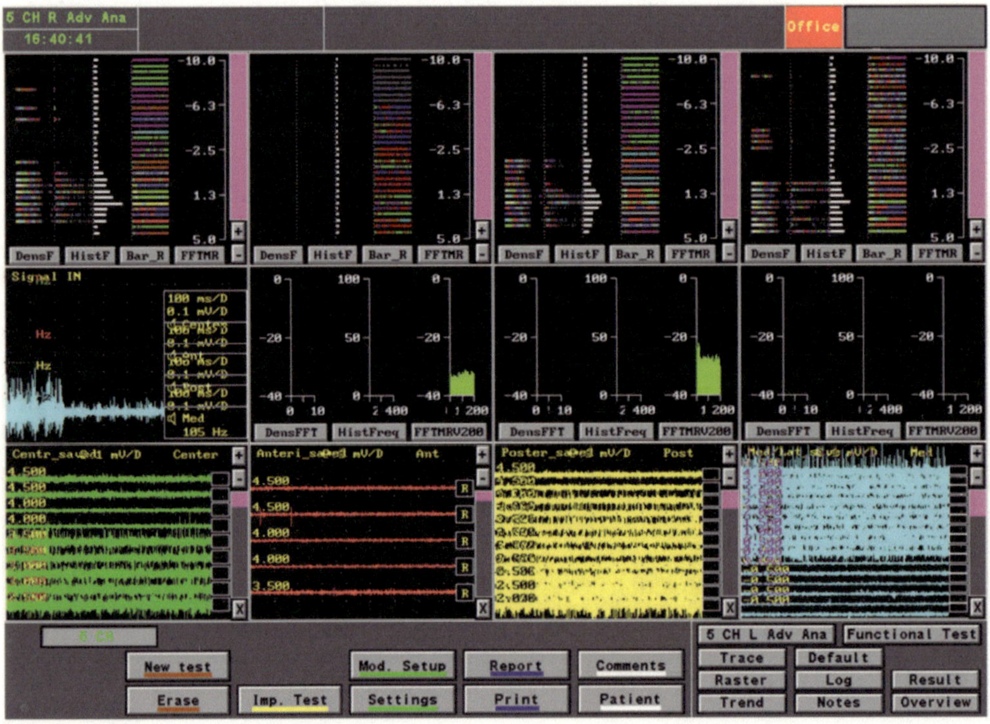


Fig. 4. Microelectrode – recoding for visualization of typical STN-signature along the z-axis

Final positioning of the permanent electrode (DBS electrode, model 3389, Medtronic, USA) was monitored on the fluoroscopy screen to avoid discrepancies between planned and real localization of the tip of the electrode. After electrode positioning the electrode was secured to the patient's skull using bone cement and miniplates for fixation (Figure 5). The same procedure was repeated on the other side. After all neurosurgical steps stereotactic frame was removed from the patient´s head and implantation of impulse generator (Kinetra Impulsgenerator, model 7428, Medtronic, Minneapolis) was done under general anaesthesia.

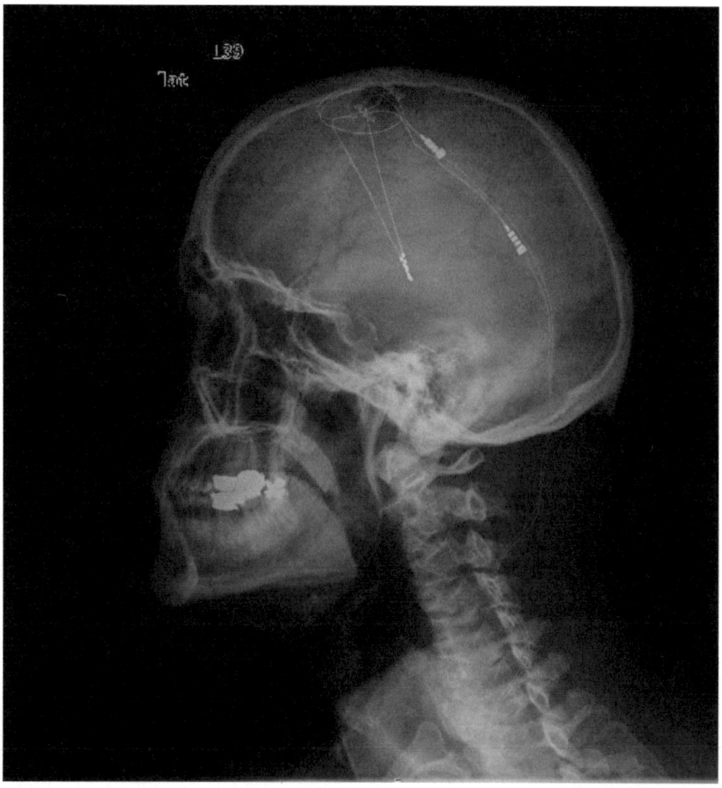

Fig. 5. Real position of the stimulation electrodes, documented by fluoroscopy

On the same or next day patients underwent postoperative MRI to rule out any surgery associated complications (Figure 6a, b). Stimulation testing and wound control took place and depending on their and the family conditions they was discharged home or to rehabilitation. In regular follow-ups, medication was checked and adjustments were made to optimise the stimulation parameters After placement of permanent electrodes, a pulse generator (Kinetra Impulsgenerator, model 7428, Medtronic, Minneapolis) was implanted in the infraclavicular fossa and connected to the electrodes. The following stimulation consisted of continuous square-wave pulses (frequency: 130 Hz, pulse duration: 120 µs, amplitude: 2.5 V). Clinical examination was performed to rule out any postoperative complications, motor, especially oculomotor and speech abnormalities. Postoperative MRI confirmed the electrode position.

## 2.3 Results

Planning procedure for following STN-DBS using preoperative acquired 1.5T and 3T MRI data is a reliable tool for successful stereotaxic treatment of PD. Using T1w image date after injection of contrast media an excellent visualization of anatomical details (ventricle structures, sulci and gyri) as well as passing vessels could be guaranteed. High resolution 3 Tesla MRI (T2w) allowed brilliant identification of the typical almond-shaped STN and the Nc. rubber with their typical hypointense shape. Image fusion was realized manually using

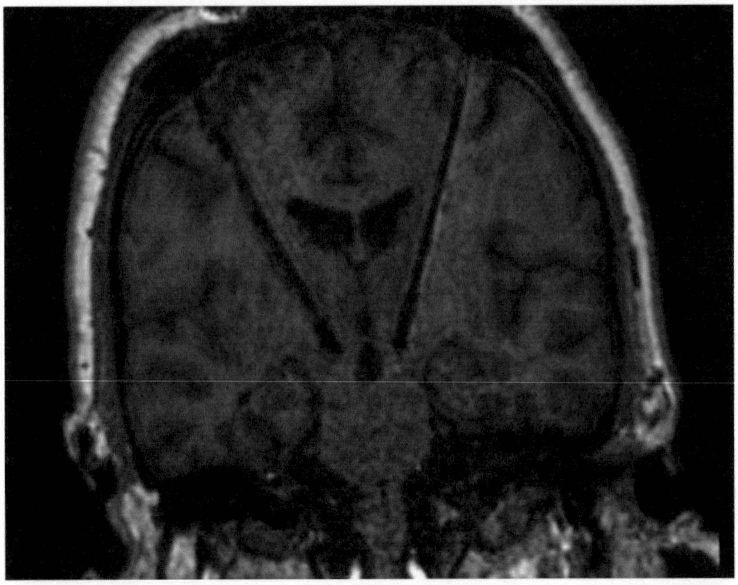

a

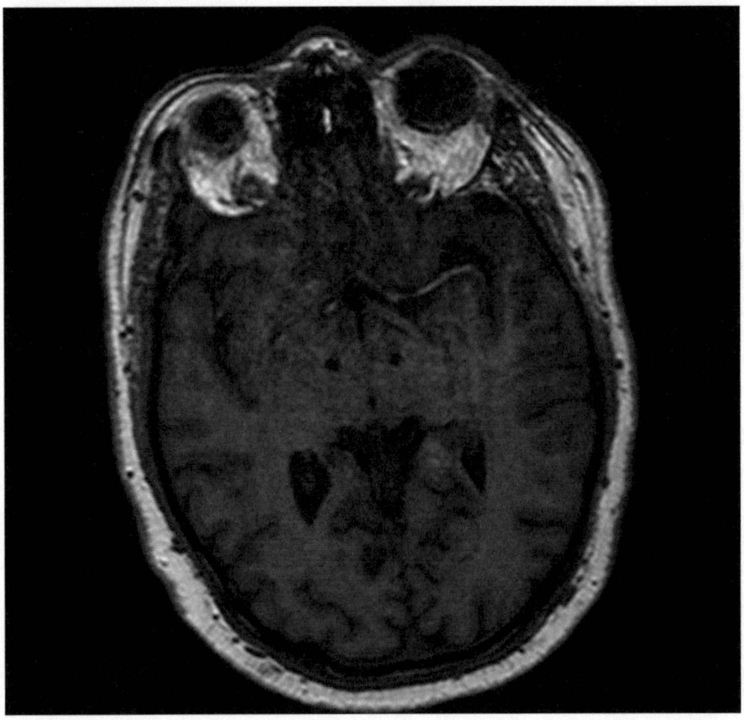

b

Fig. 6. a, b: Postoperative control of electrode positioning in different planes (a: coronar, b: axial), confirmed by small metal artefacts anatomical landmarks with an accuracy of 0.9 mm, ranging from 0.4-1.1 mm. Corresponding to the anatomical markers and the theoretical target coordinates the STN position was superior to the substantia nigra, lateral to the anterior portion of the red nucleus and medial to the internal capsule: The longest medial-lateral and ventral-posterior diameter of STN was aimed and located immediately lateral to the anterior aspect of the Nc. rubber in the axial plane. With the help of ben gun system five electrodes were implanted simultaneously in the target region to validate target region electrophysiologically. Typical STN signature, representing neuronal activity could be documented in implanted microelectrodes. After microrecording macrostimulation was performed using electrodes with the best STN signal to confirm correct electrode placement using common stimulation parameter In both groups the image fusion accuracy was with 0.37 (group I) and 0.40 (group II) nearly the same and allowed a precise and slice identical correlation of both, T1w and T2w image series in both modalities (1.5 T, 3 T)(Table 1). The number of microelectrodes which detected a typical STN signature during MER of both sites increased from 6.7 (group I) to 7.1 (group II) averagely and showed a tendency of a safer localization of the expected target point basing on preoperative acquired image data in the second group. Further data of planning (functional coordinates) and surgical (surgical time) procedures are summarized in Table 1 and correspond with planning data of other studies (Okun et al., 2005).

| radiological and surgical data | Group I (n=13)<br>T1-w (1.5 Tesla)<br>T2-w (1.5 Tesla) | Group II (n=14)<br>T1-w (1.5 Tesla)<br>T2-w (3.0 Tesla) |
|---|---|---|
| **fusion accuracy, mean (min - max)** | 0.37 (0.2 – 0.6) | 0.40 (0.2 – 0.7) |
| **surgical time (min) mean (min - max)** | 267 (202 – 313) | 247 (160 – 302) |
| **functional coordinates** | | |
| x | ± 11.25 | ± 10.4 |
| y | - 1.95 | - 2.05 |
| z | - 4.15 | - 4.45 |
| **active electrodes, mean (min - max)** | 6.7 (2 – 9) | 7.1 (4 – 9) |

Table 1. Summarized radiological, planning and surgical data

As a result of this, the functional coordinates have the biggest differences in the x-coordinates, but were comparable in the others. Interestingly, in group I the central track (48%) dominated as the best traject for the placement of the permanent stimulation electrode, which is followed by the medial one's (20%)(Figure 7). Contrary to this, in group II predominated the anterior track with 41.7%, compared to 37% of the central track (Figure 8).

In the comparison of both groups we found a domination of the central (group I) and anterior and central position of the active electrode (group II, Figure 9).

In the postoperative course the mean administered dose of L-dopa decreased significantly in group I from 698.1 mg/day to 200.0 mg/day twelve months later, that means 28.7 % of the initial mean dosage and in group II from 686.5 mg/day to 183.3 mg/day (24.9%)(Table 2,

Figure 10). The reduction of L-dopa dose one, two, three and twelve months postoperatively differed not significantly between both groups.

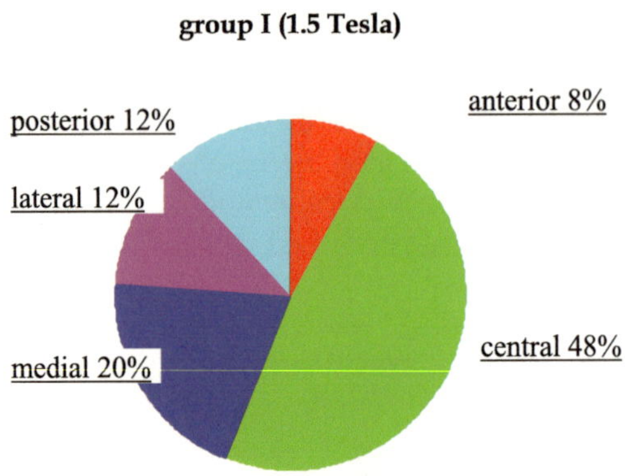


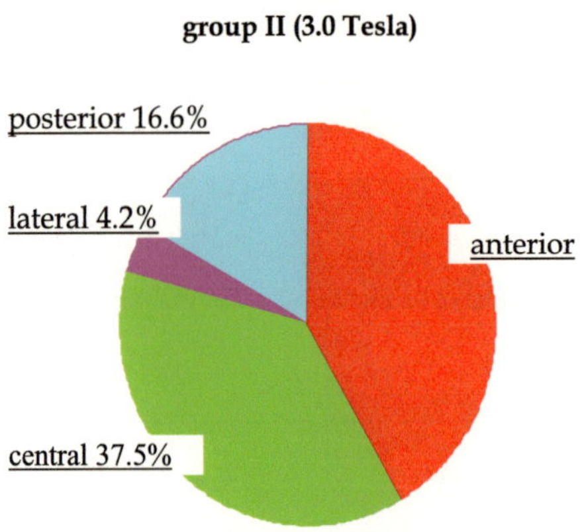


Fig. 8. Distribution of active electrodes in group II (3 Tesla MRI)

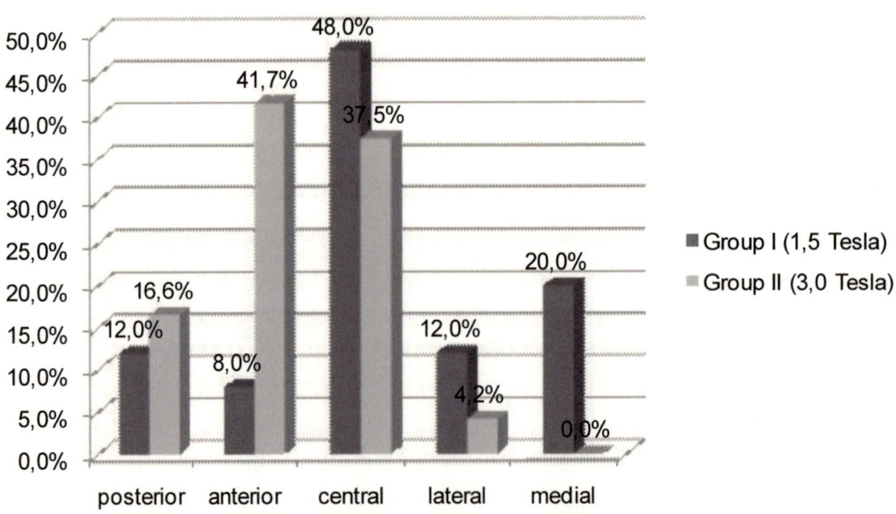


Fig. 9. Distribution of "active" electrodes with typical STN signature, detected by microrecording

| L-dopa (daily dose, mg-values given as mean) | Group I (n=13) T1-w (1.5 Tesla) T2-w (1.5 Tesla) | Group II (n=14) T1-w (1.5 Tesla) T2-w (3.0 Tesla) |
|---|---|---|
| **Preoperative** | 698.1 SD ± 251 | 686.5 SD ± 469 |
| **Postoperative - one month** | 170.8 SD ± 151** | 170.8 SD ± 123** |
| **Postoperative - two months** | 112.5 SD ± 210** | 187.5 SD ± 131** |
| **Postoperative - three months** | 155.5 SD ± 212** | 212.5 SD ± 75** |
| **Postoperative - twelve months** | 200.0 SD ± 115** | 183.3 SD ± 177** |

Table 2. Comparison of preoperative and postoperative L-dopa-medication in both groups. In spite of some irregularities in the course of twelve months the final dose reduction in both groups is comparable and no criteria for the used image modality. (** $p < 0.01$)

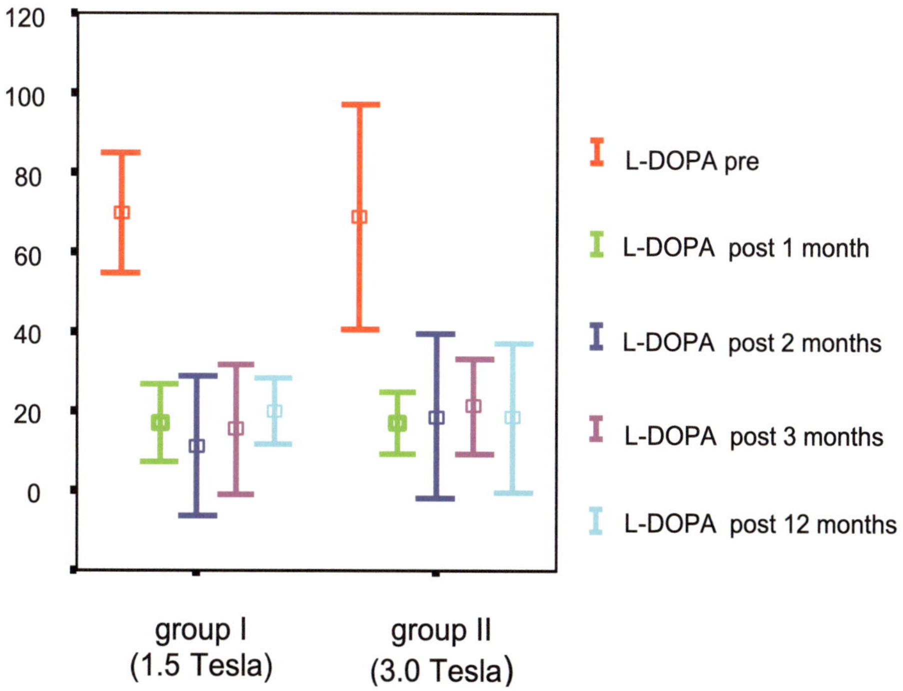


Fig. 10. Pre- and postoperative L-DOPA medication in both groups, depending on time course (preoperative, one, two, three and twelve months after STN-DBS)

The motor ratings improved significantly ($p \leq 0.01$) from the preoperative (medication-off) to the stimulator-on (medication-on) conditions in both groups (Table 3, Figure 11). Mean improvement were 70.4% (group I) and 55.4% (group II), respectively, for UPDRS, part III (Table 3, Figure 11). No significant differences between the two groups were seen.

| UPDRS ( III ) | Group I (n=13)<br>T1-w (1.5 Tesla)<br>T2-w (1.5 Tesla) | Group II (n=14)<br>T1-w (1.5 Tesla)<br>T2-w (3.0 Tesla) |
|---|---|---|
| **Preoperative** | 43.9 SD ± 20.0 | 42.6 SD ± 10.0 |
| **Postoperative - one month** | 13.4 SD ± 10.0** | 13.6 SD ± 6.2** |
| **Postoperative - twelve months** | 13.0 SD ± 6.3** | 19.0 SD ± 4.5** |

(** $p < 0.01$)

Table 3. Improvement of UPDRS (part III) in both groups up to one year after functional neurosurgery.

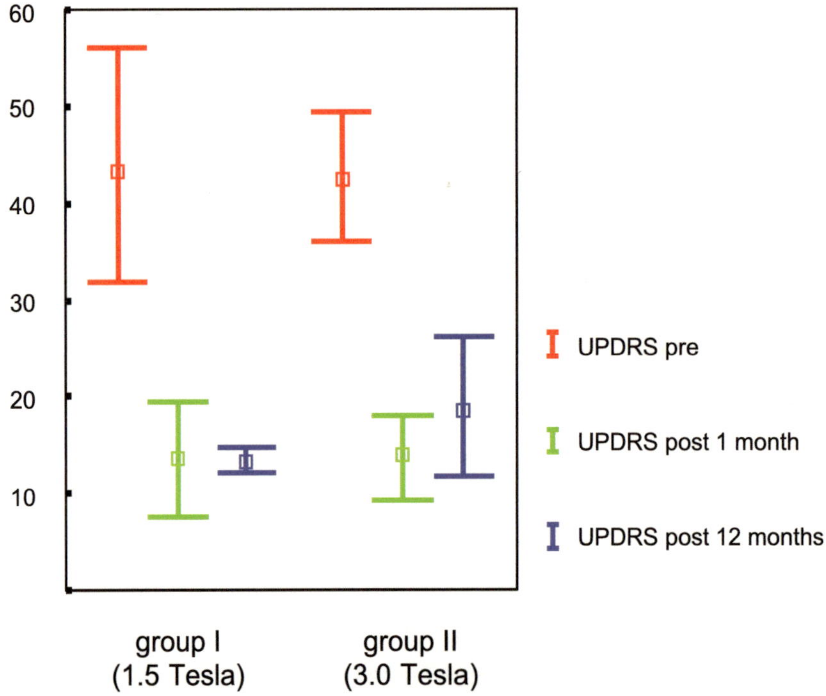


Fig. 11. Clinical effect (UPDRS (part III) up to one year after deep brain stimulation

## 3. Discussion

The principle of stereotaxic surgery was created by Horsley and Clarke as well as Spiegel, Wycis and Leksell. Stereotaxic surgery is a well established and accurate method and offers increasing possibilities for diagnosis and therapy. Today, stereotaxic localization based on

CT and MRI data is mostly used to guide the neurosurgeon during biopsy and functional neurosurgery with an accuracy of less than one millimetre, which is an essential advantage of used high precision stereotaxic frames. Former studies confirmed the high accuracy of stereotaxic devices despite system associated errors.

The beneficial effect of bilateral STN stimulation for neurosurgical treatment of PD is confirmed by countless studies and groups and should not be the focus of this article. At present time many neurosurgical concepts exist making the functional neurosurgery for PD via STN-DBS safe for patients and surgeons as well. The clinical results with traditional ventriculography, CT-guidance, MR-imaging and combined techniques are comparable. In this STN-DBS study for treatment of idiopathic PD we performed microrecording and macrostimulation as routinely used steps during the stereotaxic procedure, but practiced different MR planning modalities for electrode placement : 1.5 and 3 Tesla MR (T1w and T2w). Differences in both techniques and both groups as well as clinical and surgical data are the initial points for the following discussion.

In this study we used different MR modalities to define the target point and used MER and macrostimulation for electrophysiological respectively clinical validation of chosen trajectories for final electrodes.

The great appeal of 3T MRI is the improvement in image quality and an increased signal-to-noise ratio (SNR). Many are excited about the opportunity to not only use the increased SNR for clearer images, but also the chance to exchange it better resolution and contrast - a fact already well known from comparisons of images obtained at 0.5T, 1T, and 1.5T MRI. In the case of 3T MRI the SNR correlates in approximately linear fashion with field strength, it is roughly twice as great at 3T as at 1.5T. The magnetic susceptibility is exacerbated and the time necessary to acquire satisfactory images can be substantially reduced and motion artifacts can be minimized. Among other benefits, higher contrast may permit reduction of gadolinium doses and, in some cases, earlier detection of disease, a possible stimulus to use higher field systems. These possibilities makes the 3T MRI attractive especially for brain imaging.

Nevertheless, significant obstacles to 3T MRI presented by the physics at higher field strengths. 1. especially the T1 relaxation times are prolonged with increasing magnet field strength, the chemical shift is larger and the susceptibility is stronger. 2. There are safety concerns. The energy deposited in the patient's tissues is fourfold higher at 3T than at 1.5T. Especially with the use of fast spin echo and fluid attenuation inversion recovery (FLAIR), the limit on the specific absorption rate (SAR) power deposition prescribed by the FDA can easily be reached compared to 1.5T MR protocols. Scanner manufacturers are incorporating modified pulse sequences to avoid this problem, which can also be solved by restricting the volume of tissue that is studied in detail.

In our study we couldn´t observe, that the application of 3T MRI could avoid multiple passes of microelectrodes for electrophysiologic confirmation of correct target location as a possible reason to decrease the overall time of the surgical intervention and to reduce the risk of possible complications related to brain tissue trauma.

Corresponding to this surgical concept we found a sustained improvement in PD-associated motor disability (UPDRS), a reduction of postoperative L-Dopa respectively L-Dopa-equivalent medication and a minimizing of levodopa-induced motor complications, which is confirmed by other study results. Despite of other surgical concepts of target definition, which published elsewhere, the MR-based STN localization leads to comparable results in both groups.

The STN is a biconvex lens-shaped structure, which can be visualized as a hypointense region by T2w MRI. Described by Yelnik and Percheron, 1979, STN as a relatively small region of approximately 735 $mm^3$ is obliquely oriented along the three anatomical axis of the space, which means approximately 20° oblique to the horizontal plane, 35° to the sagittal plane, and approximately 55° to the frontal plane (Yelnik & Percheron, 1979). As a consequence the STN has three anatomical characteristics, which make its localization difficult: it is lens shaped, relatively small, and oblique. For these reasons, the position of STN cannot be simply determined by viewing a single planar plane, but rather requires a precise and reproducible 3D reconstruction of its entire extent and a clear differentiation from the surrounding tissue. Besides the anatomical peculiarities the STN shows interindividual variations in size, shape and dimension, which complicated the positioning of electrodes basing on statistical and anatomical coordinates. In this study we used different MR modalities (T1w, T2w, 1.5mT vs. 3mT) to define the target point. Following postprocessing allowing a detailed visualization in all three sections of the space and perpendicularly along the planned trajectories, using excellent contrast between hypointense structure of STN and Nc. ruber and the hyperintense tissue in the surrounding. With the use of 3mT MRI a high resolution of basal cerebral structures, including the target area of STN and its neighbouring structures, could be achieved. Criteria for the following placement of microelectrodes were the longest medial-lateral and ventral-posterior diameter of STN and the ventral border of the red nucleus. The central trajectory was aimed and located immediately lateral to the anterior aspect of the Nc. ruber in the axial plane with regard to the patient's anatomy. MER and macrostimulation were used for electrophysiological respectively clinical validation of chosen trajectories for final electrodes. MER obtained by electrophysiological examination were consistent with other reports of bursting and non-bursting activities (Hutchison et al., 1998; Raeva & Lukashev, 1993) and correlated in the majority of tested trajectories with the typical STN signature in frequency and amplitude. Microrecording results were limited by the typical activity patterns of neighbouring structures of the zona inserta, substantia nigra and the background activity of the basal cerebral structures as well.

The image guided placement of micro- and final electrodes implicates the preoperative fixation of the stereotaxic frame just before image acquisition hours before surgery. Unfortunately most of these classic stereotaxic frames (weight: 2000 to 2500 g) are really heavy and uncomfortable during it´s fixation on the patients skull. During image acquisition, planning and surgical procedure all patients are free of L-Dopa medication to guarantee a reliable neurological testing during electrode positioning and following clinical testing. Stress, medication free interval and tremor-associated disability enforce possible motion artefacts in the acquisition of planning image data sets. This movement theoretically reduces the accuracy of image coregistration between image modalities.

Following preoperative postprocessing procedure including image fusion and definition of electrode trajectories is time consuming - to be just in time on the day of surgery is stressfull for patients and surgeons and can be a logistic problem, which is difficult to measure.

Beside the fixation of the patient´s head on the table via special head holders conventional functional neurosurgery requires the adjustment of all axis of the space corresponding to the target and entry coordinates using the microdrive and a special target arcl. A re-checking is following using by the target arch simulator, which gives additional safety, but which is time consuming. After finishing the dominant side all the equipment has to be removed, readjusted and readapted for the second side, which delay the surgery additionally and which implicates moments of inaccuracies. In the consequence, the accuracy of "static" image guided devices decreases with the time of surgery secondary to the intraoperative brain shift as a result of a) loss of cerebrospinal fluid (CSF), b) gravity, c) anaesthesiological procedure and d) brain-immanent characteristics. Confirmed by own experiences a tissue shift even in the region of STN could be documented exemplarily in the end of a hours lasting routine DBS procedure by vectorshift deformation analysis, which expressly underline the requirement of a stringent surgery. As a result of diverse shift studies it´s accepted, that long lasting procedures can dipose progressive CSF loss via burr hole trepanation and brain shift associated inaccuracies even in the middle of the brain. In the consequence, all factors, disposing shift associated inaccuracies should be prevented strictly. Microrecording and macrostimulation are relatively standardised steps and can help to compensate the mentioned inaccuracies electrophysiologically. Both neurosurgical steps are the preconditions for the following positioning of the final electrode.

In this series the mean number of active electrodes was with 6.7 (group I) and 7.1 (group II) per patient should be very good, but is confirmed by other studies. In our opinion the slight difference of the mean number of active electrodes between both groups is a possibly result of a better resolution of anatomical structures and improved signal-to-noise ratio by 3 T MRI, especially in the target region and can be the reason for a shorter surgical time. In our study intraoperative MER was an essential tool to find an optimal target point for the macrostimulation, which can reduce the surgeon's uncertainty and increases the procedure's safety. Macrostimulation was performed only in this macroelectrode, in which the cellular activity characteristics of the STN have been identified. The criteria for changing stimulation electrode were the missing motor effect of macrostimulation and persistent stimulation-induced side effects, including paresis, sensible sensations or dyskinesia. Correct anatomical and functional target - namely where the best clinical result with a partial or complete relief of symptoms - were the base for the actual placement of the permanent electrode.

As a consequence of preoperative postprocessing and following planning procedure the functional coordinates were comparable in both groups and differed only slightly, especially the x-coordinates, which were ± 11.25 in group I and ± 10.4 in group II. This correlates possibly with a changed selection of the best track for the permanent electrode placement from the central position (48%) in group I to the anterior (41.7%) and central (37.5%) position in group II. Maybe this is an indication for the phenomenon that a smaller distance from the target point to the AC-PC line correlates with a good clinical response stimulating the anterior part of the Nc. subthalamicus. However, both study groups are too small to conclude a strict and reliable tendency.

Corresponding to this surgical concept we found a sustained improvement in PD-associated motor disability (UPDRS, part III), which is confirmed by Pollo et al., 2007, and Kleiner-Fisman et al., 2006, presenting meta-analysis of outcomes from 1993 until 2004.

The medication doses could be reduced to the same extent in both groups and were in the range reported in the literature (Beric et al., 2001; Limousin et al., 1998; Minguez-Castellanos et al., 2005; Okun et al., 2005; Russmann et al., 2004). Differences in preoperative image acquisition (1.5 T, 3 T), postprocessing and defined target coordinates and chosen electrode tracks were not associated with a definite improvement of motor response and drug reduction, which would justify the use of 3 T MRI absolutely.

## 4. Conclusions

Acquisition of T2w 3 T MRI for following planning procedure is a useful tool to visualize the target region and anatomical landmarks with a high fidelity of detailed information. Microrecording is an excellent and reliable method to validate the target area intraoperatively by registration of typical STN signatures. Over and above that, it allows an identification of the longest segment of STN, which we preferred as the electrode position for macrostimulation and for placement of permanent STN-electrode. With the use of 3 T MRI data for image postprocessing and planning procedure the visualization of the target point - the STN - could be improved and allowed a high precision in the definition of target and entry coordinates of the virtual trajectory. Macrostimulation via macroeletrodes confirmed the target point and was used to detect any side effects for further stimulation. The macrostimulation and intraoperative testing guaranteed a proper placement of both electrodes, expecting a high rate of successful surgeries and permanent functional effects.

With our study we could confirm an encouraging response of PD-associated movement disorders. Besides the neuroradiological, physiological and neurosurgical techniques and procedures, the most important prerequisite is the optimal visualization of the target area, which can be achieved by high-resolution MRI. In the consequence using 3 T MRI series is one way to increase the surgeons and patients safety and to support an optimal electrode placement.

But, this study is not suitable to conclude, that a better visualization of the STN is also associated with a further clinical improvement of motor response and reduction of L-dopa, which is known in conventional functional neurosurgery using 1.5 T MRI. Further studies should be initiated to find a better conclusion. Up to this point, the choice of method should depend on the technical resources, preferences and experiences of each centre.

## 5. References

Agid Y: Continuous high frequency stimulation of deep brain structures in brain pathology. Brain Res Bull 1999, 50:475

Anderson VC, Burchiel KJ, Hogarth P, Favre J, Hammerstad JP: Pallidal vs subthalamic nucleus deep brain stimulation in Parkinson disease. Arch Neurol 2005, 62:554-560

Benabid AL, Benazzouz A, Hoffmann D, Limousin P, Krack P, Pollak P: Long-term electrical inhibition of deep brain targets in movement disorders. Mov Disord 1998, 13:119-125

Benazzouz A, Hallett M: Mechanism of action of deep brain stimulation. Neurology 2000, 55:13-16

Beric A, Kelly PJ, Rezai A et al.. Complications of Deep Brain Stimulation Surgery. Stereotact Funct Neurosurg2001;77:73-78

DeLong MR, Wichmann T: Deep brain stimulation for Parkinson's disease. Ann Neurol 2001, 49:142-143

Dowsey-Limousin P, Fraix V, Benabid AL, Pollak P: Deep brain stimulation in Parkinson's disease. Funct Neurol 2001, 16:67-71

Dujardin K, Defebvre L, Krystkowiak P, Blond S, Destèe A. Influence of chronic bilateral stimulation of the subthalamic nucleus on cognitive function in Parkinson's disease. J Neurol. 2001; 248,603-611

Hariz MI, Bergenheim AT (1993) Clinical evaluation of computed tomography-guided versus ventriculography-guided thalamotomy for movement disorders. Acta Neurochir 58 : 53-55

Hariz MI, Fodstad H: Deep brain stimulation in Parkinsons's disease. N Engl J Med 2002, 346:452-453

Hariz, MI, Bergenheim, AT (1990) A comparative study on ventriculographic and computerized tomography-guided determinations of brain targets in functional stereotaxis. J Neurosurg 73 : 565-571

Hutchison WD, Allan RJ, Opitz, H et al: Neurophysiological identification of the subthalamic nucleus in surgery for Parkinson's disease. Ann Neurol 44:622-628, 1998

Kleiner-Fisman G, Herzog J, Fisman DN, Tamma F, Lyons KE, Rahwa R, Lang AE, Deuschl G: Subthalamic nucleus deep brain stimulation: summary and meta-analysis of outcomes. Mov Disord 2006, 21:290-304

Koller WC, Lyons KE, Wilkinson SB, Troster AI, Pahwa R: Longterm safety and efficacy of unilateral deep brain stimulation of the thalamus in essential tremor. Mov Disord 2001, 16:464-468

Kopper F, Volkmann J, Müller D, Mehdorn M, Deuschl G. High-frequency deep brain stimulation in the treatment for Parkinson's disease, tremor and dystonia. Der Nervenarzt. 2003;74:709-725

Krack P, Pollak P, Limousin P et al.. Subthalamic nucleus or internal pallidal stimulation in young onset Parkinson's disease Brain. 1998; 121, 451 - 457

Krause M, Fogel W, Heck A, Hacke W, Bonsanto M, Trenkwalder C, Tronnier V: Deep brain stimulation for the treatment of Parkinson's disease: subthalamic nucleus versus globus pallidum internus. J Neurol Neurosurg Psychiatry 2001, 70:464-470

Kupsch A, Earl C (1999) Neurosurgical intervention in the treatment of ideopathic Parkinson disease: neurostimulation and neural implantation. J Mol Med 77 : 178-84

Limousin P, Krack P, Pollack P et al.. Electrical stimulation of the subthalamic nucleus in advanced Parkinson's disease. N Engl J Med. 1998;339:1105-1111

Lopiano L, Rizzone M, Bergamasco B et al.. Deep brain stimulation of the subthalamic nucleus in PD: an analysis of the exclusion causes. Journal of the Neurological Sciences. 2002;195;167-170

Lopiano L, Rizzone M, Bergamasco B, Tavella A, Torre E, Perozzo P, Valentini MC, Lanotte M: Deep brain stimulation of the subthalamic nucleus: clinical effectiveness and safety. Neurology 2001, 56:552-554

Martinez-Martin P, Valldeoriola F, Tolosa E et al.. Bilateral Subthalamic Nucleus Stimulation and Quality of Life in Advanced Parkinson's Disease. Movement Disorders. 2002;17, 372 - 377

Minguez-Castellanos A, Escamilla-Sevilla F, Katati MJ, Martin-Linares JM, Meersmans M, Ortega-Moreno A, Arjona V: Different patterns of medication ch'ange after subthalamic or pallidal stimulation for Parkinson's disease: target related effect or selection bias? J Neurol Neurosurg Psychiatry 2005, 76:34-39

Okun MS, Tagliati M, Pourfar M, Fernandes HH, Rodriguez RL, Alterman RL, Foote KD: Management of referred deep brain stimulation failures: a retrospective analysis from 2 movement disorders centers. Arch Neurol 2005, 62:1250-1255

Pollo C, Vingerhoets F, Pralong E, Ghika J, Maeder P, Meuli R, Thiran JP, Villemure JG: Localization of electrodes in the subthalamic nucleus on magnetic resonance imaging. J Neurosurg 2007, 106:36-44

Raeva S, Lukashev A, Lashin A: Unit activity in human thalamic reticularis neuron. I. Spontaneous activity. Electroencephalogr Clin Neurophysiol 79:133-140, 1991

Raeva S, Lukashev A: Unit activity in human thalamic reticularis neuron. II. Activity evoked by significant and non-significant verbal or sensory stimuli. Electroencephalogr Clin Neurophysiol 86:110-122, 1993

Russmann H, Ghiera J, Combrement P, Villemure JG, Bogousslavsky J, Burkhard PR, Vingerhoets FJ: L-dopa-induced dyskinesia improvement after STN-DBS depends upon medication reduction. Neurology 2004, 63:153-155

Vesper J, Klostermann F, Stockhammer F, Funk T, Brock M: Results of chronic subthalamic nucleus (STN) stimulation for Parkinson's disease - a one-year follow-up study. Surg Neurol 2002, 57:306-313

Volkmann J, Allert N, Voges J, Weiss PH, Freund HJ, Sturm V: Safety and efficacy of pallidal or subthalamic nucleus stimulation in advanced PD. Neurology 2001, 56:548-551

Yelnik J, Percheron G: Subthalamic neurons in primates: a quantitative and comparative analysis. Neuroscience 4:1717-1743, 1979

# Section 6

# Advanced Techniques in Neurosurgery

# 19

# An Assistive Surgical MRI Compatible Robot – First Prototype with Field Tests

Tapio Heikkilä[1], Sanna Yrjänä[2], Pekka Kilpeläinen[1], John Koivukangas[2] and Mikko Sallinen[1]
[1]*VTT Technical Research Centre of Finland*
[2]*Department of Neurosurgery, University of Oulu, Oulu, Finland*

## 1. Introduction

### 1.1 Overview

Magnetic Resonance Imaging (MRI) is superior to other imaging modalities in detecting diseases and pathologic tissue in the human body. The excellent soft tissue contrast allows better delineation of the pathologic and surrounding structures. For example, brain surgery requires exact three-dimensional orientation to piece together anatomical and pathological locations inside the brain. The target location can be seen in the preoperative MRI and neuroradiologists can give assessments, e.g., of tumor nature. Still, factors affecting the resection technique e.g. density of neovasculature and consistency of tumor tissue cannot always be evaluated beforehand. Intraoperative MRI (IMRI) - complementing preoperative MRI - is continuously being developed to give additional information to the neurosurgeon (Tuominen et al., 2002, Yrjänä, 2005).

Robot technology can contribute to working conditions and efficiency of IMRI operations and robots that are compatible with MRI devices represent a new and promising special field in robotics, which can improve clinical diagnostics and treatment for internal diseases, including neurologic ones (Gassert et al., 2008). There are several commercial solutions in operation for surgical robots such as Da Vinci, Minerva, NeuroMate and PathFinder just to mention few but not yet for operation in MRI devices (Zhijiang & Lining, 2003), (Dasgupta & Henderson, 2010), (Jaara, 2007). One solution for assistive surgery is the minimally surgically invasive (MIS) robot which is a large, multi-arm system (Zoppi et. al., 2010). Such kinds of systems are expensive which makes them difficult to reach common use.

### 1.2 State-of-the-art

Development of MRI compatible robots implies multidisciplinary work. Solutions from conventional robotics are not applicable as such even if the development of such a system is similar to design of a mechatronic device (Cleary & Nguyen, 2001). Strong static and coupling magnetic fields and radio frequency pulses produced by the MRI devices make for a challenging and potentially hazardous environment. Magnetic fields exert forces and eddy currents on materials that are magnetically incompatible or conduct electricity. This may lead to wrong signal information, uncertainties in actuator control and dangerous forces in the construction if they are located in too strong a magnetic field (Virtanen, 2006). Limited working space, limited access to this space, need for line of sight to MR images and comfort of patients and surgeons set additional constraints.

Analysis for optimal design for MRI compatible robots has been proposed by (Gasparetto & Zanotto, 2010). Many MRI compatible robotic devices have also been reported, for biopsies according to the target [for brain (Masamune et al., 1995), breast (Larson et al., 2004), prostate (Susil et. al., 2003)] and also to the structure of the MRI device (Chinzei & Miller, 2001), (Tsekos et al., 2005). To solve the challenge of operation in limited space, a manipulator with several degrees of freedom seems to be best solution, as also proposed in this paper. One solution for that has also been introduced by (Chinzei et. al, 2000). It has good reach by using two manipulator arms but compared to our solution, accuracy is more limited due to lack of efficient calibration. Development of a general purpose device has also been reported (Tsekos et al., 2008).

In comparison, if very high accuracy is needed, also parallel kinematic structures have been presented (Plante et. al., 2009). By constructing the manipulator using dielectric elastomer actuators, here 6 parallel, absolute position accuracy of 1,8mm Root Mean Square (rms) can be reached. Use of this kind of robot structure is limited typically to a volume of a 80x70mm$^2$ ellipse which limits its use. Operation accuracy has been improved by developing advanced human-robot co-operation where the robot guides the human during the surgery by virtual fixtures which are controlled by using force control, i.e. 6 Degrees-of-Freedom (DOF) force and torque sensor attached to the wrist of the robot (Castillo-Cruces & Wahrburg 2010).

The manipulators developed make use of different methods of actuation, mainly according to four main categories (Elhawary et. al., 2005): transmission by hydraulic or pneumatic actuators, ultrasonic motors based on the piezoceramic principle and remote manual actuation. Progress in materials, position sensing, different actuation techniques, and design strategies have contributed to the technical feasibility in MRI environments, but still most systems lack clinical validation, which is needed for commercial products (Elhawary et. al., 2005), (Gassert et al., 2008). Most advanced example is the NeuroArm (Pandya et al., 2009) which has been developed for open neurosurgical procedures in IMRI environments. NeuroArm is an image-guided, MRI compatible robotic system that is capable of both microsurgery and stereotaxy. However, it is still a manipulator type device where the robot motion control is based on surgeon's manual operations of the joystick type control devices supported by on-line visual information of the MRI device.

Our goal has been a device with portable and readily locatable kinematic structure enabling a variety of applications, like assisting biopsies, tumor operations, and installing automatic dosage implants. Especially requirements from brain surgery, originating from the IMRI guided operations at the Oulu University Hospital (Yrjänä, 2005) have been guiding our work. Semiautomatic operation was targeted where the tool, e.g., a biopsy needle is taken automatically very close to the target location ("entry point"), and final adjustment and needle motions are carried out by the surgeon or at least with tight supervision by the surgeon. The requirement for accuracy of automatic motions is at the level of +/- 1-2 mm for the needle. Finally, we sought to achieve optimal performance within a volume corresponding to that of the human head, our "region of surgical interest" (Koivukangas et al., 2003).

The dimensions of the MRI device and characteristics of the changing magnetic field sets constraints to the robot constructs and dimensions as well as the robot controller hardware (HW), as the robot should not disturb the imaging within IMRI operations, and on the other hand the imaging should not disturb the robot operation. We have developed an MRI compatible robot prototype. MRI compatibility has been introduced in (Virtanen, 2005) and robot control and calibration methods in (Heikkilä et. al, 2009). In the following we give further details about the mechanics, kinematics, calibration, control system and especially results from field tests in the IMRI premises of the Oulu University Hospital. We report to our knowledge on the first robot to repeatedly perform a preprogrammed exercise in the magnetic field of an IMRI scanner in a safe noncollision manner.

## 2. Mechanical structure and control system

The requirements for the robot prototype were derived based on the experiences of the neurosurgery group at Oulu University Hospital, acquired with IMRI premises with low field horizontally open resistive magnet 0.23 Tesla (T) scanner (Philips, 2011) with a 44 cm patient gap and optical tool navigation devices. During operations while the patient is being imaged, regular operating room products and devices are moved outside a 0.5-mT line (1.5 m from the MR image center point), or out of the imaging room so as not to disturb the imaging (Yrjänä, 2005). The robot controller should be at least outside this 0.5 mT line, or outside the operating room so that the imaging does not induce disturbances to the cables and robot controller HW and vice versa. Correspondingly, the robot main body should be located outside a 2 mT line (1 m from the image center point) to prevent disturbances from imaging to actuators and vice versa.

The MRI compatibility of the robot prototype is designed for the part of the robot which is close to or inside the MRI device during its operation. We have defined, for purposes of neuronavigation (Koivukangas et al., 1993a, b) and robot development, the "region of surgical interest" (ROSI) as the part of the human body that needs to be imaged and then operated using an image guidance method that ensures a suitable minimally invasive surgical approach followed by delineation and treatment of the tumor or other lesion (Koivukangas et al., 2003). Following this principle, our robot has similar kinematic structure as common industrial robots, but with link lengths adjusted to comply with the operation space in the ROSI. The 4th link introduces the needed MRI compatible reach into the working space close to the MR imaging center with its 1000 mm length. The 4th, 5th and 6th links and related joints are made from MRI compatible material, i.e., carbon fiber and aluminium (Virtanen & Nevala, 2007). The bearings in the two last joints are AISI 316 Stainless ball bearings (Virtanen, 2006). The base and the first three links are also made from aluminium.

Joint position sensors for the first four joints are optical encoders and for the last two joints are optical (Harja et al., 2007). The motors are located at the joints, except for the last two joints, for which they are located at the 3rd link with power transmission by nylon strings. The encoder resolutions of the joints were 0.005625 degrees (joint 1), 0.09 degrees (joint 2), 0.09 degrees (joint 3), 0.00625 degrees (joint 4), 0.06 degrees (joint 5), and 0.0125 degrees (joint 6). The repeatability of the tool position (e.g., needle) – as calculated from the encoder resolutions - is at the level of +/- 0.26 mm, +/- 0.24 mm and +/- 0.37 mm in x, y and z directions, respectively. The mechanical outlook of the robot prototype is shown in fig. 1.

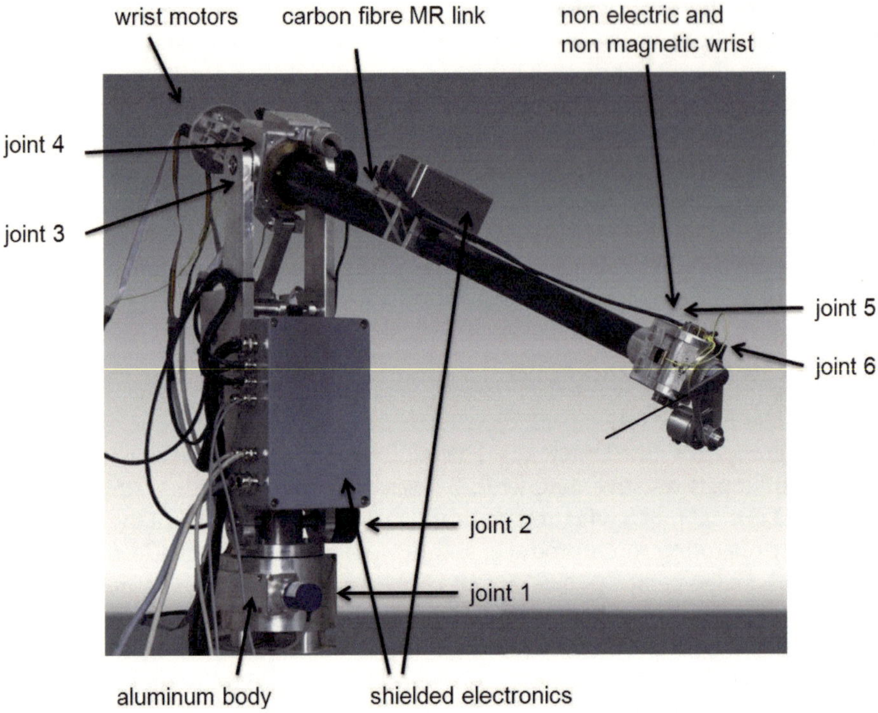


Fig. 1. Structure of the MRI compatible robot prototype.

The working space inside the MRI device is limited and accordingly there are limitations also in the 2nd and 3rd joint motions, +/- 20 degrees and +/- 42 degrees respectively. For other joints the joint limits are looser, i.e. +/- 75 degrees (6th joint) or more. In the wrist there is also a 3 DOF joystick (fig 2.) for the surgeon to control the final adjustment motions. The joystick is made from aluminum and uses fiber-optic sensors (Harja et al., 2007).

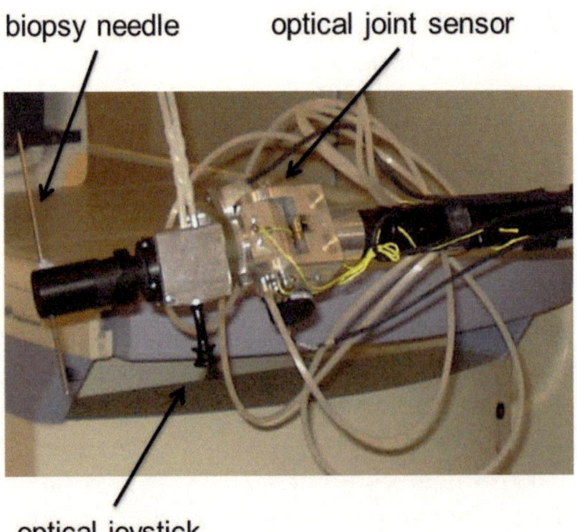


Fig. 2. Optical joystick in the robot wrist

The robot control system is based on a PC/104 controller, with integrated motor drives, and I/O cards for joint measurements and motor controls. The PC/104 controller runs a RT/Linux operating system. The control system is enclosed in RF shielded housing (Rittal Vario-Case iS; fig 3).

The robot control SW is based on RCCL (Robot Control C Library) running on the RT/Linux. The RCCL library [RWRCCL version (Stein, 2004)] implements the joint servo control, trajectory control in joint spaces as well as coordinated motion control in Cartesian space, including inverse kinematic solutions.

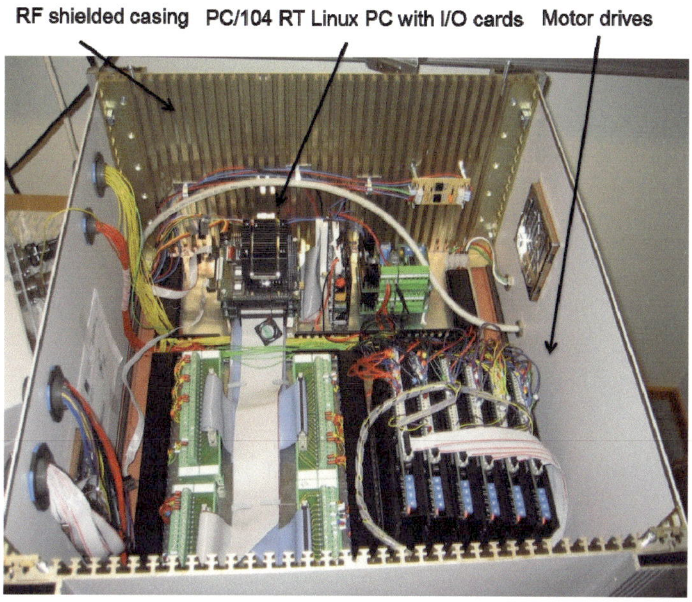


Fig. 3. Control system HW.

## 3. Work space of assistive surgical tasks

The assistive surgical tasks include presentation of surgical instruments to the surgeon in a proper location with respect to the patient. An exemplary target task goes in two phases:

1. the robot presents the biopsy tool in a proper orientation and location as defined by the surgeon based on the MRI image, and
2. the surgeon carries out the final positioning of the biopsy tool by interactive control, optionally with a redundant axis coincident with the needle axis.

The gross motion paths up to and within the ROSI are carried out by the robot automatically and the fine motions into the contact are guided by the surgeon, either by direct visual feedback from the target or supported by the MRI device. The task space for carrying out the fine motions interactively is limited, and the Cartesian paths of the interactive motions vary little by orientations and a few centimeters by translation.

A simulation model was constructed in the IGRIP simulation tool for studying the paths for brain biopsies in the robot joint space. A simulation model with the MRI compatible robot,

MRI device, and patient is illustrated in fig 4. The robot presents the biopsy tool within a few mm distance from the patients head surface (the "entry point"). In the simulations the nominal interactive paths are following the surface normal of the upper head surface of the patient. In practice the entry point and the target location finally determine the entry orientation.

Because of limitations in the joint motions and the kinematic structure of the robot, the robot base has to be located carefully to avoid singularities in joint space during the interactive motions. With simulations it was confirmed, that a feasible location is on either side of the patient. In other assistive surgical tasks the task space is similar, e.g., above the abdomen.

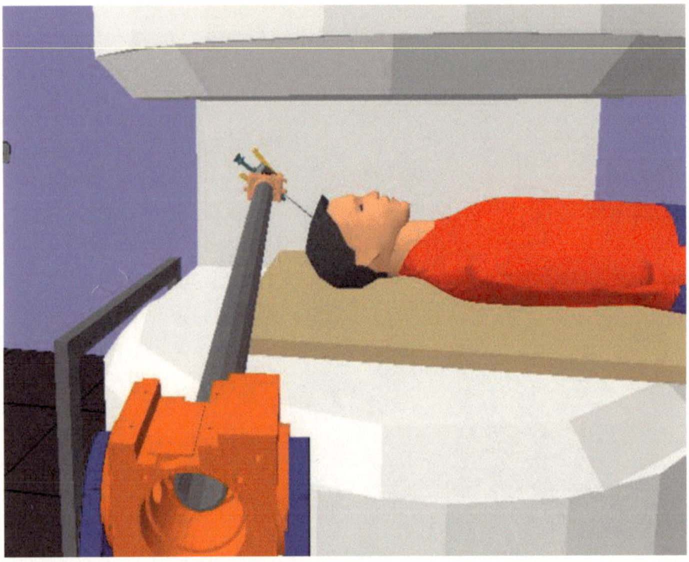

Fig. 4. A feasible entry point location of the MRI compatible robot.

## 4. Robot calibration

Robot calibration considers internal robot features like joint-axis geometries, joint angle off-sets, actuator/link compliances, actuator transmission and coupling factors (Bernhardt & Albright 1993). With precise models for these factors the absolute positioning accuracy can be brought to the level of robot repeatability. Geometric characteristics are concerned by kinematic calibration and kinematic models are usually described by the Denavit-Hartenberg (DH) convention, where the joint axis and link geometry is described as homogeneous transformations with 2 rotational and 2 translational variables. For nominally parallel axis so called modified DH model has been used (Hayati's modified model) with three rotational and 1 translational variable per axis/joint (Zuang & Roth, 1996). The kinematic model is non-linear, and model parameters are typically estimated all at the same time iteratively using the Jacobian of a measurement model. The robot tool positions are recorded together with corresponding joint values and compared to expected positions as calculated by the nominal kinematic model. With linearized error models between the expected and real poses the deviations from the models can be correlated into the form of estimated small corrections, which are added to the nominal parameter values. All independent model parameters can be calculated at the same time and the result is an optimal estimate for the parameter increments with regard to the measurements. Doing this calculation iteratively the parameter values should converge to optimal ones with regard to the measurements.

Another way to estimate the model parameters is to model the joint axis as lines in space and by measuring the robot end point motions while moving joints one-by-one, estimate the axis line models in a joint by joint manner and then calculate the kinematic model parameters from the pairs of estimated line models. The MRI compatible surgery assistant robot operates in very limited joint velocities and it has special geometric structure due to the MRI compatibility requirements - long 3rd link - and so has a special form of work space, which is additionally very limited for the second joint. Considering optimal estimation with all DH parameters estimated at the same time this introduces challenges to compose a proper sample set and fine tune the iterative estimation, e.g., in the Levenberg-Marquardt (LM) form [for details about LM estimation, see, e.g. (Manolis, 2005)]. Because of the robot characteristics and requirements we decided to go for axis-by-axis calibration and compose the DH models for the axis/links subsequently. This resulted in an intuitive calibration procedure and allowed to readily focus on improving sample sets on a joint/axis basis. Although the resulting set of parameter values is not finally optimal, based on extensive simulations it seems satisfactory in the sense of reaching the required kinematic accuracy. It should also be noted, that if finally optimal calibration is required, this kind of sequential axis-by-axis calibration can be used to acquire reliable initial values for truly optimized estimation of the kinematic parameters, e.g., by linearized kinematic models and the LM estimation.

Within the kinematic calibration each joint/link has a local coordinate system attached to the rotating axis. The transformations between the joints and links are modeled following the Denavit-Hartenberg (DH) principle with 2 rotations and 2 translations per axis (rot-trans-trans-rot) with the exception between joints 2 and 3, where modified DH is used (Hayati modification: rot-trans-rot-rot) (Zuang & Roth, 1996). The initial orientations of the local coordinates are here - for our own convenience - slightly different from the original DH convention and are aligned with the base coordinates. The rotations around different joint axes are done as follows: rot-z for the joint 1, rot-x for joints 2,3 and 5, and rot-y for joints 4 and 6 (see fig 5). There are 24 independent parameters, including the transformation from base (world) to the 1st axis and 2nd axis and excluding the tool transformation within the last link.

The calibration is based on observing a point of a calibration target in 3D space while the joint makes a circular motion. Two solutions for measuring the target 3D point were considered: a real multi camera system and a simulated high accuracy laser tracker. The real measurements were carried out with a multi-camera system, where three cameras were located around the working space of the robot (fig 5). Two cameras were located behind the robot with 2 m distance and optical axis towards robot tool and with 90 degrees angles to each other. These were used to observe motions for joints 3, 4, 5 and 6. A third camera was located on the other side of the robot with 1.5 m distance, focusing on motions of joints 1 and 2, and all three cameras were used to observe calibration motions for joints 2 and 3. The voxel accuracies for detecting the calibration target point with Basler Scout scA1400 cameras (1392x1040 pixels) and considering careful camera to camera calibrations, can be estimated to be at the level of +/- 0.5 mm for observing joints 1 and 2, and +/- 1.0 to +/- 1.4 mm for other joints. A fourth camera was used in simulations to test how it can contribute to the calibration accuracy.

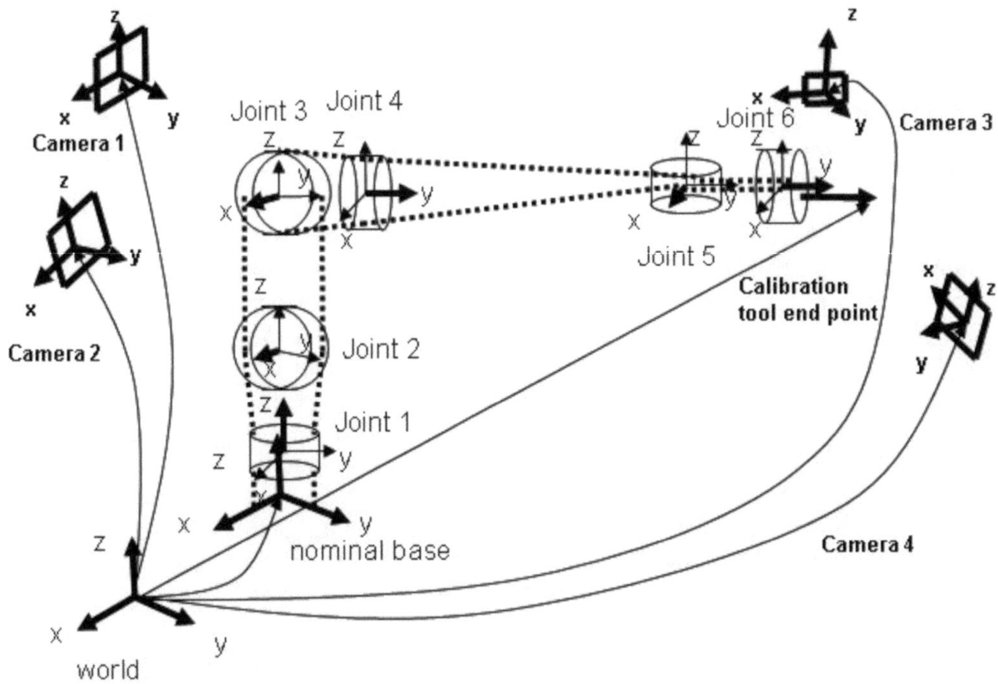


Fig. 5. Overview of the robot joint coordinate systems and a multi-camera system for kinematic calibration measurements

Radial distortion of the lenses was found to be at the level of 0.5 %, and it was corrected in the images before applying image data to the calibrations. The cameras were calibrated to a world frame - and each other - using a flat calibration "world" grid and by estimating the six pose parameters for each camera in the world coordinates. The location of the conic calibration target was measured with different cameras and a corresponding 3D point was constructed based on corrected location in image plane, the pin hole camera model and calibration data (position and orientation) of the cameras.

In the real tests a simple calibration target was observed with the multiple cameras located around the working space of the robot. The image processing routines were simple and based on background lighting and tresholding. This is robust and readily implemented, but repeating precisely same motions (same calibration object locations) will not increase the accuracy in statistical sense. Locating the calibration target object under static lighting conditions results always to a same binary image, because the robot repeatability is much better than the resolution of the camera system.. We added statistical property to the samples by taking three good base positions (fig 6.) for each joint, and added small random variation to the positions. In this way the statistical nature of the samples could be maintained while keeping the best calibration positions, and accuracy improved by increasing the size of sample sets.

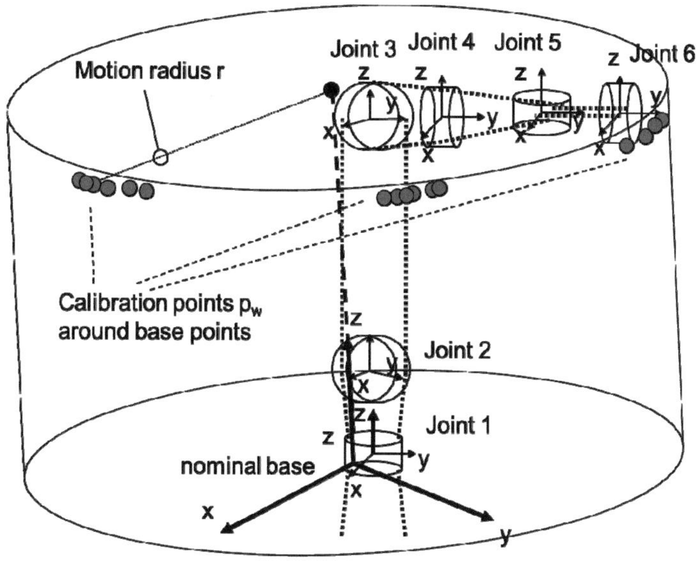


Fig. 6. Base points and their variation for the joint 1 measurements.

The line estimations were done as limited pose estimations, comparable to the pose estimation of paper rolls in (Vähä et al., 1994), with five parameters per joint axis 3D line (2 translation and 2 rotation parameters and the radius of the rotational motion). Jacobians were derived using two fitting criteria: distance of calibration point from the cylindrical surface and distance of calibration point from the plane surface of the rotational motion (circle of the calibration motion). As expected, the convergence in the estimation was in all cases very good, with max 7 to 8 iteration steps. After all the line models for all joints were measured and estimated, the related DH parameters were calculated. Details about the line estimations are given in appendix I and about deriving the DH parameters from the estimated line models are given appendix II.

The sample sets were composed based on the joint motion limits, and the goodness of sample sets was estimated with Matlab simulations. The sizes of sample sets were varied and the tresholding within the voxel accuracy and inaccuracy of the joint servos were taken into consideration; additional white noise ranging with -1, 0 or +1 times the corresponding encoder resolution, was added to the joint values. The simulated sample sizes were 21, 42, 98, and 182 points. In addition, the largest sample set was simulated with a voxel noise corresponding to a more accurate camera (Basler Scout scA1600, with pixel resolution 1628 x 1236) (samples 182/0.75). Simulated results for the DH parameter variation after joint axis estimation are shown in fig 7.

Clearly for all parameters except one it is possible to reach a standard deviation less than 0.1 mm. Bias remains in all parameters independent of the sample sizes; for the translation across the second link axis it is comparably large because of the strict limitation in the joint 2 motions. It was also easily found in the simulations that the bias can be removed if the base points for the axis can be symmetrically spread over the rotation space, with 120 degrees angles between the base points. This is, however, not possible as the joint limits are hard for joints 2, 3, and 5.

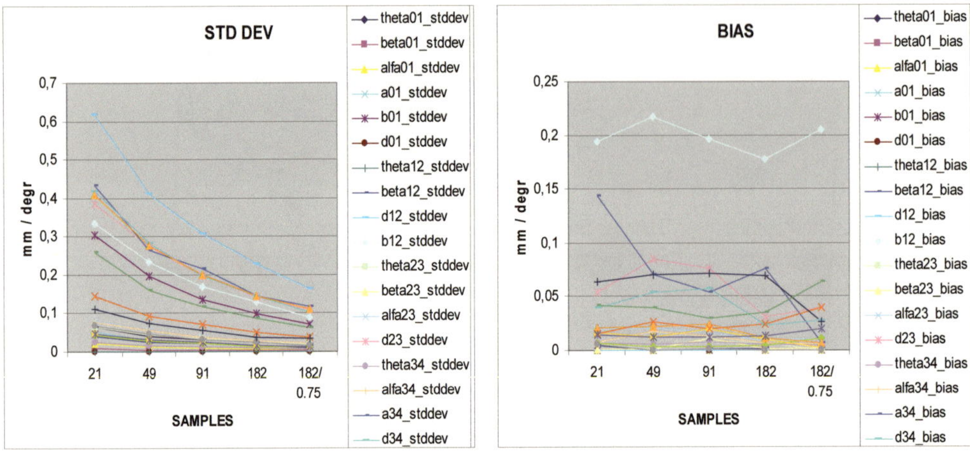


Fig. 7. Standard deviations and bias of the DH parameters

In addition, the tool positioning accuracy was estimated based on the variations of the DH parameters and joint uncertainties (+/- 1 joint encoder pulse). The variation of the end tip location of a biopsy needle (150 mm) was calculated by propagating the covariances of the link/joint transformations from robot base to last link, based on the variances of the DH parameters. Bias was taken as an additive factor to the mean of the corresponding parameters. It was seen, that +/- 1 mm standard deviation is achievable, comparable to +/- 3 mm maximum variation. Lowest estimation accuracy is clearly for the translations parameters between joints 2 and 3, and 3 and 4. The reason is in the limits of the joint 2 motions. The calibration procedure was carried out also with the real robot and a multi-camera system. The results were in expected limits (max deviations from nominal parameter values were less than 1.5 mm), though more thorough testing would give more reliable results and especially details concerning different parameters.

Simulation tests were also carried out using the target tracking accuracy of a Leica Lasertracker (Leica, 2003), for which the absolute measurement accuracy is +/- 0.036 mm. In this case the sample size was 42 points for joints 1 and 2, and 21 points for other joints. The standard deviations were less than 0.08 mm for the translation parameters and 0.0095 degrees for the rotation parameters. Maximum deviations were less than +/- 0.21 mm for the translation parameters and +/- 0.035 degrees for rotation parameters. Cumulative maximum translation deviation was at the level of +/- 0.6 mm for translation parameters, and +/- 0.085 degree for the rotations of the 3 first joints; these are dominating rotations from the point of view of tool locating accuracy because of the long links from the joints up to the tool end tip. This means that with high-end calibration sensors the required kinematic accuracy can readily be achieved.

## 5. Tests in the IMRI premises

The robot prototype was tested in the 0.23 T intraoperative MRI environment. The used scanner has a C-shaped open configuration with a vertical magnetic field. The premises has been routinely used for neurosurgical operations. The biopsy tool tracking has been achieved using optical 3D tracking devices (Northern Digital, 2011) and registration tags to integrate the patient location and the MR images (Tuominen et al., 2002).

The prototype was fixed to a floor worktop which was set over two props for the tests. Using this arrangement the prototype could be moved to desired points around the scanner. The tests had the following endpoints:

1. Test functionality of the prototype in the magnetic field.
2. Test MR safety and compatibility of the prototype, and
3. Test capability of the robot to move a biopsy needle guide to the correct configuration to allow the surgeon to pass a biopsy needle through the guide to a target

The functionality of the 6 DOF surgical robot was confirmed. It was found capable of positioning an instrument to the desired point and orientation, thus indicating the surgical trajectory from the surface of a target inside the target in the magnetic field. The joystick could be used to move the pointing instrument from the surface of the target inside the target under visual control. Motions of the prototype were fluent except at the margins of the motion ranges (fig. 8).

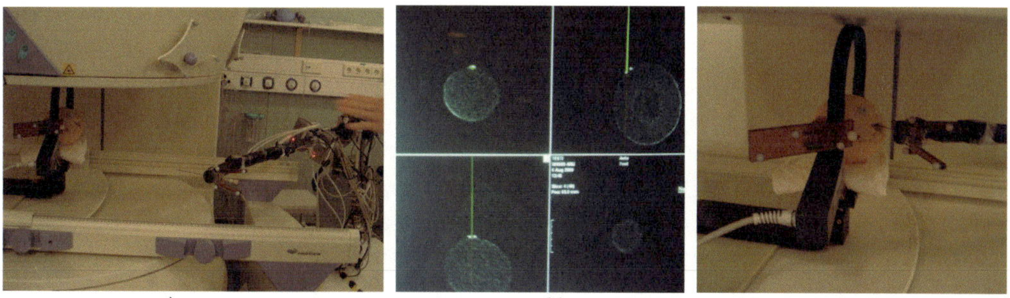

a) b) c)

Fig. 8. The surgical robot driven to desired position simulating a biopsy procedure: a) motion towards a target (melon) entry point, b) control view with an custom made optical neuronavigator UI, c) biopsy needle inserted to the target (melon).

The prototype entity was found to be MR safe, but 5th and 6th joints interfered with imaging because of temporarily used incompatible fasterner screws. These joints were removed before continuing to the test biopsy. Motors 1 and 4 also malfunctioned when the main body of the robot was within the 20 mT (200 Gauss) fringe field, but the robot could be repositioned to avoid malfunction. All control electronics functioned inside the imaging room but the robot was controlled without displays to minimize electromagnetic noise. The keyboard caused disturbances and needed to be turned off during imaging. Servo motors caused some noise in the MR images despite the EMC shielding box.

The capability of the prototype to pass a biopsy needle guide to a correct configuration was tested with a melon (cucumis melo) fixed to an intraoperative RF coil integrated head holder A fatty vitamin capsule was inserted inside the melon before it was placed for the MR imaging and scanned using a fast field echo imaging sequence. The needle guide was fixed to a 10 cm long extension piece which was applied to the robot arm in place of the 5th and 6th joints. The robot prototype was then programmed to drive the needle guide to a distance 10 mm from the surface of the melon. The tip of the biopsy needle was driven into correct position first using the joystick controls. The robot was then programmed to repeat a series of non-collision steps to reposition the needle correctly to aforementioned position. The actual biopsy procedure was then simulated by passing the biopsy needle by hand through the guide until the tip of the needle hit the vitamin capsule inside the melon. A tag of the optical tool tracking system was connected to the biopsy needle and the tool tracking was used to guide and verify the insertion successfully, including the entry and final locations of the needle tip inside the melon (fig 8 b).

## 6. Discussion

A working readily maneuverable robot prototype has been constructed. The working space is generally limited, but suitable for IMRI related operations in the region of surgical interest. Motion control based on the RCCL library was quick to implement and was easily used as far as robots paths needed to be programmed. Because the Cartesian speed of a tool (e.g., a biopsy needle) can be very low (ca. 5 cm / sec), the feasibility of joint trajectories has been achieved in test runs.

The kinematic calibration was carried out in a simple and straightforward way. The limitations of joints, especially for joint 2, clearly caused the largest estimation uncertainties in the related DH parameters. Based on simulations the required accuracy is still achievable if the laser tracker is used for tracking the calibration target. A multi camera system can be used as well, but usability with the ordinary cameras we have been using is limited for cross checking the kinematic parameter values. Still, for interactive control of fine motions with tight integration of the surgeon this is enough. For more advanced automatic motion control the remaining uncertainties would require laser tracker based calibration.

From the presented ROSI principle it follows, that the surgical guidance device must be optimized for functionality in the volume of the ROSI, which in neurosurgery means that of the human head. This involves dividing the tasks of the robot into gross and local movements. This was achieved in the present tests by robotic movement of the needle guide to a predetermined position 10 mm from the target followed by manual passage of the needle to the target.

The longer term goal is to integrate the robot and its usage tighter with MR images. This will lead to integration of the MRI device with respect to the robot coordinate system and then using the same technology for tracking the tool attached to the robot end tip. This will substantially loosen the accuracy requirements of the robot: global accuracy will be taken care by the optical tracking tool [currently at the level of +/- 0.7 mm (Katisko, 2007)] after which local accuracy of the robot becomes critical, just like in the case of interactive control. It is also noteworthy that there are varying IMRI practices for imaging and operating, e.g., the following (Yrjänä, 2005):

- Imager lowered for surgery
- Surgery in fringe field
- Surgery in adjacent Operation Room
- Magnetic field turned off for surgery
- Surgery in imaging space
- Surgery adjacent to the imaging space
- Imager moved away for surgery

Depending on the case, the requirements for the robot may vary quite much. We have reached the level of a prototype principally compatible with the IMRI premises and optimized for the ROSI. However, the varying imaging and operating practices create challenges for deciding the next stages of development.

The present robot project was a logical continuation in our research community of early experience with the development of neuronavigation based on a 6 DOF passive mechatronic arm (Koivukangas et al., 1993a, b). This device was routinely clinically used for image-guided procedures, guiding a variety of instruments in the same way as optical tracking systems. The mechatronic arm had joints that were designed to house both electromagnetic clutch brakes and servo motors.

The rationale for developing an active robot arose from the need to transfer the result of presurgical planning directly to the surgical field, like by the Robodoc (Bargar et. al. 1998), which can be preprogrammed to create an optimal boney fit for prostheses in hip and knee replacement surgery. From the other reported IMRI developments the present robot differs in that it was specified to perform safe preprogrammed movement of a needle guide to the target in the region of surgical interest and to act as a stative, or needle guide holder, while the surgeon passes the biopsy needle or forceps to the target--all of this in the magnetic field of an IMRI scanner. It was a necessary first step to confirm the functionality and accuracy of our robotic solution. With continued experience in both robotics and image-guided surgery, our group plans on extending the functionality of the robot.

## 7. Conclusions

A prototype robot for assisting surgery operations in IMRI environments was described in this paper. We reported on the robot to repeatedly perform a preprogrammed exercise in the magnetic field of an IMRI scanner in a safe noncollision manner. The target was a fatty vitamin pill placed inside a melon. The robot brought the end effector into the region of surgical interest and positioned the tip of the needle guide holder 10 mm from the object, serving as a stereotactic device to enable the passage of the biopsy instrument to its exact final target.

The mechatronic structure, calibration and experimental tests in an IMRI environment were explained in more details. Simulations showed that expected locating accuracy from the point of view of joint sensors and calibrations sensors can be achieved. The robot could be operated in a semiautomatic manner, either running paths or interactively using joystick, in joint space or Cartesian space. Field tests in the hospital IMRI unit confirmed the applicability of the system in the region of surgical interest even under MRI conditions.

## 8. Appendix I: Estimation of the axis as a line in space

The calibration is carried out in a joint by joint manner. Each joint is moved one by one, and the end tip 3D coordinates of the calibration object is recorded in world frame. For each joint motion a 3D line model of the joint is calculated, which results to six 3D line models in the world frame. From these line models the DH parameters are further calculated.

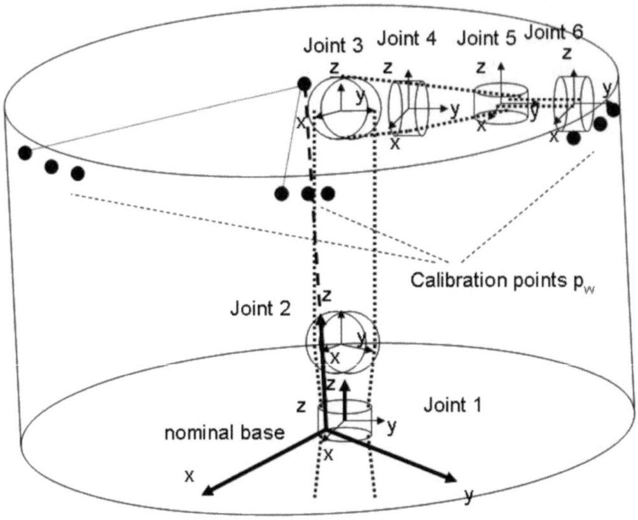


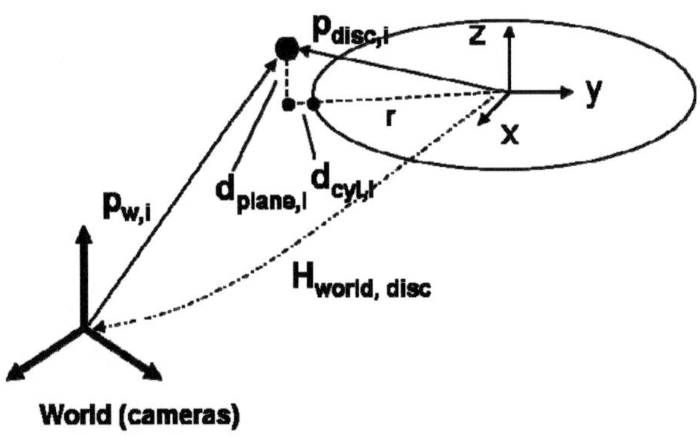


The robot makes a rotary calibration motion around the calibrated axis, where the measured end point of the arm tip forms a "disc" in space. Then the parameters of the calibrated axis are given as a pose $\overline{H}_{world,disc}$ which is presented in a homogeneous matrix form in zyx Euler form:

$$\overline{p}_{i,disc} = \overline{H}_{world,disc} * \overline{p}_{i,world}$$

for which

$$\overline{H}_{world,disc} = f\left(\overline{\theta}\right)$$

Let the state vector $\overline{\theta}_{all}$ all be composed of the parameters of the calibrated axis and related calibration data:

$$\overline{\theta}_{all} = \left[\overline{\theta} \quad r\right]$$

where

$\theta$ is the vector of pose parameters and,
$r$ is the radius of the rotation "disc", i.e., around the axis.

The pose parameters of the "disc" are then

$$\bar{\theta} = \begin{bmatrix} \alpha & \beta & \chi & x & y & z \end{bmatrix}^T$$

where
$\alpha$ is rotation around x axis,
$\beta$ is rotation around y axis
$\chi$ is rotation around z axis, here undefined,
$x$ is x coordinate,
$y$ is y coordinate,
$z$ is z coordinate,

We have nominal values for the "disc" pose parameters, to which the measured 3D points are matched. Because the rotational part of the "disc" pose are non-linear, we define two error measures, related to which we linearize the measurement model.

Let the error measure for point *i* be

$$\bar{e}_i = \begin{bmatrix} d_{plane,i} \\ d_{cyl,i} \end{bmatrix}$$

where $d_{plane,i}$ is distance from the measured point to the disc plane and

$d_{cyl,i}$ is distance from the measured point to the cylindrical surface set by the disc

The nominal disc location is always in origin, so the distance from the measured point to the disc plane is the z coordinate of the measured point in the disc pose:

$$d_{plane} = \bar{p}_{disc,z}$$

The distance from the cylindrical surface of the disc is in a similar way

$$d_{cyl} = \sqrt{p_{s,disc,x}^2 + p_{s,disc,y}^2} - r$$

Now we derive the linear relationship between the error measure and the state parameters:

$$\frac{\partial \bar{e}}{\partial \bar{\theta}} = \frac{\partial \bar{e}}{\partial \bar{p}_{disc}} * \frac{\partial \bar{p}_{disc}}{\partial \bar{\theta}}$$

for which

$$\frac{\partial d_{plane}}{\partial \bar{p}_{disc}} = \frac{\partial \bar{p}_{disc,z}}{\partial \bar{p}_{disc}} = \begin{bmatrix} 0 & 0 & 1 \end{bmatrix}$$

and

$$\frac{\partial d_{cyl}}{\partial \bar{p}_{disc}} = \left[ \frac{p_{disc,x}}{\sqrt{p_{s,disc,x}^2 + p_{s,disc,y}^2}} \quad \frac{p_{disc,y}}{\sqrt{p_{s,disc,x}^2 + p_{s,disc,y}^2}} \quad 0 \right]$$

The partial derivatives of the measured point in the disc pose are

$$\frac{\partial \bar{p}_{disc}}{\partial \bar{\theta}} = \begin{bmatrix} 0 & p_{disc,z} & -p_{disc,y} & 1 & 0 & 0 \\ -p_{disc,z} & 0 & p_{disc,x} & 0 & 1 & 0 \\ p_{disc,y} & -p_{disc,x} & 0 & 0 & 0 & 1 \end{bmatrix}$$

The 3rd column will be omitted, because the rotation around the calibrated axis, i.e., around the z-axis of the disc pose cannot be estimated.

For the radius of the disc we get

$$\frac{\partial d_{cyl}}{\partial r} = -1$$

Finally the estimate the parameter increments for the updated 6 parameters (rotation around z axis omitted):

$$\Delta\bar{\theta} = \begin{pmatrix} \Delta\alpha \\ \Delta\beta \\ \Delta x \\ \Delta y \\ \Delta z \\ \Delta r \end{pmatrix} = -\left(\bar{J}^T * \bar{J}\right)^{-1} * \bar{J}^T * \bar{e}$$

where the Jacobian

$$\bar{J} = \frac{\partial \bar{e}}{\partial \bar{\theta}}$$

The complete estimation algorithm is as follows:

0. set initial disc pose and radius
1. calculate nominal calibration point positions in disc frame
2. calculate error measures for each calibration point
3. calculate the Jacobian, i.e., the partial derivatives
6. calculate parameters increments for the state parameters
7. update the state parameters
8. if increments not 'small enough', go to 1, otherwise end.

## 9. Appendix II: From line models to DH parameters

Measured axis lines are given as an arbitrary point in the line $p_i$ and a normalized direction vector $n_i$. From a pair of these the DH parameters or modified DH parameters will be derived.

**DH parameters**

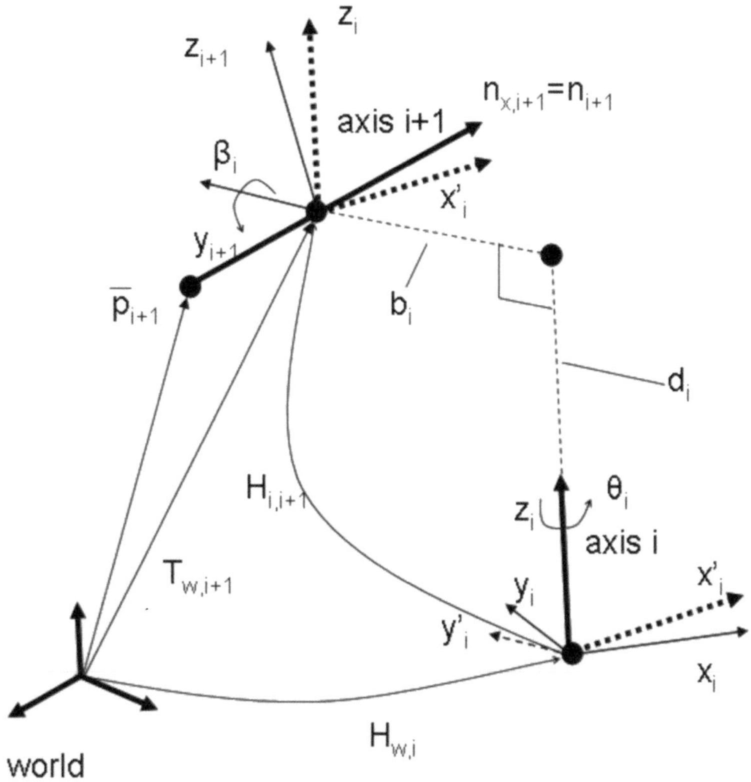


Transformation from the joint *i* coordinates to joint *i+1* coordinates goes, according to the DH parameters, in four steps:

- rotate $H_i$ around $z_i$ with $\theta_i$ so that $x_{i+1}$ aligns with the $zx_i$ plane
- transfer $H_i$ along $z_i$ with $d_i$ to a point where distance from $x_{i+1}$ is shortest
- transfer $H_i$ along $y_i$ with $b_i$ to an intersection point with $x_{i+1}$
- rotate $H_i$ around $y_i$ with $\beta_i$ so that $x_{i+1}$ aligns with $x_i$

The transformation from world/base coordinates, in which the lines are measured, to the local coordinates of joint I can be divided to rotation and translation parts:

$$H_{w,i} = \begin{bmatrix} \overline{R}_{w,i} & \overline{T}_{w,i} \end{bmatrix}$$

For the rotation between the joint coordinates *i* and *i+1* we start from the unit vectors of the transformation.

$$R_{i,i+1} = \begin{bmatrix} \overline{n}_{x,i,i+1} & \overline{n}_{y,i,i+1} & \overline{n}_{z,i,i+1} \end{bmatrix}$$

Unit vector of x is aligned with the axis of joint *i+1*, and so we can derive the unit vectors for y and z:

$$\overline{n}_{y,i+1} = \frac{\overline{n}_{z,i} \times \overline{n}_{x,i+1}}{\left\| \overline{n}_{z,i} \times \overline{n}_{x,i+1} \right\|}$$

$$\overline{n}_{z,i+1} = \overline{n}_{x,i+1} \times \overline{n}_{y,i+1}$$

Axis of joint *i+1*, i.e., $n_{x,i+1}$ in joint *i* coordinates is then

$$\overline{n}_{x,i+1,i} = \overline{H}_{w,i}^{-1} * \overline{n}_{x,i+1}$$

and as coordinates

$$\overline{n}'_{x,i+1,i} = \begin{bmatrix} x_{n,x,i+1,i} \\ y_{n,x,i+1,i} \\ z_{n,x,i+1,i} \end{bmatrix}$$

Then we get for the angle $\theta_i$

$$\theta_i = a\tan(\frac{y_{n,x,i+1,i}}{x_{n,x,i+1,i}})$$

and for the angle $\beta_i$

$$\beta_i = -a\sin(z_{n,x,i+1,i})$$

For the translation in direction of $y_{i,i+1}$ we get the same as the distance $b_i$ between the axis i and axis i+1:

The point of axis *i+1* after rotation by $\theta_i$ as $H_{i,\theta}$

$$\overline{H}_{\theta,i} = \begin{bmatrix} \cos(\theta) & -\sin(\theta) & 0 & 0 \\ \sin(\theta) & \cos(\theta) & 0 & 0 \\ 0 & 0 & 1 & 0 \\ 0 & 0 & 0 & 1 \end{bmatrix}$$

and

$$\overline{p}_{1,i,i+1} = \overline{H}_{w,i}^{-1} * \overline{H}_{\theta,i}^{-1} * \overline{p}_{1,w,i+1}$$

Then we get

$$b_i = \overline{p}_{i,i+1,y}$$

Axis $i+1$ is located in the direction of the rotated $xz$ plane, with the distance of $b_i$ from this plane. The point in axis $i+1$ which is closest to axis $i$ is also located in rotated $yz$ plane. From point $p$ this closest point locates to the direction of $x_{i+1}$ with the following coefficient

$$k = -\frac{p_{i,i+1,x}}{n_{x,i,i+1}}$$

and then the point gets the z coordinate and also the translation along the $z$-axis of $H_{w,i}$ as

$$d_i = p_{i,i+1,z} + k * z_{nxi,i+1}$$

**Modified DH parameters**

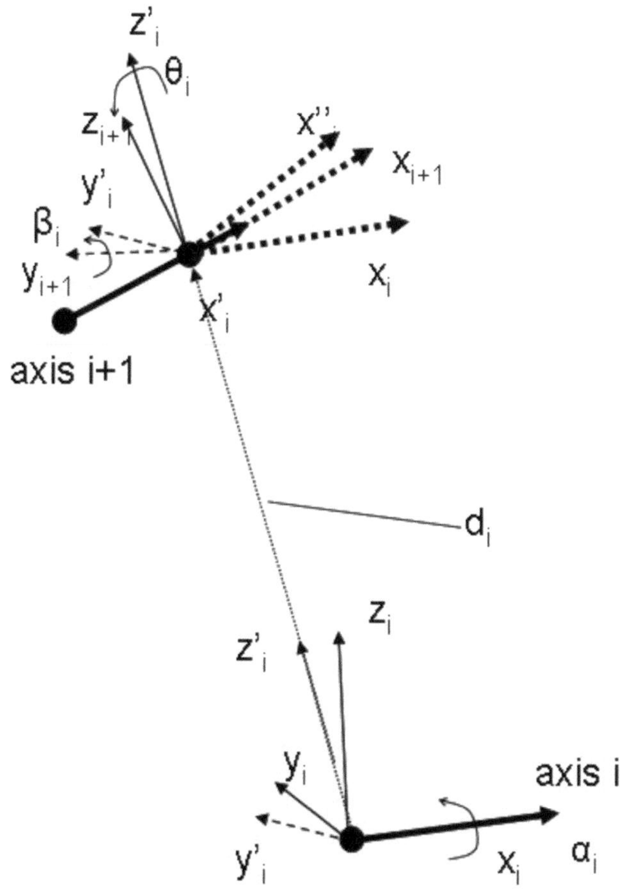


Transformation from the joint $i$ coordinates to joint $i+1$ coordinates goes, according to the modified DH parameters, in four steps:

- rotation around $x$ axis $i$ with $a_i$ to direct $z$ axis towards axis $i+1$
- translation of $H_i$ with $d_i$ to intersect the axis $i+1$
- rotate around $z$ with $\theta_i$ and
- rotate around $y$ with $\beta_i$ so that the coordinate systems are aligned

The distance of the point of axis *i+1* in the *zy* plane of the frame $H_i$ is the *x* coordinate of point $p_{i+1}$ in the axis *i+1*. The intersection point of the axis *i+1* with the *zy* plane - and the origin of the frame $H_{i+1}$ becomes then

$$H_{w,i} = \begin{bmatrix} \overline{R}_{w,i} & \overline{T}_{w,i} \end{bmatrix}$$

For the translation between the joint coordinate systems we get

$$\overline{T}_{i,i+1} = \overline{p}_{i,i+1} + \frac{p_{i,i+1,x}}{n_{i,i+1,x}} * \overline{n}_{i,i+1}$$

and the rotation angle $a_i$ becomes then

$$\alpha_{i,i+1} = a\tan\left(\frac{T_{i,i+1,y}}{T_{i,i+1,z}}\right)$$

The link transformation after rotation $a_i$ becomes then

$$\overline{H}_{\alpha,i} = \begin{bmatrix} 1 & 0 & 0 & T_{i,i+1,x} \\ 0 & \cos(\alpha) & -\sin(\alpha) & T_{i,i+1,y} \\ 0 & \sin(\alpha) & \cos(\alpha) & T_{i,i+1,z} \\ 0 & 0 & 0 & 1 \end{bmatrix}$$

and further

$$\overline{H}_{\alpha,i} = \begin{bmatrix} \overline{R}_{i,i+1,\alpha} & T_{i,i+1} \\ 0 \ \ 0 \ \ 0 & 1 \end{bmatrix}$$

where

$$\overline{R}_{i,i+1,\alpha} = \begin{bmatrix} \overline{n}_{x,i,i+1,\alpha} & \overline{n}_{y,i,i+1,\alpha} & \overline{n}_{z,i,i+1,\alpha} \end{bmatrix}$$

For the *y* and *z* axis for the frame $H_{i+1}$ we get then

$$\overline{n}_{y,i+1} = \frac{\overline{n}_{z,i,i+1,\alpha} \times \overline{n}_{x,i+1}}{\left\| \overline{n}_{z,i,i+1,\alpha} \times \overline{n}_{x,i+1} \right\|}$$

$$\overline{n}_{z,i+1} = \overline{n}_{x,i+1} \times \overline{n}_{y,i+1}$$

The direction vector of the axis i+1 becomes after the rotation $a_i$ around *x* axis *i*

$$\overline{n}_{1,i,i+1,\alpha} = \overline{H}_{a,i}^{-1} * \overline{n}_{i,i+1}$$

The rotation angle $\theta_i$ around $z$ axis is then

$$\theta_{i,i+1} = a\tan\left(\frac{n_{i,i+1,\alpha,y}}{n_{i,i+1,\alpha,x}}\right)$$

The link transformation after rotation $\theta_i$ becomes then

$$\overline{H}_{\alpha,\theta,i} = \overline{H}_{\alpha,i} * \overline{H}_{\theta,i}$$

where

$$\overline{H}_{\theta,i} = \begin{bmatrix} \cos(\theta) & -\sin(\theta) & 0 & 0 \\ \sin(\theta) & \cos(\theta) & 0 & 0 \\ 0 & 0 & 1 & 0 \\ 0 & 0 & 0 & 1 \end{bmatrix}$$

The transformation can be given also with the rotation and translation parts

$$\overline{H}_{\alpha,\theta,i} = \begin{bmatrix} \overline{R}_{i,i+1,\alpha,\theta,i} & T_{i,i+1} \\ 0 \quad 0 \quad 0 & 1 \end{bmatrix}$$

where

$$\overline{R}_{i,i+1,\alpha,\theta} = \begin{bmatrix} \overline{n}_{x,i,i+1,\alpha,\theta} & \overline{n}_{y,i,i+1,\alpha,\theta} & \overline{n}_{z,i,i+1,\alpha,\theta} \end{bmatrix}$$

Finally the rotation angle $\beta_i$ around y axis is

$$\beta_{i,i+1} = -a\tan\left(\frac{n_{i,i+1,\alpha,\theta,z}}{n_{i,i+1,\alpha,\theta,x}}\right)$$

## 10. Acknowledgements

The Oulu medical robotics community has over 20 years of experience in the field of medical applications, and some earlier contributions of it are also referred to in the text. The authors would like to acknowledge many colleagues who contributed to the realization of the robot prototype: Yrjö Louhisalmi LicTech (ME), Prof. Kalervo Nevala PhD (ME), Jani Virtanen PhD, Jani Katisko LicTech (biophysics), Pekka Isto PhD, Tapani Koivukangas MS (ME), Pirkka Tukeva MS (ME), Matti Annala engineer, and Jari Hämeenaho technician.

## 11. References

Bargar W. L., Bauer A., Börner M. Primary and revision total hip replacement using the Robodoc system. Clin Orthop Relat Res. 1998, Sep;(354):82-91.

Bernhardt R. & Albright S. (1993). Introduction. In Bernhardt R., Albright S (eds.): *Robot Calibration*, Chapman & Hall, Cambridge 1993, 311 p.

Castillo-Cruces R. & Wahrburg J. (2010). Virtual fixtures with autonomous error compensation for human-robot cooperative tasks. *Robotica* (2010) Vol 28, 2, pp. 267-277.

Chinzei K. & Miller K. (2001). MRI guided surgical robot, In: *Proceedings of the Australian Conference of Robotics and Automation*, Sydney 2001, pp. 50–55.

Chinzei K., Hata N., Jolesz F.A., Kikinis R. (2000). MR Compatible Surgical Assist Robot: System Integration and Preliminary Feasibility Study. In: *Proceedings of the 3rd International Conferece of Medical Image Computing and Computer-Assisted Intervention*, Pittsburg, Pennsylvenia, USA, 11-14 October. 2000; pp. 921-930.

Cleary K. & Nguyen C. (2001). State of the Art in Surgical Robotics: Clinical Applications and Technology Challenges. *Computer Aided Surgery*, November 2001. 26p

Dasgupta P., Henderson A., (2010). Robotic urological surgery. *Robotica* (2010) Vol 28, pp. 235-240.

Elhawary H., Zivanovic A., Davies B. & Lamperth M. (2005), A review of magnetic resonance imaging compatible manipulators in surgery. *Proceedings of IMechE*, Vol. 220 Part H: Journal of Engineering in Medicine, pp. 413 - 424.

Gasparetto A., Zanotto V. (2010). Toward an optimal performance index for neurosurgical robot's design. *Robotica* (2010) Vol 28, pp. 279-296

Gassert R., Burdet E, & Chinzei K. (2008). MRI-Compatible Robotics. A Critical Tool for Image-Guided Interventions, Clinical Diagnostics, and Neuroscience. *IEEE Engineering in in Medicine and Biology Magazine*, May/June 2008, pp. 12 - 14.

Harja J., Tikkanen J., Sorvoja H. & Myllylä, R. (2007). Magnetic resonance imaging-compatible, three-degrees-of-freedom joystick for surgical robot. *The International Journal of Medical Robotics and Computer Assisted Surgery*, Vol.3, Issue 4, (December 2007), 7 p.

Heikkilä T., Isto P., Järviluoma M., Kilpeläinen P., Sallinen M. (2009). A Prototype for an Assistive Surgical MRI Compatible Robot. *The 14th IASTED International Conference on Robotics and Applications - RA 2009*. November 4 – 6, 2009, Cambridge, Massachusetts, USA.

Jaara J. (2007). *Designing surgical robot for clinical robot for MR-imaging environment.* Diploma thesis, University of Oulu (in finnish). 60p + 12p appendixes.

Katisko J & Koivukangas J (2007) Optically neuronavigated ultrasonography in an intraoperative magnetic resonance imaging environment. *Neurosurgery* 60(4 Suppl 2): 373–381.

Koivukangas J., Louhisalmi Y., Alakuijala J., Oikarinen J. (1993a) Ultrasound-controlled neuronavigator-guided brain surgery. *J Neurosurg* 79: 36-42.

Koivukangas J., Louhisalmi Y., Alakuijala J., Oikarinen J. (1993b) Neuronavigator-guided cerebral biopsy. *Acta Neurochir Suppl* 58: 71-74.

Koivukangas J, Katisko J, Yrjänä S, Tuominen J, Schiffbauer H, Ilkko E (2003) Successful neurosurgical 0.23T intraoperative MRI in a shared facility. Neurosurgery 2003. Monduzzi Editore Medimond: 439-444.

Larson B. T., Erdman A. G., Tsekos N. V., Yacoub E., Tsekos P. V. & Koutlas I. G. (2004). Design of an MRI-compatible robotic stereotactic device for minimally invasive interventions in the breast, *Journal of Biomechanical Engineering*, vol. 126, pp. 458–465.

Leica Geosystems (2003). *Leica Absolute Tracker™ With PowerLock Active Vision Technology.* Available from http://www.leica-geosystems.com/en/Laser-Tracker-Systems-Leica-Absolute-Tracker_69047.htm

Manolis I. (2005). A. A brief description of the Levenberg-Marquardt algorithm implemented by levmar. *Foundation for research and technology,* Heraklion, 2005.

Masamune, K., Kobayashi E., Masutani Y., Suzuki M., Dohi T., Iseki H. & Takakura K.(1995). Development of an MRI-compatible needle insertion manipulator for stereotactic neurosurgery. *Journal of Image Guided Surgery*, vol. 1, pp. 242–248.

Northern Digital Inc. (2011). *Polaris Family of Optical Tracking Systems.* Available from: http://www.ndigital.com/medical/polarisfamily.php

Ojala, R. (2002). *MR-guided interventions at 0.23T. Facilities, user interface, guiding technology and musculoskeletal applications.* PhD Thesis, University of Oulu, 73 p.

Pandya S., Motkoski J. W., Serrano-Almeida C., Greer A. D., Latour I., Sutherland G. R., Advancing Neurosurgery with Image-Guided Robotics. *Journal of Neurosurgery* 111:1141-1149, 2009.

Philips, Panorama 0.23T R/T Manufacturer Specifications (2011). Available from http://www.medwow.com/med/mri/philips/panorama-0-23t-r-t/28837.model-spec

Plante J-S., Lauren M., DeVita K., Kacher D., Roebuck J., DiMaio S., Jolesz F. & Dubowsky S. An MRI-Compatible Needle Manipulator Concept Based on Elastically Averaged Dielectric Elastomer Actuators for Prostate Cancer Treatment: An Accuracy and MR-Compatibility Evaluation in Phantoms. *Journal of Medical Devices*, Sep. 2009, Vol 3. 10p.

Stein, M. (2004). RWRCCL: *A New RCCL Implementation Using Real-Time Linux And A Single CPU.* Available from:
http://faculty.rwu.edu/mstein/verbiage/RWRCCL.pdf

Susil R. C., Krieger A., Derbyshire J. A., Tanacs A., Whitcomb L. L., Fichtinger G. & Atalar E. (2003). System for MR image-guided prostate interventions: Canine study, *Radiology*, vol. 228, pp. 886–894.

Tsekos N. V., Ozcan A. & Christoforou E. (2005). A prototype manipulator for MR-guided interventions inside standard cylindrical MRI scanners. *Journal of Biomechanical Engineering*, vol. 127, pp. 972–980.

Tsekos N., Christoforou E. & Özcan, A. (2008). A General-Purpose MR-Compatible Robotic System - Implementation and Image Guidance for Performing Minimally Invasive Interventions. *IEEE in Engineering and Biology Magazine*, May/June 2008, pp. 51 - 58.

Tuominen, J., Yrjänä S. K., Katisko J. P., Heikkilä J., Koivukangas J (2002) Intraoperative imaging in a comprehensive neuronavigation environment for minimally invasive brain tumor surgery. *Acta Neurochir Suppl* 85: 115-120.

Virtanen, J. (2006). *Enhancing the compatibility of surgical robots with magnetic resonance imaging.* PhD Thesis, University of Oulu, 2006. 196 p.

Virtanen, J. & Nevala, K. (2007). MR- compatibility of an intraoperative robot. *12th IFToMM Word Congress*, Besancon, France, June 18-21, 2007. 6 p.

Vähä P., Heikkilä T., Röning J. & Okkonen J. (1994). Machine of the Future: An Intelligent Paper Roll Manipulator. *Mechatronics*, Vol. 4, No. 8, pp. 861 - 877.

Yrjänä S. (2005). *Implementation of 0.23 T magnetic resonance scanner to perioperative imaging in neurosurgery*. PhD Thesis, University Of Oulu, 2005, 71 p.

Zhijiang D., Lining S. Review of Surgical Robotics and Key Technologies Analysis. In: *Proceedings of the IEEE International Conference on Robotics, Intelligent Systems and Signal Processing*. Changsha, China, October 2003, pp. 1041 – 1046.

Zoppi M., Khan M., Schäfer F., Molfino R. (2010). Toward lean minimally invasive robotic surgery. *Robotica* (2010) Vol 28, pp. 185-197.

Zuang H. & Roth Z. (1996). *Camera-Aided Robot Calibration*. CRC Press Inc., Florida, USA, 1996, 353 p.

# 20

# Robotic Catheter Operating Systems for Endovascular Neurosurgery

Shuxiang Guo, Jian Guo, Nan Xiao and Takashi Tamiya
*Kagawa University*
*Japan*

## 1. Introduction

With the quickening pace of modern life, the brain diseases of people are increasing, such as cerebral aneurysm and infarction and so on. The traditional surgery spends patients a lot of operation time and has long recovery time, the burden on patients is heavy. Intracavity intervention is expected to become increasingly popular in the medical practice, both for diagnosis and for surgery. A lot of diagnosis and medical surgery with an endoscope or a catheter are performed for minimally invasive surgery recently. There are a lot of advantages as earliness etc. However, it requires a lot of skills for the operation so that this may do the operation in the inside of the body that cannot be watched directly.

Such surgery presents many challenges:

1. Doctors must be very well trained and possess the skills and experience to insert catheters. Intravascular neurosurgery is much more difficult than traditional surgery and there are few skilled doctors who can perform this type of operation. To keep pace with the growing number of patients, a mechanism is required to allow the training of sufficient numbers of doctors.
2. During the operation, doctors check the position of the catheter tip using the X-ray camera. Although they wear protective suits, it is very difficult to shield the doctor's hands and face from the effects of the X-ray radiation, which may result in radiation-related illness after long periods of exposure. The skilled surgeons operate the catheter using their hands directly, the conceptional scheme is shown in Fig.1.
3. In intravascular neurosurgery, catheters are inserted into the patient's blood vessels, which in the brain are very sensitive. When operating in this area, extreme care is required to avoid damaging the fragile vessels. An experienced neurosurgeon can achieve an accuracy of about 2 mm. However, as the contact force between the blood vessel and the catheter cannot be judged accurately by the doctor, so how to measure the contact force and feedback to the surgeon become significant.
4. Sometimes doctors cannot be physically present to operate on patients. Therefore, Internet-based master-slave systems are required for such cases so that the operation can be proceeded.

According to the above background, we developed two kinds of novel robotic catheter operating systems with danger avoiding method respectively, using the developed danger avoiding method it can not only help surgeons to know the situation inside blood vessel, but also can support surgeon to improve safety of operating process during intravascular neurosurgery. They can also provide the force feedback to the surgeon. We did experiment "In Vitro" to prove the feasibility of the developed first robotic catheter system, and we did evaluation for the second developed robotic catheter system.

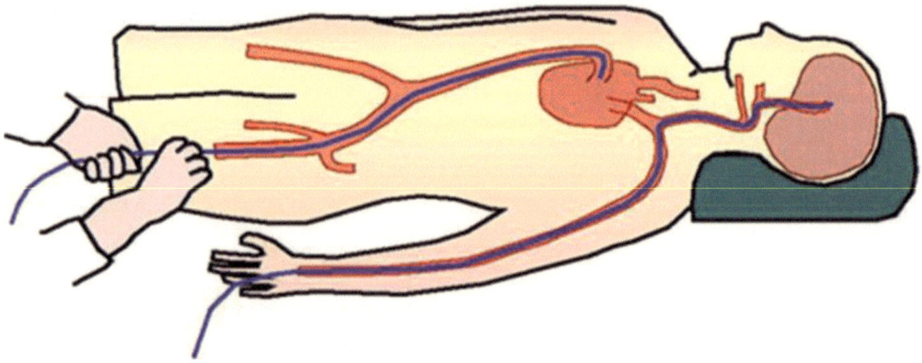

Fig. 1. Operating catheter with surgeon's hand

## 2. Relative products and researches on robotic catheter systems

In the past, there were a lot of researches and products on robotic catheter system. One of the more popular products is ANGIO Mentor endovascular surgical training simulator [OKB Medical], which is shown in Fig.2, it is a virtual reality (VR) simulator system, which can be used to train unskilled surgeon to do the operation of intravascular neurosurgery. However, it lacks of force feedback to the surgeons.

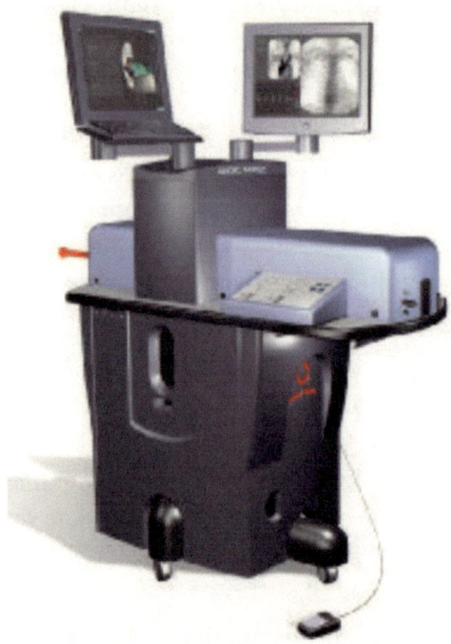

Fig. 2. ANGIO Mentor endovascular surgical training simulator

Another popular product is the Sensei robotic catheter system offered by Hansen Medical [Hansen Medical], which is shown in Fig.3, it can provide more precise manipulation with less radiation exposure to the doctor, however, force detection at the distal tip is very hard.

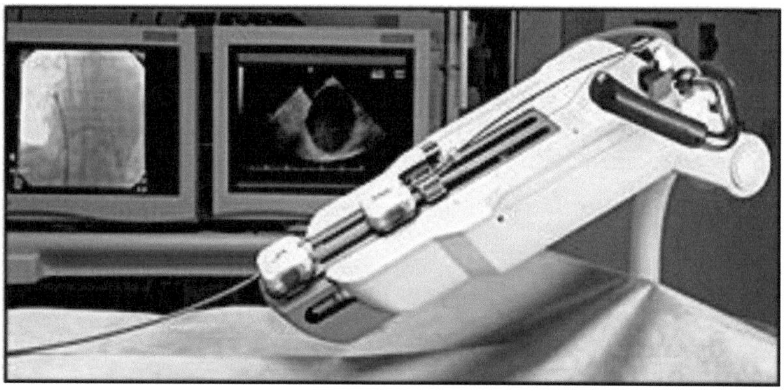

Fig. 3. Sensei robotic catheter system

Active catheter systems with SMA and ICPF as actuators were developed [S.Guo1996], new catheter driving method using linear stepping mechanism for intravascular neurosurgery has been developed [F.Arai2002], remote catheter navigation systems have been reported by [G. Srimathveeravalli2010], [Yogesh Thakur2009], [T.Goto2009], [E. Marcelli2008], and so on. Furthermore, the master-slave catheter systems were also developed [Y.Fu2011]. Although these products and catheter system have been developed, most concern is still the safety of the system. Force information of the catheter during the operation is very important to insure the safety of the surgery. A potential problem with a remote catheter control system is the lack of mechanical feedback. However, detection of the force on catheters is very hard to solve in these systems. In order to solve the problems, in this paper we proposed two kinds of novel robotic catheter systems with force feedback and monitoring image. They can provide the force feedback to the surgeon in real time.

## 3. Design of intelligent force sensors system

During the operation of intravascular neurosurgery, it is significant to obtain the contact force information between catheter and blood vessel [Christopher R. Wagner2002]. How to get it? And how to transmit it to the surgeon? In order to detect the contact force information between catheter and blood vessel, we developed an intelligent force sensors system for robotic catheter systems. By using the developed force sensors system, we can obtain the contact force information and feedback it to the surgeon. If there are no force sensors on the catheter, it is easy to damage the blood vessel during operating, because the blood vessel is fragile. The Fig.4 shows the comparison of safety between without force sensors on catheter and with force sensors on catheter.

### 3.1 Development of micro force sensors

The state-of-the-art in force and tactile sensing for minimally invasive surgery (MIS) has been reported [P. Puangmali2008], it presents the significance of the tactile sensor in MIS. Some tactile force sensors have been reported for the application of intravascular neurosurgery [R. Sedaghati2005], [K. Takashima2005, 2007], a micro force sensor on the catheter tip has been used in previous studies [Jan Peirs2004], and so on. However, these could only detect the contact force between the catheter head and the blood vessels, the frictional force and contact force between the side of catheter and blood vessel wall were not been paid attention. In order to solve above existed problems, in this paper, novel micro tactile force sensors were developed to measure the frictional force and contact force between blood vessel and the side of the catheter. The prototype of the developed tactile force sensors are shown in Fig.5, which are made of pressure sensitive rubber, their sizes are 4.0x4.0x0.5 mm and are fixed on the side wall of catheter by a linking shape.

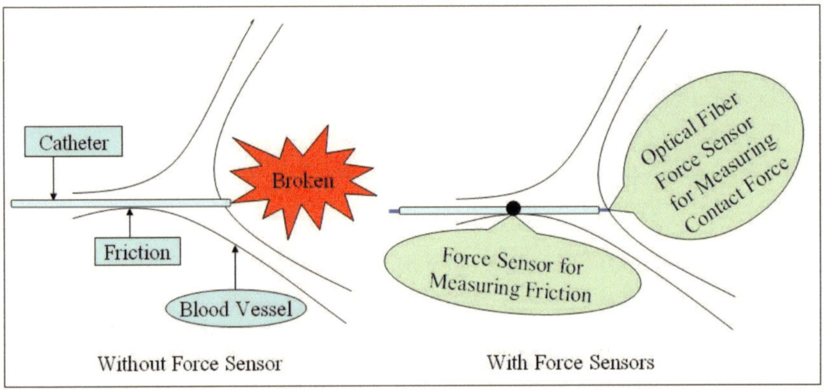


Fig. 4. Comparison of safety between two situations (Without force sensors and with force sensors)

A micro optical force sensor was used to measure front end force of the catheter, meanwhile, the optical fibre force sensor was served as guide wire to lead the catheter for inserting and rotating. The FOP-M optical fibre force sensor of FISO Technologies Inc. was used this time in our research.

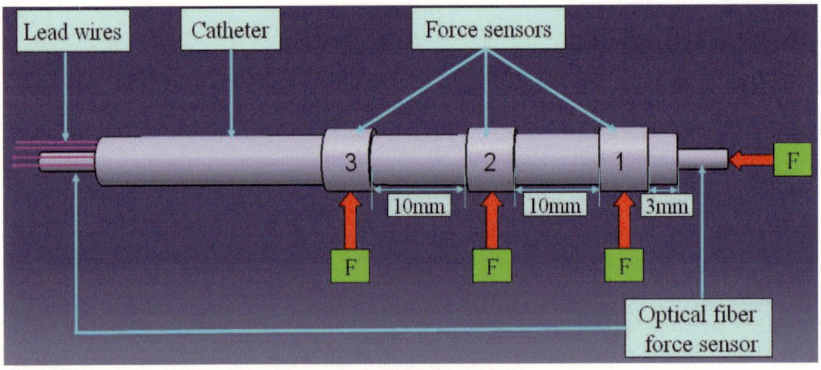


Fig. 5. Prototype of developed force sensors system

### 3.2 Calibration for the developed tactile force sensors

The calibration of the developed tactile force sensors was done, the calibration system is shown in Fig. 6, which consists of an electronic balance, a serial electric circuit, an oscilloscope, a power supply and a force load, we adjust the force load to different scale, the electronic balance will become different value, the tactile force sensor is loaded different value with force load, the tactile sensor output is different, the calibration results are shown in Fig.7, they indicated the relationship between load force and sensor output, based on the calibration results, we can obtain the concrete force output information of tactile sensors during the operation.

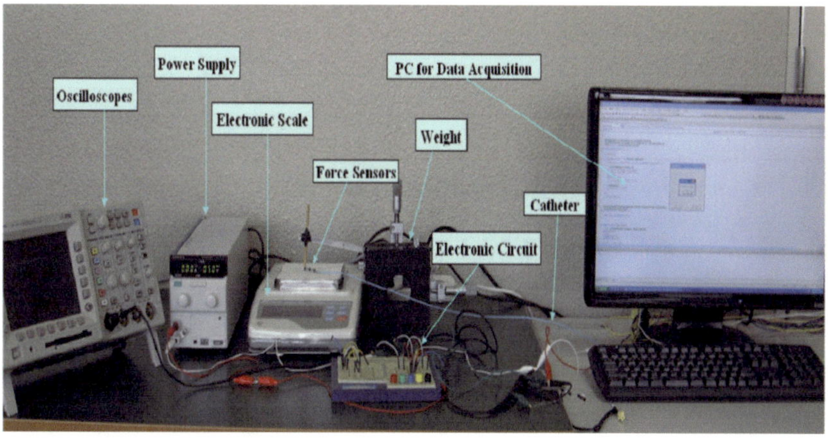


Fig. 6. Calibration system for the developed force sensors

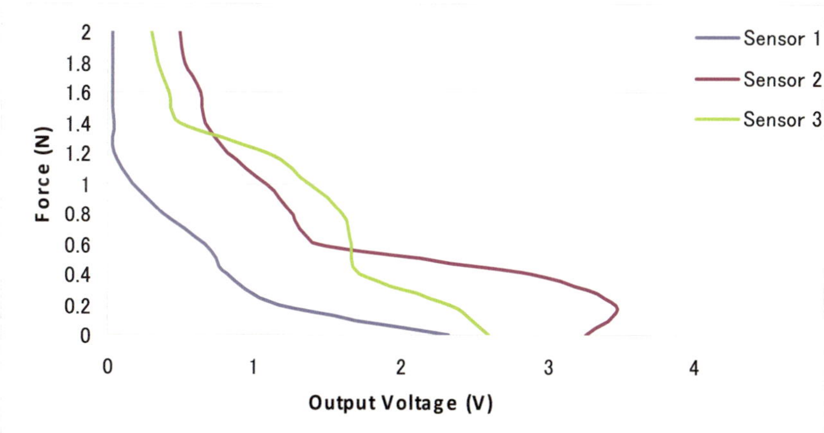


Fig. 7. Calibration results for the developed force sensors

### 3.3 Curve fitting equation for the calibration results

Based on the calibration results, we establish an equation between sensor outputs and load force using Matlab curve fitting tool, it is shown in equation (1), and we can also obtain the coefficient of equation for sensor1, sensor2 and sensor3, it is shown in table 1. Matlab curve fitting results for tactile force sensors are shown in Fig.8.

According to this equation, we can get the detail force output value of developed tactile force sensors if the tactile force sensors touch the blood vessel wall. Through the concrete force output value, surgeon can monitor the situation which catheter contact with the blood vessel sidewall.

$$f = c_{i3}v^3 + c_{i2}v^2 + c_{i1}v + c_{i0} \quad (i = 1,2,3) \tag{1}$$

| Coefficient | Sensor 1 | Sensor 2 | Sensor 3 |
|---|---|---|---|
| Ci3 | -0.4762 | -0.1874 | -0.03155 |
| Ci2 | 2.075 | 1.368 | 0.2049 |
| Ci1 | -2.97 | -3.406 | -1.15 |
| Cio | 1.668 | 3.25 | 2.145 |

Table 1. Coefficient of proposed cubic equation

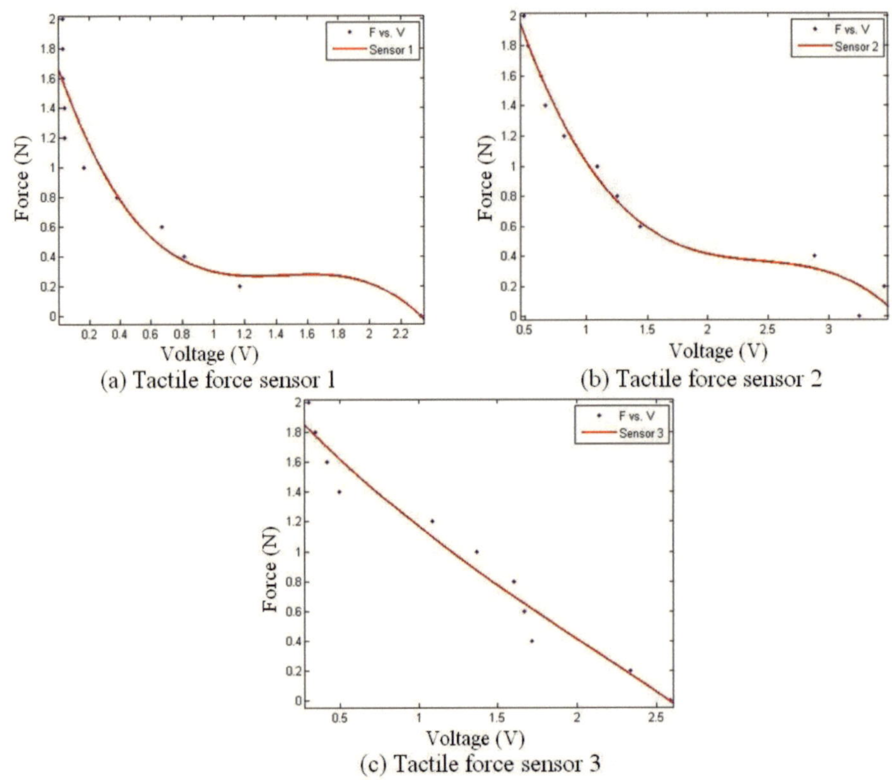


(a) Tactile force sensor 1 (b) Tactile force sensor 2 (c) Tactile force sensor 3

Fig. 8. Matlab curve fitting results for tactile force sensors

### 3.4 Force monitoring system

A force display method for a catheter operating system has been developed [J.Guo et al 2010], this method distinguished the force from developed force sensors to three ranges, safe range, danger warning range and dangerous range, however, this force display method did not show the detail force information at any moment, so surgeons could not know the concrete force information at any time, therefore, we improved the force information monitoring method so that surgeon can know the detail information at any moment during the operation, Fig.9 shows the force information monitoring system on the master side.

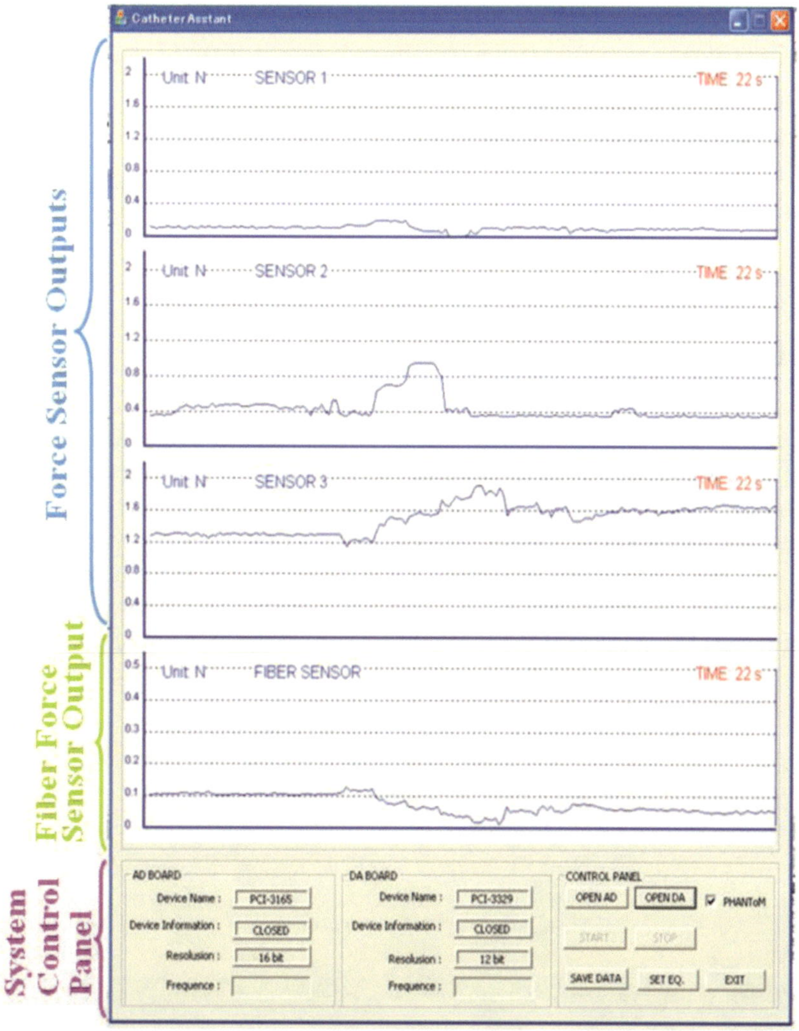


Fig. 9. Force information monitoring system

The novel force information monitoring method consists of two parts, sensor outputs part and system control panel part, which can monitor the changed force that catheter contact with blood vessel wall real time during the operation, in the sensor outputs part, it is divided four areas, three developed tactile force sensor outputs display areas and an optical fibre force sensor output display area. We can control the master-slave system in the system control panel part. Three tactile force sensors were used to measure the side force of catheter, and an optical force sensor was used to detect the front end force of catheter, if the force sensors touch the blood vessel, the output of force sensors will be shown in the force monitoring system real time, at the same time, the force feedback signals will be sent to the Phantom Omni, further more, The situation of operation can be monitored using web camera. In the master side, surgeons can not only monitor the force variation real time, but also they can feel the force feedback through Phantom Omni, when the contacted force is exceeded safe value, the Phantom Omni will be locked, so the developed system can automatically avoid the danger, and it can help surgeon improve the safety effectively during the operation.

## 4. Robotic catheter operating systems

Our research group developed two kinds of robot-assisted catheter system in the past, one kind is with haptic device called Phantom Omni as master manipulator, the other kind is with the master manipulator which can imitate surgeon's operating skill to insert and rotate catheter, we will introduce them as follows:

### 4.1 The first developed robotic catheter operating system

The first developed robotic catheter operating system is shown in Fig.10, at master side, the surgeon sees the monitoring image and operates the Phantom Omni, at the same time, the controlling instructions were transmitted to the slave side, after receiving the controlling instructions from master side, the slave manipulator drives the catheter to insert and rotate. Bu using the web camera to monitor the situation of operation, and by using force sensors to measure the contact force between catheter and blood vessel, the monitoring image and feedback force were transmitted to the surgeon in real time, based on the feedback force and monitoring image, the surgeon decides whether to insert the catheter or not. The flow chart of control signals is shown in Fig.11.

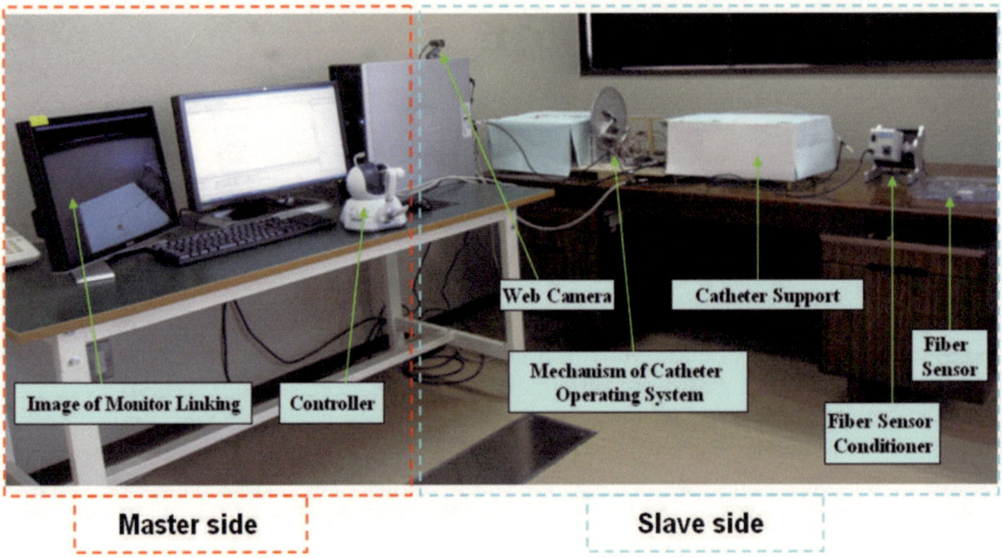


Fig. 10. The first developed master-slave robotic catheter system

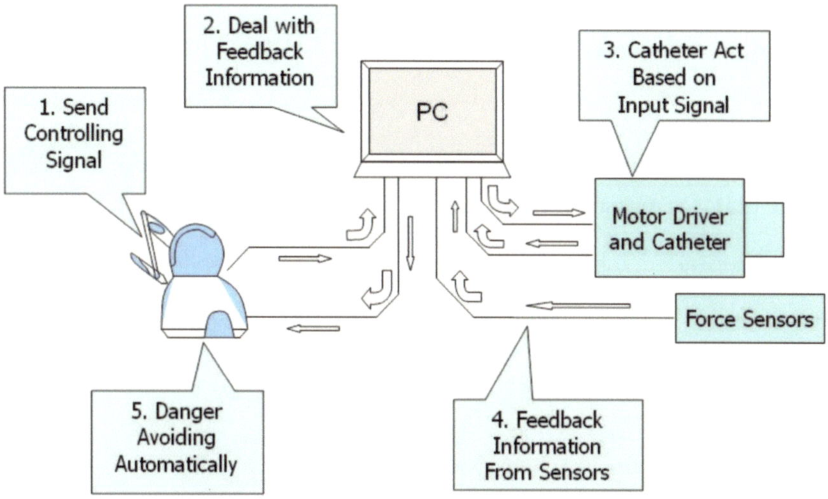


Fig. 11. Flow chart of control signals for first kind of catheter system

#### 4.1.1 Master manipulator

The master manipulator is shown in Fig.12, called Phantom Omni, it is a haptic device, in this research, it was used to control the action of catheter, including inserting motion and rotating motion, we also use it to realize force feedback to avoid danger during operation of intravascular neurosurgery, when the force sensors contacted with blood vessel, the force feedback will be transmitted to the surgeon's hand in real time, if the contact forces exceeded warning force value, the Phantom Omni will be locked, so the developed catheter operating system can avoid the danger automatically, and it can help surgeon improve the safety effectively during the operation.

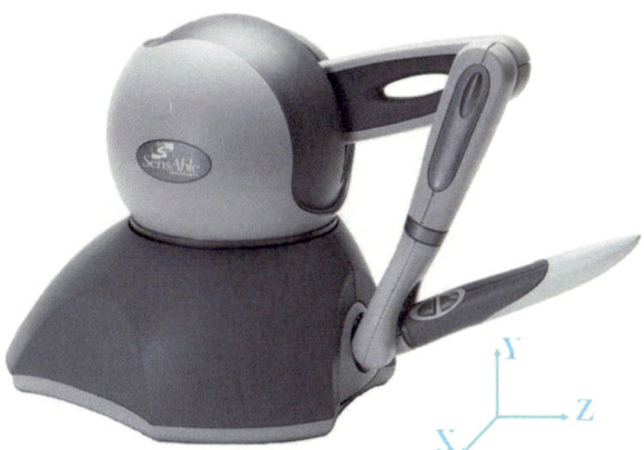


Fig. 12. Coordinate system of Phantom Omni

In order to realize the force feedback using Phantom Omni, the mechanical model of Phantom Omni was established, it is as follows:

The Phantom Omni output force $\vec{F}$ is:

$$\vec{F} = xi + yj + zk \tag{2}$$

Z direction is the inserting direction.
X direction is the rotating direction.

$$x \cdot z \equiv 0 \tag{3}$$

$f_1, f_2, f_3$ is the forces that were measured by the developed force sensors.
$f_4$ is the force that was measured by the optical fibre force sensor.

When catheter is inserted, the Phantom Omni output force is as follows:

$$\vec{F} = 0 \cdot i + 0 \cdot j + A_i k$$
$$A_i = \begin{cases} 0 & (f_4 < C_0) \\ k \cdot f_4 & (f_4 > C_0) \end{cases} \quad (k < 0) \tag{4}$$

When catheter is rotated, the Phantom Omni output force is as follows:

$$\vec{F} = A_r \cdot i + 0 \cdot j + 0 \cdot k$$
$$f_{\max} = \max(f_1, f_2, f_3) \tag{5}$$
$$A_r = \begin{cases} 0 & (f_{\max} < C_1) \\ k \cdot f_{\max} & (f_{\max} > C_1) \end{cases} \quad (k < 0)$$

Based on the mechanical model of Phantom Omni, the force feedback output from Phantom Omni can be obtained, the value of the Phantom Omni force feedback is the force that surgeon feels. So the haptic force feedback can be realized by Phantom Omni and force sensors.

### 4.1.2 Slave manipulator

The conception of slave manipulator is shown in Fig.13, it can realize two motions for catheter, one is axial motion (moving forward and back-ward), and the other is radial motion (rotation). The catheter mostly moves forward and backward. When meeting the branch of blood vessel or moving difficulty, the catheter must rotate in order to enter the branch of blood vessel or get across block.

The mechanism of slave manipulator is shown in Fig.14, we make use of stepping motors as the actuators for driving the catheter. They can control the catheter moving to different directions. Considering the weight of mechanism, the whole mechanism is made of aluminium. The base of mechanism is made of stainless steel in order to increase the stabilization.

### 4.1.3 Experimental set up

We carried out the remote operating simulation experiment "in Vitro" using developed master-slave system in the simulator of blood vessel with an aneurysm, the simulator of blood vessel is made by silicon glass tube, which is shown in Fig.15. It is considered whose conditions are similar to those of a blood vessel of human brain.

Through the remote operating simulation experiment, we can measure the contact force between blood vessel wall and the catheter by developed micro tactile force sensors and optical fibre force sensor. Using the developed force monitoring system, we can obtain the outputs from micro tactile force sensors and optical fibre force sensor.

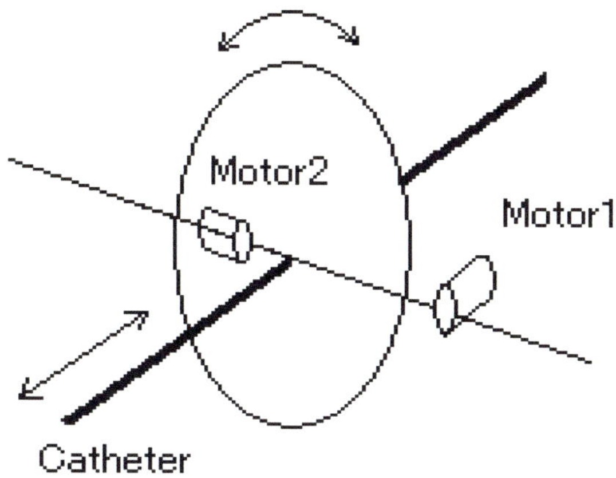

Fig. 13. Conception of slave manipulator

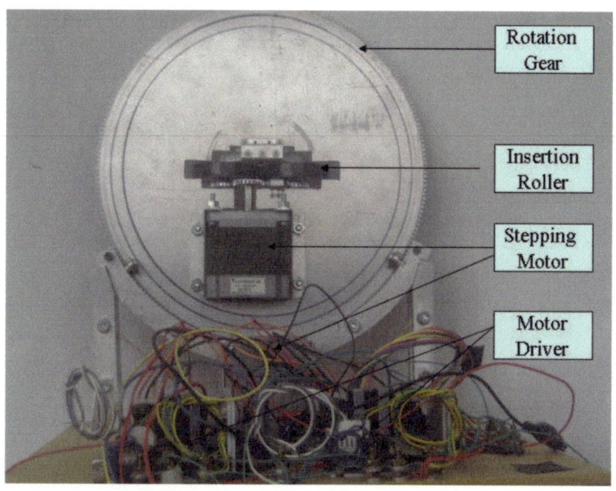

Fig. 14. Mechanism of slave manipulator

The experimental results are shown in Fig.16, Fig.17 and Fig.18. The output of developed tactile sensors are shown in Fig.16, the output of optical fibre force sensor is shown in Fig.17, making use of the mechanical model of Phantom omni, we can get the force feedback output of Phantom Omni, which is shown in Fig.18. From the graph we can know the relationship between operating time and force feedback from force sensors, and also we can know the force value when force sensors contact the simulator of blood vessel. It can also prove that the Phantom Omni is sensitive, and also it can avoid the danger automatically. The experimental results indicated that the developed novel type catheter operating system with force information monitoring method works properly, it can measure the contact force between catheter and blood vessel, also we can monitor the situation of simulation experiment using web camera, this catheter operating system can be controlled by teleoperation, and it can effectively improve the operability of aneurysm with force feedback for intravascular neurosurgery.

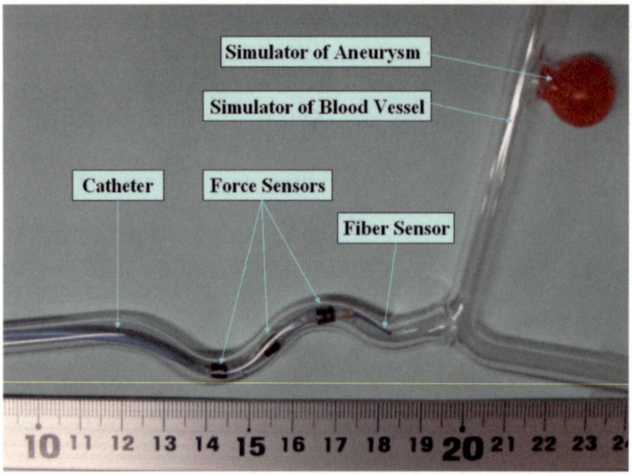


Fig. 15. Experimental set up

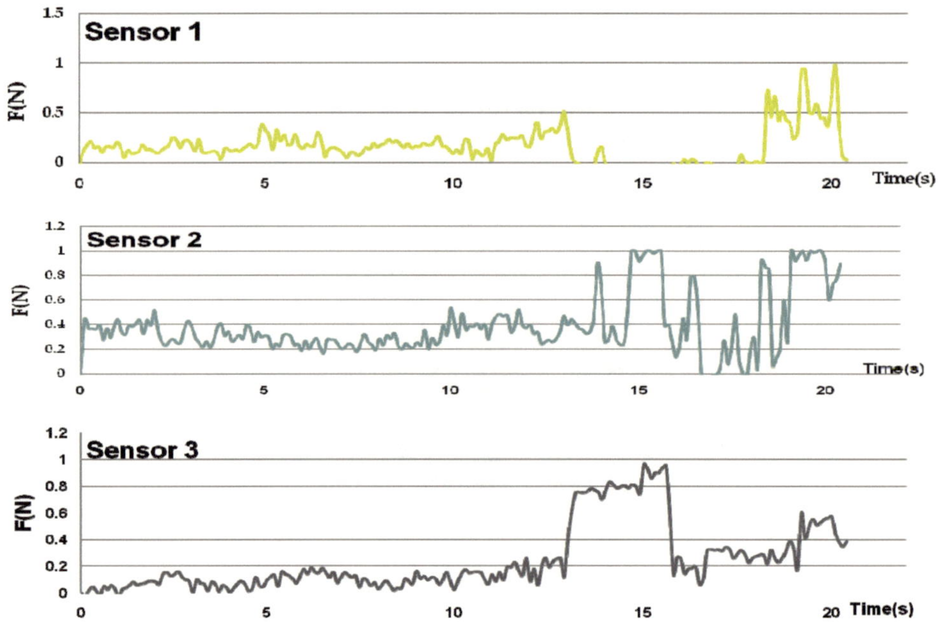


Fig. 16. Force outputs of developed tactile force sensors

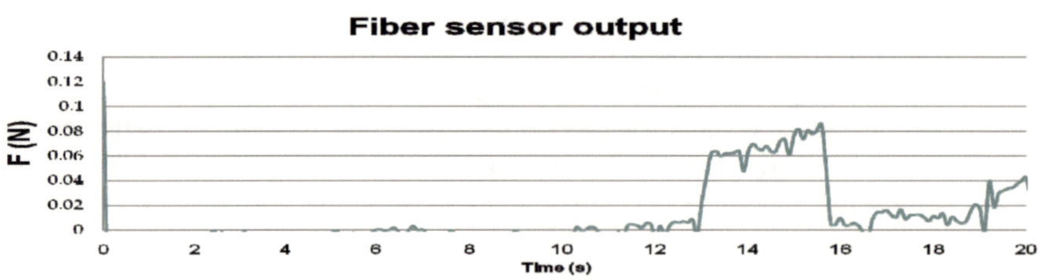


Fig. 17. Force output of optical fibre force sensor

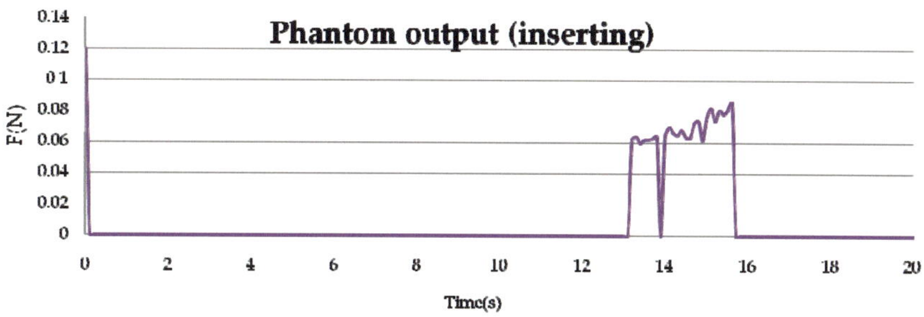


Fig. 18. Force feedback output of Phantom Omni

### 4.2 The second developed robotic catheter operating system

Because the Phantom manipulator can not imitate the operating skill of surgeon, we developed the other kind of robotic catheter system to simulate surgeon's operating skill for doing the operation of intravascular neurosurgery. Conceptual scheme of the second kind of robotic catheter system is shown in Fig.19. The flow chart of control signals for second kind of catheter system is shown in Fig.20.

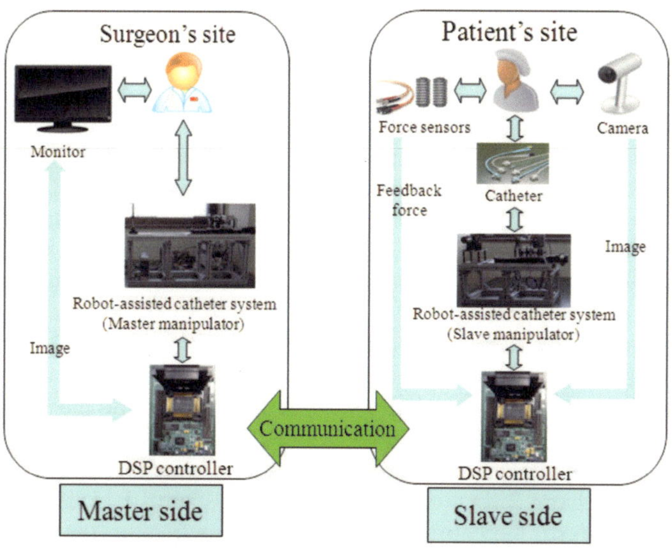


Fig. 19. Conceptual scheme of the second kind of robotic catheter system

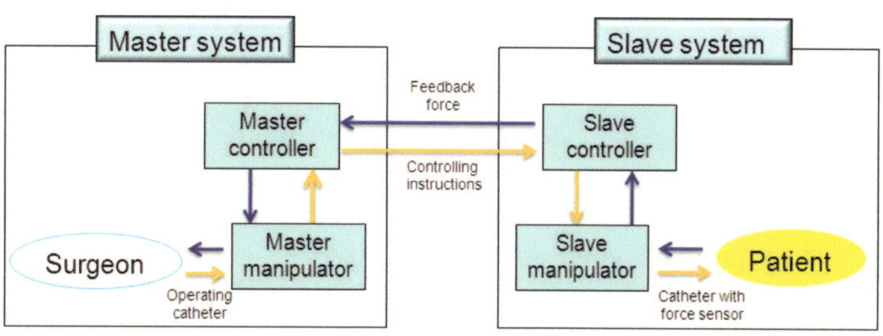


Fig. 20. Flow chart of control signals for second kind of catheter system

### 4.2.1 Master manipulator

On the master side, the slide platform is fixed on the supporting frame (Fig.21). The master system devices, including a left handle with one switch, a right handle, step motor, load cell, and maxon motor, are on the slide platform. The step motor is used to drive the slide platform forward and backward, the load cell is used to measure the operating force of surgeon's hand.

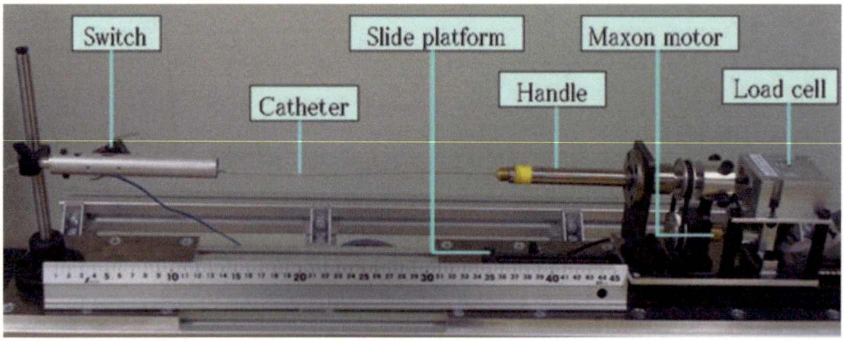


Fig. 21. Master manipulator

### 4.2.2 Slave manipulator

The slave side consists of a catheter clamping device, two DC motors, a slide platform, step motor, maxon motor, load cell, torque sensor, and support frame. The slave side mechanism shown in Fig.22 is similar to the master side; a slide platform is fixed on the supporting frame. The devices of the slave system are on the slide platform. The step motor is used to the drive slide platform forward and backward and the maxon motor is used to rotate the catheter. The two DC motors are used to control the catheter clamp. The load cell is used to measure the force between the catheter and blood vessel wall and the torque sensor and maxon motor are used to measure the force of catheter rotation. The measured force information is transmitted to the surgeon's hand, so that the surgeon can feel the feedback information from the slave side. A switch on the left handle on the master side controls the catheter clamp. When the surgeon wants to insert or rotate the catheter, clamp 2 is raised and clamp 1 clamps the catheter. The catheter navigator moves forward with the catheter for insertion or rotation. Clamp 2 then clamps the catheter; clamp 1 is raised and the catheter navigator moves backward. Repeating these actions, the actions of the slave side follow the commands of the master side in real time. If the catheter contacts the blood vessel wall, the force information is detected and transmitted to the surgeon's hand.

### 4.2.3 Mechanism control

In order to ensure the consistency and stability of the robotic catheter system, for both the rotating and inserting motions, a proportional-integral-derivative (PID) control method was developed for the robotic catheter operating system. A numerical simulation indicated that the response of the system was good using the PID control method. Furthermore, we did a simulation experiment using the robotic catheter system with the PID control strategy. The experimental results show that the response and consistency were good, enabling a surgeon to perform intravascular neurosurgery.

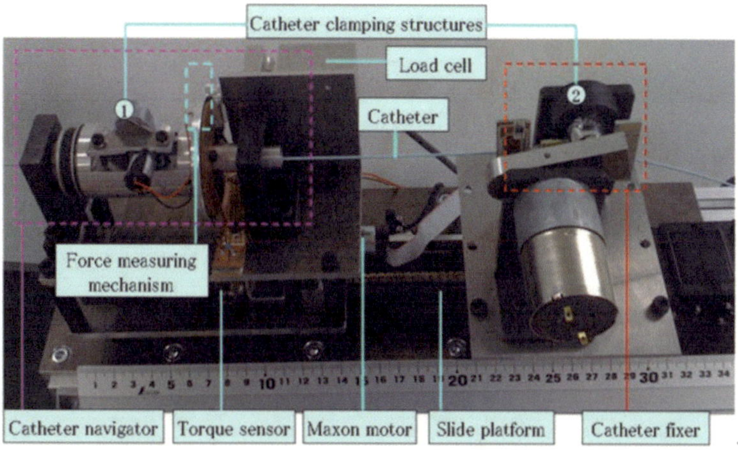


Fig. 22. Slave manipulator

#### 4.2.3.1 Control strategy for inserting motion

We used the PID algorithm to assure accurate inserting motion, while reducing the hysteresis in real time. The following dynamic equation represents the control in the inserting direction:

$$F(t) = \mathrm{m}\ddot{x}(t) + c\dot{x}(t) + kx(t) \tag{6}$$

Where F(t) is the force applied by the operator, $x(t)$, $\dot{x}(t)$, and $\ddot{x}(t)$ are the displacement, velocity, and acceleration of the operator's hand, respectively, m is the quality of the robotic catheter operating system (on the slide platform on the master side), c is the viscous damping coefficient, and k is the stiffness.

When the operator operates the right handle on the master side, the load cell measures the force. Using a dynamic equation based on the relationship between the operating force and resistance, the PID control strategy is used to adjust the consistency of the operating force in order to avoid overshoot. Fig.23 outlines the control of the inserting motion. The parameters of the operating system are as follows:

$$m = 2kg, c = 0.02N/(m/s), k = 10N/m$$

As on the master side, based on the input and output of the step motor, we used the same PID control strategy on the slave side to control the consistency and response of the slave mechanism during insertion.

#### 4.2.3.2 Control strategy for rotating motion

Equation (7) represents the torque balance for the rotating motion on the master side, where m is the quality of the catheter operating system (on the slide platform on the master side), c is the viscous damping coefficient, $m = 2kg, c = 0.02N/(m/s)$, θ is the angle of rotation, u(t) is the variation in the torque, which is the torque of the maxon motor, $\dot{\theta}$ is the angular velocity, and $\ddot{\theta}$ is the angular acceleration. The control of rotation is shown in Fig.24.

$$m\ddot{\theta}+c\dot{\theta}=u(t) \tag{7}$$

As on the master side, based on the input and output of the maxon motor, we used the same PID control strategy on the slave side to ensure the consistency and response of the slave mechanism for rotation.

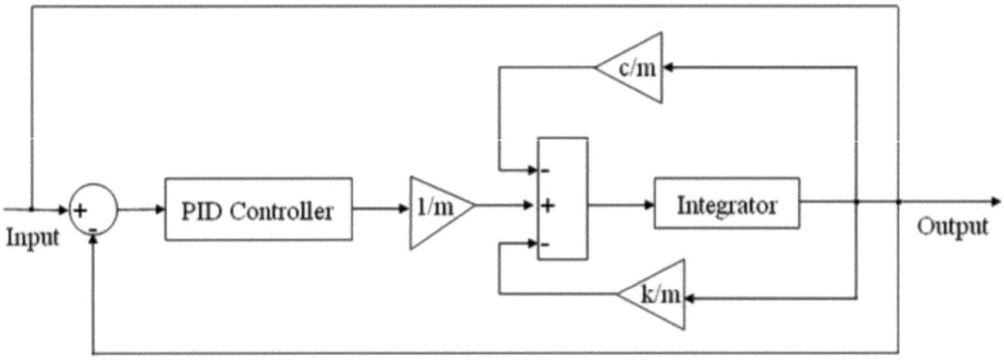


Fig. 23. The control of the insertion

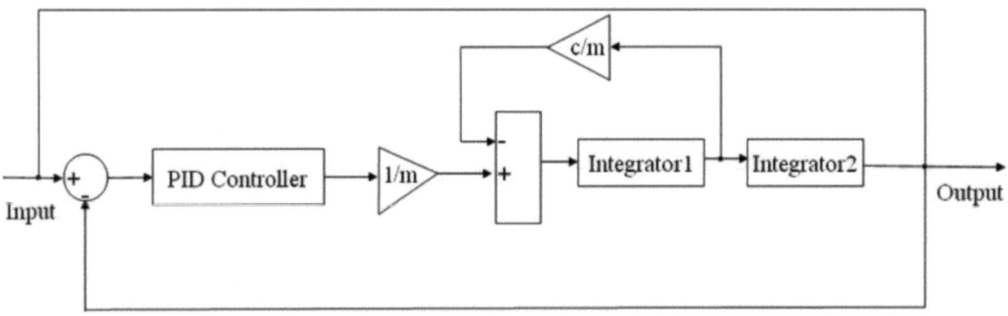


Fig. 24. The control of rotation

### 4.3 Catheter inserting experiment in vitro

In order to validate the robotic catheter operating system, we performed a simulation experiment to evaluate the characteristics of the master-slave robotic catheter operating system using an endovascular evaluator (EVE) (Fig. 25), which consisted of a fluid control unit and blood pressure monitoring instrument. The bending angles and radii of the tubes in the EVE are close to those of human arteries. The tubes were made of silicon rubber. The elasticity of the tubes was similar to that of a blood vessel wall. In order to keep the blood pressure of the EVE close to the blood pressure of a human, the fluid control unit was used to adjust the blood pressure, which was monitored with the blood pressure monitoring instrument. The operator operates the right handle on the master side to insert and rotate the catheter, which is inserted into the EVE from the femoral artery, controlling the speed and position of the catheter. The simulation experiment is shown in Fig. 26.

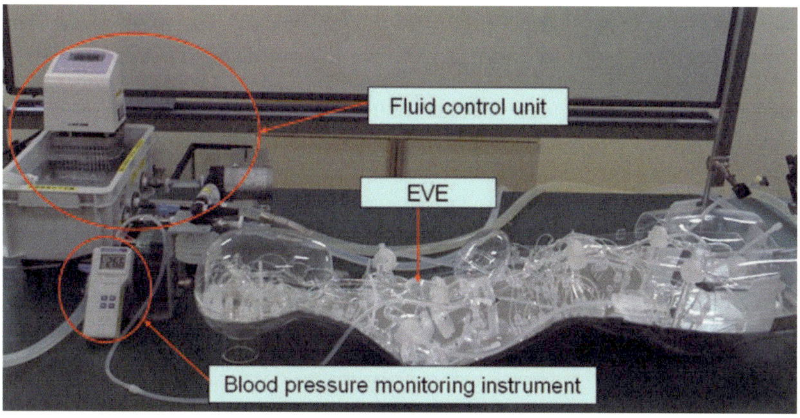


Fig. 25. The fluid control unit and blood pressure monitoring instrument of EVE

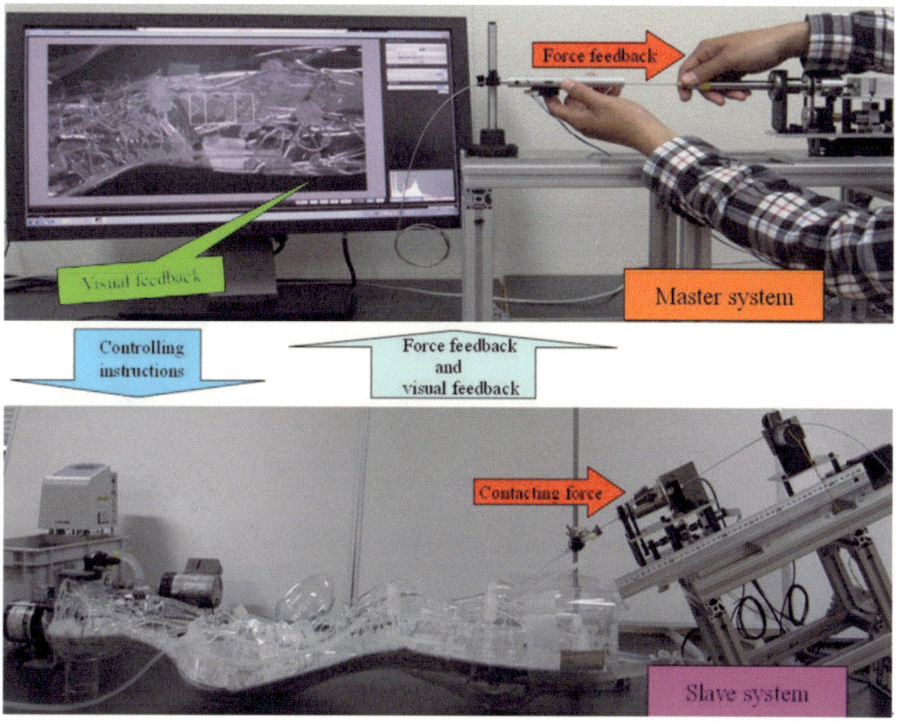


Fig. 26. Simulation experiment using EVE

#### 4.3.1 Experimental results

We evaluated the robotic catheter system in a simulation experiment. Fig. 27 shows the results for the inserting motion, where the x-axis is the time axis and the y-axis is the displacement of the right handle on the master side (blue curve) and the catheter on the slave side (red curve). An upward slope is forward movement and a downward slope is backward movement. Fig. 28 shows the evaluation of rotation, where the x-axis is the time axis and the y-axis is the rotation of the right handle on the master side (blue curve) and the catheter on the slave side (red curve). From Figs. 27 and 28, the motions of the slave side follow the operating motions of the master side coincide very well in real time.

The measured insertion force is shown in Fig. 29, and this is also the feedback force transmitted to the operator's hand. The force sensors measure the contact force between the catheter and blood vessel wall. The fibre force sensor measures the force between the tip of the catheter and the blood vessel wall, the output of the fibre force sensor is shown in Fig. 30.

The experimental results indicate that our robotic catheter system can be used to perform VIS, without risk. The insertion force of the catheter is measured and fed back to the operator's hand, as is the contact force measured by the force sensors.

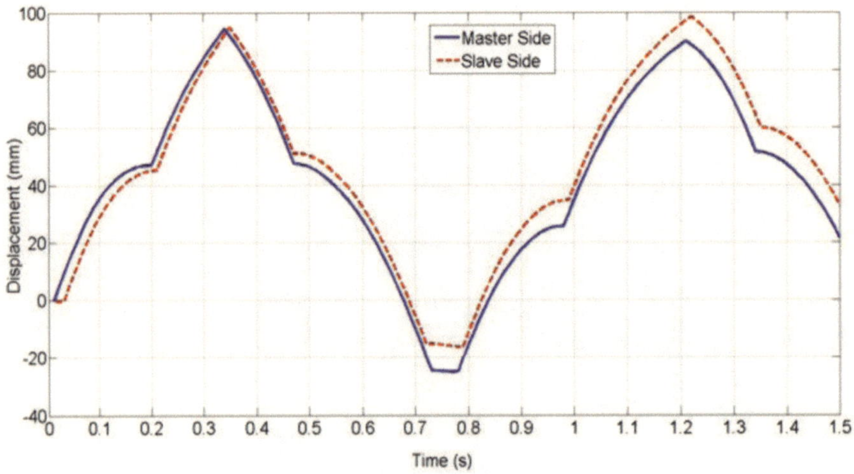


Fig. 27. Evaluated results for catheter insertion

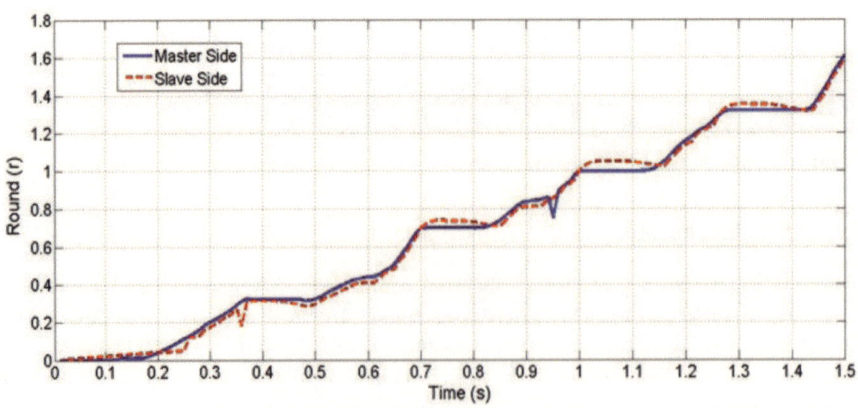


Fig. 28. Evaluated results for catheter rotation

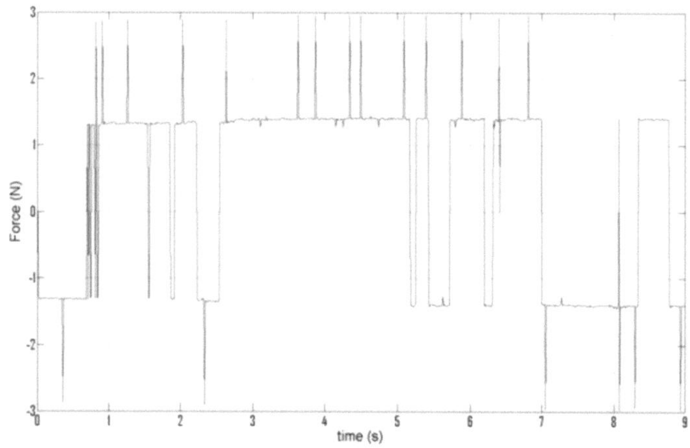


Fig. 29. The feedback force from the slave side

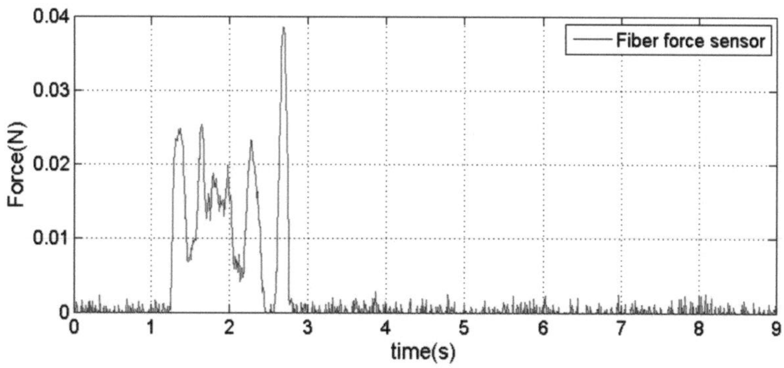


Fig. 30. The output of the fibre force sensor

### 4.3.2 Discussion

A simulation experiment was performed to validate our robotic catheter system. In order to enhance the stability and consistency of the robotic catheter system, we used a PID control strategy. The experimental results indicate that the response and consistency of the system were good, enabling a surgeon to perform VIS. It can also be used to train surgeons to insert and rotate a catheter for VIS smoothly. Nevertheless, due to the accuracy of the measuring device, the robotic catheter system is not ideal. In the future, we will improve the system. In addition, in the simulation experiment we used distilled water with a lubricant to simulate blood. Since the viscosity of distilled water differs from that of blood, the experimental results will differ slightly from an actual operation. We plan to improve the system by conducting animal experiments.

## 5. Conclusions

This paper presents two kinds of robotic catheter operating systems, they can assist surgeons to do the operation of intravascular neurosurgery, in addition, we designed a intelligent force sensors system to detect the contact force information between catheter and blood vessel, and also, we have done the simulation experiment "In Vitro" by using first developed robotic catheter system, the experimental results indicated that the first developed robotic catheter system work well, it can avoid danger automatically. We evaluated the second robotic catheter operating system via experiment in vitro by using EVE model, the evaluated results present that the second robotic catheter system can imitate the surgeon's operating skill to insert and rotate catheter, it is suitable for training unskilled surgeons to do the operation of intravascular neurosurgery. In the future, we will do some experiment in vivo by using the robotic catheter system.

## 6. Acknowledgment

This research is supported by Kagawa University Characteristic Prior Research fund 2011.

## 7. References

C. Preusche, T. Ortmaier, G. Hirzinger.(2002), Teleoperation concepts in minimal invasive surgery. Control Engineering Practice, 2002; 10:1245-1250.

C.R. Wagner, Nicholas Stylopoulos, Robert D. Howe(2002), The role of force feedback in surgery: analysis of blunt dissection, the Tenth Symposium on Haptic Interfaces for Virtual Environment and Teleoperator System, 2002.

E. Marcelli, L. Cercenelli, G. Plicchi.(2008), A novel telerobotic system to remotely navigate standard electrophysiology catheters, Computer in Cardiology 2008; 35:137-140.

F. Arai, R. Fujimura, T. Fukuda, M. Negoro.(2002), New catheter driving method using linear stepping mechanism for intravascular neurosurgery. Proceedings of the 2002 IEEE International Conference on Robotic & Automation, 2002; pp. 2944-2949.

G. Srimathveeravalli, T. Kesavadas, X. Li.(2010), Design and fabrication of a robot mechanism for remote steering and positioning of interventional devices, International Journal of Medical Robotics and Computer Assisted Surgery 2010; 6:160-170.

Hansen Medical, http://www.hansenmedical.com/sensei

J. Wang and S. Guo, H. Kondo, J. Guo and T. Tamiya.(2008), A Novel Catheter Operating System with Force Feedback for Medical Applications, International Journal of Information Acquisition, Vol.5, No.1, pp.83-91, 2008.

J. Peirs, Joeri Clijnen, Dominiek Reynaerts, Hendrik Van Brussel, Paul Herijgers, Brecht Corteville, et. al.(2004), A micro optical force sensor for force feedback during minimally invasive robotic surgery, Sensors and Actuators, Vol.115, No.2-3, pp.447-455, 2004.

J. Guo, N. Xiao, S. Guo.(2010), A force display method for a novel catheter operating system, Proceedings of the 2010 IEEE International Conference on Information and Automation, 2010; pp. 782-786.

J. Guo, N. Xiao, S. Guo, T. Tamiya.(2010), Development of a force information monitoring method for a novel catheter operating system, Information: An International Interdisciplinary Journal, 2010; 1(6):1999- 2009.

K. Takashima, K. Yoshinaka, T. Okazaki, K. Ikeuchi.(2005), An endoscopic tactile sensor for low invasive surgery. Sensors and Actuators A 2005; 119:372-383.

K. Takashima, R. Shimomura, T. Kitou, H. Terada, K. Yoshinaka, K. Ikeuchi.(2007), Contact and friction between catheter and blood vessel. Tribology International 2007; 40:319-328.

OKB Medical, http://www.okbmedical.com/angio

P. Puangmali, K. Althoefer, L.D. Seneviratne, D. Murphy, P. Dasgupta.(2008), State-of-the-art in force and tactile sensing for minimally invasive surgery. IEEE Sensors Journal, 2008; 8(4):371-381.

P. Polygerinos, T. Schaeffter, L. Seneviratne, K. Althoefer.(2009), Measuring tip and side forces of a novel catheter prototype: a feasibility study, Proceedings of the 2009 International Conference on Intelligent Robots and System, 2009; pp. 966-971.

Q. Pan, S. Guo, T. Okada.(2011), A novel hybrid wireless microrobot, International Journal of Mechatronics and Automation, 2011; 1(1):60-69.

R. Sedaghati, J. Dargahi, H. Singh.(2005), Design and modeling of an endoscopic piezoelectric tactile sensor, International Journal of Solids and Structures, Vol.42, No.21-22, pp.5872–5886, 2005.

S. Abdulla, P. Wen.(2011), Robust internal model control for depth of anaesthesia, International Journal of Mechatronics and Automation, 2011; 1(1):1-8.

S. Guo, Hidekazu Kondo, Jian Wang, Jian Guo, Takashi Tamiya.(2007) A New Catheter Operationg System for Medical Applications. Proceedings of the 2007 IEEE/ICME International Conference on Complex Medical Engineering, pp. 82-87, 2007.

S. Guo, Tatsuya Nakamtra, Toshio Fukuda, Keisuke Oguro, and Makoto Negoro. (1996), Micro Active Catheter Using ICPF Actuator Characteristic Evaluation, Proceedings of IEEE the 22nd Annual International Conf. on Industrial Electronics, Control, and Instrumentation, pp.1312-1317, 1996.

T. Fukuda, S. Guo, K. Kosuge, F. Arai, M. Negoro, and K. Nakabayash. (1994), Micro Active Catheter System with Multi Degree of Freedom, Proceedings of 1994 IEEE International Conference on Robotic and Automation, Vol.3, pp. 2290-2295, 1994.

T. Goto, T. Miyahara, K. Toyoda, J. Okamoto, Y. Kakizawa, J. Koyama, M. G. Fujie, K. Hongo.(2009), Telesurgery of microscopic micromanipulator system "NeuRobot" in neurosurgery: Interhospital Preliminary Study, Journal of Brain Disease 2009; 1:45-53.

X. Wang, M. Meng.(2011), Perspective of active capsule endoscope: actuation and localization, International Journal of Mechatronics and Automation, 2011; 1(1):38-45.

Y. Fu, A. Gao, H. Liu, S. Guo.(2011), The master-slave catheterization system for positioning the steerable catheter, International Journal of Mechatronics and Automation, 2011; 1(3), in press.

Y.C. Wu, J.S. Chen.(2011), Toward the identification of EMG-signal and its bio-feedback application, International Journal of Mechatronics and Automation, 2011; 1(2):112-120.

Y. Thakur, Jeffrey S. Bax, David W. Holdsworth and Maria Drangova.(2009), Design and performance Evaluation of a remote catheter navigation system, IEEE Transactions on Biomedical Engineering, Vol.56, No.7, July 2009, pp:1901-1908.

# 21

# The Role of Neural Stem Cells in Neurorestoration

E.O. Vik-Mo, A. Fayzullin, M.C. Moe, H. Olstorn and I.A. Langmoen
*Vilhelm Magnus Laboratory,*
*Department of Neurosurgery and Institute of Surgical Research, Oslo University Hospital*
*Norway*

## 1. Introduction

Many neurological diseases have a poor prognosis. Most neurological treatment is primarily based on minimizing secondary - or further damage - and to optimize the remaining neurological function. Even a highly successful treatment like deep brain stimulation for Parkinson's disease improves neurological function through conditional lesioning. Several neurodegenerative diseases have no established treatments[1].

The complex electrochemical, molecular and anatomical structure of the central nervous system is established during prenatal and early postnatal development. Thus, it was long considered impossible to heal or substitute destroyed nervous tissue. The adult human brain used to be viewed as static, as it was a common perception that no new neurons could be generated after birth. This has been referred to as the "no new neurons"-dogma[2], and it goes back to the early neuronanatomist and Nobel Prize laureate Santiago Ramon y Cajal, who stated that "nothing may regenerate in the brain or central nervous system, everything may die"[3]. This axiom was challenged in the 1960s, but the work by Joseph Altman and co-workers was met with skepticism and was generally not accepted by the scientific community[4, 5].

During the 1970`s and 80`s Fernando Nottebohm and his colleagues made some very important discoveries. They found that the vocal centers in the brain of male canaries increase in size prior to the breeding season when vocal activities escalate to play pivotal roles in mating. In a series of studies they found no proliferation in the vocal centers, but showed that cell divisions took place in the ventricular wall. The newborn neurons then migrated to the vocal centers where they were integrated in neuronal circuits[6].

Evidence for neurogenesis in the mammalian brain was first presented by Reynolds and Weiss in 1992. They isolated cells from the striatum of adult mice and induced proliferation by epidermal growth factor[7]. Subsequently subsets of the cells developed the morphology and antigenic properties of neurons and astrocytes. Some of the newly generated cells also expressed immunoreactivity for the neurotransmitters typically found in that area of the adult mouse brain. In 1998 Eriksson et al. identified cells with stem cell characteristics *in situ* in the brain of adult humans post mortem[37, 152].

Through a steadily improving knowledge, primarily over the last 20 years, we have found that the central nervous system harbors cells with the ability to divide, mature and restore function after damage. Through manipulation it is even possible to differentiate cells derived from other organs into functioning neural cells that could be used as treatments.

A new approach, based on regeneration of central nervous tissue, might allow for better treatments for several of these devastating diseases. Although awaited with great hope, the translation of this basic research into tested treatments for patients is still wanting.

## 2. Definition of neural stem cells

Stem cells (SC) can loosely be described as cells that (I) have capacity for self-renewal (symmetric division), and (II) can give rise to cells other than themselves through asymmetric cell division[8]. SCs give rise to more differentiated progeny; **progenitor cells**. These cells have a more restricted ability for proliferation and differentiation.

The development from a multipotent stem cell to a variety of differentiated progeny has been most thoroughly examined in the hematopoietic system[9]. Here a detailed set of surface markers and transcription factors has been described to identify stem cells and different subsets of progenitor and differentiated cells[10]. Such a molecular phenotyping of the hierarchical organization allows for a detailed functional description, and to form hypothesis readily testable. However, even in this relatively well characterized cellular hierarchy controversies exist both on the stem cell nature and on the correct phenotype of such cells.

Cells with SC characteristics that can give rise to neural tissue **or** are derived from the central nervous system (CNS) are called neural stem cells (NSC). NSC can be derived from several sources. In principal such cells can be classified according to the sources of origin. Cells can be isolated from embryos, fetal, or the adult CNS. Neural stem cells are multipotent, giving rise to the three major cell types of the mammalian CNS: neurons, astrocytes and oligodendrocytes. Adult stem cells, also referred to as somatic stem cells, are undifferentiated cells found among mature and specialized cells in a tissue or organ, and reside in various tissues in the human body, including the central nervous system. It is the stem cells of the adult brain that drive adult neurogenesis.

The hierarchy of somatic stem cell differentiation in solid tissue is however much less clear[11, 12]. In addition, little is known about the differentiation pathways from such stem cells into the main groups of cells comprising brain stroma. Suggested progenitor cell phenotypes may differ between different parts of the brain[13, 14]. The fact that there exist thousands of different types of neurons in the CNS adds magnitudes of complexity. The impact of *in vitro* cultural artifacts confuses available data even further. Similar problems of stem- and progenitor-cell identification are present in several other organ systems where somatic stem cells have been described (breast, lung, prostate, skin, and gut). With such an uncharted landscape, defining a definitive SC population clearly poses a great problem.

Several approaches have been used to isolate and identify potential NSC. After the successful use of flow cytometry for identification of SC in the hematopoietic system, surface markers have been sought for NSC. The marker CD133 (also termed prominin-1 or AC133) was initially identified on a subset of human hematopoietic stem and progenitor cells [15]. Antibodies directed at this protein were shown to prospectively identify a population of progenitor cells isolated from fetal human brain tissue[16]. CD133 is also expressed by the slow-dividing fraction of human umbilical cord progenitor cells[17]. This marker has been identified in the subventricular zone (SVZ) and rostral migratory stream [18] and even cortex [19] in human post-mortem derived tissue. Conflicting data exist however[20, 21], where a group identified CD133 positive cells in cells derived from embryonic SC, ependymal cells and brain tumor cells - but not in neurogenic cells derived from the adult human subventricular zone. This discrepancy may be due to technical issues, but could also be related to the plasticity of these cells in vitro as CD133 levels seems to be affected by bioenergetic stress[22-24]. Due to the discrepancy between studies, other adult human neural stem cell (ahNSC) or precursor markers have been suggested (SSEA1, CXCR4, A2B5, peanut-agglutinin ++)[21, 25]. These are less explored, but all seem to struggle with the level of variability and heterogeneity.

SCs are more robust than differentiated cells. The fact that NSC can be isolated from human brain >48 hrs post mortem exemplifies this fact[26]. Another well known example is the regrowth of hair lost during chemotherapy treatment. During chemotherapy patients loose hair one to three weeks after initiation of therapy. However, the SC of hair follicles survive, and usually hair grow back from three to six months after termination of therapy[27]. The molecular machinery behind increased DNA-repair mechanisms, free-radical scavengers systems and membrane pumps to expel toxic substances have been described in a range of cancers[28]. The presence of the same molecular machinery in a variety of malignancies implies that such mechanisms are based on activation of intrinsic cellular properties and signaling events. The molecular machinery allowing protection of somatic stem cells could be used to prospectively identify and enrich for such cells. The efflux of toxic substances by ABC (ATP Binding Cassette Transporter) membrane pumps was used to identify a population of cells with high efflux of the DNA-binding dye Hoechst 33342 with stem cell properties in murine hematopoietic system [29]. This functional phenotype was identified in fractions of cells isolated from developing mouse brain [30] and brain tumor cell lines [31]. Similarly, the ability to metabolize aldehydes has been used to identify stem cells in developing and adult murine brain[32]. Whether this approach will overcome the problems described above for surface markers is still unknown.

A third approach is to enrich for stem cells using culturing conditions selectively allowing for these cells to proliferate. This has been shown to effectively allow NSC proliferation in a range of species (murine[33], canine[34], porcine[35], monkey[36] and human[37]). Similarly, non-adherent, serum-poor culturing conditions have been shown to be applicable for SC in colon[38, 39], breast[40, 41], prostate[42,43], heart[44], skin[45, 46], pancreas[47, 48], and liver[49]. Under these conditions SC can proliferate extensively, while cells lacking this ability are eliminated. The demonstration of extensive self-renewal and generation of differentiated progeny by a large number of groups have shown this to be a robust method of isolating SC.

## 3. Neurogenesis and biology of endogenous NSCs

### 3.1 Neurogenesis and neurogenic regions

Stem cells differentiating into neurons (neurogenesis) have been identified in both the dentate gyrus of the hippocampus and in the walls of the lateral ventricles in the subventricular zone (SVZ) and the rostral migratory stream (RMS) - the main pathway by which newly born neurons from SVZ reach the olfactory bulb. Cells in both neurgenic niches seem to translate through similar cellular development, but the anatomical organization is quite different.

In the dentate gyrus cells migrate only a few micrometers, from the subgranular zone to the granule cell layer. Cells develop from a precursor cell type in which mitotic events are found. Most of the newly formed cells are eliminated, and only few cells are able to establish axons, dendrites and functional synapses (postmitotic maturation phase). During the late survival phase characteristic electrophysiological patterns develop, receiving glutamatergic input from the entorhinal cortex and sending out axons to the hippocampal CA3 region. After a maturation period of several weeks the newly developed neurons establish characteristics identical to the other preexisting neurons[2].

The SVZ, in the walls of the lateral ventricles, contains the largest concentration of dividing cells in the adult mammalian brain[4, 50]. In the human brain there seems to be far more proliferating cells in the SVZ compared to the hippocampus[51, 52]. The cellular composition and organization of this region differs somewhat amongst species[53, 54]. In mammals the SVZ contains three cell populations important for stem cell proliferation. The proper stem cell population is maintained through slowly dividing astrocyte-like neural stem cells known as type B cells. These cells give rise to actively proliferating type C cells, which in turn give rise to immature neuroblasts, called type A cells. These neuroblasts, not yet neuronally committed, migrate to the olfactory bulb via chain migration by cell-cell contacts. Neuroblast chains are ensheathed by the processes of type B cells. In the anterior and dorsal SVZ, these chains condense to form the RMS [55-57]. After reaching the olfactory bulb cells migrate radially along blood vessel, and differentiate into interneurons incorporated into the functional circuitry of olfactory bulb and forebrain[50, 57].

In the adult brain, rodent and human studies reveal that neurogenesis continues in the SVZ throughout adult life[4, 56, 58-60]. The SVZ-RMS structure of the human brain contains $10^5$ dividing cells, a number that is high compared with the rodent[51, 61]. As age increases in rodents, the number of neurogenic cells decreases[62, 63]. Early data based on magnetic resonance spectroscopy suggests that this may also be the case in humans[64].

Under normal circumstances the function of the SVZ is to produce neuroblasts for the RMS[51, 53, 56]. More recent experiments have demonstrated that the progenitors of the SVZ are capable of producing oligodendrocytes in addition to olfactory interneurons[65]. After experimental injury in animal models of Huntigton disease and stroke, the SVZ not only supplies the RMS with neuroblasts but SVZ progenitor cells also migrate toward the site of injury and cell death[66, 67]. Thus, the proliferation and migration from the SVZ responds to injury, suggesting a more important role for this region in neurorestoration.

### 3.2 Regulatory signaling of the NSC pool

The proliferation and differentiation of the NSC pool is highly regulated. The microenvironment maintaining this function is called the stem cell niche. This is a combination of signaling through extracellular matrix (ECM), cell-cell contacts, secreted substances, innervation and physical factors.

The niche is embedded in extensions of the vascular basal lamina that extends around NSCs and progenitors[68]. These laminin and collagen I-rich ECM structures can be observed under the electron microscope and have been named fractones. These structures has been suggested to bind secreted growth factors, like Fiborblast growth factor (FGF), regulating concentrations and signaling strength of secreted factors[69, 70], tenascin-C[70-72], osteopentin[73], chondroitin/dermatan sulfate proteoglycans[74, 75].

Ependymal cells, lining the ventricles, exert a supporting/ regulatory function in the niche, since they can modulate the transport of ions and other factors from the cerebrospinal fluid (CSF)[76]. They secrete neurogenic factors like pigment epithelium-derived factor (PEDF)[77] and the pro-neurogenic bone morphogenic protein (BMP) signaling substances[78, 79]. These cells also form gap junctions with SVZ astrocytes[80], allowing controlled transfer of substances from the CSF to the niche. NSC adapt close contacts to blood vessels both in the subgranular zone and the SVZ[69, 81]. This connection is suggested to be central in neurogenesis[82]. This could be through cell-cell-contact mediated signaling or through secreted factors like PEDF, leukemia-inhibitory factor (LIF) and brain-derived neurotrophic factor (BDNF) [83].

Several studies have shown effect on SVZ progenitor proliferation through infusion of growth factors into the ventricles. FGF, epidermal growth factor (EGF) and transforming growth factor alpha (TGFalpha)[62, 84, 85] have no identified source within the niche, but may originate from the choroid plexus and transported through CSF. Platelet derived growth factor (PDGF), PEDF and Vascular endothelial growth factor (VEGF) derived from endothelial cells regulate NSC and progenitor proliferation[77, 86-88], and PDGF also have effects on the differentiational balance between neurons and oligodendrocytes[86]. Several other secreted factors contributes to this orchestra of regulation like LIF[87, 89], BDNF[90, 91] and BMPs[78, 92].

Of special interest are the three stem cell related signaling pathways; Hedgehog-, Wnt- and Notch- pathways. Sonic hedgehog (Shh) is a morphogen known to regulate neurogenesis and gliogenesis during development. This signaling increase precursor and NSC proliferation both in the hippocampus and the SVZ[94-96] and Shh is essential for their maintenance[97]. Genetic manipulation by knocking-down the Shh signaling results in depletion of SVZ neurogenesis, while increased signaling leads to upregulation of proliferation[98]. Wnt-pathway signaling is orchestrated through a number of secreted Wnt ligands and a range of Frizzled receptors, and their interaction mediates the possibility for fine tuning of a proliferation-differentiation signal[99-102]. The combination of FGF and b-catenin signaling might be a requisite for neuronal differentiation[103]. Notch signaling is based on binding of ligands and receptors that are membrane bound, and thus acts through cell-cell interaction. This signaling is essential for niche maintenance, and again regulates both the size of the NSC pool and differentiation[104, 105], and differences in Notch signaling distinguish NSC from progenitors[106].

The convergence of synaptic input by classical neurotransmitters like γ-amino-butyric acid (GABA) and serotonin (5-HT) modulates the NSC niche. GABA is the principle inhibitory neurotransmitter in the adult CNS but has an excitatory action in the SVZ and the subgranular zone of the hippocampus[107, 108]. This effect is similar to its effect during brain development [109]. Isolated rat neuroblasts also express the GABA-A receptor. GABA has been found to decrease neuroblast migration[110] and to cause cell cycle exit[111], suggesting that the number of dividing neuroblasts could be regulated by a feedback loop between NSCs and neuroblasts[112]. Major focus has been put on the serotonergic systems effect on the niche due to its importance in psychiatric diseases [113]. Early studies depleting serotonin (5-HT) in prenatal stages showed a reduction in cell proliferation in both neurogenic niches[114]. The effects of 5-HT are mediated on receptor level on NSC population might, however, differ in the SVZ and the subgranular layer[115, 116].

In Huntington's disease (HD) the SVZ increases in size, and has increased number of progenitor cells, while the mature cells present are altered. In Parkinson disease, on the other hand, the number of proliferating progenitors is almost halved compared to the normal situation[66, 67, 117-119]. This is believed to be related to the loss of dopamine stimulation of NSC proliferation.

Gas composition also affects NSC regulation. Processes of nitrergic neurons intercalate with neuroblasts in the SVZ [120]. Inhibitors of Nitirc oxide (NO) signaling affects cell proliferation and NO synthase deficient mice also exhibit higher levels of proliferation in the SVZ[120-122]. Oxygen tension highly affects the potency and proliferative potential of NSC[123, 124], and can switch the neurogenesis from differentiation of GABA-positive to glutamate positive neurons[125].

### 3.3 Cancer stem cells and their relation to NSC

The phenotype of neural stem cells is mirrored in several aspects of malignant tumor biology[126-128]. Several of the intrinsic molecular pathways and extracellular signaling systems identified in regulation of NSC have also been identified in cancer cells. Such cells, termed cancer stem cells (CSC) have been suggested to be essential in tumor growth and therapy resistance. Since NSC harbor the molecular machinery to respond to signals of proliferation and defense mechanisms to extrude toxic substances[129, 130], it has been suggested that NSC are the cell of origin for brain neoplasms[131]. By using conditionally targeted gene knock down of the tumor suppressor p53 in neural progenitor cells (Nestin +) and astrocytes (GFAP+), it has been demonstrated that both populations of cells can give rise to tumors[132, 133]. The induction of tumors however seem to be at lesser threshold by RAS and AKT transformation in Nestin+ cells, suggesting greater risk of tumor development from less differentiated cells. Similarly, different cell populations of NSCs, neural progenitor cells (NPCs) and more differentiated cells can all be candidates for malignant transformation[131]. In two subgroups of medulloblastomas different cells of origin and different molecular pathways seem to be important in tumorigenesis. Midline medulloblastomas present in the brain stem seem to develop from dorsal brainstem progenitors and be dependent on the Wnt- pathway. More laterally situated, cerebellar tumors seem to develop from granule neuron progenitors and be stimulated through SHH-pathway signaling[134].

The NSC pool and niche is highly controlled through a range of factors, underscoring the biological importance of these cell populations. Manipulating the signaling pathways for NSC homeostasis could thus be potential therapeutic intervention in brain tumors. Conversely, it is apparent that molecular signals or drugs that induce NSC proliferation could potentially be tumorigenic.

## 4. Challenges for the generation of NSCs

Several stem cell types have neural capabilities: 1. pluripotent self-renewing embryonic stem cells, 2. multipotent stem cells with broad potential and self-renewing capacity from embryonic, fetal or adult brain, 3. neural progenitors with limited potential and self-renewal capacity from adult brain or spinal cord, 4. committed neural progenitors (neuronal and glial) from brain subregions [135].

Embryonic stem cells (ESCs) have an almost unlimited capacity to self-renew. On the other hand, ESCs also have a considerable teratogenic potential after implantation into host tissue, and it is not yet clear how long chromosomal stability can be maintained[136]. In addition, immense ethical concerns exist regarding the use of human ESCs as well as government restrictions that continue to limit clinical applications [137].

Human fetal mesencephalic NSCs fulfill some important requirements for the use in cell replacement strategies. They can be generate high yields of functional neurons from a small starting population, representing on-demand availability of cells without major logistical problems and the possibility to standardize the cell source in a clinical setting. In contrast to ES cells, tumorigenicity seems to be a minor problem with fetal NSCs. These cells are less flexible with regards to multiplication and differentiation, but there is increasing evidence that it is more beneficial to use cells that are already committed to becoming a particular cell type[138].

More recently, induced pluripotent stem cells (iPS) were generated, and such cells offer another source of autologous neural stem cells[137]. It has been known that differentiated cells can be reprogrammed to an embryonic-like state by nuclear transfer to oocytes, fusion with ES cells or molecular reprogramming of somatic cells into induced pluripotent stem cells using genetic factors[138]. Most of the current reprogramming methods are using expression of putative oncogenes by retroviral vectors. The factors used are involved in carcinogenesis, posing a risk for clinical translation. Important questions regarding safety and genetic stability must be solved before iPS can be used in clinical trials[139].

Brain-derived ahNSC are very attractive because of the clear logistical benefits if the therapeutic stem cells can be derived from a patient's own body. Technical obstacles (obtaining fetal and embryonic tissue, immune graft rejection in hetero- and xenotransplantation, potential tumor formation after grafting of induced pluripotent cells) as well as ethical issues (in contrast to embryonic, fetal, hetero- or xenotransplantations of cells) can be avoided. Despite this, there are limited data concerning the application of adult human-derived neural stem cells in clinical trials and very limited number of experimental data[140].

Adult human neural stem cells can be isolated from a range of sources. Cells derived from the two neurogenic regions of the brain have been the most thoroughly examined, but cells with neurogenic potential in vitro can be derived from subcortical white matter[141], spinal cord[142], filum terminale[143, 144] and hypothalamus[145]. Also cells derived from the olfactory mucosa, found in the nasal cavity, contain ahNSC[146]. Several of these regions allow for harvesting of autologous NSC with minimal risk and morbidity for the patient[143, 146, 147].

Multipotent adult stem cells have also significant advantages with regard to autologous transplantation approaches without immunological graft rejection. Hematopoietic stem cells

(HSCs) and mesenchymal stem cells (MSCs) are valuable sources for cell transplantation and cell therapy. Although recent *in vitro* as well as *in vivo* studies suggested that multipotent adult stem cells, or their pro-neurally converted derivatives, could display protective or regenerative effects in experimental models of CNS diseases[138], more experimental data to translate the application of this type of cells to clinical trial is needed[137].

The discovery of multipotent stem and progenitor cells in the adult human brain has opened the possibility of treating central nervous system disorders through replacement of the injured tissue by transplanted cells or by stimulating recruitment of endogenous repair mechanisms. We have previously shown that in principle adult human neural progenitor cells (ahNPCs) could be transplanted to ischemically damaged brain for in vivo maturation into neurons[93,148]. The latter can be achieved both by infusion of growth factors or by transplanting progenitors delivering neurogenic factors to the injured brain. .

To obtain such a goal, one must have culturing protocols with the ability to obtain enough cells resulting in a clinically significant effect in one or more patients. In addition, the cells must survive long enough for quality testing and possible genetic manipulation before transplantation. One of the main obstacles when culturing ahNPCs has been that the cells seem to stop proliferating after a limited number of passages and also lose their ability for proper differentiation with repetitive passages[151]

The problem may however not apply to all ahNSC, as olfactory mucosa derived SC show higher propencity for proliferation and have been shown to be effective in an animal model of PD[195]. Also, it has been reported that ahNPCs can be propagated *in vitro* for as long as 20 months (12 to 15 passages) and have shown differentiation into cells expressing neuronal and astrocytic markers[149]. Together with a publication by Walton et al.[150], this article provides further evidence that the limitations upon continued propagation of ahNPCs previously reported by others may be surmounted.

Finally, when an adequate number of cells have been produced in vitro, the cells must be documented to have the appropriate ability to differentiate into mature neurons with the ability to produce synapses and generate functional action potentials. While we have documented this in cells cultivated short term in vitro[151-153], similar data on long term cultivated cells are lacking. We are looking forward to future experiments we hope will evaluate the ability of these long-term propagated progenitors for normal functional differentiation in vitro and in vivo.

## 5. NSC treatment strategies

Concerning the techniques of NSC application, regardless of the cell source, there are several treatment strategies that are explored in restorative approach.

### 5.1 Stimulation of endogenous NSC

It is evident that the adult brain contains a pool of NSC that have the ability to proliferate- and that can respond to extrinsic signals[154, 155].

Recent data suggests that NSCs and NPCs can migrate from their site of birth to other parts of the brain and contribute to the replacement of specific cell types lost due to injury or disease[156-158]. In animal stroke models striatal neurons can be derived from endogenous NSC and progenitors [157, 159-161]. Similarly, compensatory neurogenesis exists in Huntington's and Alzheimer's disease patients. Compensatory neocortical neuron production have been demonstrated after targeted ablation of both interneurons and corticospinal neurons[162-165]. This neurogenesis is, however, quite modest and not associated with clinically significant functional effects. This is probably due to the limited number of stem cells recruited and/or the unfavorable environment of the injured adult brain for supporting efficient production of new neurons and glia.

Thus, the current challenge is to understand how to modify the molecular basis of compensatory neurogenesis in order to overcome its limiting factors in the pathological and aged CNS, while supporting those that accentuate its' influence.

Several of the described factors that affects the NSC pool are potentially tumor inducing when administered systemically, thus a major obstacle in developing this type of therapy is how to deliver the factor- or rather- the sequence of factors needed at high temporal and anatomical precision. Animal models have primarily used intraventricular injections or viral delivery methods to achieve this. Intraventricular injection of TGFAlpha activates endogenous neurogenesis in the SVZ of Parkinson's disease (PD) model rats [166, 167]. Similarly, the injection of the Notch receptor ligand angiopoietin2 or DII4 growth factors can induce widespread stimulation of endogenous neural precursors, and in a PD rodent model rescue injured dopamine neurons and stimulate improvement of motor function. Adenoviral co-delivery of BDNF and BMP signaling molecule Noggin induces striatal neuron replacement from endogenous precursors and delays motor impairment in a Huntington's disease model[168]. Intraventricluar injection of EGF and erythropoietin in combination can mobilize endogenous adult neural stem cells to promote cortical tissue re-growth and functional recovery after stroke[169]. Systemic erythropoietin is already in clinical use for the stimulation of erythropoiesis, thus allowing a rapid translation of this approach to clinical investigation. In a combination with the neurotrophic hormone β-human chorionic gonadotropin (hCG) this was found to be safe, and potentially beneficial in a phase II trial for the stimulation of neurogenesis after stroke[170].

### 5.2 Cell replacement by transplantation

As several obstacles remain regarding how to stimulate the correct cells with the correct sequence of stimulatory factors within the complex NSC niche, most therapeutic strategies are based on the transplantation of in vitro or ex vivo manipulated cells.

Most groups have favored the transplantation of immature cells. The idea is to let grafted cells differentiate under the influence of the host environment, integrate into the local neuronal network and thus become a functional unit of the brain or spinal cord. Immature cells are believed to be more robust than differentiated cells, and could contain the necessary plasticity to overcome pathological scar formation and inhibitory signals of relocation and differentiation. This approach is the most common in animal models of neurorestoration[2]. Also, the transplanted cells must have the ability to form the correct cells needed, and must stop proliferation when the proper cell types have been formed.

Better control of the developed progeny could be achieved by grafting of mature or at least partly differentiated cells. It is supposed that predifferentiation may help the processes of functional integration of transplanted cells. We have shown that in selective injury of hippocampal CA1 region by global ischemia both ahNSC and predifferentiated cells preferentially migrate into the damaged area[93,148]. The predifferentiated cells develop more markers of differentiated neurons at an earlier time point. Thus, ahNSC can be manipulated *in vitro* to yield a greater neuronal differentiation after transplantation. In approaches where potential tumor forming cells are used, a controlled differentiation could reduce the risk of adverse tumor formation[165]. Similar in-vitro predifferentiation has been tested for generation of dopaminergic neurons in PD[169]. Further modification of the transplanted cells could be genetically manipulated cells that secret anti-apoptotic or pro-differentiation signal or a combination of NSC and stromal cells.

### 5.3 Microenvironmental modification

A third approach facilitates the ability of transplanted cells to affect the environment which the cells are transplanted into. Autocrine and paracrine factors derived from NSC can modulate the niche and stem-, progenitor and differentiated cells after transplantation. In rats it has been found that secreted growth factors from transplanted NSCs stimulated proliferation of endogenous NSC[171], called "bystander effect". In several transplantation studies functional recovery is far greater than the number of identified transplanted cells would indicate. This has been suggested to be a result of synergistic effects of the NSC on the host microenvironment.

Furthermore, transplanted NSC can secrete factors not present in the host. Infantile neuronal ceroid lipofuscinosis is a fatal neurodegenerative disease caused by a deficiency in the lysosomal enzyme palmitoyl protein thioesterase-1 (PPT1). The lack of this enzyme leads to pathological lipofuscin-like material accumulating in cells, leading to progressive loss of vision, decreasing cognitive and motor skills, epileptic seizures and premature death. Normally functioning cells produce surplus of this enzyme, and some of this is secreted to the extracellular environment. This secreted enzyme can be absorbed by other cells, also cells not producing this enzyme on their own. This can be done in quantities high enough to stop lysosomal sequestering. In a mouse model lacking the gene for PPT1 transplanted NSC could reduce lipofuscine levels, provide neuroprotection and delay loss of motor function [172].

## 6. Towards using NSC to treat neurological disorders

Although NSC therapy have been suggested as a therapy for a range of neurological diseases, here we highlight the results for the most studied diseases; PD, stroke, and spinal cord injury.

### 6.1 Parkinson's disease

Over the past 30 years, neural transplantation has emerged as a possible therapy for PD. It was shown that grafted neural cells from different sources can survive for over 20 years and exert beneficial effects in PD patients[173]. Different types of cell have been tested both in experimental and clinical trial. Embryonic derived stem cells have been suggested the cell of choice, since they promise to be made in high quantities and to hold large amounts of the desired cell type [138]. Clinical testing of transplants to patients with PD of primary human embryonic dopaminergic neurons or tissue using double-blind, placebo-controlled protocols have shown positive results. The patients displayed impressive improvements of symptoms and restoration of dopaminergic neurotransmission, but also demonstrated several clinical limitations. Only subpopulations of patients showed significant clinical benefits. Moreover, a significant proportion of patients (with up to 56%) suffered from dyskinesias after a twelve-hour drug-free period[174-176].

Whether, these early results could be transferable to the use of ESC is uncertain. Also, the use of ÈSC harbors problems of controlling cell growth and differentiation, including brain tumor and teratoma formation[138, 177-179]. In contrast, there are no reports of tumor formation in fetal NSCs transplantations, what makes the usage of fetal tissue-specific be a safer way to establish a transplantation protocol in PD. Open-label clinical studies continued through the 1990s have shown that fetal ventral mesencephalic allografts could survive in patients with advanced PD, become functionally integrated, and produce sustained clinical benefits; however, it also soon became clear that transplants of this type produced very variable responses, with some patients showing only little improvement or transient benefits[173]. In patients receiving grafts post mortem studies have demonstrated that also transplanted cells display Lewy bodies, a sign of PD[180, 181].

Overall several issues hinders the further development of a cellular replacement approach for PD[176]. Ethical issues and technical problems (i.e. obtaining fetal and embryonic tissue, immune graft) are slowing down the clinical application in PD patients. New candidate for cell replacement are needed, but the role of other types of potential sources for transplantations - brain-derived adult neural stem cells, adult multipotent stem cells, induced pluripotent cells is still not clear. One case-report describes the effect of autologous transplantation of SVZ derived NSC[140]. Although effects on several clinical aspects were reported, these only lasted 36 months and weaned off after 4-5 years. Based on this result, a phase II study has been approved, but later put on hold due to demands put on cell production facilities (neurogeneration.com).

### 6.2 Stroke

Stroke is another severe pathology where significant loss of neural tissue is the major factor of the illness. No current therapies promote neuronal recovery following ischemic insults. As mentioned above, endogenous NSC proliferate as a response to both ischemic stroke and subarachnoid hemorrage[182, 183], and stimulation of this endogenous neurogenesis has been tried using a combination with of erythropoietin and hCG as mentioned above.

Based on work in animal models, transplantation of exogenous cells into the injured brain to replace the lost cells or support the remaining cells is one of promising direction[184]. There is a significant experimental background that supports the idea that the grafting of exogenous stem cells from multiple sources can generate neural cells that survive and form synaptic connections after transplantation in the stroke-injured brain[185]. The world's first fully regulated clinical trial of a neural stem cell therapy for disabled stroke patients - PISCES study (Pilot Investigation of Stem Cells in Stroke) – has been started in Scotland at the Institute of Neurological Sciences in 2011. Stem cell therapy (purified population of human neural stem cells, derived from human fetal brain tissue) is being administered to a total of 12 patients. The obtained data is planned to be announced in 2012.

### 6.3 Spinal cord injury

Cell replacement in spinal cord injury (SCI) is also a field of great interest for neurobiologist and clinicians. A large number of different cells including embryonic and adult stem cells have been transplanted into animal models of spinal cord injury, and in many cases these procedures have resulted in modest sensorimotor benefits[186]. Also a range of clinical experiments involving administration of stem cells for SCI patients have already taken place. Early studies in nine patients showed that unselected human fetal neural tissue transplanted to progressively developing posttraumatic syringomyelia could safely be used to obliterate the syrinx[187, 188]. No tumor developed, but the clinical effect of this obliteration was however limited.

A Portuguese study have reported using unselected olfactory mucosa transplanted into SCI damage site in twenty patients with complete medullary lesions[189, 190]. Treatment resulted in a filling at the transplant site. Urodynamic responses improved in five patients. Two of the patients regained voluntary control of anal sphincter. Eleven patients improved while one patient declined in ASIA impairment scale. The authors concluded that olfactory mucosa autografts are feasible, safe and possibly beneficial.

Geron Corporation (Menlo Park, CA, USA) was in 2009 given a US Food and Drug Administration (FDA) approval for the first test of human embryonic stem cell derived oligodendroglial cells in patients for SCI. Although high controversy existed regarding cell source, safety and patient selection, several patients were included into the study. After an early stop in the study because of worries regarding cyst development at injection sites in preclinical studies, recruitment started in 2010. In the first four patients included in the study, the treatment appeared safe. Sadly, the study was recently stopped due to financial reasons[191].

## 7. Future directions

Through the last two decades the presence and potential of NSC has become apparent. NSC are used to understand developments of pathology and new based treatments are explored in a range of neurological disease

Although we clearly are at a very early stage of translating the basic biological understanding of NSC into possible therapies, several phase I and II studies have been reported using cell based approaches to treat neurological conditions. However several obstacles affect the translation of promising preclinical studies. Laws, regulation and public understanding of this research are poorly developed. While ethical concerns have develop into regulations that forces restrictive use on a broad range of new technologies in some regions, lack of established safety and quality parameters have led to unsafe and dangerous trials other places[192]. It is a story as old as it is unfortunate, in which opportunistic individuals and companies may manipulate hype and hope for financial gain[193]. Already reports exist on patient developing tumors after ill-designed and unsafe treatment based on NSC[194]. Certainly, at this early stage NSC based therapies should be part of a well designed and publically reported clinical trial (http://www.isscr.org/clinical_trans/pdfs/ISSCRPatientHandbook.pdf).

## 8. References

[1] Gogel S, Gubernator M, Minger SL. Progress and prospects: stem cells and neurological diseases. Gene Ther 2011; 18(1):1-6.

[2] Kempermann G. Adult Neurogenesis. Stem Cells and Neuronal Development in Adult Brain. New York: Oxford University Press; 2006.
[3] Cajal R. Degeneration and Regeneration Nervous System. Oxford University Press; 1913.
[4] Altman J. Proliferation and migration of undifferentiated precursor cells in the rat during postnatal gliogenesis. Exp Neurol 1966; 16(3):263-278.
[5] Kornblum HI. Introduction to neural stem cells. Stroke 2007; 38(2 Suppl):810-816.
[6] Nottebohm F. Neuronal replacement in adulthood. Ann N Y Acad Sci 1985; 457:143-161.
[7] Reynolds BA, Weiss S. Generation of neurons and astrocytes from isolated cells of the adult mammalian central nervous system. Science 1992; 255(5052):1707-1710.
[8] Morrison SJ, Shah NM, Anderson DJ. Regulatory mechanisms in stem cell biology. Cell 1997; 88(3):287-298.
[9] Kawamoto H, Wada H, Katsura Y. A revised scheme for developmental pathways of hematopoietic cells: the myeloid-based model. Int Immunol 2010; 22(2):65-70.
[10] Giebel B, Punzel M. Lineage development of hematopoietic stem and progenitor cells. Biol Chem 2008; 389(7):813-824.
[11] Vickaryous MK, Hall BK. Human cell type diversity, evolution, development, and classification with special reference to cells derived from the neural crest. Biol Rev Camb Philos Soc 2006; 81(3):425-455.
[12] Croft AP, Przyborski SA. Formation of neurons by non-neural adult stem cells: potential mechanism implicates an artifact of growth in culture. Stem Cells 2006; 24(8):1841-1851.
[13] Alvarez-Buylla A, Kohwi M, Nguyen TM, Merkle FT. The heterogeneity of adult neural stem cells and the emerging complexity of their niche. Cold Spring Harb Symp Quant Biol 2008; 73:357-365.
[14] Stancik EK, Navarro-Quiroga I, Sellke R, Haydar TF. Heterogeneity in ventricular zone neural precursors contributes to neuronal fate diversity in the postnatal neocortex. J Neurosci 2010; 30(20):7028-7036.
[15] Yin AH, Miraglia S, Zanjani ED et al. AC133, a novel marker for human hematopoietic stem and progenitor cells. Blood 1997; 90(12):5002-5012.
[16] Uchida N, Buck DW, He D et al. Direct isolation of human central nervous system stem cells. Proc Natl Acad Sci U S A 2000; 97(26):14720-14725.
[17] Wagner W, Ansorge A, Wirkner U et al. Molecular evidence for stem cell function of the slow-dividing fraction among human hematopoietic progenitor cells by genome-wide analysis. Blood 2004; 104(3):675-686.
[18] Kam M, Curtis MA, McGlashan SR, Connor B, Nannmark U, Faull RL. The cellular composition and morphological organization of the rostral migratory stream in the adult human brain. J Chem Neuroanat 2009; 37(3):196-205.
[19] Schwartz PH, Bryant PJ, Fuja TJ, Su H, O'Dowd DK, Klassen H. Isolation and characterization of neural progenitor cells from post-mortem human cortex. J Neurosci Res 2003; 74(6):838-851.
[20] Pfenninger CV, Roschupkina T, Hertwig F et al. CD133 is not present on neurogenic astrocytes in the adult subventricular zone, but on embryonic neural stem cells, ependymal cells, and glioblastoma cells. Cancer Res 2007; 67(12):5727-5736.
[21] Sun Y, Kong W, Falk A et al. CD133 (Prominin) negative human neural stem cells are clonogenic and tripotent. PLoS One 2009; 4(5):e5498.

[22] Bar EE, Lin A, Mahairaki V, Matsui W, Eberhart CG. Hypoxia increases the expression of stem-cell markers and promotes clonogenicity in glioblastoma neurospheres. Am J Pathol 2010; 177(3):1491-1502.

[23] Griguer CE, Oliva CR, Gobin E et al. CD133 is a marker of bioenergetic stress in human glioma. PLoS One 2008; 3(11):e3655.

[24] Platet N, Liu SY, Atifi ME et al. Influence of oxygen tension on CD133 phenotype in human glioma cell cultures. Cancer Lett 2007; 258(2):286-290.

[25] Pfenninger CV, Roschupkina T, Hertwig F et al. CD133 is not present on neurogenic astrocytes in the adult subventricular zone, but on embryonic neural stem cells, ependymal cells, and glioblastoma cells. Cancer Res 2007; 67(12):5727-5736.

[26] Palmer TD, Schwartz PH, Taupin P, Kaspar B, Stein SA, Gage FH. Cell culture. Progenitor cells from human brain after death. Nature 2001; 411(6833):42-43.

[27] Trueb RM. Chemotherapy-induced alopecia. Curr Opin Support Palliat Care 2010; 4(4):281-284.

[28] Hanahan D, Weinberg RA. The hallmarks of cancer. Cell 2000; 100(1):57-70.

[29] Goodell MA, Brose K, Paradis G, Conner AS, Mulligan RC. Isolation and functional properties of murine hematopoietic stem cells that are replicating in vivo. J Exp Med 1996; 183(4):1797-1806.

[30] Murayama A, Matsuzaki Y, Kawaguchi A, Shimazaki T, Okano H. Flow cytometric analysis of neural stem cells in the developing and adult mouse brain. J Neurosci Res 2002; 69(6):837-847.

[31] Kondo T, Setoguchi T, Taga T. Persistence of a small subpopulation of cancer stem-like cells in the C6 glioma cell line. Proc Natl Acad Sci U S A 2004; 101(3):781-786.

[32] Corti S, Locatelli F, Papadimitriou D et al. Identification of a primitive brain-derived neural stem cell population based on aldehyde dehydrogenase activity. Stem Cells 2006; 24(4):975-985.

[33] Reynolds BA, Weiss S. Generation of neurons and astrocytes from isolated cells of the adult mammalian central nervous system. Science 1992; 255(5052):1707-1710.

[34] Milward EA, Lundberg CG, Ge B, Lipsitz D, Zhao M, Duncan ID. Isolation and transplantation of multipotential populations of epidermal growth factor-responsive, neural progenitor cells from the canine brain. J Neurosci Res 1997; 50(5):862-871.

[35] Dyce PW, Zhu H, Craig J, Li J. Stem cells with multilineage potential derived from porcine skin. Biochem Biophys Res Commun 2004; 316(3):651-658.

[36] Tonchev AB, Yamashima T, Sawamoto K, Okano H. Enhanced proliferation of progenitor cells in the subventricular zone and limited neuronal production in the striatum and neocortex of adult macaque monkeys after global cerebral ischemia. J Neurosci Res 2005; 81(6):776-788.

[37] Kukekov VG, Laywell ED, Suslov O et al. Multipotent stem/progenitor cells with similar properties arise from two neurogenic regions of adult human brain. Exp Neurol 1999; 156(2):333-344.

[38] Carpentino JE, Hynes MJ, Appelman HD et al. Aldehyde dehydrogenase-expressing colon stem cells contribute to tumorigenesis in the transition from colitis to cancer. Cancer Res 2009; 69(20):8208-8215.

[39] Ricci-Vitiani L, Lombardi DG, Pilozzi E et al. Identification and expansion of human colon-cancer-initiating cells. Nature 2007; 445(7123):111-115.
[40] Dontu G, Al-Hajj M, Abdallah WM, Clarke MF, Wicha MS. Stem cells in normal breast development and breast cancer. Cell Prolif 2003; 36 Suppl 1:59-72.
[41] Liu S, Dontu G, Mantle ID et al. Hedgehog signaling and Bmi-1 regulate self-renewal of normal and malignant human mammary stem cells. Cancer Res 2006; 66(12):6063-6071.
[42] Lawson DA, Witte ON. Stem cells in prostate cancer initiation and progression. J Clin Invest 2007; 117(8):2044-2050.
[43] Duhagon MA, Hurt EM, Sotelo-Silveira JR, Zhang X, Farrar WL. Genomic profiling of tumor initiating prostatospheres. BMC Genomics 2010; 11:324.
[44] Davis DR, Zhang Y, Smith RR et al. Validation of the cardiosphere method to culture cardiac progenitor cells from myocardial tissue. PLoS One 2009; 4(9):e7195.
[45] Le RH, Zuliani T, Wolowczuk I et al. Asymmetric distribution of epidermal growth factor receptor directs the fate of normal and cancer keratinocytes in vitro. Stem Cells Dev 2010; 19(2):209-220.
[46] Toma JG, Akhavan M, Fernandes KJ et al. Isolation of multipotent adult stem cells from the dermis of mammalian skin. Nat Cell Biol 2001; 3(9):778-784.
[47] Gaviraghi M, Tunici P, Valensin S et al. Pancreatic cancer spheres are more than just aggregates of stem marker-positive cells. Biosci Rep 2010; 31(1):45-55.
[48] Seaberg RM, Smukler SR, Kieffer TJ et al. Clonal identification of multipotent precursors from adult mouse pancreas that generate neural and pancreatic lineages. Nat Biotechnol 2004; 22(9):1115-1124.
[49] Uchida Y, Tanaka S, Aihara A et al. Analogy between sphere forming ability and stemness of human hepatoma cells. Oncol Rep 2010; 24(5):1147-1151.
[50] Lois C, varez-Buylla A. Proliferating subventricular zone cells in the adult mammalian forebrain can differentiate into neurons and glia. Proc Natl Acad Sci U S A 1993; 90(5):2074-2077.
[51] Curtis MA, Kam M, Nannmark U et al. Human neuroblasts migrate to the olfactory bulb via a lateral ventricular extension. Science 2007; 315(5816):1243-1249.
[52] Lucassen PJ, Meerlo P, Naylor AS et al. Regulation of adult neurogenesis by stress, sleep disruption, exercise and inflammation: Implications for depression and antidepressant action. Eur Neuropsychopharmacol 2010; 20(1):1-17.
[53] Doetsch F, Garcia-Verdugo JM, varez-Buylla A. Cellular composition and three-dimensional organization of the subventricular germinal zone in the adult mammalian brain. J Neurosci 1997; 17(13):5046-5061.
[54] Quinones-Hinojosa A, Sanai N, Soriano-Navarro M et al. Cellular composition and cytoarchitecture of the adult human subventricular zone: a niche of neural stem cells. J Comp Neurol 2006; 494(3):415-434.
[55] Lois C, varez-Buylla A. Long-distance neuronal migration in the adult mammalian brain. Science 1994; 264(5162):1145-1148.
[56] Lois C, Garcia-Verdugo JM, varez-Buylla A. Chain migration of neuronal precursors. Science 1996; 271(5251):978-981.
[57] Peretto P, Merighi A, Fasolo A, Bonfanti L. Glial tubes in the rostral migratory stream of the adult rat. Brain Res Bull 1997; 42(1):9-21.

[58] Benraiss A, Chmielnicki E, Lerner K, Roh D, Goldman SA. Adenoviral brain-derived neurotrophic factor induces both neostriatal and olfactory neuronal recruitment from endogenous progenitor cells in the adult forebrain. J Neurosci 2001; 21(17):6718-6731.
[59] Eriksson PS, Perfilieva E, Bjork-Eriksson T et al. Neurogenesis in the adult human hippocampus. Nat Med 1998; 4(11):1313-1317.
[60] Luskin MB, Boone MS. Rate and pattern of migration of lineally-related olfactory bulb interneurons generated postnatally in the subventricular zone of the rat. Chem Senses 1994; 19(6):695-714.
[61] Kam M, Curtis MA, McGlashan SR, Connor B, Nannmark U, Faull RL. The cellular composition and morphological organization of the rostral migratory stream in the adult human brain. J Chem Neuroanat 2009; 37(3):196-205.
[62] Kuhn HG, ckinson-Anson H, Gage FH. Neurogenesis in the dentate gyrus of the adult rat: age-related decrease of neuronal progenitor proliferation. J Neurosci 1996; 16(6):2027-2033.
[63] Luo J, Daniels SB, Lennington JB, Notti RQ, Conover JC. The aging neurogenic subventricular zone. Aging Cell 2006; 5(2):139-152.
[64] Manganas LN, Zhang X, Li Y et al. Magnetic resonance spectroscopy identifies neural progenitor cells in the live human brain. Science 2007; 318(5852):980-985.
[65] Menn B, Garcia-Verdugo JM, Yaschine C, Gonzalez-Perez O, Rowitch D, varez-Buylla A. Origin of oligodendrocytes in the subventricular zone of the adult brain. J Neurosci 2006; 26(30):7907-7918.
[66] Arvidsson A, Collin T, Kirik D, Kokaia Z, Lindvall O. Neuronal replacement from endogenous precursors in the adult brain after stroke. Nat Med 2002; 8(9):963-970.
[67] Tattersfield AS, Croon RJ, Liu YW, Kells AP, Faull RL, Connor B. Neurogenesis in the striatum of the quinolinic acid lesion model of Huntington's disease. Neuroscience 2004; 127(2):319-332.
[68] Mercier F, Kitasako JT, Hatton GI. Anatomy of the brain neurogenic zones revisited: fractones and the fibroblast/macrophage network. J Comp Neurol 2002; 451(2):170-188.
[69] Kerever A, Schnack J, Vellinga D et al. Novel extracellular matrix structures in the neural stem cell niche capture the neurogenic factor fibroblast growth factor 2 from the extracellular milieu. Stem Cells 2007; 25(9):2146-2157.
[70] Jaworski DM, Fager N. Regulation of tissue inhibitor of metalloproteinase-3 (Timp-3) mRNA expression during rat CNS development. J Neurosci Res 2000; 61(4):396-408.
[71] de CA, Lemasson M, Saghatelyan A, Sibbe M, Schachner M, Lledo PM. Delayed onset of odor detection in neonatal mice lacking tenascin-C. Mol Cell Neurosci 2006; 32(1-2):174-186.
[72] Kazanis I, Belhadi A, Faissner A, Ffrench-Constant C. The adult mouse subependymal zone regenerates efficiently in the absence of tenascin-C. J Neurosci 2007; 27(51):13991-13996.
[73] Sailor KA, Dhodda VK, Rao VL, Dempsey RJ. Osteopontin infusion into normal adult rat brain fails to increase cell proliferation in dentate gyrus and subventricular zone. Acta Neurochir Suppl 2003; 86:181-185.

[74] Akita K, von HA, Furukawa Y, Mikami T, Sugahara K, Faissner A. Expression of multiple chondroitin/dermatan sulfotransferases in the neurogenic regions of the embryonic and adult central nervous system implies that complex chondroitin sulfates have a role in neural stem cell maintenance. Stem Cells 2008; 26(3):798-809.

[75] von Holst A, Sirko S, Faissner A. The unique 473HD-Chondroitinsulfate epitope is expressed by radial glia and involved in neural precursor cell proliferation. J Neurosci 2006; 26(15):4082-4094.

[76] Bruni JE. Ependymal development, proliferation, and functions: a review. Microsc Res Tech 1998; 41(1):2-13.

[77] Ramirez-Castillejo C, Sanchez-Sanchez F, ndreu-Agullo C et al. Pigment epithelium-derived factor is a niche signal for neural stem cell renewal. Nat Neurosci 2006; 9(3):331-339.

[78] Lim DA, Tramontin AD, Trevejo JM, Herrera DG, Garcia-Verdugo JM, varez-Buylla A. Noggin antagonizes BMP signaling to create a niche for adult neurogenesis. Neuron 2000; 28(3):713-726.

[79] Peretto P, Dati C, De MS et al. Expression of the secreted factors noggin and bone morphogenetic proteins in the subependymal layer and olfactory bulb of the adult mouse brain. Neuroscience 2004; 128(4):685-696.

[80] Zahs KR. Heterotypic coupling between glial cells of the mammalian central nervous system. Glia 1998; 24(1):85-96.

[81] Palmer TD, Willhoite AR, Gage FH. Vascular niche for adult hippocampal neurogenesis. J Comp Neurol 2000; 425(4):479-494.

[82] Shen Q, Goderie SK, Jin L et al. Endothelial cells stimulate self-renewal and expand neurogenesis of neural stem cells. Science 2004; 304(5675):1338-1340.

[83] Riquelme PA, Drapeau E, Doetsch F. Brain micro-ecologies: neural stem cell niches in the adult mammalian brain. Philos Trans R Soc Lond B Biol Sci 2008; 363(1489):123-137.

[84] Craig CG, Tropepe V, Morshead CM, Reynolds BA, Weiss S, van der KD. In vivo growth factor expansion of endogenous subependymal neural precursor cell populations in the adult mouse brain. J Neurosci 1996; 16(8):2649-2658.

[85] Wagner JP, Black IB, Cicco-Bloom E. Stimulation of neonatal and adult brain neurogenesis by subcutaneous injection of basic fibroblast growth factor. J Neurosci 1999; 19(14):6006-6016.

[86] Jackson EL, Garcia-Verdugo JM, Gil-Perotin S et al. PDGFR alpha-positive B cells are neural stem cells in the adult SVZ that form glioma-like growths in response to increased PDGF signaling. Neuron 2006; 51(2):187-199.

[87] Jin K, Mao XO, Sun Y, Xie L, Greenberg DA. Stem cell factor stimulates neurogenesis in vitro and in vivo. J Clin Invest 2002; 110(3):311-319.

[88] Jin K, Zhu Y, Sun Y, Mao XO, Xie L, Greenberg DA. Vascular endothelial growth factor (VEGF) stimulates neurogenesis in vitro and in vivo. Proc Natl Acad Sci U S A 2002; 99(18):11946-11950.

[89] Mi H, Haeberle H, Barres BA. Induction of astrocyte differentiation by endothelial cells. J Neurosci 2001; 21(5):1538-1547.

[90] Leventhal C, Rafii S, Rafii D, Shahar A, Goldman SA. Endothelial trophic support of neuronal production and recruitment from the adult mammalian subependyma. Mol Cell Neurosci 1999; 13(6):450-464.
[91] Scharfman H, Goodman J, Macleod A, Phani S, Antonelli C, Croll S. Increased neurogenesis and the ectopic granule cells after intrahippocampal BDNF infusion in adult rats. Exp Neurol 2005; 192(2):348-356.
[92] Colak D, Mori T, Brill MS et al. Adult neurogenesis requires Smad4-mediated bone morphogenic protein signaling in stem cells. J Neurosci 2008; 28(2):434-446.
[93] Olstorn H, Varghese M, Murrell W, Moe MC, Langmoen IA. Predifferentiated brain-derived adult human progenitor cells migrate toward ischemia after transplantation to the adult rat brain. Neurosurgery 2011; 68(1):213-222.
[94] Ahn S, Joyner AL. In vivo analysis of quiescent adult neural stem cells responding to Sonic hedgehog. Nature 2005; 437(7060):894-897.
[95] Palma V, Lim DA, Dahmane N et al. Sonic hedgehog controls stem cell behavior in the postnatal and adult brain. Development 2005; 132(2):335-344.
[96] Wechsler-Reya RJ, Scott MP. Control of neuronal precursor proliferation in the cerebellum by Sonic Hedgehog. Neuron 1999; 22(1):103-114.
[97] Balordi F, Fishell G. Hedgehog signaling in the subventricular zone is required for both the maintenance of stem cells and the migration of newborn neurons. J Neurosci 2007; 27(22):5936-5947.
[98] Han YG, Spassky N, Romaguera-Ros M et al. Hedgehog signaling and primary cilia are required for the formation of adult neural stem cells. Nat Neurosci 2008; 11(3):277-284.
[99] Bonnert TP, Bilsland JG, Guest PC et al. Molecular characterization of adult mouse subventricular zone progenitor cells during the onset of differentiation. Eur J Neurosci 2006; 24(3):661-675.
[100] Garcia-Castro MI, Marcelle C, Bronner-Fraser M. Ectodermal Wnt function as a neural crest inducer. Science 2002; 297(5582):848-851.
[101] Lie DC, Colamarino SA, Song HJ et al. Wnt signalling regulates adult hippocampal neurogenesis. Nature 2005; 437(7063):1370-1375.
[102] Yu JM, Kim JH, Song GS, Jung JS. Increase in proliferation and differentiation of neural progenitor cells isolated from postnatal and adult mice brain by Wnt-3a and Wnt-5a. Mol Cell Biochem 2006; 288(1-2):17-28.
[103] Israsena N, Hu M, Fu W, Kan L, Kessler JA. The presence of FGF2 signaling determines whether beta-catenin exerts effects on proliferation or neuronal differentiation of neural stem cells. Dev Biol 2004; 268(1):220-231.
[104] Alexson TO, Hitoshi S, Coles BL, Bernstein A, van der KD. Notch signaling is required to maintain all neural stem cell populations--irrespective of spatial or temporal niche. Dev Neurosci 2006; 28(1-2):34-48.
[105] Chapouton P, Skupien P, Hesl B et al. Notch activity levels control the balance between quiescence and recruitment of adult neural stem cells. J Neurosci 2010; 30(23):7961-7974.
[106] Mizutani K, Yoon K, Dang L, Tokunaga A, Gaiano N. Differential Notch signalling distinguishes neural stem cells from intermediate progenitors. Nature 2007; 449(7160):351-355.

[107] Ge S, Pradhan DA, Ming GL, Song H. GABA sets the tempo for activity-dependent adult neurogenesis. Trends Neurosci 2007; 30(1):1-8.

[108] Wang DD, Krueger DD, Bordey A. GABA depolarizes neuronal progenitors of the postnatal subventricular zone via GABAA receptor activation. J Physiol 2003; 550(Pt 3):785-800.

[109] Owens DF, Liu X, Kriegstein AR. Changing properties of GABA(A) receptor-mediated signaling during early neocortical development. J Neurophysiol 1999; 82(2):570-583.

[110] Bolteus AJ, Bordey A. GABA release and uptake regulate neuronal precursor migration in the postnatal subventricular zone. J Neurosci 2004; 24(35):7623-7631.

[111] Overstreet WL, Bromberg DA, Bensen AL, Westbrook GL. GABAergic signaling to newborn neurons in dentate gyrus. J Neurophysiol 2005; 94(6):4528-4532.

[112] Liu X, Wang Q, Haydar TF, Bordey A. Nonsynaptic GABA signaling in postnatal subventricular zone controls proliferation of GFAP-expressing progenitors. Nat Neurosci 2005; 8(9):1179-1187.

[113] Santarelli L, Saxe M, Gross C et al. Requirement of hippocampal neurogenesis for the behavioral effects of antidepressants. Science 2003; 301(5634):805-809.

[114] Brezun JM, Daszuta A. Depletion in serotonin decreases neurogenesis in the dentate gyrus and the subventricular zone of adult rats. Neuroscience 1999; 89(4):999-1002.

[115] Banasr M, Hery M, Printemps R, Daszuta A. Serotonin-induced increases in adult cell proliferation and neurogenesis are mediated through different and common 5-HT receptor subtypes in the dentate gyrus and the subventricular zone. Neuropsychopharmacology 2004; 29(3):450-460.

[116] Radley JJ, Jacobs BL. 5-HT1A receptor antagonist administration decreases cell proliferation in the dentate gyrus. Brain Res 2002; 955(1-2):264-267.

[117] Curtis MA, Penney EB, Pearson AG et al. Increased cell proliferation and neurogenesis in the adult human Huntington's disease brain. Proc Natl Acad Sci U S A 2003; 100(15):9023-9027.

[118] Curtis MA, Waldvogel HJ, Synek B, Faull RL. A histochemical and immunohistochemical analysis of the subependymal layer in the normal and Huntington's disease brain. J Chem Neuroanat 2005; 30(1):55-66.

[119] Curtis MA, Penney EB, Pearson J, Dragunow M, Connor B, Faull RL. The distribution of progenitor cells in the subependymal layer of the lateral ventricle in the normal and Huntington's disease human brain. Neuroscience 2005; 132(3):777-788.

[120] Moreno-Lopez B, Romero-Grimaldi C, Noval JA, Murillo-Carretero M, Matarredona ER, Estrada C. Nitric oxide is a physiological inhibitor of neurogenesis in the adult mouse subventricular zone and olfactory bulb. J Neurosci 2004; 24(1):85-95.

[121] Packer MA, Stasiv Y, Benraiss A et al. Nitric oxide negatively regulates mammalian adult neurogenesis. Proc Natl Acad Sci U S A 2003; 100(16):9566-9571.

[122] Pinnock SB, Balendra R, Chan M, Hunt LT, Turner-Stokes T, Herbert J. Interactions between nitric oxide and corticosterone in the regulation of progenitor cell proliferation in the dentate gyrus of the adult rat. Neuropsychopharmacology 2007; 32(2):493-504.

[123] Morrison SJ, Csete M, Groves AK, Melega W, Wold B, Anderson DJ. Culture in reduced levels of oxygen promotes clonogenic sympathoadrenal differentiation by isolated neural crest stem cells. J Neurosci 2000; 20(19):7370-7376.

[124] Studer L, Csete M, Lee SH et al. Enhanced proliferation, survival, and dopaminergic differentiation of CNS precursors in lowered oxygen. J Neurosci 2000; 20(19):7377-7383.

[125] Horie N, So K, Moriya T et al. Effects of oxygen concentration on the proliferation and differentiation of mouse neural stem cells in vitro. Cell Mol Neurobiol 2008; 28(6):833-845.

[126] Galli R, Binda E, Orfanelli U et al. Isolation and characterization of tumorigenic, stem-like neural precursors from human glioblastoma. Cancer Res 2004; 64(19):7011-7021.

[127] Singh SK, Clarke ID, Terasaki M et al. Identification of a cancer stem cell in human brain tumors. Cancer Res 2003; 63(18):5821-5828.

[128] Varghese M, Olstorn H, Sandberg C et al. A comparison between stem cells from the adult human brain and from brain tumors. Neurosurgery 2008; 63(6):1022-1033.

[129] Bao S, Wu Q, McLendon RE et al. Glioma stem cells promote radioresistance by preferential activation of the DNA damage response. Nature 2006; 444(7120):756-760.

[130] Salmaggi A, Boiardi A, Gelati M et al. Glioblastoma-derived tumorospheres identify a population of tumor stem-like cells with angiogenic potential and enhanced multidrug resistance phenotype. Glia 2006; 54(8):850-860.

[131] Visvader JE. Cells of origin in cancer. Nature 2011; 469(7330):314-322.

[132] Alcantara LS, Chen J, Kwon CH et al. Malignant astrocytomas originate from neural stem/progenitor cells in a somatic tumor suppressor mouse model. Cancer Cell 2009; 15(1):45-56.

[133] Marumoto T, Tashiro A, Friedmann-Morvinski D et al. Development of a novel mouse glioma model using lentiviral vectors. Nat Med 2009; 15(1):110-116.

[134] Gibson P, Tong Y, Robinson G et al. Subtypes of medulloblastoma have distinct developmental origins. Nature 2010; 468(7327):1095-1099.

[135] Gage FH. Mammalian neural stem cells. Science 2000; 287(5457):1433-1438.

[136] Erdo F, Buhrle C, Blunk J et al. Host-dependent tumorigenesis of embryonic stem cell transplantation in experimental stroke. J Cereb Blood Flow Metab 2003; 23(7):780-785.

[137] Schwarz SC, Schwarz J. Translation of stem cell therapy for neurological diseases. Transl Res 2010; 156(3):155-160.

[138] Meyer AK, Maisel M, Hermann A, Stirl K, Storch A. Restorative approaches in Parkinson's Disease: which cell type wins the race? J Neurol Sci 2010; 289(1-2):93-103.

[139] Belmonte JC, Ellis J, Hochedlinger K, Yamanaka S. Induced pluripotent stem cells and reprogramming: seeing the science through the hype. Nat Rev Genet 2009; 10(12):878-883.

[140] Levesque F, Neuman T, Rezak M. Therapeutic Microinjection of Autologous Adult Human Neural Stem Cells and Differentiated Neurons for Parkinson's Disease: Five-Year Post-Operative Outcome. The Open Stem Cell Journal 2009; 1:20-29.

[141] Nunes MC, Roy NS, Keyoung HM et al. Identification and isolation of multipotential neural progenitor cells from the subcortical white matter of the adult human brain. Nat Med 2003; 9(4):439-447.

[142] Akesson E, Piao JH, Samuelsson EB et al. Long-term culture and neuronal survival after intraspinal transplantation of human spinal cord-derived neurospheres. Physiol Behav 2007; 92(1-2):60-66.

[143] Varghese M, Olstorn H, Berg-Johnsen J, Moe MC, Murrell W, Langmoen IA. Isolation of human multipotent neural progenitors from adult filum terminale. Stem Cells Dev 2009; 18(4):603-613.

[144] Arvidsson L, Fagerlund M, Jaff N et al. Distribution and Characterization of Progenitor Cells within the Human Filum Terminale. PLoS One 2011; 6(11):e27393.

[145] Sousa-Ferreira L, Alvaro AR, Aveleira C et al. Proliferative hypothalamic neurospheres express NPY, AGRP, POMC, CART and Orexin-A and differentiate to functional neurons. PLoS One 2011; 6(5):e19745.

[146] Murrell W, Feron F, Wetzig A et al. Multipotent stem cells from adult olfactory mucosa. Dev Dyn 2005; 233(2):496-515.

[147] Westerlund U, Svensson M, Moe MC et al. Endoscopically harvested stem cells: a putative method in future autotransplantation. Neurosurgery 2005; 57(4):779-784.

[148] Olstorn H, Moe MC, Roste GK, Bueters T, Langmoen IA. Transplantation of stem cells from the adult human brain to the adult rat brain. Neurosurgery 2007; 60(6):1089-1098.

[149] Sun Y, Pollard S, Conti L et al. Long-term tripotent differentiation capacity of human neural stem (NS) cells in adherent culture. Mol Cell Neurosci 2008; 38(2):245-258.

[150] Walton NM, Sutter BM, Chen HX et al. Derivation and large-scale expansion of multipotent astroglial neural progenitors from adult human brain. Development 2006; 133(18):3671-3681.

[151] Moe MC, Varghese M, Danilov AI et al. Multipotent progenitor cells from the adult human brain: neurophysiological differentiation to mature neurons. Brain 2005; 128(Pt 9):2189-2199.

[152] Moe MC, Westerlund U, Varghese M, Berg-Johnsen J, Svensson M, Langmoen IA. Development of neuronal networks from single stem cells harvested from the adult human brain. Neurosurgery 2005; 56(6):1182-1188.

[153] Westerlund U, Moe MC, Varghese M et al. Stem cells from the adult human brain develop into functional neurons in culture. Exp Cell Res 2003; 289(2):378-383.

[154] Eriksson PS, Perfilieva E, Bjork-Eriksson T et al. Neurogenesis in the adult human hippocampus. Nat Med 1998; 4(11):1313-1317.

[155] Kukekov VG, Laywell ED, Suslov O et al. Multipotent stem/progenitor cells with similar properties arise from two neurogenic regions of adult human brain. Exp Neurol 1999; 156(2):333-344.

[156] Carlen M, Cassidy RM, Brismar H, Smith GA, Enquist LW, Frisen J. Functional integration of adult-born neurons. Curr Biol 2002; 12(7):606-608.

[157] Parent JM, Vexler ZS, Gong C, Derugin N, Ferriero DM. Rat forebrain neurogenesis and striatal neuron replacement after focal stroke. Ann Neurol 2002; 52(6):802-813.

[158] Zhang B, Wang RZ, Yao Y et al. Proliferation and differentiation of neural stem cells in adult rats after cerebral infarction. Chin Med Sci J 2004; 19(2):73-77.

[159] Lichtenwalner RJ, Parent JM. Adult neurogenesis and the ischemic forebrain. J Cereb Blood Flow Metab 2006; 26(1):1-20.

[160] Lindvall O, Kokaia Z. Recovery and rehabilitation in stroke: stem cells. Stroke 2004; 35(11 Suppl 1):2691-2694.

[161] Thored P, Arvidsson A, Cacci E et al. Persistent production of neurons from adult brain stem cells during recovery after stroke. Stem Cells 2006; 24(3):739-747.

[162] Chen J, Li Y, Zhang R et al. Combination therapy of stroke in rats with a nitric oxide donor and human bone marrow stromal cells enhances angiogenesis and neurogenesis. Brain Res 2004; 1005(1-2):21-28.

[163] Curtis MA, Connor B, Faull RL. Neurogenesis in the diseased adult human brain--new therapeutic strategies for neurodegenerative diseases. Cell Cycle 2003; 2(5):428-430.

[164] Jin K, Sun Y, Xie L, Childs J, Mao XO, Greenberg DA. Post-ischemic administration of heparin-binding epidermal growth factor-like growth factor (HB-EGF) reduces infarct size and modifies neurogenesis after focal cerebral ischemia in the rat. J Cereb Blood Flow Metab 2004; 24(4):399-408.

[165] Magavi SS, Leavitt BR, Macklis JD. Induction of neurogenesis in the neocortex of adult mice. Nature 2000; 405(6789):951-955.

[166] Cooper O, Isacson O. Intrastriatal transforming growth factor alpha delivery to a model of Parkinson's disease induces proliferation and migration of endogenous adult neural progenitor cells without differentiation into dopaminergic neurons. J Neurosci 2004; 24(41):8924-8931.

[167] Fallon J, Reid S, Kinyamu R et al. In vivo induction of massive proliferation, directed migration, and differentiation of neural cells in the adult mammalian brain. Proc Natl Acad Sci U S A 2000; 97(26):14686-14691.

[168] Cho SR, Benraiss A, Chmielnicki E, Samdani A, Economides A, Goldman SA. Induction of neostriatal neurogenesis slows disease progression in a transgenic murine model of Huntington disease. J Clin Invest 2007; 117(10):2889-2902.

[169] Kolb B, Gibb R. Brain plasticity and recovery from early cortical injury. Dev Psychobiol 2007; 49(2):107-118.

[170] Cramer SC, Fitzpatrick C, Warren M et al. The beta-hCG+erythropoietin in acute stroke (BETAS) study: a 3-center, single-dose, open-label, noncontrolled, phase IIa safety trial. Stroke 2010; 41(5):927-931.

[171] Park HW, Lim MJ, Jung H, Lee SP, Paik KS, Chang MS. Human mesenchymal stem cell-derived Schwann cell-like cells exhibit neurotrophic effects, via distinct growth factor production, in a model of spinal cord injury. Glia 2010; 58(9):1118-1132.

[172] Tamaki SJ, Jacobs Y, Dohse M et al. Neuroprotection of host cells by human central nervous system stem cells in a mouse model of infantile neuronal ceroid lipofuscinosis. Cell Stem Cell 2009; 5(3):310-319.

[173] Brundin P, Barker RA, Parmar M. Neural grafting in Parkinson's disease Problems and possibilities. Prog Brain Res 2010; 184:265-294.

[174] Freed CR, Greene PE, Breeze RE et al. Transplantation of embryonic dopamine neurons for severe Parkinson's disease. N Engl J Med 2001; 344(10):710-719.

[175] Hagell P, Piccini P, Bjorklund A et al. Dyskinesias following neural transplantation in Parkinson's disease. Nat Neurosci 2002; 5(7):627-628.

[176] Olanow CW, Goetz CG, Kordower JH et al. A double-blind controlled trial of bilateral fetal nigral transplantation in Parkinson's disease. Ann Neurol 2003; 54(3):403-414.

[177] Dihne M, Bernreuther C, Hagel C, Wesche KO, Schachner M. Embryonic stem cell-derived neuronally committed precursor cells with reduced teratoma formation after transplantation into the lesioned adult mouse brain. Stem Cells 2006; 24(6):1458-1466.

[178] Lensch MW, Schlaeger TM, Zon LI, Daley GQ. Teratoma formation assays with human embryonic stem cells: a rationale for one type of human-animal chimera. Cell Stem Cell 2007; 1(3):253-258.

[179] Robinson AJ, Meedeniya AC, Hemsley KM, Auclair D, Crawley AC, Hopwood JJ. Survival and engraftment of mouse embryonic stem cell-derived implants in the guinea pig brain. Neurosci Res 2005; 53(2):161-168.

[180] Kordower JH, Chu Y, Hauser RA, Freeman TB, Olanow CW. Lewy body-like pathology in long-term embryonic nigral transplants in Parkinson's disease. Nat Med 2008; 14(5):504-506.

[181] Li JY, Englund E, Widner H et al. Characterization of Lewy body pathology in 12- and 16-year-old intrastriatal mesencephalic grafts surviving in a patient with Parkinson's disease. Mov Disord 2010; 25(8):1091-1096.

[182] Oya S, Yoshikawa G, Takai K et al. Attenuation of Notch signaling promotes the differentiation of neural progenitors into neurons in the hippocampal CA1 region after ischemic injury. Neuroscience 2009; 158(2):683-692.

[183] Sgubin D, Aztiria E, Perin A, Longatti P, Leanza G. Activation of endogenous neural stem cells in the adult human brain following subarachnoid hemorrhage. J Neurosci Res 2007; 85(8):1647-1655.

[184] Burns TC, Verfaillie CM, Low WC. Stem cells for ischemic brain injury: a critical review. J Comp Neurol 2009; 515(1):125-144.

[185] Miljan EA, Sinden JD. Stem cell treatment of ischemic brain injury. Curr Opin Mol Ther 2009; 11(4):394-403.

[186] Thomas KE, Moon LD. Will stem cell therapies be safe and effective for treating spinal cord injuries? Br Med Bull 2011; 98:127-142.

[187] Falci S, Holtz A, Akesson E et al. Obliteration of a posttraumatic spinal cord cyst with solid human embryonic spinal cord grafts: first clinical attempt. J Neurotrauma 1997; 14(11):875-884.

[188] Wirth ED, III, Reier PJ, Fessler RG et al. Feasibility and safety of neural tissue transplantation in patients with syringomyelia. J Neurotrauma 2001; 18(9):911-929.

[189] Lima C, Pratas-Vital J, Escada P, Hasse-Ferreira A, Capucho C, Peduzzi JD. Olfactory mucosa autografts in human spinal cord injury: a pilot clinical study. J Spinal Cord Med 2006; 29(3):191-203.

[190] Lima C, Escada P, Pratas-Vital J et al. Olfactory mucosal autografts and rehabilitation for chronic traumatic spinal cord injury. Neurorehabil Neural Repair 2010; 24(1):10-22.

[191] http://www.isscr.org/ISSCR_Optimistic_on_Future_of_Stem_Cell_Treatments_Despite_Geron_s_Discontinued_Program.htm

[192] Hyun I, Lindvall O, hrlund-Richter L et al. New ISSCR guidelines underscore major principles for responsible translational stem cell research. Cell Stem Cell 2008; 3(6):607-609.

[193] Lench MW. Public perception of stem cell and genomic research. Genome Medicine 2011; 3:44.

[194] Amariglio N, Hirshberg A, Scheithauer BW et al. Donor-derived brain tumor following neural stem cell transplantation in an ataxia telangiectasia patient. PLoS Med 2009; 6(2):e1000029.

[195] Murrell W, Wetzig A, Donnellan M, Féron F, Burne T, Meedeniya A, Kesby J, Bianco J, Perry C, Silburn P, Mackay-Sim A. Olfactory mucosa is a potential source for autologous stem cell therapy for Parkinson's disease. Stem Cells 2008; 26(8):2183-92

# Section 7

## Appendix

# 22

# Hemostatic Agents in Neurosurgery

F. Lapierre, S. D'Houtaud and M. Wager

## 1. Introduction

Adequate hemostasis is a prerequisite in neurosurgery, to prevent dramatic postoperative bleedings and their consequences. Different sorts of local hemostatic agents have been developed, with a variable efficacy. Some of them have been used for years, none being perfect.

The residual presence of these agents may behave as foreign bodies, and induce inflammation, infection, and even delayed bone growth.

Safety is an other concern since most of modern agents contain more or less human and animal components.

We are going to review the history of those agents, their different categories, compare them and try to establish some guidelines when using them, with their different indications.

## 2. Hemostasis (basis)

Hemostasis comes from the coordinated activation of platelets and plasma clotting factors to form a platelet fibrin clot. Two processes, primary and secondary hemostasis activation of the clotting cascade id done by collagen for the intrinsic pathway, and the extrinsic pathway is activated by the release of tissue factors from the damaged zone. The two converge ento the common pathway which begins with the conversion of Factor X to Xa, the conversion of prothrombin to thrombin, which is integral in clot stabilization via fibrin. This common pathway is facilitated by Factor V (Hawiger 1987).

## 3. History

From the beginning of the neurosurgical practice, local hemostatic agents have proved to be very useful completing the more classical use of the electrocoagulation whatever its type, mono or bipolar or sometimes laser.

### 3.1 First attempts

#### 3.1.1 Auto or hetero-muscle application

Until the early 1950, neurosurgeons used as topical hemostatic agents fresh chicken breast which was delivered to the operative theatre just before the beginning of the operation. Electrocoagulation device was not very good, and they often had to apply the chicken flesh on the brain during ten minutes while washing the field with warm serum, and removed it before closing the dura.

Fresh muscle harvested from the temporal site or the thigh is still commonly used for extradural dural hemostasis and may be left in situ.

At the same times, bone wax was used and is still used for bone hemostasis (Grant 2007). Bone wax was created by Sir Victor Haden Horsley (1857-1916) from beewax in 1892. Since this period different components were added to wax, but the common name remained "Horsley wax".

### 3.2 Hydrogen peroxide

It has been used for decades as a hemostatic agent and is believed to establish hemostasis through its vasoconstrictive properties, and is also credited to create a disruption of the blood-barrier and an aggregation of the platelets and neutrophils leading to thrombus formation. The free diffusion of H2O2 through the vessel walls and its conversion to water and 02 leads to intra-luminal bubbles, micro-embolisms and vessels obstruction.

### 3.3 Modern evolution

Multiple local hemostatic agents now exist (Abaut & Basle 2003, Grant 2007)

#### 3.3.1 Fibrin sealants

The better understanding of hemostasis mechanisms brought new perspectives for the conception of other local agents. The first discussion for topical agents is due to Bergen who emphasized the role of fibrin in hemostasis. Secundary, this will move to the preparation of fibrin sealants, the first combination of bovine thrombin with human plasma for topical use. In 1938, purified thrombin became available, with obtention of new fibrin sealants used in 1940, as reported in the literature, even for nerve repair. In 1944, their use was reported to optimize skin-grafts survival and adhesion of skin grafts, in severe burn injury during the war by Cronkite. Richard Upjohn Light 1945 reviews the different existing helps to improve hemostasis in neurosurgery, and Fincher 1946 reports the uses of gelatin foam .

But the technics used in those times only led to preparations being the potential source of transmission of viral hepatitis. So bovine thrombin was substituted for human thrombin to minimize the risk of viral transmission. But some patients developed coagulopathies due to the use of bovine thrombin related to immune-mediated production of thrombin and factorV inhibitors.

All these difficulties led to abandon the fibrin sealants for years.

In the late 1960, isolation and concentration of clotting factors from human plasma became possible, and in 1972, Matras produced the first item of modern fibrin sealants. The first commercially fibrin sealant was approved in Europe in 1982, and Later in USA in 1990.

In 1998, Tisseel and Hemascel sealants were approved by FDA, and the firs sealant with entirely human components called Crosseals was made in 1993. Surgical use widely spread in nearly all specialities.

### 3.3.2 Gelatin hemostatic agents

They were introduced in 1940 such as Gelfoam and Surgifoam.

Gelfoam is a purified pork skin gelatine with hemostatic properties which may come from its physical features, and not from an effect on the clotting cascade. It may be used with saturated thrombin.

They exist as sponges and have a capacity to expand up to 200% in vivo, which may be a negative property in some deep fields specially in neurosurgery.

Floseal combines human derivated thrombin with bovine derivated gelatin matrix granules which are mixed at the time of use, and also exists as a liquid device minimizing the expansion property, allowing its application in minimal invasive surgery and neurosurgery.

### 3.3.3 Cyanoacrylate adhesives

They were developed by Dr H Coover in 1942. It consists cyanoacrylate monomers which polymerize in long chains in the presence of hydroxyl ions.

### 3.3.4 Oxyfied regenerated glucose

Is a plant -based topical hemostatic introduced in 1960. It is made by regenerating a pure plant-derived cellulose secondary knitted and oxidized. It acts as a scaffold for clot formation. On post-operative imaging, it may mimic an abcess or some residual tumor.

### 3.3.5 Microfibrillar collagen

This substance (Avitene) was introduced in 1970. Microfibrillar applied collagen products come from the purification of bovine collagen, followed by microcristallisation. It is presented as a powder, and is more effective than gelatine based hemostasis, since it is able to activate the clotting cascade.

### 3.4 Thrombin and fibrinogen (fibrin glue)

Are the most recently appeared.

Fibrin glues contain thrombin and fibrinogen: when combined, the fibrinogen is activated by thrombin and converted into fibrin monomere which form an adhesive glue at the tissues applied.

The fibrin monomere interacts with the patient's own factor VIII and calcium to convert the final product into a fibrin polymer that allows for platelets activation and aggregation with subsequent hemostasis.

They are presented with a dual chamber syringe that allows for the combination of the thrombin and fibrinogen when the plunger is depressed. They also can be used in spray. Many commercial products are now on the market: Tisseel (Baxter), Evicel formerly called Crosseal (Johnson and Johnson)...Tisseel is now bovine free.

## 4. Classification of existing products

### 4.1 Surgical local hemostatic agents with an aspecific effect on the clotting cascade

*Hemostatic agents with a natural origin*

Are medical devices of Class III, and may be extracted from animals (calf, ox, pig or horse) or plants (wood, cotton, alga, potatoe-starch)

*Mecanism of efficacy*

Collagen and gelatine induce the platelet aggregation leading to a clot when in contact with blood

Oxidized cellulosis allows absorption of blood. Glycuronic acid diminishes the PH, induces vasoconstriction, and the creation of hematin film, and in vitro shows an bactericid effect.

Alginates release the Ca++ ions , with a platelet activation followed by a fibrinoformation. Alga fibers reinforce the clot structure.

Starch acts like a filter which concentrate the blood cells and the proteins such as thrombin, albumin and fibrinogen, with an hemostasis occurring in a few minutes.

*Different products*

| **Composition** | **origin** | **product** | **presentation** |
|---|---|---|---|
| Collagen | Calf | Pangen | compress |
| | Ox | Avitene | |
| | Pig | Surgicol | |
| | Horse | Antema (Biomet) | |
| | | Tissufleece (Baxter)<br>Gentafleece (Baxter)<br>Septocoll ( Biomet) + gentamycin<br>Collatemp (Inocoll) | |
| Gelatin | Ox | Floseal (Baxter) + Thrombin<br>Gelitaspon (Caps recherche) | Gel<br>powder, gel, pad |
| | Pig | Surgiflo Johnson & Johnson) | gel |
| | | Spongostan (Johnson & Johnson)<br>Gelita (Pouret) | Powder<br>Plugs |
| Oxidized cellulosis | Wood | Surgicel (Johnson&Johnson ) | Compress |
| | Cotton | Gelitacel (Caps recherché) | |
| Alginates | Laminaria Hyperborea | Algosterile | Compress |
| Starch | Potatoe | Arista (Medafor) | Powder |

*Hemostatic agents with a synthetic origin*

Their classification depends on their chemical category

- Aldehyds associated with gelatine (GRF) or albumin (Bioglue -Gamida-)
- Glycol polyethylens (Coseal -Baxter- and pleuraseal)
- Cyanoacrylates (Glubran and Omnex)

*Mechanism of efficacy*

Their aim is the constitution of a film to obtain water tightness and prevent the risk of hemorrage

They won't be developed here their use being contraindicated in neurosurgery.

### 4.2 Hemostatic agents with a specific effect on hemostasis cascade

Concern four products containing all fibrinogen and thrombin, their difference is due to the different associated coagulating factors leading to product the last stage of the coagulation (Silver, Wang & AL 1995, Jackson 2001). Experimental studies have compared the properties and efficacy of the different fibrin sealants (Dickneite, Metzner & Al 2003) in correlation with their components. They emphasized the necessity of Factor XIII as the key of a good efficacy for clotting. All tested fibrin sealants performed well on individual parameters, but Beriplast (Aventis Behring) was the foremost fibrin sealant in consistently providing early hemostasis.

These products are the Tissucol, the Beriplast, the Quixil and the Tachosyl.

Each one contains other coagulation factors (Factor XIII, fibronectin,plasminogen), and an antifibrinolytic.

The Quixil contains no substance from animal origin, but transnenamic acid and subsequently must never be in contact with nervous tissues.

**Tissucol (Baxter)**

- Can exist as a solution or a spray
- *Powder and reconstitution solution I
- Contains human components: fibrinogen (90mg/ml), Factor XIII(10UI/ml), fibronectin(5,5mg/ml), plasminogen0,08mg/ml), bovine aprotinin (3000 UIK/ml)
- *Powder and reconstitution solution II
- Contains human thrombin (500 UI/ml)
- *The excipient of powder and reconstitution I
- Contains glycin, human albumin, sodium nitrate, tyloxapol
- *The excipient of powder and reconstitution solution IIContains Glycin, Sodium chlorure, reconstitution solution EPPI, Calcium chlorure
- Must be kept in refrigerator, can be kept for 2 years
- After reconstitution remains stable for 4 hours

**Beriplast (Nycomed)**

- Same presentation
- *Powder and reconstitution solution I

- Contains human components: Fibrinogen (90mg/ml), Factor XIII( 60UI/ml), with bovine aprotinin (1000UIK/ml)
- *Powder and reconstitution II
- Contains human thrombin (500UI/ml)
- *Powder and reconstitution solution
- Contains human thrombin (500UI/ml)
- *Powder and reconstitution solution I
- Contains Isoleucin, Arginin, Sodium glutamate, human albumin, Sodium citrate, reconstitution EPPI, Sodium chlorure
- Can be kept for one year at room temperature, and 2 in refrigerateur
- Remains stable for 24 hours after preparation.

**Quixil (Johnson &Johnson)**

We don't detail its composition for the previously related reason.

**Tachosil (Nycomed)**

Presents as compress

- *The white side is covered with human fibrinogen( 5,5mg/cm2
- * The yellow side with human thrombin (2UI/cm2
- The excipients associate horse collagen, human albumin, Riboflavin, sodium chlorure, sodium citrate, L-Arginin.
- Can be kept for three years at room temperature

**Autolog fibrin:Vivostat system (Vivolution)**

- Is a medical device whose the European autorisation has been given in 2000.
- This automatized system can provide autolog from the patient blood in 23 minutes.
- It associates a processor, a Kit preparation and a spray system.
- It contains no animal component so it eliminates all risks of viral transmission
- Nowadays, it is mainly used in cardiac and thoracic surgery, in vascular and abdominal surgery, but not in neurosurgery.

## 5. Patches and pads

Those non-invasive hemostatic closure devices as described by Hirsch, Reddy & Al 2003 are mainly used to obtain hemostasis of percutaneous arteriotomy sites of arterial catheterization. This type of patch comes from the studies confirming the hemostatic properties of a high-molecular -weight polysaccharide the poly-N-acetyl-glucosamine (p-Glc-Nac).

Its use is mostly in cardiac surgery and and in interventional radiology.

### 5.1 Choice of the device and indications

First we shall remind that some specialities are contra-indicated in neurosurgery: cyanoacrylates, Quixil, alginates. $H_2O_2$ must only be used out of the dura mater.

The choice of the product and the strategy for local hemostasis are correlated with the type of neurosurgery, the sources of the bleeding, and the neurosurgeon practice, and the financial supplies.

No one must expect from local hemostatic products whatever their quality to be a substitute for the classical bipolar electrocoagulation hemostasis, and more widely for the respect of the tissues.

### 5.1.1 Type of bleeding

*Arterial bleeding*

Bipolar coagulation must be used and gives a perfect adequacy to the needs if associated with irrigation.

*Bleeding from a venous sinus*

The suture remains the best mean when possible, possibly reinforced with a muscle or aponevrotic patch. If the bleeding is close to the vault, the suspension of the dura mater to the bone with interposition of a patch of muscle, oxidized cellulosis or both is the solution.

Anterior cavernous sinus bleeding can be controlled by injection of fibrin glue with a good hemostasis. However of the series reported by Sekhar, Natarajan & Al 2007, of the 20 patients who had an injection in the superior petrosal sinus, 2 experienced complications caused by occlusion of veins draining the brainstem. The 46 whose anterior cavernous sinus had been injected had no complications.

*Diffuse bleeding "cloth-bleeding"*

A global hemostasis disturbance must be searched.

Local hemostatic agents are indicated, the most often oxidized cellulosis (surgical) will be applied, as well as tissucol (solution or spray).

*Bone bleeding*

Bone wax remains the most commonly used device, with a good efficacy. However, large amounts must be avoided for they will stay there for ever as a foreing body, and may be the cause of chronic infection, and a secondary removal.

When skull base surgery is performed, surgical, muscle can be on the bleeding site. According to the concerned neurosugeons, the most effective product is the Floseal (powder).

*Dura mater water-proof*

Prevention of cerebro-spinal fluid (CSF) leaks must be done by the tight closure of the dura mater, reinforced if necessary by application of Surgicel.

Large defects require a graft which can also be sutured, the suture of which may be reinforced in the same way.

In large defects of the dura mater or on the skull base, most of the neurosurgeons will fill the defect with autolog fat tissue (easily indentified on post-operative CT-scan or MRI pictures) associated with glue (Tissucol or Bioglue). An external lumbar CSF derivation will be added in the most difficult cases.

N-B: A local hemostatic agent will never by itself be sufficient to give a definitive water-proof security.

### 5.2 Main uses in daily practical practice

*Skull and brain injuries*

The surgery of the skull base defects requires in most of the cases the filling of bone defects with tailed bone grafts, followed by the suture and/or grafting of the dura mater and as previously described the application of a local agent, Surgicel being the most widely used.

Brain contusions require after excision of the necrotic tissues to apply some Surgicel if any small bleeding goes on, the best option being to obtain a very good hemostasis with nothing left in the remaining cavity.

Opened cranio-cerebral wounds must be cleaned with a non-aggressive product, and H2O2 is still indicated in such circumstances.

*Transphenoidal surgery*

Bleeding during pituitary surgery with a transphenoidal approach can lessen visibility, and this confined narrow route does not allow the use of electrocoagulation. The use of oxidized cellulose or glue is very useful. Ellgala, Maartens & Al 2002 have tested the use Floseal during 293 with a satisfying result.

*Endoscopic surgery*

The endoscopic treatment of CSF leaks of the anterior skull base whatever their a aetiology, includes the identification of the defect, the filling of the defect with a fragment of the medial turbinate fixed with bioglue followed by appliance of the rest of the pedicled turbinate below and oxidized cellulose (Surgicel) packing.

Same procedures using muscle or turbinate may be used if a leak occurs during an hypophysis surgery procedure, Surgicel being commonly used to maintain the devices and /or to reinforce hemostasis.

Some devices such as catheters are very useful in those deep tight fields.

*Spine and spinal cord surgery*

Vertebral plexus are better controlled with local hemostatic agents. Fibrin glue is effective when the more common appliance of Surgicel is not effective (Sekhar, Natarajan & Al 2007)

Spinal cord tumors must be approached through laminotomy, the lamina section being done with a craniotomy. After retraction of the posterior arch flap, the extradural hemostasis must be perfect sometimes difficult due to epidural veins. Bipolar coagulation of the veins will be completed by appliance of small fragments of Surgicel, and bone wax on bone section the opening of the spinal cord is done under magnification. Surgicel application will help for hemostasis, the coagulation use being as restricted as possible.

After the tumour removal, no hemostatic agent should be left intradurally. The closing of the dura mater is seldom absolutely waterproof, and Surgicel and glue are commonly used to improve its quality (Lapierre 2009).

In other intra-dural spinal surgery one must avoid to let in situ any agent.

*Brain surgery*

From the extra-dural stage to the ending of the extradural hemostasis after the dura mater closure, local hemostatic agents have their place all along the procedure, to protect the brain, and to complete local hemostasis (Federspiel, Josephson &Al). In brain tumours, oxidized cellulose (surgical) is widely used, during the ablation of the tumour and at the end of the procedure to prevent and stop any bleeding in the remaining cavity whatever the type of tumor. One must be aware that it is still illegal to let products like Surgicel inside brain cavities, and inside the dura mater. Many physicians however will not take this in account considering the appliance of local agents on previously bleeding walls a better security for the patient. Tschan & Al 2010 have also evaluated the efficacy and safety of micropolysaccaride hemispheres (MPH) with no reported adverse effect. As soon as postoperative day 1, MPH were not detected anymore. There was no tumor mimicking enhancement. Many publications and everyone experience however report signal anomalies on post operative imagery mimicking residual tumour or early recurrence, or even an abcess, or a cotton pad when using Surgicel or gelatine sponge (Maurer, Ekholm & Al 1986)...This has led to some iterative unuseful surgery and even legacy. The histologic study only shows granuloma.

In aneurisms surgery, before the development of interventional radiology, aneurisms who could not be clipped were wrapped with muscle and hemostatic agents, unsuccessfully. Nowadays, surgery of aneurisms only requires hemostatic agents during the procedure to protect the brain and stop the faint bleedins coming from the neighbouring. Appliance of some small Surgicel pieces to the aneurism neck and clip may help to maintain the clip parallel to the vessel direction when releasing the retractors.

*Spinal surgery*

Local hemostatic agents have many indications in spinal surgery of all types, especially to ensure the epidural veins hemostasis.

They must not be left in contact with nerve roots intra or extradurally, due to the possibility of granuloma formation. Their presence is credited of the appearance of post-operative pain.

In case of epidural spontaneous hematomas they are very useful particularly if they are due to anti-coagulant accidents.

A randomized study performed in 127 patients by Renkens, Payner & Al 2001 comparing Floseal, microfibrillar collagen (Aviten) and fibrin glue showed the control of hemostasis in ten minutes for 97% of the cases with Floseal, and for 71% with the other agents.

## 6. Listing of main complications

*Stroke*

Is only reported when using hydrogen peroxide (H2O2). Mut, Yemisci & al 2009 reported one case in a patient, after which they performed an experimental study on mice brains using 3% H2O2 solution. When H2O2 was applied on the cortex, a vasoconstrictive response of all arteries and arterioles of the treated zone was observed, and after 15 seconds of exposure to H2O2, multiple bubbles were observed within the lumen of all subpial arteries when pial layer had been destroyed, or not.

Histology revealed the production of peroxynitrite, and the diffusion of H2O2 through the superficial cortical layers. The addition of peroxide and H2O2 resulted in platelet aggregation and acute thrombus formation. The combination of NO and H2O2 is cytotoxic, and mediated by generated NO radicals. Among them, peroxinitrite is a potent and destructive oxdant, which may disrupt the blood-brain barrier.

Those data confirm that H2O2 must only be used in the extra-dural space.

*Peripheral nerve impairment*

The potential effect of hemostatic agents of peripheral nerve function was suspected by clinical experience of postoperative local deficit or pain after the appliance of hemostatic agents in situ.

Experimental studies heve been performed by Nagamatsu, Podratz & al 1996 and Alkan, Inat & al 2007.

The first used oxicel (OC) (Deseret medical, Becton Dickinson and Company, Sandy, Utah) for studies in vitro and in vivo in rats. In vitro, neurite outgrowth of the dorsal root ganglion neuron was inhibited after 15 minutes exposure

In vivo, the Ph was lowered in the subperineurium, and remained low for 2 hours. The acidity of the oxidised cellulose is involved in the development of experimental neuropathy by OC. The direct application of OC to peripheral nerves must be avoided.

The second studied the effect of oxidized regenerated cellulose, gelatine sponge, bone wax and bovine collagen on the sciatic nerve of the rat, embedded in each substance. The compound action potential (CAP), and the nerve conduction velocity (NCV) were studied one hour and four weeks after the operation. In the bovine collagen and bone wax groups they were no statistically significant differences compared with initial control group.

In the gelatine sponge group, CAP was increased statistically significantly 4 weeks after surgery.

In the oxidized regenerated cellulose, NCV was significantly reduced, and the CAP increased 1 hour after surgery. No significant difference was seen after 4 weeks, but partial necrosis and walking disturbances were seen on the operated legs after 1 to 3 weeks.

Bovine collagen seems the most adapted for direct appliance to the nerves.

Intra-spinal retained Surgicel can induce radiculopathy (Partheni, Kalogheropouplou & Al 2006) and MRI studies could not exclude a post-operative hematoma, leading to reoperate the patient

*Granulomatous formations*

When left in the operative field, hemostatic agents may induce early or late tissue reactions and the formation of granulomas especially oxidized cellulose ( Voormolen, Ringers & Al 1987) . Kaymaz, Tokgoz & al 2005, in an experimental study in the rabbit brain report the modifications due to the application of oxidized cellulose and gelatine sponge. They observe on MRI a perilesional oedema in both series, while histopathology a tissue-degeneration more marked with the gelatine sponge use 24 hours after operation. In a rat brain neurosurgical model (228 animals), Ereth, Schaff & Al 2008 studied Arista, Surgicel, Avitene,

Floseal or Kaolin (positive control) and showed the presence of residual material in all animals with Avitene, Surgicel and Floseal at day 14. Avitene and Floseal demonstrated a propensy for causing granuloma formation.

Apel-Sarid, Cochrane &Al 2010 report a pediatric case series of 3 patients: the 3 cases had intra cerebral surgery (2 for tumors ablations, and one focal dysplasy treatment). The local hemostatic used agent was microfibrillar collagen haemostat (Avitene). The three had a second surgery for new or recurrent seizures, and MRI exploration suspected either a tumour recurrence or an abscess. Histologically, the mixed inflammatory infiltrate was typified by the presence of Avitene-centric necrotizing granulomas surrounded by a palisade of macrophages and often several eosinophils.

So long, one must remain aware that the best behaviour is to remove any local hemostatic agent before closing the dura, if possible.

*Viral transmission*

With purified products, the risk of viral transmission has become very weak but is not totally missing, since all the products contain bovine components except for Vivostat. No recent report has been published yet. Virally inactivated human thrombin has replaced now bovine thrombin in most European products. (Buttusil 2003)

*Antibodies formation and immunologic concerns*

In the series of Renkens, Payner & Al 2001, at 6-8 weeks post operative evaluation of antibodies again bovine thrombin and bovine FactorVa demonstrated no stastical significance in the differences between treatment and control groups.

There was no evidence of antibody-related coagulopathy in either group. However, immunology mediated coagulopathy associated with exposure to bovine thromin or to fibrin sealants containing this component is widely recognized. This component had to be replaced by human thrombin (Buttusil 2003). Bovine aprotinin (BA) may induce severe anaphylactic reactions, especially in patients previously treated with such products, suggesting that the use of a test dose should be proposed.

Crosseal A containing traneximic acid (TA) eliminates this risk, but is contraindicated for neurosurgery.

## 7. Financial point of view for hemostatic agents

The most sophisticated they are, the most expansive. Anyway, the most daily used of all remain the oxidized cellulose, and the coast remains important. I should dare to add considering the glues that during the 15 years of my practice they did not exist. When they were available I have been using them for the ten following years.

After some warning about security, I stopped. The results remain identical during these three consecutive periods.

In developing countries, the price remains prohibitive, and in other countries, the local hemostatic agents are probably widely over-used. The indispensable devices remain electrocoagulation, Horsley wax, associated with a cautious and accurate surgery. The indication of local hemostatic agents must be evaluated in terms of rik-benefit for the patient, and not considered as a comfort for the surgeon. Of course local hemostatic agents are useful in some cases, but must not considered as compulsory in the daily practice.

## 8. Disclosure

The authors report no conflict of interest concerning the materials ad devices described in this paper.

## 9. References


Abaut, A-Y, Basle, B. 2008, Les agents hémostatiques chirurgicaux, *Pharm Hosp* 43, 2-8

Alkan, A, Inal, S, Yildirim, M, Bas, b, Agar, E. 2007. The effects of hemostatic agents on peripheral nerve function: An experimental study. *J oral maxillofac Surg* 65, 6306-634

Apel-sarid, L, Cochrane, D, D, Steinbok, P, Byrne, A, T, Dunham, C.2010. Microfibrillar collagen haemostat-induced necrotizing granulomatous inflammation developing after craniotomy: a pediatric case series. *J Neurosurg Pediatrics* 6, 385-392

Busuttil, R, W. 2003. A comparison of antifirinolytic agents used in hemostatic fibrin sealants. *J Am Coll Surg,* 197, 6 , 1021-1028

Dickneite, G, Metzner, H, Pfeifer, T, Kroez, M, Witzke, G. 2003. A comparison of fibrin sealants in relation to their in vitro and in vivo properties.¸*Thrombosis research* 112, 73-82

Dona, C, Vaccino.C. 2009. Topical hemostasis: a valuable adjunct to control bleeding in the operating room, with a special focus on thrombinand fibrin sealants. *Informa Phamaceutical Science* 2. 243-247

Ellegala, D, B, Maartens, N, F, Laws, E, R. 2001. Use of floseal hemostatic sealant in transphenoidal pituitary surgery: Technical note. *Neurosurgery* 51, 513-516

Ereth-Mark, H, Schaft, M, Ericson, E, Wetgen, N, Nuttal, G, Oliver, W, C, 2008. Comparative safety and efficacy of topical hemostatic agents in a rat neurosurgical model. *Neurosurgery,* 63, 369-372

Federspiel, F, Josephson, A, Dardelle, D, Gaillard, S, Letailleur, M. 2008. Utilisation des agents hémostatiques en neurochirurgie. *Pharm Hosp* 43, 9-13

Fincher, E, 1946. Further uses of gelatine foam in neurosurgeryPresented at the meeting of the Harvey Cushing Society, October 12, Boston MasschussettsHarvey *Cushing Society Reports* 97-104

Grant, G. 2007. Update on hemostasis: neurosurgery. *SurgeryS55,* 142, 4S, S55-S60

Hawiger, j. 1987. Formation and regulation of platelet and fibrin hemostatic Plug. *Human pathology* 18, 2, 111-122

Hirsch, J, A, Reddy, S, A, Capasso, W, E, Linfante, I. 2003. Non-invasive hemostatic closure devices: "Patches and Pads". *Techniques in Vascular and Interventional Radiology,* 6, 2, 92-95

Ito, H, Onishi, H, Shoin, K, Nagatani, H. 1989. Granuloma caused by oxidized cellulose following craniotomy. *Acta Neurochirurgica,* 100, 1-2

Jackson, M, R. 2001. Fibrin sealants in surgical practice: an overview. *The American Journal of surgery* 182 1S-7S

Kaymaz, m, Tokgoz, N, Kardes, O, Özköse, z, Özogui, c, Orbay, t. 2005. Radiological and histopathological examination of early tissue reactions to absorbable hemostatic agents in the rabbit brain. *Journal of clinical neuroscience.* 12, 4, 445-448

Kothbauer, K, R, Jallo, G, I, Siffert, J, Jimenez, E, Allen, J, C, Epstein, F, J. 2001. Foreing body reaction to hemostasis materials mimicking recurrent brain tumor. *J Neurosurg*, 95, 0503

Krause, D.2008. Regulatory history of adsorbable hemostatic agents and dressings. *Le pharmacien hospitalier(hors série1)*, 84, 3716

Lapierre, F. 2009. Les agents hémostatiques locaux en neurochirurgie: note technique. *Neurochirurgie*, 55 Hors série 1, 40-44

Light Upjohn Richard 1945. Hemostasis in neurosurgery Harvey *Cushing Society Reports* 414-434

Maurer, P, K, Ekholm, S, E, Mac Donald, J, V, Sands, M, Kido, D. 1986. Postoperative radiographic appearance of intracranial hemostatic gelatine sponge. *Surgical Neurology* 26, -, 562-566

Mut, M, Yemisi, m, Gursov-Ozdemir, Y, Ture, U. 2009. Hydrogen peroxide induced stroke: elucidation of the mechanism in vivo. *J Neurosurg* 110, 94-100

Nagamatsu, M, Podratz, j, Windebank, A, J, Low, P, A. 1997, Acidity is involved in the development of neuropathy caused by oxidized cellulose. *Journal of the neurological sciences* 146, 97-102

Partheni, m, lalogheropoulou, C, Karageorgos, N, Paniagiotopoulos, V, Voulgaris, S, Tzortzidis, F. 2006. Radiculopathy after lumbar discectomy due to intraspinal retained surgical: clinical and magnetic resonance imaging evaluation. *The spine Journal* 6, 455- 458

Peng, C, W, Chou, B, T, Bendo, J, A. 2009. Vertebral artery injury in cervical spine surgery: anatomical considerations, management and preventive measures. *The spine Journal* , 9, 70-76.

Renchengary, S, S. 1993 . Principles of neurosurgery. Wilkins R.H, 1;18-19

Renkens, K, L Jr, Payner, T, D, Leipzig, T, J, Feuer, H, Morone, M, A, Koers, J, M, Lawson, K, J, Lentz, R, Shuey, H Jr, Conaway, G, L, Andersson, G, B, An, A, S, Hickey, m, Rondinone, J, F, Shargill, N, S. 2001. A multicenter, prospective, randomized trial evaluating a new agent for spinal surgery. *Spine* , 26, 1645-1650

Rousou, J, Levitsky, S, Gonzalez-Lavin, L, Cosgrove, D, Magilligan, D, Weldon, C, Hiebert, c, Hess, P, Joyce, L, Bergsland, J. 1989? Randomized clinical trial of fibrin sealant in patients undergoing resternotomy or reinterventional cardiac operations: a multicenter study. *J Thoracic Cardiovasc surgery* , 97, 687-693

Satkunurath, K, Royston, D, 2008. Hemostatic drugs in trauma and orthopaedic practice. *Traumacare*, 1, 24-29

, D, 2007.The use of fibrin glue to stop venous bleeding in the epidural space, vertebral venous plexus, and anterior cavernous sinus: technical note. *Operative neurosurgery I*, 61,

Seyednejad, H, Imani, M, Jamieson, T, Seifalian, A, M. 2008. Topical hemostatic agents. *Br J Surg* 95, 1195-1225

Spiller, M, Tenner, M, S, Couldwell, W, T. 2001. Effect of absorbable hemostatic agents on the relaxation time blood: An in vitro study with implications for post-operative MRI. *J neurosurg* 95, 687-693

Silver, F, H, Wang M-C, Pins, G, D, 1995. Preparation and use of fibrin glue in surgery. *Biomaterials* 16, 891-903

Tschan, W, T, 2010, Rahmen Der Neurowoche, GMS Publishing House, Doc P 1740. http//creative commons, org/licenced/by-nc-nd/30/deed.de-

Voormolen, J, H, C, Ringers, J, Bots, G, A, M, Van Der Heide, A, Hermans, J. 1987. Hemostatic agents: Brain tissue reaction and effectiveness. *Neurosurgery* 20, 5, 702-709

# 23

# Use of Physical Restraints in Neurosurgery: Guide for a Good Practice

Ayten Demir Zencirci
*Ankara University, Faculty of Health Sciences, Nursing Department*
*Turkey*

## 1. Introduction

Physical restraints are widely used in hospitals in many countries, especially during critical care, against a range of difficult clinical situations. They are intended to protect patients and their relatives from any harm to themselves: falling from beds, removing tubes, drains, and medical equipments from their bodies, and to ease patients' control (Bower & McCullough, 2000).

Weaning from artificial ventilation, recovering from acute illness can be a long and difficult process. The problem with critically ill patients is re-sedation, often needed to handle agitation and avoid treatment interference (Cohen et al., 2002). Sedatives lengthen hospitalization and complicate recovery (Westcott, 1995); therefore, the management of these patients can often be a dilemma (Hine, 2007).

### 1.1 What is a restraint?

Physical restraint is (American Nurses Assosication, 2001) "any chemical or physical involuntary method restricting an individual's movement, physical activity, or normal access to the body."

Physical restraint is also defined as any device, material, or equipment attached to or near a person's body, neither controlled nor easily removed by a patient and that deliberately prevents or intended to prevent free body movement to a position of choice or patients normal access to their body (Retsas, 1998).

### 1.2 History of physical restraint

Physical restraint use in acute and intensive cares dates back long. While actions -against restraint were taken in England and France during the 19th century, its use in acute care settings in the US was assumed as a therapeutic and morally correct approach against accidents and injures (Bower & McCullough, 2000). In the 1980s, physical restraint applications in acute care settings were on general medical-surgical units (Frengley & Mion, 1986; Lofgren et al., 1989; Mion et al., 1989; Robbins et al., 1987).

Restraint use has become a legal issue with individual rights becoming paramount in the society. First in the USA, federal restraint standards were implemented in 1984 (U.S.

Department of Health and Human Services, 1984). The Mental Health Act of 1983, Wales, (Department of Health and Welsh Office, 1999) named five common reasons to use the restraint, of which three were the most relevant in critical care settings: noncompliance with treatment, self-harm, and risk of a physical injury by an accident. Canada and British Columbia have legislations (Currie, 1997). While the UK, however, does not accept physical restraint use at all, it is common in the US, Australia, and Europe (Maccioli et al., 2003; Royal College of Nursing, 2004; Van Norman & Palmer, 2001). Nurses and scientists from other disciplines tried to agree on physical restraint use starting in 1988 no consensus reached yet on its use in hospitals (Bower & McCullough, 2000).

## 2. Alternative procedures

Other strategies to manage agitation include :

- Sedation: agitation is often managed with the use of sedatives or antipsychotic drugs ; however, drugs could ultimately lead to further agitation and a vicious circle ensues. The overuse of sedatives could also complicate a patient's recovery by causing hypotension and apnea and by exposing the patient to risks associated with immobility (Westcott, 1995; Woodrow, 2000).
- Communication with patients, relatives
- Touch
- Involvement of family
- Massage
- Acupuncture (Bray et al., 2004)

### 2.1 Barriers hindering restraint elimination

Research has clearly established that physical restraints can be injurious both physically and mentally for inhabitants, cost more resources, and increase serious injuries.

Barriers to shortening the restraint use included: fear of patient injury, staff and resource restrictions, lack of education and information about alternatives to restraints, policy and management issues, beliefs and expectations (of staff, family and residents), inadequate review practices and statement barriers (Moore & Haralambous 2007).

Perceived barriers to individualized care identified were insufficient staff, safety and authoritarian concerns, lack of team collaboration and phone call, lack of participation by the nursing assistants for care planning, and staff and family attitudes (Walker et al., 1999).

Staff or family attitudes and fears can stop success with restraint elimination measures. The restraint team should be practical and provide education and resources, permit individuals to express their fears and suspicions, and encourage active involvement in designing the plan of care. Approaching restraint decline with an incremental plan allows caregivers to conquer their fears and resistance. Beginning with one unit at a time or starting with the easiest residents and working toward the more difficult may make the task of restraint reduction more reasonable (Castle & Mor, 1998). The successful interventions will allow staff and family members to become more relaxed and convinced with the removal of restraints.

## 3. Indications and contraindications

Physical restraints are indicated for patient safety and avoiding falls, but the most widespread reason is to put off the taking away of invasive tubes and devices (Fletcher, 1996; Cruz et al., 1997; Minnick et al., 1998; Happ, 2000; Choi and Song 2003). Patients might need repeatedly to be self-extubated while patients was physically restrained (Balon 2001) and restrained patients of self-extubation rate were 77% (Birkett et al, 2005) .

Delirium and agitation been the most frequent hospital complications in 'older' patients, resulting in poor hospital outcomes and increased morbidity and death (Ely et al., 2001), physical restraints are frequently used in this setting, ranging in the literature between 8-68% for hospitalized elderly people (Hamers & Huizing 2005).

### 3.1 The use of physical restraint in critical care

The intensive care environment itself may grow added stress and agitation, caused by mechanical ventilation, invasive procedures, pain, fear, anxiety, sensory overload and sleep cycle disruptions (Haskell et al., 1997). Incidence of agitation rose because of higher number of of older and more severely ill patients in intensive care units (ICU) (Cohen et al., 2002). However, the prevalence of agitation and delirium in ICU varied between 15 - 87% of patients (Sanders et al., 1992; Ely et al., 2001; Roberts, 2001). This variation could be due to numerous factors and definitions utilized to describe altered mental status: delirium, acute confusional state, sundown syndrome, ICU psychosis and ICU delirium (Haskell et al., 1997).

Agitated patients exhibits constant fidgeting and movement; pulling at bed sheets, invasive devices and catheters; trying to get out of bed; shouting and hitting and were disorientated to the time and the place (Haskell et al., 1997; Cohen et al., 2002). The agitations in critically ill adults are associated with potentially dangerous complications: self-extubation (self-removal of endotracheal tube), removal of arterial and venous lines and non-compliance with life-saving treatment (Cohen et al., 2002; Nirmalan et al., 2004). Ultimately, the presence of agitation delayed weaning from ventilation and lengthened ICU stay (Westcott, 1995; haskell et al., 1997; Cull & Inwood, 1999; Cohen et al., 2002).

Systematically reviewed physical restraint use ranged 3.4- 21% in acute care patients, who were physically restrained for 2.7 to 4.5 days during their hospitalization. The range in residential care settings was between 12%, 47%, and 32%, respectively. The restraint applied was 20 days at least in each month (Evans et al., 2002). Patients were restrained at 6-13%, with higher rates (18- 22%) as well for people 65 years or older. The most common reason for physical restraint was to prevent falls (up to 77%) and disruption of therapy (up to 40%) (MacPherson et al., 1990; Mion et al., 1989). Rates varied in different countries: less than 9% in Denmark, Iceland, and Japan; between 15- 17% in France, Italy, Sweden, and the US, the highest use, almost 40% in Spain (Ljunggren et al., 1997).

However, physical restraint is contraindicated edema and cyanosis, pressure ulcers, aspiration and breathing problems, agitation, contractures, fractures, paralyz and most importantly if the informed consent is not obtained from patients or surrogates (Demir, 2007a; Demir, 2007b).

## 4. Key step of the procedure

### 4.1 Types of physical restraints

There are a number of kinds of restraints. The most common restraint devices are wrist restraints (Minnick et al., 1998, Happ, 2000), ankle restraint (Demir, 2007a) and chest or waist restraints (Carrion et al., 2000; Demir, 2007a). Boxing gloves or mittens, involved wrapping the hands in bandages to prevent free use of the fingers (Fletcher, 1996; Nirmalan et al., 2004), therefore preventing the patient from grabbing and pulling at tubes and lines (Demir, 2007a), are also popular. Among the most frequent for adults are jacket restraints, belt restraints, mit for hand restraints, and limb restraints. Restraints for infants and children include mummy restraints, elbow restraints and crib nets (Kozier et al., 2004).

**Jacket (body restraint):** A sleeveless vest with straps that cross in front or back of the patient and are tied to the bed edge or chair legs.

**Belt:** Straps or belts applied transversely the patient to save him or her to the stretcher, bed, or wheelchair.

**Mitten or hand:** Enclosed cloth fabric applied over the patient's hand to put off injury from scratching

**Elbow:** A combination of cloth and plastic or wooden tongue blades that halt the elbow to prevent flexion.

**Limb or extremity:** Cloth devices that stop one or all limbs by firmly tying the restraint to the bed frame or chair.

**Mummy:** A blanket or sheet that is folded around the child to bound the movement. Mummy restraints are used to execute procedures on children.

### 4.2 General principles for the care of restrained patients

- The purpose of restraint is to provide optimal care of the patient,
- Use of restraint must not be an alternative to insufficient human or other resources
- Restraint should only be used when alternative therapeutic measures have seemed ineffective to acquire the desired outcome,
- Decisions regarding use or non-use of after a detailed patient assessment, by an interdisciplinary team,
- Critical care areas must develop and implement protocol/guidelines in order to aid nurses and others,
- Whatever form of restraint is used there must be suitable, continual evaluation tools used and the findings acted upon,
- Clear, concise documentation of decisions, plans and treatment must be kept within the patients' record,
- The patient and their family should be engaged within discussions to inform them of the reason for choice of the restraint method,
- Schooling all staff regarding chemical, physical and psychological restraint must take in training and competency programs in critical care units (BACCN position in Bray et al., 2004).

### 4.3 Application guidelines

- Obtain consent from the patient and surrogate,
- Enlighten rationale for application of restraint,
- Select the appropriate type of restraint,
- Assess skin for discomfor,
- Apply restraint to patient assuring some movement of body part. One to two fingers should slide between restraint and patient's skin. Tie straps securely with clove hitch knot,
- Lock restraint to bed frame; do not tie the straps to the side rail,
- Assess restraints and skin integrity every 30 minutes,
- Discharge restraints at least every 2 hours,
- Continually appraise the need for restraints (at least every 4-8 hours),
- Guarantee that a physician's order has been provided or, in an emergency, obtain one within 24 hours after applying the restraint,
- Assure the patient and the patient's people that the restraint is impermanent and protective,
- Apply the restraint in a way that the patients can move as freely as possible without defeating the idea of the restraint,
- Ensure that limb restraints are applied securely but not so tightly that they obstruct blood flow to anybody area or extremity,
- Pad bony prominence (e.g., wrist and ankles) before applying a restraint over them. The movements of a restraint without stuffing over such prominences can quickly erode the skin,
- Constantly tie a limb restraint with a knot (e.g., a clove hitch) that will not tighten when pulled,
- Tie the ends of a body restraint to the part of the bed that moves to lift the head. Never tie the ends to a side rail or to the set frame of the bed if the bed position is to be altered,
- Asses the restraint every 30 minutes. Some services have specific forms to be used to document ongoing assessment,
- Free all restraints at least every 2 to 4 hours, and provide range-of-motion train and skin care,
- Reassess the continued requirement for the restraint at least every 8 hours. Embrace an assessment of the fundamental source of the behavior necessitating use of the restraints,
- When a restraint is momentarily removed, do not leave the client alone,
- Instantly report to the nurse in charge and record on the client's chart any constant reddened or broken skin areas under the restraint,
- At the first sign of cyanosis or pallor, coldness of a skin area, or a client's complaint of a tingling feeling, pain, or numbness, release the restraint and exercise the limb,
- Apply a restraint so that it can be freed quickly in an emergency and with the body part in a typical anatomic position,
- Offer emotional support verbally and through touch (Kozier et al., 2004, Taylor et al., 1997).

### 4.4 JCAHO restraint standards for non-psychiatric patients

*Special Conditions When Restraint Is Applied:*

- Based on important alteration in the patient's state with the physician notified immediately and written orders obtained within 24 hours

- Initiated by a registered nurse
- Based on protocols customary for situations where patients may hurt themselves if staff initiate, maintain, and terminate restraint without an order from autonomous practitioner

*Organizational Perspective:*

- Be specific for each institution
- Exhibit clinical justification
- Exhibit the use of innovative alternatives
- Outline preventive strategies
- Name ways to reduce risks associated with restraint use

*Policies/Procedures/Protocols:*

- Be clearly declared
- Advocate use of least limiting measures

*Preventive Strategies:*

- Identify potentially risky patient behaviors
- Identify efficient and tried alternatives

*Plan of Care*

- Individualized and guarantee patient's assessed needs are met
- Conserve patient's rights, dignity, and well-being

*Education:*

- Be continuing for staff and patient
- Be provided to families when fitting

*Initiation and Monitoring of Restraint Use:*

- Based on state law
- Initiated based on individual orders or approved
- Protocols with written physician order obtained within 12 hours
- Applied/monitored/assessed/reassessed by qualified staff
- Monitored at least every 2 hours
- Obtained a new permission for every 24 hours when continuous restraint is used

*Documentation:*

- Incorporate all restraint episodes according to organizational policies and procedures
- Record , at a minimum, every 2 hours
- Specify alternatives tried before restraints were applied
- Write in into the patient's medical record

*Key elements of restraint documentation*

- Reason for the restraint
- Method of restraint
- Application: Date, time, and patient's response

- Duration
- Frequency of observation and patient's response
- Safety: Release from restraint with periodic, routine exercise and assessment for flow and skin integrity
- Assessment of the continuous demand for restraint
- Patient outcome

## 5. Complications of physical restraint

Increasing awareness of its negative effects and its limited efficacy in the last decade reduced the use of physical restraint. One hundred deaths in the USA occur annually in addition to higher hospital infection rates and injuries by improper physical restraint. Moreover, patients under physical restraint lost muscle strength, had pressure ulcers, incontinence, strangulation (Taylor et al., 1997), and were severely agitated, confused, depressed, angry, fearful, confused, panicked, and experienced sleeping difficulties, loss of role, shyness, body disformation, resistance or objection to daily routine activities, higher disorganized behaviours, cognitive and behavioural problems due to changes in blood chemistry, and loss of self-trust and respect (Bonner et al., 2002; Bray et al., 2004; Cannon et al., 2001; Castle, 2002; Choi & Song, 2003; Evans et al., 2002, 2003; Hem et al., 2001; Koch & Lyon, 2001; Shorr et al., 2002; Swauger & Tomlin, 2000). Avoiding physical injuries by physical restraint is only possible through improved quality of care. The rules were by the Health Care Financing Administration in 1987 and Joint Commission on Accreditation of Healthcare Organizations (JCAHO; Taylor et al., 1997). Government and accreditation organizations have supported the decisions on physical restraint use in the last 15-20 years because of increased significance of patients' rights.

Over the last 20 years there has been an increasing evidence supporting the reduction of restraints' use of. Some complications reported by Demir (2007a) were: edema and cyanosis by wrist and arm restraints, pressure ulcers, aspiration and breathing problems caused by sheet and belt pressure on chest, head hits by angry patients on bed sides, contractures of joints, and rejecting meals. Nine patients were suffocated when tied up with sheet on the chest, two had humerus fractures, two needed head skin sutures after falling out of bed, and one was paralyzed after being tied to the bed by the arms.

Atrioventricular irregularities in elderly patients on whom limb and vest restrained were observed (Evans et al., 2003). After longer periods of agitation, tachycardia and deaths were experienced. Mott et al. (2005) stated that physical restraint did not fully serve the purpose and increased agitation. Sullivan-Marx and colleagues' (1999) reported a higher risk of falls and strangulation (Lee et al., 1999) as well. Time restrained patients spent in hospitals were longer than unrestrained patients and experienced higher risks of complications, lower discharges from hospitals, and higher death risks (Arbesman & Wright, 1999; Clary & Krishnan, 2001; Paterson et al., 2003).

Asphyxiation, the most common cause of restraint related death, is termed as "restraint asphyxia" in the forensic and emergency literature by Reay (1998). Death occurred in approximately 12% of cases of a total of 214 episodes of hobble tying in agitated delirium (Stratton et al., 2001). There were various reports: 131 deaths to the FDA, USA, from 1987-1996, for the manufacturers of protective restraints (Morrison, 1997) , 58 asphyxia occurrences out of 770 cases and 44 wheel chair related fatal accidents out of 58 cases (Calder & Kirby 1990), also reported. Higher physical restraint with agitation, more complications and frequent fell down (Shorr et al., 2002).

## 6. Ethical and legal considerations on restraint use

All nurses (/health professionals) have a duty to safeguard and protect their patients from harm. The nurse's moral obligation is to do no harm (non-maleficence) and promote good (beneficence). It might also be conflicting for critical care nurses, when they are to maintain a safe environment for agitated and delirious patients and also the potentially lifesaving technological devices. The picture is even more complex by the nurse's obligation to ensure patient freedom, dignity, and autonomy (Reigle, 1996). Since everyone has the right to be free from forced restraint of movement, torture or degrading treatment (HMSO, 1998), nurses have to justify use of physical restraint (Kapp, 1996). However, the literature contained very little evidence of restraints providing protection. So researchers debates just how ethical are the use of physical restraints.

The nurse's responsibility is to respect patient autonomy, whereas the use of physical restraint violates the principles of informed consent. Since restraint is a non-validated therapy, their use is considered investigational and a higher standard of informed consent should be required (Moss & LaPuma, 1991). Providing informed consent implies that the patient is competent to take the information on board; however, if physical restraint is being considered, the patient is probably agitated and less likely to have the capacity to give informed consent (Royal College of Nursing, 2004). Although the Department of Health (2001) guidelines are clear that no one is able to give consent on behalf of another, communication with the patient and the relatives on the rationale for restraint remains paramount. The reasonable person' rule can be applied in such cases, which enables a professional to act in the best interests of the patient (Beauchamp & Childress, 2001). A reasonable person is the one who would wish to be treated for life-threatening conditions even not able to give consent (Dimond , 2002). When there are other available alternatives, however, health care professionals should not assume that a reasonable person would wish to be physically restrained. Admittedly, the alternatives include other methods of restraint in the form of sedation, which itself can prolong and complicate a patient's recovery.

The Mental Capacity Act (Deparment of Constitutional Affairs, 2005) states that anything done for or on behalf of individuals without capacity, for example restraint, must be the least restrictive of their basic rights and freedoms and be in their best interests. If restraint is to be in the patient's best interest, health care professionals must have been satisfied by all legal and ethical implications, since otherwise they might face allegations of assault (Deparment of Health, 2001). Crucial differences exist between restraint that violates rights and dignity and restraint that does not violate any autonomously expressed wishes protects the patient from self-harm and is in the patients' best interests (Nirmalan et al., 2004). However, the evidences discussed previously, exposing the patient to potential harmful effects from restraint is in their best interests is debatable.

### 6.1 Informed consent

Consent from patients or surrogates for all healthcare activities and medical treatments are a must since fundamental moral duty forbids any actions against a person's wishes and dignity. Informed consent thus entails a shared decision by both patient and health professional (Andanda, 2005). If a patient has a doubtful capacity, health care professionals have to take necessary steps against deterioration first and then consider capacity and consent matters (English et al., 2004).

Informed consent is widely recognized in international guidelines (Bandman & Bandman, 2002; International Council of Nurses, 2001) and in legislation (Department of Health and Welsh Office, 1999). There are four basic elements of informed consent, developed starting with Nuremberg trials (Andanda, 2005), which are also valid for patient care:

- "Capacity to consent;
- Full disclosure of relevant information;
- Adequate comprehension of the information by the participant;
- Voluntary decision to participate and withdraw from participation at any stage without prejudice of the participant. Participant withdrawal should be accepted and withdrawing participants should not be expected to give any reasons for their decision."

One could evaluate informed consent well only if she has a good understanding of human rights and ethics. Human rights are defined by the American Nurses Association (ANA) as "assertions that call for treating human beings as ends in them, rather than as goals or purposes of others" (Bandman & Bandman, 2002). Ethical principles, of which three guides for all care activity used by nurses are the following: respect for persons, beneficence, and justice. These principles were at the US federal level in the Belmont Report in 1979 (The National Commission for the Protection of Human Subjects of Biomedical and Behavioral Research (NCPHS]) (Burns & Grove, 1999). The dignity and rights of the patient are before the goals of any research or anything since many medical or nursing cares, though acceptable, could be harmful or outweigh the expected benefits (English et al., 2004).

The recent studies on informed and shared decision within clinical care have revealed a pronounced tension among three competing factors:

- Paternalistic conservatism about information exposé to patients has been worn by moral arguments and largely established by the medical profession,
- While many patients may wish to be given information about available treatment options, many also emerge cognitively and psychologically too ill to understand and to hold it, and
- Even when patients do comprehend information about likely treatment options; they do not essentially wish to make such choices themselves and might prefer to leave final decisions to the clinicians.

The second and third factors apparently disagree with the first and make the case more difficult (Doyal, 2001).

Physical restraint has become a common method for difficult clinical situations in hospitals although it has been well recognized in years that nurses should obtain consent from the patient before any nursing care procedure (Bandman & Bandman, 2002; Aveyard, 2005). Similarly, informed consent has become a common method of protecting patients and health care givers as well (Kanerva, 1999) from unexpected cost of physical restraint use, because of increased concern for human and patient rights in the USA and the UK. While physical restraint is required or essential in patients with unsatisfactory mental (Bridgman & Wilson, 2000) or decision-making capacity (Harrison et al., 1997) or psychiatric patients, informed consent is still a must and be, at least, obtained from surrogates (Usher & Arthur, 1998). In other words, a patient at any stage, or under any circumstances is to agree or to disagree with a certain treatment (Beauchamp & Childress, 2001).

Some codes of ethics and regulations are in use in a variety of countries but there are few in Turkey. Only existing code is "Medicine and professional ethics", which was accepted in 1960 and later revised in 1998 (Turkish Medical Association, 1999). The Patients' Rights Regulations placed into effect by the Ministry of Health in August 1998 is the first and only regulation (The General Directorate of Development of Regulations and Publishing, 1998). The content of these is similar to the Declaration on the Promotion of Patients' Rights' in Europe (World Health Organization, 1994). More, however, has to be implemented in Turkey to avoid misguided / misused physical restraint without informed consent and its consequences of legal challenges for maltreatment, negligence, or human rights. However, Demir-Zencirci (2009) stated that most of nurses in her study (97.6%, n= 248) used physical restraint without informed consent.

The aim of informed consent is to protect the autonomous choices of vulnerable persons such as physically restrained patients. Informed consent for medical interventions should be based on size and likelihood of the risks associated with the proposed intervention. As the risks associated with the use of physical restraints are significant, consent for their use is crucial (Reigle, 1997).

## 7. Illustrative cases

### Case 1

A 21 year old male patient was hospitalized in neurosurgery because of a car accident resulted in depressed fracture on left temporal and subarachnoid hemorrhage. Three-four cm laceration existed on right deltoid anterior. When arrived to Emergency Unit via 112, he experienced extensive respiratory distress and higher arterial blood pressure. Ear Nose Throat Department failed to insert endotracheal tubes, therefore, opened tracheostomy. He was unconscious and his orientation and cooperation were not assessed. The patient had extensior on the upper extremity and flexor attracts on the lower extremity via painful stimuli. Vital signs were, later on, normalized. White blood cells were too high (29.200/L), $Sa0_2$ was 94.3%, blood ph was 7.34, Gag reflex was positive, and no neck stiffness. Patient was physically restrained on wrists and ankles.

### Aplication

- Provided a physician order.
- Explained to the surrogate what you are going to do, why it is necessary, and how they cooperate.
- Discussed with the surrogate how the results will be used in planning further care or treatments.
- Allowed time for the surrogate to express feelings about being tied/restrained.
- Provided needed emotional reassurance that the restraints will be used only when absolutely necessary and that there will be close contact with the surrogate in case assistance is required.

- Provided a written informed consent from his legal surrogate/his father.
- Washed hands and observed appropriate infection control procedures.
- Provided for patient privacy.
- Applied the wrist and ankle restraint with cotton ties.
- Pad put on bony prominences on the wrist and ankle for to prevent skin abrassion.
- Pulled the tie of the restraint through the slit in the wrist portion or through the buckle.
- Assessed restraints and skin integrity every 30 minutes.
- Discharged restraints at least every 2 hours.
- Appraised the need for restraints for every 4-8 hours.
- Stopped the restraint and applied the exercises on the limb and changed the position for there was cyanosis and pallor, coldness of a skin area.

Mr. A was discharged on foot from neurosurgery intensive care units after 29 days. Physical restraint was applied only 24 days and no complications occurred.

**Case 2**

A 51 year old female patient with headache, nausea and vomiting got in to the acute care settings. Patient has experienced lethargy and vomiting for three days. She has been brought to the hospital because of increased lethargy. Findings were confusion, lethargic, roughly intact cranial nerves. She reflected no pathologic reflex. Hiperdans parallel with subarachnoid hemorrhage on cranial ct and aneurysmal dilatation on Distal Middle Cerebral Artery were observed. Patient was hospitalized and in neurosurgery intensive care unit and anti-edema and antiepileptic therapy were inititiated.

Confusional, defective orientation and co-operation are observed. Four fifth muscle strength, no pathologic reflex, and (+) neck stiffness. Blood values: Aspartate Aminotransferase (AST) and Gamma Glutamyl Transferase (GGT), Blood urea nitrogen and Creatinine high at range, hemoglobin low at range.

Patient was physically strained on right elbow and ankle.

**Aplication**

- Provided a physician order.
- Explained to the surrogate what you are going to do, why it is necessary, and how they cooperate.
- Discussed with the surrogate how the results will be used in planning further care or treatments.
- Allowed time for the surrogate to express feelings about being tied/restrained.
- Provided needed emotional reassurance that the restraints will be used only when absolutely necessary and that there will be close contact with the surrogate in case assistance is required.
- Provided a written informed consent from her legal surrogate/her husband.
- Washed hands and observed appropriate infection control procedures.
- Provided for patient privacy.
- Applied the wrist and ankle restraint with cotton ties.
- Pad put on bony prominences on the wrist and ankle for to prevent skin abrasion.
- Pulled the tie of the restraint through the slit in the wrist portion or through the buckle.

- Assessed restraints and skin integrity every 30 minutes.
- Discharged restraints at least every 2 hours.
- Appraised the need for restraints for every 4-8 hours.
- Stopped the restraint and applied the exercises on the limb and changed the position for there was cyanosis and pallor, coldness of a skin area.

Mrs. A has been still unconscious, aphasic and agitated, and continues to physically restraint on right wrists and ankles. She was discharged on bed from neurosurgery intensive care units after 35 days. Physical restraint has been still applied at your home. Mrs. A has a stage II pressure ulcers on coccyx and abrasion and edema on your wrist and ankle.

## 8. Conclusion

Physical restraint may be highly associated with nurses' monitoring and patients may suffer serious complications. Enhancements in intensive and acute care settings and in nurse staffing and education are necessary. Like many people, we believe that using physical restraint to control disruptive patient behaviors before alternative methods are tried or to compensate for shortages in nursing staff is unethical and unacceptable. In these conditions, use of physical restraints is an anathema to best practice principles, a denial of patient autonomy and beneficent professional health care practice principles. Nurses first have to consider patients' requests and needs if they wish to provide optimal care for patients/relatives.

Professional nursing practice accepts that the use of physical restraints is occasionally unnecessary, harmful, and potentially deadly (Demir 2007a,). Physical restraint used by nurses sometimes violates patients' autonomy or self respect and causes patients to lose their trust to the nurses. One should agree that physical restraint is an unethical assault on patients' rights and should be used carefully after alternative methods are tried (Demir-Zencirci-2009).

If physical restraint is used without enough care, it might result in life-threatening conditions, some of which were reported by respondents. Therefore, physical restraint without consent should not be used without physician orders or expert consultation. Last but not the least; nurses have always to remember that their responsibility is to offer optimal care to society and humankind, and best care to patients.

## 9. References

American Nurses Association. (2001). Ethics and Human Rights Position Statements: Reduction of Patient Restraint and Seclusion in Health Care Settings. Available at: http://www.nursingworld.org/MainMenuCategories/EthicsStandards/Ethics-Position-Statements/prtetrestrnt14452.aspx (accessed 27 July 2011).

Andanda, P. (2005). Module two: informed consent. *Dev World Bioeth,* 5:14- 29, ISSN 1471-8847

Arbesman, M.C. & Wright, C. (1999). Mechanical restraints, rehabilitation therapies, and staffing adequacy as risk factors for falls in an elderly hospitalised population. *Rehabilitation Nursing,* 24, 122–128, ISSN

Aveyard, H. (2005). Informed consent prior to nursing care procedures. *Nurs Ethics,*12:19-29, ISSN 0969-7330

Balon, J. A. (2001). Common factors of spontaneous self-extubation in a critical care setting. International Journal of Trauma Nursing, 7 (3), 93-99. ISSN: 1075-4210

Bandman, E.L. & Bandman, B. (2002). Ethical Issues in the Nursing Care of Elderly. *Nursing Ethics Through the Life Span.* (4th ed). London: Prentice- Hall International, p.233-59, ISSN 0-8385-6976-5

Beauchamp, T.L. & Childress, J.F. (2001). Moral Theories. *Principles of Biomedical Ethics.* (5th ed.) New York: Oxford University Pres, p: 337-77, ISSN 0-19-514332-9

Birkett, K.M.; Southerland, K.A. & Leslie, G.D. (2005). Reporting unplanned extubation. *Intensive Crit Care Nurs,*21:65-75; ISSN 0964-3397

Bonner, G.; Lowe, T.; Rawcliffe, D. & Wellman, N. (2002). Trauma for all: A pilot study of the subjective experience of physical restraint for mental health inpatients and staff in the UK. *Journal of Psychiatric and Mental Health Nursing,* 9, 465–473. ISSN 1351-0126

Bower, F.L. & McCullough, C.S. (2000). Restraint use in acute care settings: Can it be reduced? *Journal of Nursing Administration,* 30, 592–598, ISSN 0002-0443

Bray, K.; Hill, K.; Robson, W.; Leaver, G.; Walker, N.; O'Leary, M.; Delaney, T.; Walsh, D.; Gager, M. & Waterhouse, C. (2004). British association of critical care nurses position statement on the use of restraint in adult critical care units. *Nursing in Critical Care;* 9: 199–211. ISSN: 1478-5153.

Bridgman, A.M. & Wilson, M.A. (2000). The treatment of adult patients with mental disability. Part 1: Consent and duty. *British Dental Journal,* 189: 66-8, ISSN: 0007-0610

Burns, N. & Grove, S.K. (1999). Examining Ethics in Nursing Research. In: Understanding Nursing Research. 3rd ed. Philadelphia: WB Saunders Co, p: 159-92, ISSN 0-7216-0011-5

Calder, J. & Kirby, R.L. (1990). Fatal wheelchair-related accidents in the United States. *American Journal of Physical Medicine and Rehabilitation,* 69, 184–190, ISSN 0894-9115

Cannon, M.E.; Sprivulis, P. & McCarthy, J. (2001). Restraint practices in Australasian emergency departments. *Australian and New Zealand Journal of Psychiatry,* 35, 464–467, ISSN 0004-8674

Carrion, M.I.; Ayuso, D.; Marcos, M.; Robles, M.P.; De La Cal, M.A.; Alia, I. & Esteban, A. (2000). Accidental removal of endotracheal and nasogastric tubes and intravascular catheters. *Critical Care Medicine,* 28: 63–66. ISSN: 0090-3493

Castle, N.G. & Mor, V. (1987). Physical Restraints in Nursing Homes: A Review of the Literature Since the Nursing Home Reform Act of 1987. *Medical Care Research and Review,* 55: 139-170, ISSN: 1077-5587

Castle, N.G. (2002). Nursing homes with persistent deficiency citations for physical restraint use. *Medical Care,* 40: 868–878, ISSN 0025-7079

Choi, E. & Song, M. (2003). Physical restraint use in a Korean ICU. Journal of Clinical Nursing, 12, 651–659. ISSN: 0962-1067

Clary, G. & Krishnan, R. (2001). Delirium: Diagnosis, neuropath genesis and treatment. *Journal of Psychiatric Practice,* 7, 310–323, ISSN 1527-4160

Cohen, I.L.; Gallagher, T. J.; Pohlman, A.S.; Dasta, J.F.; Abraham, E. & Papadokos, P.J. (2002). Management of the agitated intensive care unit patient. *Critical Care Medicine,* 30 (suppl.): S97-S123, ISSN 0090-3493

Cruz, V.; Abdul-Hamid, M., Heater, B. (1997). Research-based practice: reducing restraints in an acute care setting – phase I, *Journal of Gerontological Nursing,* 23: 31-40, ISSN 0098-9134

Cull, C. & Inwood, H. (1999). Weaning patients from mechanical ventilation. *Professional Nurse,* 14: 535–538, ISSN 0266-8130

Currie, H.H. (1997). Cruel and unusual? The implications of section 12 of the Canadian charter of rights and freedoms on restraint use in care facilities. *Unpublished Master of Arts Thesis.* Simon Fraser University, Burnaby, BC, Canada.

Demir, A. (2007a). Nurses' Use of Physical Restraints in Four Turkish Hospitals, *Journal of Nursing Scholarship,* 39: 38-45, ISSN: 1527-6546

Demir, A. (2007b). The Use of Physical Restraints on Children: Practices and Attitudes of Paediatric Nurses in Turkey, *International Nursing Review*, 54: 367-374, ISSN 0020-8132

Demir-Zencirci, A. (2009). Attitudes, informed consent obtaining rates and feelings about physical restraint use among nurses, *Turkiye Klinikleri Journal of Medical Sciences*, 29:1571-1581, ISSN 1300-0292

Department of Constitutional Affairs. (2005). Mental Capacity Act. http://www.dca.gov.uk/menincap/legis.htm (accessed 20/01/06).

Department of Health and Welsh Office. (1999). Mental Health Act 1983 Code of Practise. London: Department of Health.

Department of Health. (2001). Reference Guide to Consent for Examination or Treatment. London: Department of Health.

Dimond, B. (2004). *Legal Aspects of Nursing*, 4rd edn. London: Longman, ISSN 0582822785

Doyal, L. (2001). Informed consent: moral necessity or illusion? *Qual Saf Health Care*,10(Suppl I):i29-i33, ISSN 2044-5415

Ely, E.W.; Margolin, R.; Francis, J.; May, L.; Truman, B.; Dittus, R.; Speroff, T.; Gautam, S.; Bernard, G.R. & Inouye, S.K. (2001). Evaluation of delirium in critically ill patients: validation of the confusion assessment method for the intensive care unit (CAM-ICU). *Critical Care Medicine*, 29: 1370–1379, ISSN 0090-3493

English, V.; Romano-Critchley, G.; Sheather, J. & Sommerville, A. (2004). Treatment without Consent: Incapacitated Adults and Compulsory Treatment. Medical Ethics Today The BMA's Handbook of Ethics and Law. 2nd ed. London, BMJ Publishing Group, p:99-126, ISBN: 978-0-7279-1744-7

Evans, D.; Wood, J. & Lambert, L. (2003). Patient injury and physical restraint devices: A systematic review. *Journal of Advanced Nursing*, 41: 274–282, ISSN 0309-2402

Evans, D.; Wood, J., Lambert, L. & FitzGerald, M. (2002). Physical restraint in acute and residential care: A systematic review. Adelaide, Australia: *The Joanna Briggs Institute*.

Fletcher, K. (1996). Use of Restraints in the Elderly. *AACN Clinical Issues*, 7: 611-620, ISSN 15597768

Frengley, J. D. & Mion, L. C. (1986). Incidence of physical restraints on acute general medical wards. *Journal of the American Geriatrics Society*, 34: 565-568, ISSN 1532-5415

Hamers, J.P.H. & Huizing, A.R. (2005). Why do we use physical restraints in the elderly? *Zeitschrift für Gerontologie und Geriatrie*, 38:19–25, ISSN 0948-6704

Happ, M. B. (2000). Preventing treatment interference: the nurse's role in maintaining technologic devices. *Heart and Lung*, 29: 60-69, ISSN: 0147-9563

Harrison, C.; Kenny, N.P.; Sidarous, M. & Rowell, M. (1997). Bioethics for clinicians: 9. Involving children in medical decisions. *CMAJ*,156(6):825-8, ISSN 0820-3946

Haskell, R.B.; Frankel, H.L. & Rotondo, M.F. (1997). Agitation. *AACN Clinical Issues*; 8: 335–350, ISSN 1079-0713

Hem, E.; Steen, O. & Opjordsmoen, S. (2001). Thrombosis associated with physical restraints. *Acta Psychiatrica Scandinavica*, 103, 73–76, ISSN 0001-690X

Hine, K. (2007). The use of physical restraint in critical care. *Nursing in critical care*, 12: 6-11, ISSN 1478-5153

HMSO. (1998). Human Rights Act. London: HMSO, ISSN 0-10-544298-4.

International Council of Nurses. The ICN code of ethics for nurses. Nurs Ethics 2001;8(4): 375-9, ISSN 0969-7330

Jensen, B.; Hess-Zak, A.; Johnston, S.K.; Otto, D.C.; Tebbe, L.; Russell, C. & Waller, A. (1998). Restraint reduction: A new philosophy for a new millenium. *Journal of Nursing Administration*, 28: 32–38, ISSN 0002-0443

Kanerva, A.M.; Suominen, T.& Leino-Kilpi H. (1999). Informed consent for short-stay surgery. *Nurs Ethics*, 6:483-93, ISSN 0969-7330

Kapp, M.B. (1996). Physical restraint use in critical care: legal issues. *AACN Clinical Issues*; 7: 579–584, ISSN 1079-0713

Koch, S. & Lyon, C. (2001). Case study approach to removing physical restraint. *International Journal of Nursing Practice*, 7:156–161, ISSN 1322-7114

Kozier, B.; Erb, G.; Berman, A. & Snyder, S. (2004). Safety. In, *Fundamentals of nursing* (7th ed.) Upper Saddle River, NJ: Prentice Hall, ISSN 0-13-114229

Lee, D.T.F.; Chan, M.C.; Tam, E.P.Y. & Yeung, W.S.K. (1999). Use of physical restraints on elderly patients: An exploratory study of the perceptions of nurses in Hong Kong. *Journal of Advanced Nursing*, 29, 153–159, ISSN 0309-2402

Ljunggren, G.; Phillips, C. & Sgadari, A. (1997). Comparisons of restraint use in nursing homes in eight countries. *Age and Ageing*, 16, 43-47, ISSN 0002-0729

Lofgren, R. P.; MacPherson, D. S.; Granieri, R.; Myllenbeck, S. & Sprafka, J. M. (1989). Mechanical restraints on the medical wards: Are protective devices safe? *American Journal of Public Health*, 79, 735-738, ISSN 0090-0036

Maccioli, G.A.; Dorman,T. & Brown, B.R. (2003). Clinical practice guidelines for the maintenance of patient physical safety in the intensive care unit: Use of restraining therapies—American College of Critical Care Medicine Task Force 2001–2002. *Critical Care Medicine*, 31: 2665–2676, ISSN 0090-3493

Macpherson, D.S.; Lofgren, R.P.; Cranieri, R. & Myllenbeck, S. (1990). Deciding to restrain medical patients. *Journal of the American Geriatrics Society, 38*,516-520, ISSN: 0002-8614

Martin, B. (2002). Restraint use in acute and critical care settings: changing practice. *AACN Clinical Issues*; 13: 294–306, ISSN 1079-0713

Minnick, A.F.; Mion, L.C.; Leipzig, R.; Lamb, K. & Palmer, R. (1998). Prevalence and patterns of physical restraint use in the acute care setting. *Journal of Nursing Administration*, 28: 19–24. ISSN 0002-0443

Mion, L. (1996). Establishing alternatives to physical restraint in the acute care setting: a conceptual framework to assist nurses' decision making. *AACN Clinical Issues*, 7: 592–602, ISSN 1079-0713

Mion, L. C.; Frengley, J. D.; Jakovcic, C. A. & Marino, J. A. (1989). A further exploration of the use of physical restraints in hospitalized patients. *Journal of the American Geriatrics Society*, 37, 949-956, ISSN 1532-5415

Moore, K. & Haralambous, B. (2007). Barriers to reducing the use of restraints in residential elder care facilities, *JAN*, 58(6), 532-540, ISSN 0309-2402

Morrison, A. (1997). Device errors. Incorrect restraint use: Deadly protection. *Nursing*, 27: 32, ISSN 0360-4039

Moss, R.J. & La Puma, J. (1991). The ethics of mechanical restraints. *Hastings Cent Rep*, 21:22-5, ISSN 0093-0334

Mott, S.; Poole, J. & Kenrick, M. (2005). Physical and chemical restraints in acute care: Their potential impact on the rehabilitation of older people. *International Journal of Nursing Practice*, 11, 95–101, ISSN 1322-7114

Nirmalan, M., Dark, P.M.; Nightingale, P. & Harris, J. (2004). Physical and pharmacological restraint of critically ill patients: clinical facts and ethical considerations. *British Journal of Anaesthesia*, 92: 789–792, ISSN 0007-0912

Paterson, B.; Bradley, P.; Stark, C.; Saddler, D.; Leadbetter, D. & Allen, D. (2003). Restraint related deaths in health social care in UK: Learning the lessons. *Mental Health Practice*, 6, 10–17,

Reay, D.T. (1998). Death in custody. *Clinics in Laboratory Medicine*, 18, 1–22, ISSN 0272-2712

Reigle, J. (1996). The ethics of physical restraints in critical care. *AACN Clinical Issues*, 7: 585–591, ISSN 1079-0713

Retsas, A.P. & Crabbe, H. (1998). Use of physical restraints in nursinghomes in New South Wales, Australia. *International Journal of Nursing Studies*, 35, 177–183, ISSN 0020-7489

Robbins, L. J.; Boyko, E.; Lane, J.; Cooper, D. & Jahnigen, D. W. (1987). Binding older persons: A prospective study of the use of mechanical restraints in an acute care hospital. *Journal of the American Geriatrics Society*, 35, 290-296.949-956, ISSN 1532-5415

Roberts, B. L. (2001). Managing delirium in intensive care patients. *Critical Care Nurse*, 21: 48–54, ISSN 0279-5442

Royal College of Nursing. (2004). Complementary therapies in nursing, midwifery and health visiting practice. RCN guidance on integrating complementary therapies into critical care. London: Author, Publication code 002 204

Sanders KM, Stern TA, O'Gara PT, Field TS, Rauch SL, Lipson RE, Eagle KA. (1992). Delirium during intra-aortic balloon pump therapy. Incidence and Management. Psychosomatics; 33: 35–44. ISSN 0033-3182

Shorr, R.I.; Guillen, M.K.; Rosenblaff, L.C.; Walker, K.; Caudle, C.E. & Kritchevsky, S.B. (2002). Restraint use, restraints orders, and the risk of falls in hospitalized patients. *Journal of the American Geriatrics Society*, 50, 526–529, ISSN 0002-8614

Stratton, S.J.; Rogers, C. & Brickett, K. (2001). Factors associated with sudden death in individuals requiring restraint for excited delirium. *American Journal of Emergency Medicine*, 19, 187– 191, ISSN 0735-6757

Sullivan-Marx, E.M.; Strumpf, N.E.; Evans, L.K.; Baumgarten, M. & Mailsin, G. (1999). Predictors of continued physical restraint use in nursing home residents following restraint reduction efforts. *Journal of the American Geriatrics Society*, 47, 342–348, ISSN 1532-5415

Swauger, K.C. & Tomlin, C.C. (2000). Moving toward restraint-free patient care. *Journal of Nursing Administration*, 30: 325–329, ISSN 0002-0443

Taylor, C.; Lillis, C. & LeMone, P. (1997). Safety. In, Fundamentals of nursing (3rd ed.; pp. 525–554). Philadelphia: Lippincott.

The General Directorate of Development of Regulations and Publishing. Patients' Rights Regulations. TC Resmi Gazete 1998;23420: 67-76.

Turkish Medical Association. (1999). Medicine and professional ethics. *Tıp Dünyası* 45:1-2:(col 1-7).

U.S. Department of Health and Human Services. (1984). Use of restraints: Federal standards. Washington, DC: Author.

Usher, K.J. & Arthur, D. (1998). Process consent: a model for enhancing informed consent in mental health nursing. *J Adv Nurs*, 27:692-7, ISSN: 0309-2402

Van Norman, G. & Palmer, S. (2001). The ethical boundaries of persuasion: Coercion and restraint of patients in clinical anaesthesia practice. *International Anaesthesiology Clinical*, 39, 131–143, ISSN: 0952-8180

Walker, L., Porter, M., Gruman, C. & Michalski, M. (1999). Developing Individualized Care in Nursing Homes: Integrating the Views of Nurses and Certified Nurse Aides. *Journal of Gerontological Nursing*, 25: 30-5, ISSN: 0098-9134

Westcott, C. (1995). The sedation of patients in intensive care units: a nursing review. *Intensive and Critical Care Nursing*, 11: 26-31, ISSN 0964-3397

Woodrow, P. & Roe, J. (2006). Intensive Care Nursing: A framework for practice. London: Routledge, ISSN: 0-415-37322-0

World Health Organization. (1994). A Decleration on the Promotion of Patients' Rights in Europe. European Consultation on the Rights of Patients. Amsterdam: WHO Regional Office for Europe, p:10-17.